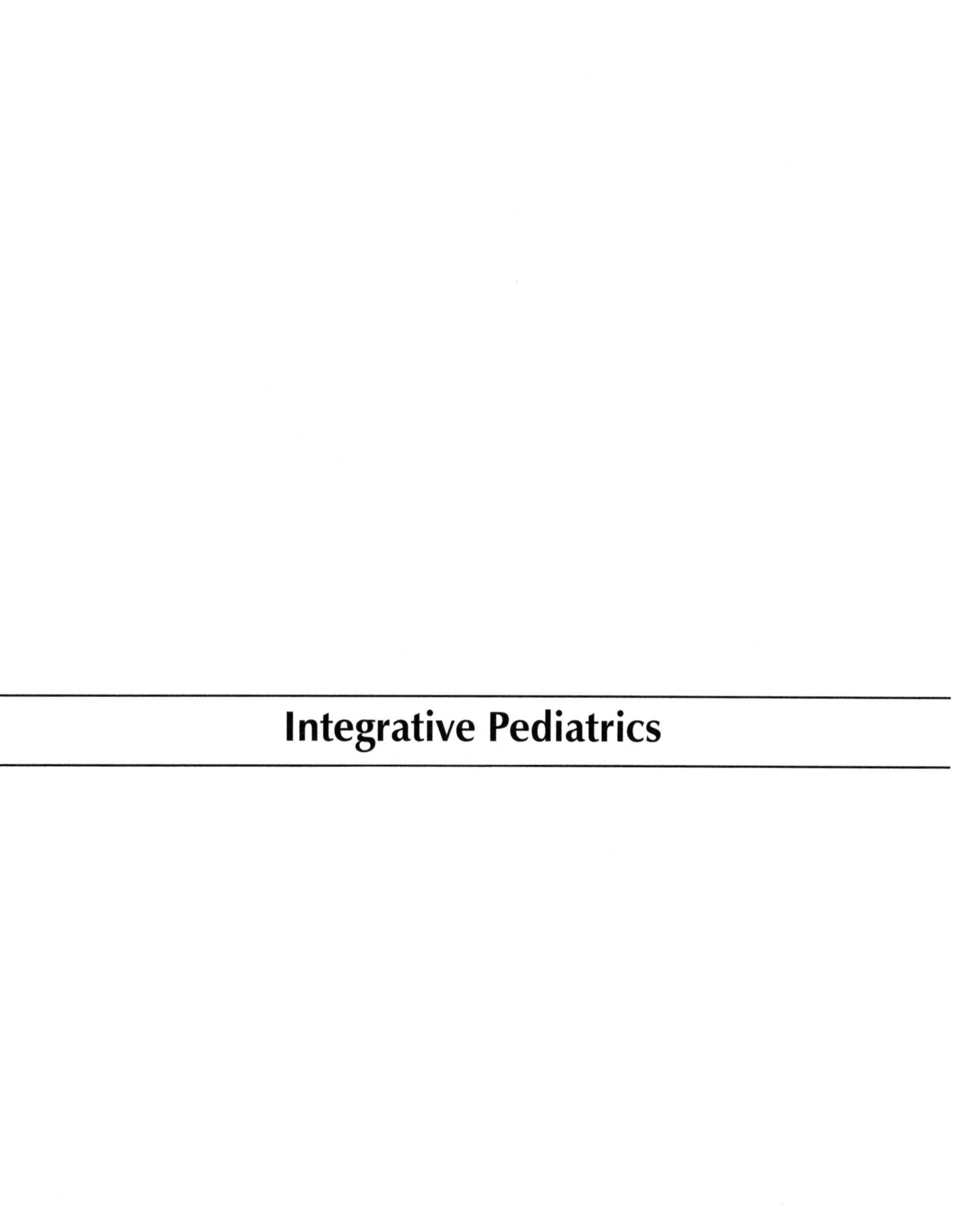

Integrative Pediatrics

Integrative Pediatrics

Editor: Alice Kunek

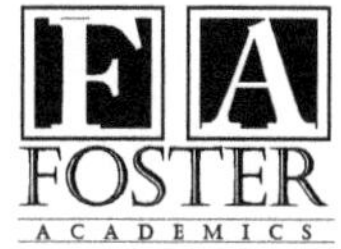

www.fosteracademics.com

www.fosteracademics.com

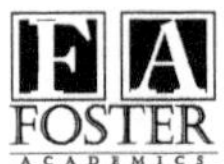

Cataloging-in-Publication Data

Integrative pediatrics / edited by Alice Kunek.
p. cm.
Includes bibliographical references and index.
ISBN 978-1-63242-471-6
1. Pediatrics. 2. Children--Diseases--Alternative treatment. 3. Integrative medicine.
4. Children--Health and hygiene. I. Kunek, Alice.
RJ47 .I58 2017
618.92--dc23

Foster Academics,
118-35 Queens Blvd., Suite 400,
Forest Hills, NY 11375, USA

ISBN 978-1-63242-471-6 (Hardback)

Printed and bound in the United States of America.

Contents

Preface

Every book is initially just a concept; it takes months of research and hard work to give it the final shape in which the readers receive it. In its early stages, this book also went through rigorous reviewing. The notable contributions made by experts from across the globe were first molded into patterned chapters and then arranged in a sensibly sequential manner to bring out the best results.

This book traces the progress of pediatrics and highlights some of its key concepts and applications. It aims at providing knowledgeable insights to the readers about the various methods and theories related to this field. Pediatrics is the practice of giving medical care to infants, children and adolescents. It is concerned with the study of identifying and treating diseases affecting children. The various studies that are constantly contributing towards advancing technologies and evolution of this field are examined in detail in the text. Some of the diverse topics covered herein address the varied branches that fall under this category. It covers in detail some existent theories and innovative concepts revolving around pediatrics. It aims to serve as a resource guide for students and experts alike and contribute to the growth of the discipline.

It has been my immense pleasure to be a part of this project and to contribute my years of learning in such a meaningful form. I would like to take this opportunity to thank all the people who have been associated with the completion of this book at any step.

Editor

1

Associations between Childhood Body Size, Composition, Blood Pressure and Adult Cardiac Structure: The Fels Longitudinal Study

Roy T. Sabo[1]*, Miao-Shan Yen[1], Stephen Daniels[2], Shumei S. Sun[1]

1 Department of Biostatistics, School of Medicine, Virginia Commonwealth University, Richmond, Virginia, United States of America, **2** Department of Pediatrics, School of Medicine, University of Colorado, Aurora, Colorado, United States of America

Abstract

Objectives: To determine whether childhood body size, composition and blood pressure are associated with adult cardiac structure by estimating childhood "age of divergence."

Methods: 385 female and 312 male participants in the Fels Longitudinal Study had echocardiographic measurements of left ventricular mass, relative wall thickness, and interventricular septal thickness. Also available were anthropometric measurements of body mass index, waist circumference, percentage body fat, fat free mass, total body fat, and systolic and diastolic blood pressures, taken in both childhood and adulthood. The age of divergence is estimated as the lowest age at which childhood measurements are significantly different between patients with low and high measurements of adult cardiac structure.

Results: Childhood body mass index is significantly associated with adult left ventricular mass (indexed by height) in men and women (ages of divergence: 7.5 years and 11.5 years, respectively), and with adult interventricular septal thickness in boys (age of divergence: 9 years). Childhood waist circumference indexed by height is associated with left ventricular mass (indexed by height) in boys (age of divergence: 8 years). Cardiac structure was in general not associated with childhood body composition and blood pressure.

Conclusions: Though results are affected by adult body size, composition and blood pressure, some aspects of adult cardiac structure may have their genesis in childhood body size.

Editor: Carmine Pizzi, University of Bologna, Italy

Funding: The research was funded by a grant from the National Heart Lung and Blood Institute (R01HL072838-05). The funders had no role in study design, data collection and analysis, decision to publish, or preparation of the manuscript.

Competing Interests: The authors have declared that no competing interests exist.

* Email: rsabo@vcu.edu

Introduction

A recent review of echocardiographic studies shows that the incidence of left ventricular hypertrophy (LVH) remains high in most races and both genders despite advances in hypertension management over the past two decades.[1] This high LVH incidence has coincided with an increase in the prevalence of childhood obesity over the previous three decades in the United States,[2] across all gender, race and socioeconomic groups.[3] Several studies have found associations between obesity,[4–10] body size,[11–13] adiposity[14,15], and blood pressure[10,16,17] and left ventricular mass (LVM), mass index (LVMI), or hypertrophy (LVH), while others have linked obesity and adiposity to relative wall thickness (RWT)[18] and other measures of cardiac structure.[14,15] LVM has also been shown to independently predict the incidence of several clinical events – including fatality – attributable to cardiovascular disease.[19]

The ability to predict cardiac structure in adults by measuring body size, composition and blood pressure in childhood is of clinical and public health importance, as such predictions might suggest corrective interventions that can be implemented in early childhood or adolescence. While some studies have linked childhood body size measurements with certain cardiovascular outcomes (such as mortality and hypertension), [20,21] fewer studies have focused on associations between childhood body size and adulthood cardiac structure. Notably, as part of the Bogalusa Heart Study (BHS), Toprak *et al.* found that childhood body mass index (BMI) was a significant factor in determining eccentric left ventricular hypertrophy in adulthood. [22] Urbina *et al.* – also from the BHS – similarly found associations between childhood body size and LVMI in young adults. [23]

In this manuscript we focus on associations between childhood body size, composition and blood pressure with adult cardiac structure. Using longitudinal data from the Fels Longitudinal Study, we estimate "ages of divergence" in childhood growth trends of BMI, waist circumference (WC), percentage body fat (%BF), fat free mass (FFM), total body fat (TBF), systolic (SBP) and diastolic (DBP) blood pressure, based on adult measures of LVMI, RTW, and interventricular septal wall thickness (IVST). We define

Table 1. Data Summary of FLS Participant Measurements.

	Males				Females			
	N	Mean	SD	95% CI	N	Mean	SD	95% CI
Adult Age	312	38.7	19.86	20.0, 96.6	385	41.5	19.66	20.0–92.4
LVMI	312	29.6	9.04	28.7, 30.5	385	28.1	8.98	27.2, 28.9
RWT	312	0.29	0.060	0.28, 0.30	385	0.29	0.056	0.28, 0.30
IVSTs	312	0.80	0.190	0.78, 0.81	385	0.72	0.152	0.71, 0.74
IVSTd	312	1.04	0.269	1.02, 1.07	385	0.94	0.222	0.92, 0.96
BMI	330	27.0	4.78	26.5, 27.5	411	26.3	5.53	25.7, 26.8
WCHt	327	55.5	7.88	54.6, 56.3	411	55.7	8.39	54.9, 56.5
%BF	143	23.5	9.00	22.0, 25.0	165	34.6	8.75	33.2, 35.9
FFM	304	66.2	8.86	65.2, 67.2	397	46.5	6.70	45.9, 47.2
TBF	304	19.9	7.90	19.0, 20.8	397	25.3	9.65	24.3, 26.2
SBP	329	121.9	13.74	120.4, 123.4	411	116.1	18.71	114.3, 117.9
DBP	181	82.6	11.42	81.0, 84.3	189	77.8	14.14	75.7, 79.8
ALC	244	0.7	0.92	0.6, 0.9	296	0.3	0.56	0.3, 0.4
SMK	192	3.5	8.22	2.4, 4.7	197	3.2	6.34	2.3, 4.1
PA	246	2.6	0.41	2.5, 2.6	296	2.5	0.43	2.4, 2.5

Sample sizes (N), means, SDs, 95% CIs (minimum and maximum provided for Adult Age) for adulthood cardiac structure, body size and composition, and lifestyle measurements. Cardiac Structure includes LVMI, RWT, and IVST (both systolic and diastolic). Body size, composition and blood pressure measurements include BMI, WCHt, %BF, FFM, TBF, SBP and DBP. Lifestyle measurements include ALC, SMK and PA.
SD: standard deviation.
Min, Max: Minimum and Maximum.
CI: Confidence Interval.
LVMI: Left-ventricular mass index, $g/m^{2.7}$.
RWT: Relative wall thickness, cm.
IVSTs: interventricular septum thickness – systolic, cm.
IVSTd: interventricular septum thickness – diastolic, cm.
BMI: Body mass index, kg/m^2.
WCHt: Waist circumference divided by height, %.
%BF: Percentage body fat, %.
FFM: Fat-free mass, kg.
TBF: Total body fat, kg.
ALC: Number of servings of alcohol consumed per day.
SMK: Number of cigarettes smoked per day.
PA: Physical activity index (scale 1–5).

Table 2. Distribution of Number of Childhood Measurements.

	Males				
Measure	**# of Subjects**	**Average # of Measurements**	**SD**	**Min**	**Max**
BMI	305	19.9	9.98	1	33
WCHt	229	11.9	6.60	1	26
%BF	177	5.0	2.88	1	11
FFM	149	5.0	2.84	1	12
TBF	149	5.0	2.86	1	12
SBP	304	12.6	6.34	1	27
DBP	200	5.6	3.73	1	15
	Females				
Measure	**# of Subjects**	**Average # of Measurements**	**SD**	**Min**	**Max**
BMI	335	19.3	10.17	1	33
WCHt	251	11.0	7.20	1	27
%BF	181	4.7	2.88	1	11
FFM	140	4.9	2.97	1	11
TBF	140	4.9	2.97	1	11
SBP	332	12.0	6.09	1	24
DBP	193	4.9	3.49	1	16

Number of subjects with at least one childhood measurement for each of body size (BMI, WCHt), body composition (%BF, FFM, TBF), and blood pressure (SBP, DBP) for each gender. Average number of childhood measurements per participant, standard deviation (SD) and minimum (Min) and maximum (Max) are also reported.

age of divergence as the age at which the difference in a particular childhood body size, composition or blood pressure measurement (between participants with low and high adult cardiac structure values) becomes significant and generally remains significant throughout the remainder of the growth trajectory [21]. For our purposes, we define high and low as the third and first quartiles, respectively, of the adult echocardiographic measurement in question. We also adjust (in separate analyses) for adult body size, composition and blood pressure, as well adult lifestyle measurements, such as alcohol use, smoking status, and level of physical activity.

Methods and Procedures

Ethics Statement

All participants provided written informed consent to participate in this study, and all procedures were approved by the Institutional Review Boards at Wright State University and Virginia Commonwealth University.

Participants

This study examined a non-random subsample of European-American male and female participants of the Fels Longitudinal Study (FLS) who were selected to undergo a echocardiographic examination. All FLS participants who were at least 20 years old and – for females – were not pregnant were approached during their routine FLS visits between 12/1/1999 and the end of data collection on 6/30/2009 to participate. Out of a total of 1,215 active FLS participants, 471 females and 405 males agreed to undergo echocardiographic measurement. Among those, 385 females and 312 males were greater than 20 years of age. Among those participants meeting the selection criteria: seven men and seven women had been diagnosed with cardiovascular disease (including stroke and heart attack); seven men and three women had type 2 diabetes mellitus (with fasting glucose exceeding 125 mg/dL); six men and two women were treated with insulin; three men and one woman had chronic obstructive pulmonary disease; 16 men and 18 women had been prescribed antihypertensive medication; and no participants had known congenital heart disease. These participants and their measurements were not removed from the study sample.

The FLS has enrolled participants continuously since 1929. Participants are generally enrolled at birth and are not selected in regard to factors known to be associated with disease, body composition or other clinical conditions. FLS subjects are examined semi-annually until 18 years of age, and biennially thereafter. Two textbooks contain more detailed information on the FLS beyond the sub-sample covered here. [24,25]

Measurements

The echocardiographic measurements were performed by a certified sonographer under the supervision of Dr. Stephen Daniels, using an ATL Philips Medical System HDI 5000 ultrasound imaging system. Two-dimensional and two-dimensional directed M-mode echocardiographic images were recorded, and measurements were made on three or more cardiac cycles according to the recommendations of the American Society of Echocardiography (ASE). [26] Left ventricular mass was calculated using the ASE formula: $LVM = 0.8(1.04\ ([LVIDd+PWTd+IVSTd]^3-[LVIDd]^3))+0.6$ g, where LVIDd is left ventricular internal dimension at end diastole, PWTd is posterior wall thickness at end diastole, and IVSTd is interventricular septal wall thickness at end diastole. Relative wall thickness was calculated as: $RWT = 2(PWTd)/(LVIDd)$. Interventricular septal wall thickness at systole (IVSTs) was also recorded. Since LVM is height-dependent, we divided LVM by height raised to the 2.7 power (LVMI) as previously suggested. [26,27]

Anthropometric body size measurements were taken following recommendations in the *Anthropometric Standardization Reference Manual.* [28] Weight was measured to 0.1 kg using a SECA scale. Height was measured to 0.1 cm using a Holtain stadiometer. BMI was then calculated as the ratio of weight to height (in meters) squared (kg/m^2). WC was measured at the level of the highest point on the right iliac crest in a plane parallel with the floor. Since WC is dependent upon height, [29] we indexed WC by dividing by height (WCHt). All measurements were taken twice, and a third measurement was taken if the difference between the first two exceeds an established tolerance (0.3 kg for weight, 0.5 cm for height, and 0.1 cm for waist circumference), and the average values were used for analysis.

Body composition measurements of FFM and TBF were made by a Lunar LPX and a DXA Hologic QDR 4500 Elite densitometer (Hologic, Waltham, MA). The coefficient of variation (CV) is 3.5**%** for soft tissue. Our DXA procedures have been compared and calibrated with those of underwater weighing (uww) [30], which is important in this study as body composition measurements for some older participants were taken using uww. To obtain consist body composition measurements across all participants, the following conversion equations were used: TBFuww = 2.1582+(1.1533xTBFdxa); FFMuww = 1.8449+(0.9329xFFMdxa); %BFuww = 2.0337+(1.1285x%BFdxa). In regard to cross-calibrating the Hologic and Lunar DXA machines, DXA data were collected from 78 FLS subjects who were scanned on the same day with both the Hologic 4500 and Lunar LPX machines. The calibration equations are: Hologic %BF = 5.6397+ 0.7908×Lunar %BF; R^2 = 0.98 and SE = 3.68; Hologic TBF = 3.0529+0.8439×Lunar TBF; R^2 = 0.98 and SE = 1.47; Hologic FFM = 0.7917+1.0349×Lunar FFM; R^2 = 0.94 and SE = 4.85. Bioelectrical impedance is proportional to total body water and to the length of the conductor or stature (stature^2/resistance).

In adults, both SBP and DBP (mmHg) were recorded as the average of three readings from a mercury sphygmomanometer with participants in a seated position. Each reading was taken by rapidly inflating the arm cuff to the maximum level and deflating at a rate of 2mmHg per second, with 30 seconds between readings. Blood pressure was measured in children in accordance with the standards of the second National Heart, Lung, and Blood Institute Task Force on Blood Pressure Control in Children [31] and the update of that report by the National High Blood Pressure Education Program. [32]

Other covariates include self-reported physical activity (PA), alcohol use (ALC), and smoking status (SMK), as each has been shown by others to affect various aspects of cardiovascular or metabolic health. [17,33–39] PA data are collected in the FLS using the Baecke Questionnaire of Habitual Physical Activity [40] and are recorded on a Likert scale. SMK is measured as the typical number of cigarettes smoked per day. ALC is defined as the typical number of alcoholic beverages consumed per day.

Statistical Analyses

All analyses were performed using SAS/STAT software version 9.4 (SAS Institute Inc., Cary, NC, USA), while all figures were produced using the R computational software (version 2.12.2). Adult measurements were summarized with means, standard deviations, and 95% confidence intervals (adult age was also summarized with minimum and maximum values); note that childhood measurements were not numerically summarized due to the large number (33 possible) of measurements taken. A linear mixed-effect repeated measures ANOVA model was used to estimate childhood body size growth trajectories. The responses for this model are one of the seven repeated-measure childhood body size or composition measurements (BMI, WCHt, %BF, FFM, TBF, SBP and DBP). Fixed effects for this model include childhood age (rounded to the nearest half year – as per the study design – and categorized), one of the four continuous adult cardiac structure measurements (LVMI, RTW, IVSTs and IVSTd), and an interaction between the two. Note that particular cardiac structure measurements for participants (159 males and 186 females) with more than one echocardiographic visit were averaged into one representative value. A participant-level random effect was included to account for within-participant dependence, which was modeled using a first-order autoregressive structure. This model allowed for testing of ages of divergence of mean childhood body size, composition and blood pressure growth profiles based on "high" and "low" values of adult cardiac structure [21], where the body size, body composition and blood pressure means predicted at the first and third quartile of the adult cardiac structure level were compared at each age (from age 2 to 18 at 0.5-year increments). First and third quartiles of adult cardiac structure were used to represent healthy (low) and unhealthy (high) values, respectively, without being too extreme. To account for multiple comparisons (there are at most 33 such comparisons and as few as 8, since not all body size and composition measures are obtained at each age in all participants), the overall significance level of 0.05 was adjusted using the step-down approach to the Bonferroni correction. [41] Models were analyzed separately for each gender since boys and girls have different growth patterns. Comparisons were made in an unadjusted manner (as stated above), and are also made adjusting for three lifestyle measurements (PA, SMK, ALC), and were then adjusted for the adult body size, composition or blood pressure measurement in question. These adjustments were made to the linear mixed-effects model described above by including these adult body size, composition, blood pressure and lifestyle measurements as fixed effects. A sensitivity analysis excluding measurements taken in participants over 65 years was also conducted (though results are not reported). Inquiries on the data used in these analyses can be made to the corresponding author.

Results

The adult echo-cardiographic measurements, as well as the adult body size, composition, and blood pressure measures are summarized in Table 1. Age, LVMI and RWT are similar between males and females, though the two IVST measures (systolic and diastolic) are on average smaller in women than in men. The two body size measurements (BMI and WCHt) are similar for men and women, while for the body composition measurements, males on average have lower %BF and TBF, and have higher FFM than females. As expected, both blood pressures are greater in males than in females. The three lifestyle measurements (ALC, SMK and PA) are similar between the sexes. For the results that follow, the sample size used for each unadjusted analysis is the minimum of the reported number of participants providing adult echocardiographic measurements in Table 1 (312 males, 385 females) and the number of participants providing at least one childhood measurement in Table 2. The sample size when adjusting for adult lifestyle measurements is the minimum of the number of participants with lifestyle measurements reported in Table 1 (ranges of 192–246 for males and 197–296 for females) and the number of participants with at least one childhood measurement reported in Table 2. The sample size when adjusting for adult body size, composition and blood pressure is the minimum of that reported for adult measurements

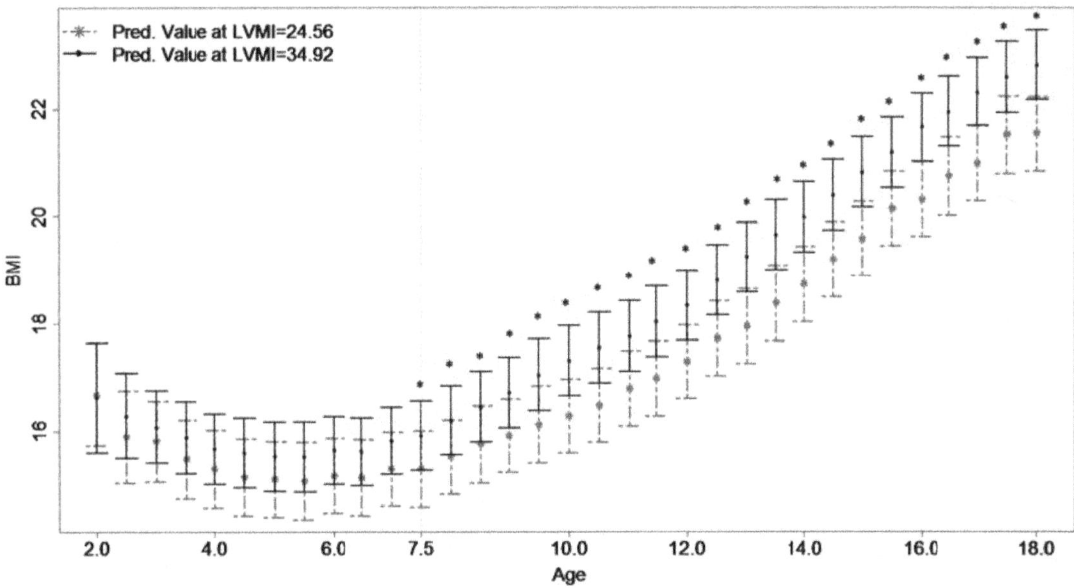

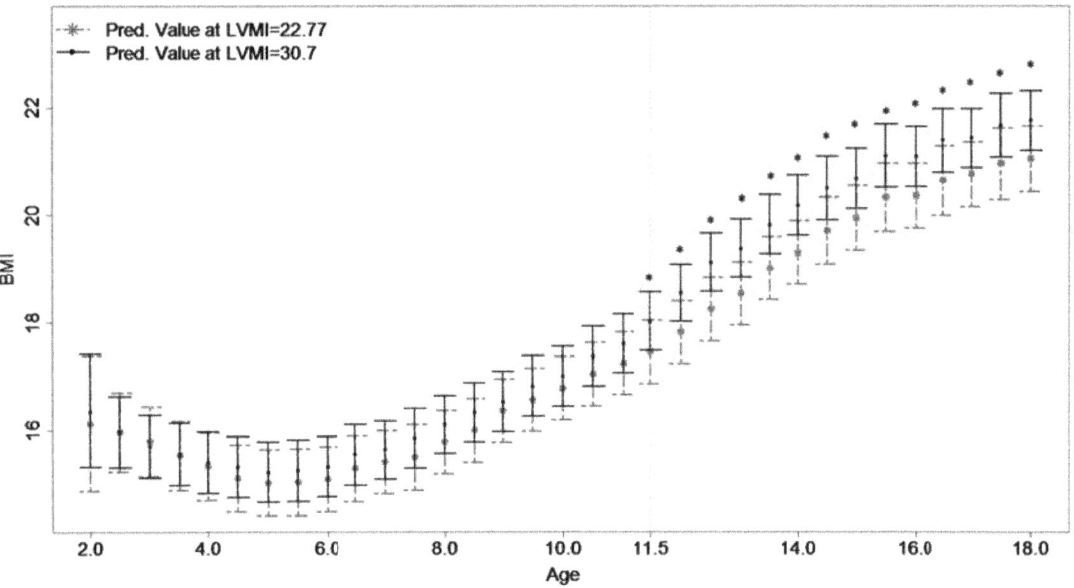

Figure 1. Childhood Body Mass Index Trajectories based upon Adulthood Left Ventricular Mass Index. *Figure 1 Legend*: Childhood growth trajectories of body mass index (BMI) are provided for men's (N = 305; high: 34.92, low: 24.56) and women's (N = 335; high: 30.70, low: 22.77) left ventricular mass index (LVMI). Asterisks indicate significant results using Bonferroni-adjusted significance levels with the step-down approach.

in Table 1 (ranges of 143–329 for males and 165–411 for females) and the number of participants reported in Table 2.

Left Ventricular Mass Index

The growth trajectories for BMI according to the first and third quartiles of adult LVMI become significantly different at age 7.5 in males (Figure 1A) and at age 11.5 in females (Figure 1B) and remain significant thereafter. In both males and females, participants with larger adult LVMI had larger childhood BMI than those adults with lower adult LVMI. After adjusting for adult lifestyle characteristics (Table 3), the age of divergence increases slightly to 8.0 in males, while the age of divergence for females remains 11.5. After adjusting for adult BMI (Table 3), no age of divergence in childhood BMI is detectable.

The growth trajectories for WCHt according to adult LVMI (Figure 2) become significantly different at age 8 in males and generally remain significant thereafter (though the differences at age 16.5 and 17.5 are not significant). There was no significant divergence in WCHt growth in females based on LVMI.

Table 3. Estimated "Age of Divergence" in Childhood Measurements.

		Males			Females		
		Unadujst	Adjusted Life	Adjusted Adult	Unadjust	Adjusted Life	Adjusted Adult
BMI	LVMI	7.5 years	8.0 years	None	11.5 years	11.5 years	None
	RWT	None			None		
	IVSTs	9.0 years	None		None		
	IVSTd	9.5 years	None		None		
WCHt	LVMI	8.0 years	8.0 years	None	None		
	RWT	None			None		
	IVSTs	None			None		
	IVSTd	None			None		
%BF		None			None		
FFM		None			None		
TBF		None			None		
SBP		None			None		
DBP		None			None		

These estimates are determined from sequential hypothesis tests of predicted childhood body size (BMI, WCHt), body composition (%BF, FFM, TBF) and blood pressure (SBP, DBP) compared at the first and third quartiles of adult cardiac structure (LVMI, RWT, IVSTs, IVSTd). These estimates are provided unadjusted for any other measurements, adjusted for adult lifestyle (Life) measurements (ALC, SMK and PA), and adjusted for the corresponding adult body size, body composition, or blood pressure measurement (Life/Adult). "None" implies that no hypotheses were rejected at any childhood age for that adult echocardiographic measurement.

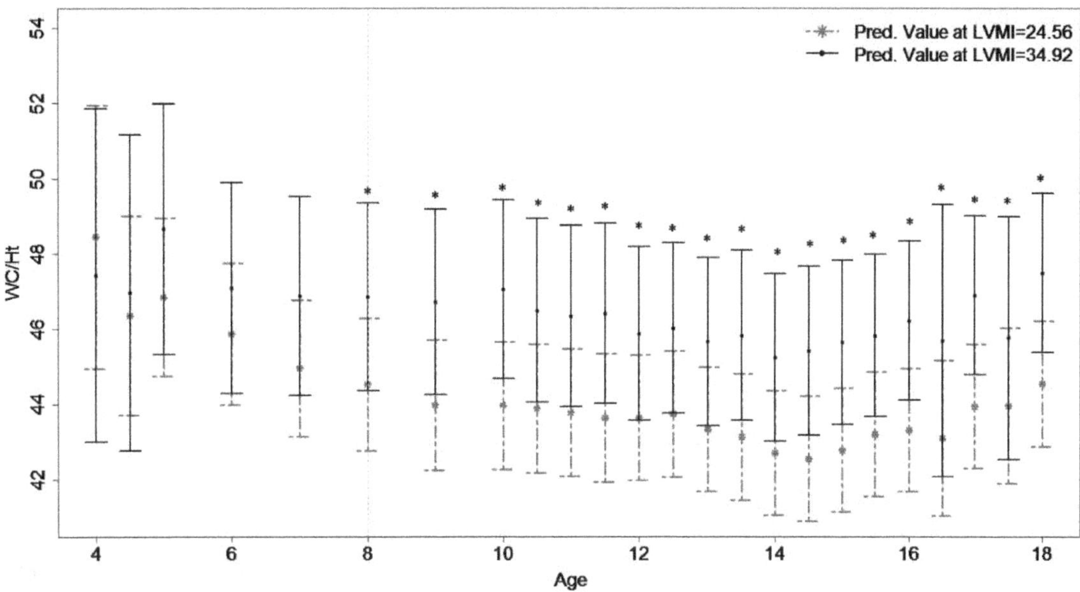

Figure 2. Childhood Waist Circumference Divided by Height Trajectories based upon Adulthood Left Ventricular Mass Index. *Figure 2 Legend*: Childhood growth trajectories of waist circumference divided by height (WCHt) are provided for men's' (N = 229; high: 34.92, low: 24.56) and women's (N = 251; high: 30.70, low 22.77) left ventricular mass index (LVMI). Asterisks indicate significant results using Bonferroni-adjusted significance levels with the step-down approach.

Participants with larger adult LVMI had larger childhood WCHt than those adults with lower adult LVMI. The age of divergence in childhood WCHt remained unchanged when adjusting for adult lifestyle measurements (Table 3), but disappeared when accounting for adult WCHt.

There were no significant differences in the childhood growth trends based on adult LVMI for the three body composition measurements (%BF, FFM, TBF) or the two blood pressures (SBP and DBP). Plots of all growth-trends based on adult LVMI are provided in Files S1, S2, S3, S4, S5, S6, and S7.

Relative Wall Thickness

The growth trends for childhood body size, body composition and blood pressure were not significantly different between adults with high and low RWT in males or females. Plots of all growth-trends based on adult RWT levels are provided in Files S1, S2, S3, S4, S5, S6, and S7.

Interventricular Septal Wall Thickness

In males, the growth trajectories for childhood BMI were significantly different according to adult IVSTs from ages 9 through 18 (Figure 3A). Adults with larger adult IVSTs had larger average childhood BMI than adults with lower IVSTs. These results were no longer significant when adjusted for adult lifestyle measurements or adult BMI. Growth trajectories for WCHt were significantly different at ages 9 and 10 but not thereafter, and thus do not constitute an age of divergence. None of the childhood body size, composition or blood pressure trends were significantly different in females based on adult IVSTs level.

In males, the childhood BMI growth trajectories were significantly different according to adult IVSTd between ages 9.5 to 18 (Figure 3B), where adults with larger IVSTd had larger childhood BMI than did adults with lower IVSTd. These differences were no longer significant when adjusted for adult lifestyle or adult BMI. Childhood %BF in males was significantly larger in adults with larger adult IVSTd than in adults with lower adult IVSTd at age 8, and childhood FFM was significantly higher in adults with larger IVSTd than in adults with lower IVSTd at ages 15 and 16. As no significant differences were observed after these ages, they did not constitute an age of divergence. None of the body size and composition trends were significantly different in females based on adult IVSTd level. Plots of all growth-trends based on adult IVSTs and IVSTd are provided in Files S1, S2, S3, S4, S5, S6, and S7.

Discussion

Our methodological approach was to treat childhood body size, composition and blood pressure measurements as the repeated measure dependent outcome, and to treat adult cardiac structure as an independent variable. While this approach is the reverse of what would seem a more natural formulation with the adult measure as the dependent variable and the childhood measure as the independent variable, it allowed us to determine associations between the childhood and adult measures. Particularly, these results show that certain aspects of cardiac structure in adults are correlated with childhood body size, with the associations showing up in some cases before age 10. This seems to imply that some childhood characteristics – whether through childhood diet, behavior, activity level, or genetic predisposition – partially explain adult cardiac health. In boys, having larger BMI or waist circumference (indexed by height) in childhood is positively associated with developing abnormal LVMI and IVST in adulthood, while in girls, having larger BMI in childhood is positively associated with developing abnormal LVMI in adulthood.

Specifically, we found that certain childhood body size measurements, such as BMI and WCHt are associated with certain adulthood cardiac structure measurements. Using the unique longitudinal data of the Fels Longitudinal Study and its sub-sample of echocardiographic measurements, we were able to show that the childhood BMI for adults with high LVMI and

A. IVSTs

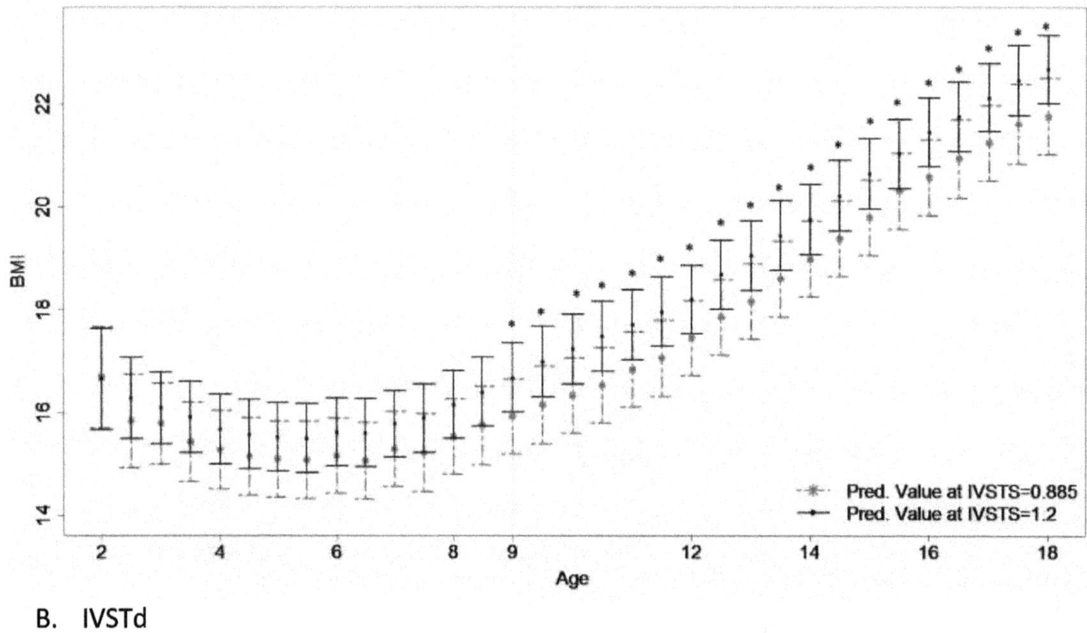

B. IVSTd

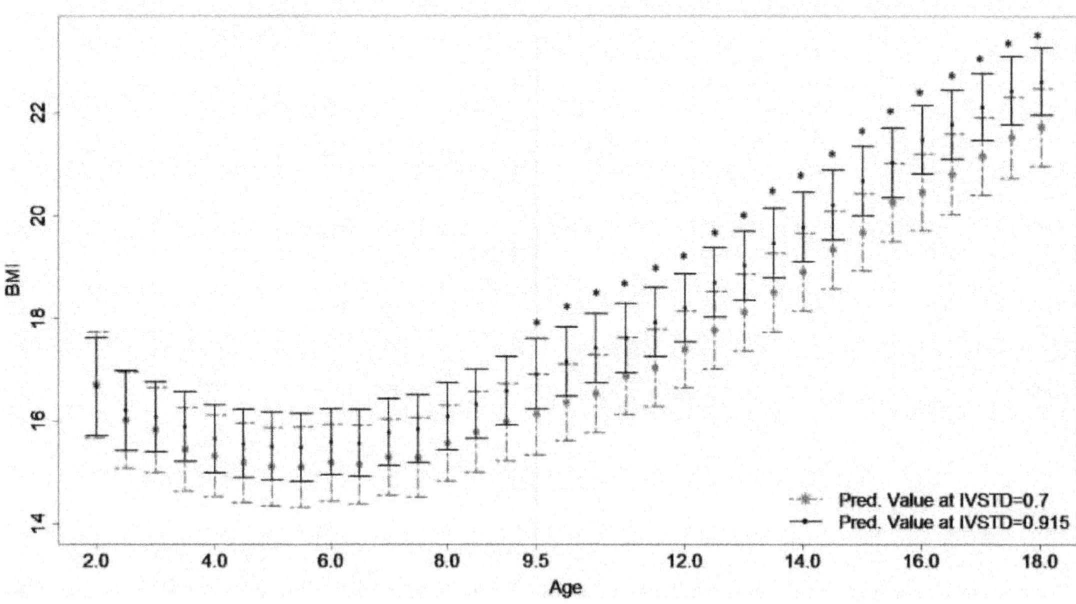

Figure 3. Childhood Body Mass Index Trajectories based upon Adulthood Interventricular Septal Thickness – Systolic and – Diastolic. *Figure 3 Legend*: Childhood growth trajectories of body mass index (BMI) are provided for men's interventricular septal thickness – systolic (N = 305; IVSTs; high: 1.200, low: 0.885) and men's interventricular septal thickness – diastolic (N = 305; IVSTd; high: 0.915, low 0.700). Asterisks indicate significant results using Bonferroni-adjusted significance levels with the step-down approach.

IVST becomes significantly different from the childhood BMI for adults with low LVMI and IVST before puberty in boys. For girls, the age of BMI divergence occurred later than that of boys for LVMI, and was non-existent based upon IVST. WCHt also experienced an early divergence in boys based upon adult LVMI, but no significant divergence was observed in girls. There were no significant associations between childhood body size with RWT, and in general there were no significant divergences in childhood body composition or blood pressure based on adult cardiac structure.

The ages of divergence were mostly independent of adult lifestyle characteristics (ALC, SMK, and PA), and were no longer significant once adult body size and/or composition were accounted for. Similar results were seen in Sabo *et al.* (2012), who estimated age of divergences in childhood body size based on adult blood pressure.[21] While this phenomenon may seem to suggest that adult obesity or adiposity are more important in the relationship with cardiac structure than are childhood growth trends, it must be remembered that both childhood obesity and adiposity track into adulthood.[42] In addition, two research teams from the Bogalusa Heart Study also found – using echocardiographic measurements – that childhood BMI was positively associated with left ventricular structure, even after accounting for (young) adult body size.[22,23] Regardless of the effects of adult body size and composition, it appears that the genesis of adult cardiac structure may be affected by body size in childhood, though earlier for boys than for girls.

Several studies have found that high blood pressure is one of the primary causes of LVH.[16,17,43] Rademacher *et al.* (2009) showed that childhood blood pressure and BMI exert independent influences on further cardiovascular risk, [10] while Malcolm *et al.* (1993) and de Simone *et al.* (1998) showed that the effect of body size on contemporaneous LVM was independent of both age and blood pressure. [12,13] Schussheim *et al.* (2007) showed that patients with subnormal left ventricular shortening fraction (LVSF) have significantly higher diastolic blood pressure and greater BMI than patients matched for age and sex with normal LVSF. [44] de Simone also found associations between blood pressure and LVSF. [45] Interestingly, we did not find any associations between childhood blood pressure and adult cardiac structure. At least with respect to DBP, this lack of association may be due to the relatively low number of FLS participants providing measurements.

One limitation of our work is that this FLS subset only contains measurements on European-American participants. Therefore, generalizations of these findings to the entire US population or to other races should be avoided. Note that Toprak *et al.* did find that African Americans had a larger incidence of concentric left ventricular hypertrophy than did European-Americans, [22] but it is unclear if that implies that there are also racial disparities in the estimated ages of divergence observed here. The FLS sub-sample studied here also varied widely in age, from 20 years over 90 years. Though echocardiographic measurements were taken on these older individuals, a sensitivity analysis excluding measurements taken when participants were over 65 years did not change the result (results not shown). We also did not account for other measurements (such as diabetes status, HDL cholesterol, triglycerides and urinary albumin-creatinine ratio), though none of these measurements were significantly associated with adult cardiac structure in the Bogalusa study [22]. The predominant strength of this work is the large average number of repeated measurements per participant, which allowed us to estimate ages of divergence for each adult cardiac structure measurement based upon childhood body size, composition and blood pressure. Also unique was the coupling of adult cardiac structure with serial childhood measures.

Supporting Information

File S1 Childhood growth trajectories of body mass index (BMI) are provided for men's and women's left ventricular mass index (LVMI), relative wall thickness (RWT), interventricular septum thickness – systolic (IVSTs), andinterventricular septum thickness – diastolic (IVSTd). Asterisks indicate significant results using Bonferroni-adjusted significance levels with the step-down approach.

File S2 Childhood growth trajectories of waist circumference divided by height (WCHt) are provided for men's and women's left ventricular mass index (LVMI), relative wall thickness (RWT), interventricular septum thickness – systolic (IVSTs), andinterventricular septum thickness – diastolic (IVSTd). Asterisks indicate significant results using Bonferroni-adjusted significance levels with the step-down approach.

File S3 Childhood growth trajectories of percentage body fat (PBF) are provided for men's and women's left ventricular mass index (LVMI), relative wall thickness (RWT), interventricular septum thickness – systolic (IVSTs), andinterventricular septum thickness – diastolic (IVSTd). Asterisks indicate significant results using Bonferroni-adjusted significance levels with the step-down approach.

File S4 Childhood growth trajectories of fat free mass (FFM) are provided for men's and women's left ventricular mass index (LVMI), relative wall thickness (RWT), interventricular septum thickness – systolic (IVSTs), andinterventricular septum thickness – diastolic (IVSTd). Asterisks indicate significant results using Bonferroni-adjusted significance levels with the step-down approach.

File S5 Childhood growth trajectories of total body fat (TBF) are provided for men's and women's left ventricular mass index (LVMI), relative wall thickness (RWT), interventricular septum thickness – systolic (IVSTs), andinterventricular septum thickness – diastolic (IVSTd). Asterisks indicate significant results using Bonferroni-adjusted significance levels with the step-down approach.

File S6 Childhood growth trajectories of systolic blood pressure (SBP) are provided for men's and women's left ventricular mass index (LVMI), relative wall thickness (RWT), interventricular septum thickness – systolic (IVSTs), andinterventricular septum thickness – diastolic (IVSTd). Asterisks indicate significant results using Bonferroni-adjusted significance levels with the step-down approach.

File S7 Childhood growth trajectories of diastolic blood pressure (DBP) are provided for men's and women's left ventricular mass index (LVMI), relative wall thickness (RWT), interventricular septum thickness – systolic (IVSTs), andinterventricular septum thickness – diastolic (IVSTd). Asterisks indicate significant results using Bonferroni-adjusted significance levels with the step-down approach.

Author Contributions

Conceived and designed the experiments: SD SSS. Analyzed the data: RTS M-SY. Wrote the paper: RTS M-SY SD SSS.

References

1. Cuspidi C, Sala C, Negri F, Mancia G, Morganti A (2012) Prevalence of left-vetnricular hypertrophy in hypertension: an updated review of echocardiographic studies. Journal of Human Hypertension 26: 343–349.
2. Singh G, Kogan M, Yu S (2009) Disparities in Obesity and Overweight Prevalence Among US Immigrant Children and Adolescents by Generational Status. Journal of Community Health 34: 271–281.

3. (2007) Health, United States, 2007 with Chartbook on trends in the health of Americans. Hyattsville, MD: US Department of Health and Human Sercies.
4. Chobanian A, Bakris G, Black H, Cushman W, Green L, et al. (2003) The Seventh Report of the Joint National Committee on Prevention, Detection, Evaluation, and Treatment of High Blood Pressure: the JNC 7 report. Journal of the American Medical Association 289: 2560–2572.
5. Coca A, Gabriel R, Figuera Mdl, Lopez-Sendon J, Fernandez R, et al. (1999) The impact of different echocardiographic diagnostic criteria on the prevalence of left ventricular hypertrophy in essential hypertension: the VITAE study. Journal of Hypertension 17: 1471–1480.
6. Gottdiener J, Reda D, Materson B, Massie B, Notargiacomo A, et al. (1994) Importance of obesity, race and age to the cardiac structural and functional effects of hypertension. The Department of Veterans Affairs Cooperative Study Group on Antihypertensive Agents. Journal of the American College of Cardiology 24: 1492–1498.
7. Lauer M, Anderson K, Kannel W, Levy D (1991) The impact of obesity on left ventricular mass and geometry. The Framingham Heart Study. Journal of the American Medical Association 266: 231–236.
8. Lauer M, Anderson K, Levy D (1992) Separate and joint influences of obesity and mild hypertension on left ventricular mass and geometry: the Framingham Heart Study. Journal of the American College of Cardiology 19: 130–134.
9. Powell B, Redfield M, Bybee K, Freeman W, Rihal C (2006) Association of obesity with left ventricular remodeling and diastolic dysfunction in patients without coronary artery disease. American Journal of Cardiology 98: 116–120.
10. Rademacher E, Jacobs D, Moran A, Steinberger J, Prineas R, et al. (2009) Relation of blood pressure and body mass index during childhood to cardiovascular risk factor levels in young adults. Journal of Hypertension 27: 1766–1774.
11. Daniels S, Morrison J, Sprecher D, Khoury P, Kimball T (1999) Association of body fat distribution and cardiovascular risk factors in children and adolescents. Circulation 99: 541–545.
12. Malcolm D, Burns T, Mahoney L, Lauer R (1993) Factors affecting left ventricular mass in childhood: the Muscatine Study. Pediatrics 92: 703–709.
13. Simone Gd, Devereux R, Kimball T, Mureddu G, Roman M, et al. (1998) Interaction between body size and cardiac workload: influence on left ventricular mass during body growth and adulthood. Hypertension 31: 1077–1082.
14. Abel E, Litwin S, Sweeney G (2008) Cardiac remodeling in obesity. Physiological Reviews 88: 389–419.
15. Lieb W, Xanthakis M, Sullivan L, Aragan J, Pencina J, et al. (2009) Longitudinal tracking of left ventricular mass over the life course: Clinical correlates of short- and long-term change in the Framingham Offspring Study. Circulation 119: 3085–3092.
16. Frohlich E (2009) The most common cause of hospitalization in Medicare patients in the United States is cardiac failure and, perhaps, the earliest involvement of the heart in hypertension and is that of left ventricular hypertrophy (LVH). Preface. Medical Clinics of North America 93: xv–xx.
17. Heckbert S, Post W, Pearson G, Arnett D, Gomes A, et al. (2006) Traditional cardiovascular risk factors in relation to left ventricular mass, volume, and systolic function by cardiac magnetic resonance imaging: the Multiethnic Study of Atherosclerosis. Journal of the American College of Cardiology 48: 2285–2295.
18. Amin R, Kimball T, Bean J, Jeffries J, Willging J, et al. (2002) Left ventricular hypertrophy and abnormal ventricular geometry in children and adolescents with obstructive sleep apnea. American Journal of Respiratory and Critical Care Medicine 165: 1395–1399.
19. Levy D, Garrison R, Savage D, Kannel W, Castelli W (1990) Prognostic implications of echocardiographically determined left ventricular mass in the Framingham Heart Study. New England Journal of Medicine 322: 1561–1566.
20. Must A, Jacques P, Dallal G, Bajema C, Dietz W (1992) Long term morbidity and mortality of overweight adolescents: a follow-up of the Harvard Growth Study of 1922 to 1935. New England Journal of Medicine 327: 1350–1355.
21. Sabo R, Lu Z, Daniels S, Sun S (2012) Serial childhood body mass index and associations with adult hypertension and obesity: the Fels Longitudinal Study. Obesity 20: 1741–1743.
22. Toprak A, Wang H, Chen W, Paul T, Srinivasan S, et al. (2008) Relation of childhood risk factors to left ventricular hypertrophy (eccentric or concentric) in relatively young adulthood (from the Bogalusa Heart Study). The American Journal of Cardiology 101: 1621–1625.
23. Urbina E, Gidding S, Bao W, Pickoff A, Berdusis K, et al. (1995) Effect of Body Size, Ponderosity, and Blood Pressure on Left Ventricular Growth in Children and Young Adults in the Bogalusa Heart Study. Circulation 91: 2400-2406.
24. Roche A, Sun S (2003) Human Growth: Assessment and Interpretation. Cambridge, United Kingdom: Cambridge University Press.
25. Roche A (1992) Growth, Maturation and Body Composition: the Fels Longitudinal Study 1929–1991. Cambridge: Cambridge University Press.
26. Lang R, Bierig M, Devereux R, Flachskampf F, Foster E, et al. (2005) Recommendations for chamber quantification: a report from the American Society of Echocardiography's Guidelines and Standards Committee and the Chamber Quantification Writing Group, developed in conjunction with the European Association of Echocardiography, a branch of the European Society of Cardiology. Journal of the American Society of Echocardiography 18: 1440–1463.
27. Daniels S, Meyer R, Liang Y, Bove K (1988) Echocardiographically determined left ventricular mass index in normal children, adolescents and young adults. Journal of the American College of Cardiology 12: 703–708.
28. Lohman G, Roche A, Martorell R (1988) Anthropometric Standardization Reference Manual. Human Kinetics. Champaign, IL.
29. Sabo R, Ren C, Sun S (2012) Comparing height-adjusted waist circumference indices: the Fels Longitudinal Study. Open Journal of Endocrine and Metabolic Diseases 2: 40–48.
30. Guo SS, Chumlea WC, Roche AF, Siervogel RM (1997) Age- and maturity-related changes in body composition during adolescence into adulthood: the Fels Longitudinal Study. Int J Obes Relat Metab Disord 21: 1167–1175.
31. Task Force on Blood Pressure Control in Children. National Heart L, and Blood Institute, Bethesda, Maryland (1987) Report of the Second Task Force on Blood Pressure Control in Children — 1987. Pediatrics 79: 1–25.
32. Adolescents. NHBPEPWGoHCiCa (1996) Update on the 1987 Task Force Report on HIgh Blood Pressure in Children and Adolescents: a working group report from teh National High Blood Pressure Education Program. Pediatrics 98: 649–658.
33. Ford E, Giles W, Dietz W (2002) Prevalence of the metabolic syndrome among US adults: findings from the third National Health and Nutrition Examination Survey. Journal of the American Medical Association 287: 356–359.
34. Guo S, Chumlea W, Cockram D (1996) Use of statistical methods to estimate body composition. American Journal of Clinical Nutrition 64: S428–S435.
35. Guo S, Chumlea W, Roche A, Siervogel R (1997) Age- and maturity-related changes in body composition during adolescence into adulthood: The Fels Longitduinal Study. International Journal of Obesity 21: 1167–1175.
36. Guo S, Zeller C, Chumlea W, Siervogel R (1999) Aging, body composition, and lifestyle: the Fels Longitudinal study. American Journal of Clinical Nutrition 70: 405–411.
37. Ross R, Janssen I (2001) Physical activity, total and regional obesity: dose-response considerations. Med Sci Sports Exerc 33: S528–S529.
38. Schubert C, Rogers N, Remsberg K, Sun S, Chumlea W, et al. (2006) Lipids, lipoproteins, lifestyle, adiposity and fat-free mass during middle age: The Fels Longitudinal Study. Int J Obes Relat Metab Disord 30: 251–260.
39. Verdecchia P, Schillaci G, Borgioni C, Ciucci A, Gattobigio R, et al. (1996) Prognostic value of left ventricular mass and geometry in systemic hypertension with left ventricular hypertrophy. American Journal of Cardiology 78: 197–202.
40. Baecke JA, Burema J, Frijters JE (1982) A short questionnaire for the measurement of habitual physical activity in epidemiological studies. Am J Clin Nutr 36: 936–942.
41. Holm S (1979) A simple sequentially rejective multiple test procedure. Scandinavian Journal of Statistics 6: 65–70.
42. Guo S, Chi E, Wisemandle W, Chumlea W, Roche A, et al. (1998) Serial changes in blood pressure from childhood into young adulthood for females in relation to body mass index and maturational age. American Journal of Human Biology 10: 589–598.
43. McNiece K, Gupta-Malhotra M, Samuels J, Bell C, Garcia K, et al. (2007) Left ventricular hypertrophy in hypertensive adolescents: Analysis of risk by 2004 national high blood pressure education program working group staging criteria. Hypertension 50: 392–395.
44. Schussheim A, Devereux R, Simone Gd, Borer J, Herrold E, et al. (1997) Usefulness of submormal midwall fractional shortening in predicting left ventricular exercise dysfunction in asymptomatic patients with systemic hypertension. American Journal of Cardiology 79: 1070–1074.
45. Simone Gd, Greco R, Mureddu G, Romano C, Guida R, et al. (2000) Relation of left ventricular diastolic properties to systolic function in arterial hypertension. Circulation 101: 152–157.

2

Multidimensional Poverty in Rural Mozambique: A New Metric for Evaluating Public Health Interventions

Bart Victor[1,2], Meridith Blevins[2,3], Ann F. Green[2], Elisée Ndatimana[6], Lázaro González-Calvo[6], Edward F. Fischer[7], Alfredo E. Vergara[2,4¤], Sten H. Vermund[2,5,6], Omo Olupona[8], Troy D. Moon[2,5,6]*

1 Owen Graduate School of Management, Vanderbilt University, Nashville, Tennessee, United States of America, **2** Vanderbilt Institute for Global Health, Vanderbilt University, Nashville, Tennessee, United States of America, **3** Department of Biostatistics, Vanderbilt University School of Medicine, Nashville, Tennessee, United States of America, **4** Department of Preventive Medicine, Vanderbilt University School of Medicine, Nashville, Tennessee, United States of America, **5** Department of Pediatrics, Vanderbilt University School of Medicine, Nashville, Tennessee, United States of America, **6** Friends in Global Health, Maputo, Mozambique, **7** Vanderbilt Center for Latin American Studies and Department of Anthropology, Vanderbilt University, Nashville, Tennessee, United States of America, **8** World Vision International, Maputo, Mozambique

Abstract

Background: Poverty is a multidimensional phenomenon and unidimensional measurements have proven inadequate to the challenge of assessing its dynamics. Dynamics between poverty and public health intervention is among the most difficult yet important problems faced in development. We sought to demonstrate how multidimensional poverty measures can be utilized in the evaluation of public health interventions; and to create geospatial maps of poverty deprivation to aid implementers in prioritizing program planning.

Methods: Survey teams interviewed a representative sample of 3,749 female heads of household in 259 enumeration areas across Zambézia in August-September 2010. We estimated a multidimensional poverty index, which can be disaggregated into context-specific indicators. We produced an MPI comprised of 3 dimensions and 11 weighted indicators selected from the survey. Households were identified as "poor" if were deprived in >33% of indicators. Our MPI is an adjusted headcount, calculated by multiplying the proportion identified as poor (headcount) and the poverty gap (average deprivation). Geospatial visualizations of poverty deprivation were created as a contextual baseline for future evaluation.

Results: In our rural (96%) and urban (4%) interviewees, the 33% deprivation cut-off suggested 58.2% of households were poor (29.3% of urban vs. 59.5% of rural). Among the poor, households experienced an average deprivation of 46%; thus the MPI/adjusted headcount is 0.27 ($=0.58\times0.46$). Of households where a local language was the primary language, 58.6% were considered poor versus Portuguese-speaking households where 73.5% were considered non-poor. Living standard is the dominant deprivation, followed by health, and then education.

Conclusions: Multidimensional poverty measurement can be integrated into program design for public health interventions, and geospatial visualization helps examine the impact of intervention deployment within the context of distinct poverty conditions. Both permit program implementers to focus resources and critically explore linkages between poverty and its social determinants, thus deriving useful findings for evidence-based planning.

Editor: Spencer Moore, University of South Carolina, United States of America

Funding: The Ogumaniha-SCIP baseline survey was supported by the United States Agency for International Development (USAID)–Mozambique (Award No. 656-A-00-09-00141-00) through a sub-grant from World Vision, Inc. Funding support for the secondary data analysis is from Vanderbilt University through the endowment of the Amos Christie Chair in Global Health. The funders had no role in study design, data collection and analysis, decision to publish, or preparation of the manuscript.

* Email: troy.moon@vanderbilt.edu

¤ Current address: US Centers for Disease Control and Prevention, Maputo, Mozambique

Background

In the last two decades, the world's governments have generated unprecedented support for a comprehensive list of global development aims, of which the Millennium Development Goals (MDGs) are an integral part. [1–4] One of the most significant outcomes of these joint efforts has been the prioritization of poverty reduction at the center of national and international policy agendas. In fact, the first goal of the MDGs is to reduce by half the global proportion of people living in extreme poverty by 2015. Three additional MDGs target public health interventions that reduce child mortality, improve maternal health, and combat HIV/AIDS, malaria and other disease [1–4]. Understanding the link between poverty and the public health interventions employed in the developing world is among the most difficult yet important problems faced today [5,6].

Increasingly the effectiveness of public health interventions is recognized as being closely tied to the impact of other efforts such as economic development, education, agriculture programs and improvements in infrastructure (including water and sanitation), shelter and security. While each intervention area brings an emphasis and focus on distinct needs, there are significant interactions and co-dependencies between areas. For example, it is generally accepted that poverty is closely associated with the availability and quality of health service, but this relationship is far from simple. There is a complex mutual causation: poor health services contribute to poverty, which in turn negatively influences the ability to access and utilize health services. To determine the impact of public health interventions on poverty reduction, it is necessary to define an appropriate framework for poverty measurement. By creating an evaluation paradigm that establishes an index of "poverty" as the primary outcome measure, yet which can be further disaggregated based on the contributions of its defined dimensions such as health, education, and living standard; we get the added value of being able to evaluate each dimension independently while simultaneously learning from the interactions and co-dependencies between areas that subsequently impact the effectiveness of the interventions employed to address them.

Traditional standards for measuring poverty are ever more criticized for their potential to both "mis-measure" and more importantly, misunderstand the true drivers of poverty. [7] Per capita income is a unidimensional measure that categorizes a person as poor if their income falls below a particular "poverty line", now frequently defined as less than $1.25 a day. [8–10] Unidimensional measures have been extensively critiqued in terms of their validity and precision and have proven inadequate to the challenge of assessing the extent and dynamics of poverty in the world. [7] Critique has been mostly directed toward use of unidimensional measurements for national policy and global comparison purposes. However, this argument is perhaps even more compelling when directed at interventions or public health programming aimed to improve well-being. An alternative approach derived from the work of Amartya Sen, introduces the idea that there are multiple dimensions of poverty [9–12].

The International Fund for Agriculture Development (IFAD) and the Sustainable Coffee Partnership, for example, have each developed sophisticated multi-criteria models that take into account many dimensions when measuring their intervention's success or not. [13] This approach for measuring many dimensions is not the same as measuring multidimensionality. In practice, extant models measure many dimensions, but most do not produce an integrated multidimensional model. One notable exception has been the work of the Oxford Poverty and Human Development Initiative (OPHI). [14] Working within the OPHI framework, Alkire and Foster have developed a method for calculating dimensional weights and cut-offs that integrate a number of dimensions into a combined metric [15].

International development organizations, researchers, and an increasing number of national governments are beginning to adopt multidimensional measures of national poverty. [14,16] The United Nations Development Program's (UNDP) Human Development Index (HDI) includes not only measures of Gross National Product (GNP) per head, but also incorporates indicators related to education and health in order to produce a composite index. Some program monitoring and evaluation efforts have also begun to incorporate multiple measures.

The three main objectives of this paper are 1) to demonstrate how multidimensional measures of poverty can be utilized in the planning and evaluation of large scale public health and development interventions; 2) to utilize the Alkire and Foster method for multidimensional poverty measurement in Zambézia Province, an extremely rural, infrastructure-depleted region of north-central Mozambique, to establish a baseline poverty index from which future comparisons will be conducted in order to measure the impact of interventions in the province; and 3) to create geospatial maps of poverty deprivation at baseline, providing program implementers a visual needs assessment that characterizes the geographic differences of each target district and aids in prioritizing program planning.

Methods

Study Context

In 2009, World Vision International was awarded a United States Agency for International Development (USAID) grant called Strengthening Communities through Integrated Programming (SCIP) for a 5-year multi-sector program aimed at improving the health and livelihoods of children, women, and families in Zambézia Province, Mozambique. Known locally as the *Ogumaniha* project, which means "united for a common purpose" in the local language of Echuabo, SCIP is based on a consortium of five international non-governmental organizations led by World Vision. The broad goals of the 5-year project are to: 1) reduce poverty in Zambézia Province by pursuing the consolidation of an integrated, innovative, and sustainable community-based program in the province; and 2) integrate current and future United States Government (USG) investments in Zambézia Province in the areas of health, HIV/AIDS, water and sanitation, income generation, and institutional capacity building.

In 2012, Mozambique ranked 185 of 187 nations on the UNDP's HDI, and the gross national income was estimated at US $906 per capita [8], with male and female life expectancies of 47 and 51 years, respectively, in 2009 [17]. Although Mozambique's health expenditure has risen substantially over the past 10 years, as a proportion of total GDP it was only 6.6% in 2011 (66 USD per capita). [18] Mozambique is one of the sub-Saharan African countries most affected by the HIV/AIDS epidemic, with a national adult HIV prevalence of 11.5% in 2009. [19] Nationally, 12% of children were considered orphans or vulnerable children, and only 43% of households had access to clean drinking water in 2009 [20].

The magnitude of poverty is especially evident in Zambézia Province, Mozambique's second largest province and home to about 4 million persons (Figure 1). [21,22] While Mozambique ranks among the poorest of the poor nations, Zambézia consistently ranks among Mozambique's lowest performing provinces with low literacy rates, poor maternal and child health (MCH) indices, high rates of tuberculosis and malaria infections, and high levels of malnutrition. [20,23,24] Zambézia Province is overwhelmingly rural and depends almost entirely on subsistence farming and fishing. The province has the highest estimated number of persons living with HIV in the country (~275,000 or nearly 20% of Mozambique's HIV-infected population) as of 2009 [19,25] and yet only 31 of Zambézia's 214 health facilities provided antiretroviral therapy (ART) as of December 2012. This is partially because Zambézia Province housed much of the armed conflict in Mozambique's 16-year civil war (1976–1992) and suffered disproportionately in destruction of its healthcare infrastructure [21,22].

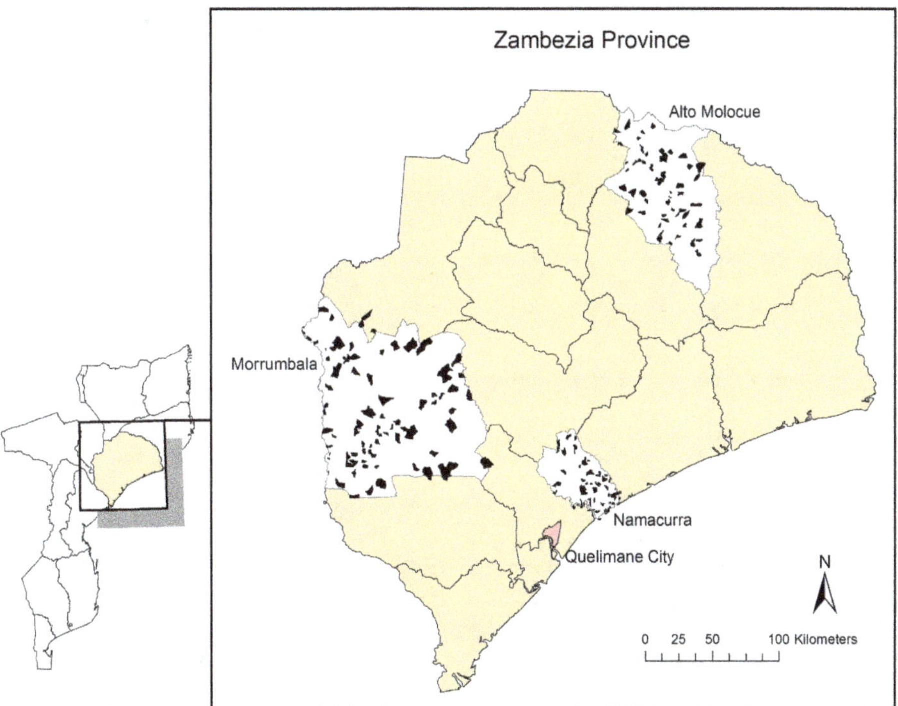

Figure 1. Map of Mozambique, Zambézia Province, with Enumeration Areas Highlighted in Three Focus Districts, Namacurra, Morrumbala, and Alto Molócuè.

Study Design

Integral to *Ogumaniha's* design is a strong monitoring system and project evaluation based on performance indicators agreed upon with USAID and the provincial government. Because the project involves multi-sectoral interventions and an interdisciplinary approach to implementation, the consortium opted for a multidisciplinary evaluation design. A survey instrument used at *Ogumaniha's* initiation (baseline survey in 2010) and at the project's end (final survey implemented June 2014) was designed based on the human development theory originated by Sen (1999) and further developed by researchers from OPHI. This instrument uses multiple dimensions to measure poverty including health, education, and income; access to goods and services; and self-empowerment. The vision of this pre-post project evaluation is that the information collected can provide a more thorough and holistic measure of the impact of this large-scale, multi-sector intervention on the overall health and well-being of the households in Zambézia Province, more so than analysis of the individual sector specific measures when viewed in isolation.

The *Ogumaniha* survey tool collects information on over 500 variables in 8 dimensions and was developed by a multidisciplinary team of researchers including staff, faculty, and graduate students from Vanderbilt University and the Universidade Eduardo Mondlane. To design the survey, we used many questions and validated scales from previous national surveys in Mozambique, including various National Institute for Statistics (*Instituto Nacional de Estatísticas* [INE]) surveys focusing on poverty and economic status; and other international surveys such as the Demographic Health Survey (DHS) and the Multiple Indicator Cluster Survey (MICS). The survey was designed to collect household information from the female head of household, defined as the principal wife of the nuclear family (polygamy is common practice), because she is thought to be most familiar with the majority of topics of interest. Survey questions covered household demographics; economic status; health knowledge, attitudes and practices; access to health and HIV-related services and products; access to improved water and sanitation; nutritional intake; and others.

The poverty index used to identify households or areas of poverty in the province following baseline survey data collection, was modeled after the Multidimensional Poverty Index (MPI) founded on the OPHI methodology which calculates the quantity of defined "poor" (the headcount), multiplied by their average amount of deprivation, called the Adjusted Headcount Ratio [15].

Data Collection

Mobile survey teams conducted interviews with 3,916 (98%) of 3,960 planned female heads of households in 259 Enumeration Areas (EAs) across 14 of Zambézia's 17 districts. Complete data for analysis was available from 3,749 (96%) of the interviews conducted. EA selection was not stratified by district, thus 3 districts were randomly excluded from the province-wide sample. Interviews were conducted either in Portuguese or in one of the five predominant tribal languages of the province (Cisena, Elomwe, Echuabo, Cinyanja, and Emakhuwa), and data were collected using mobile cell phones. Interviewers received intensive training on the use of mobile phones for data collection prior to implementation. Satellite and census maps were used to locate the EAs. Initial plans for household selection included administering questionnaires at 15 household structures identified through a color threshold algorithm and randomly selected on the satellite map; however, the actual implementation resulted in division of the EA into four quadrants and collecting 3–4 interviews starting at the household nearest the center of each quadrant (household selection paper in preparation). In a subset of 95 randomly selected EAs, anthropometric measures of a random selection of children

Table 1. Ogumaniha Multidimensional Poverty Index (MPI) adapted from the Oxford Poverty and Human Development Initiative (OPHI).

OPHI Model		*Ogumaniha* MPI			Districts of Alto Molócuè, Morrumbala and Namacurra
Dimension	**Indicator**	**Deprivation cut-off (poverty line)**	**Weight**	**Deprivation**	**Percent of households deprived per indicator (95% CI)[1]**
Education					
	Years of Schooling	Literacy score<16 and numeracy score<5	1/6	Low literacy	14.7% (11.9, 17.5)
	Child Enrollment	Child in household = "Yes"+age ">6" or age "<15"+attending school = "No"	1/6	School-aged child is not attending school	17.6% (15.5, 19.7)
Health					
	Child Mortality	Fever last 30 d = "Yes", Diarrhea last 30 d = "Yes" or Difficulty breathing last 30 d = "Yes"	1/6	Child with acute illness	21.5% (18.5, 24.6)
	Nutrition	Household dietary diversity score<4	1/12	Low dietary diversity	15.4% (13.1, 17.6)
		Lack of food episode during last month = "Yes"	1/12	Lack of food episode during last month	30.4% (27.7, 33.1)
Standard of living					
	Electricity	Electricity = "No"	1/18	No electricity	95.1% (93.7, 96.5)
	Water	Water source is river = "True", OR time to water = ">30 min", AND mode of transport to water = "On foot"	1/18	Water source is river or more than 30 minutes away on foot	29.7% (25.6, 33.8)
	Sanitation	Household uses latrine = "No"	1/18	No use of latrine	75.6% (72.4, 78.8)
	Flooring	Roof type = "grass/cane/leaves/straw"	1/18	Poor housing material (grass roof)	92.5% (90.9, 94.0)
	Cooking Fuel	Type of fuel household uses = "Wood"	1/18	Poor cooking fuel (wood)	95.9% (94.5, 97.2)
	Assets	Sum of radio = "Yes"+television = "Yes"+bicycle = "Yes" = <1	1/18	Low assets (no radio, television, bike)	43.2% (40.7, 45.8)

[1]Weighted percentages include 95% confidence intervals that incorporate the effects of stratification and clustering due to the sample design.

under 5-years residing in participating households were also included. In these EA's, households with one or more children aged 0–12 months, one child was randomly selected for weight and height measurements. Similarly, for households with one or

Table 2. Use of the Oxford Poverty and Human Development Initiative (OPHI) Method for Monitoring and Evaluation.

Advantages of the OPHI Method for Monitoring and Evaluation
-Expands dimension measures in critical areas including health
-Incorporates program specific detail in comparative evaluation
-Uses national comparisons for benchmarking and scale, and efficiency
-Isolates where the greatest impact is (and potentially unintended)
-Detects indirect benefits in poverty reduction from specific interventions
-Facilitates the collaboration between development policy makers who are increasingly measuring multidimensional poverty and development practitioners on the ground
-Allows for temporal and geographic comparisons

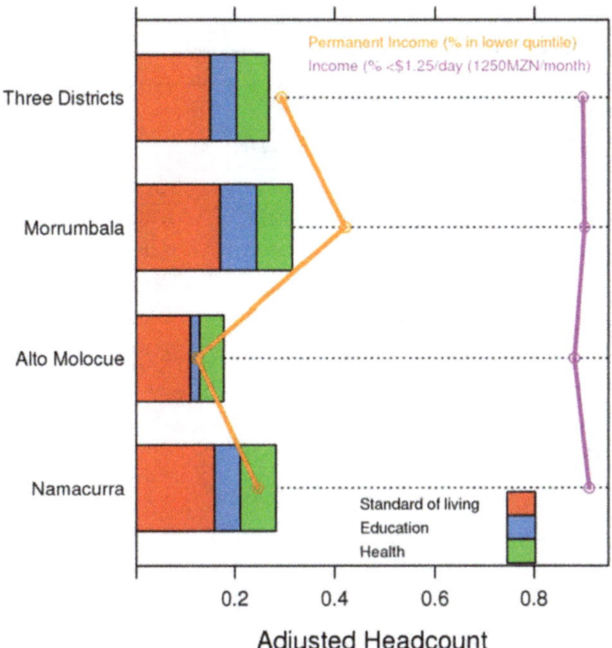

Figure 2. Decomposition by District and Broken Down by Dimension in the Three Focal Districts, *Ogumaniha* 2010. Legend: The adjusted headcount is decomposed by dimension for Morrumbala, Alto Molócuè, Namacurra and all three districts combined. Data that are overlaid include percent of households in the lowest quintile for permanent income wealth and % of households making less than USD$1.25/day. MZN = Metical.

more children aged 13–59 months, one child was randomly selected for height and weight measurements.

Baseline survey data were collected between August and September, 2010. Fourteen teams of five female surveyors were recruited, each with prior experience in survey work. The teams were assigned by language proficiency to a specific region, working under the supervision of a regional supervisor, and were trained on general aspects of survey conduct.

Mozambique's 2007 census served as the sampling frame. To appropriately capture *Ogumaniha's* public health and development interventions without increasing the sample size and survey costs, data were collected in two phases; a concentrated sample of 2,878 households in 193 EAs in three selected focal districts (Namacurra, Alto Molócuè, and Morrumbala) (Figure 1) and a smaller sample of 871 households in 66 EA from the remaining districts. These three districts were selected because they represent 3 distinct geographical regions, and *Ogumaniha* interventions were anticipated in each, allowing future analysis of intervention impact on poverty. We provide the sample size justification online: http://globalhealth.vanderbilt.edu/manage/wpcontent/uploads/Ogumaniha_SampleSize_20100613.pdf.

Alkire and Foster Method

Methods to identify and aggregate the poor using multiple dimensions have mathematical properties that allow for decomposition of poverty indices by subgroups or by indicators. [15] The Alkire and Foster method was used to construct three key poverty indices: headcount, average poverty gap, and adjusted headcount (called the *Ogumaniha* MPI). Application of this method is detailed elsewhere (see http://www.ophi.org.uk/research/multidimensional-poverty/how-to-apply-alkire-foster/); briefly, the steps for identification and aggregation of households include:

Table 3. Poverty Distribution of Zambézia Province, Districts of Morrumbala, Namacurra, and Alto Molócuè.

Poverty cut-off (Minimum deprivation)	Headcount (95% CI) (n = 2,878)
11.1%	99.2% (98.5, 99.8)
16.7%	97.7% (96.6, 98.8)
22.2%	91.4% (89.8, 93.0)
25%	77.4% (75.0, 79.8)
27.8%	75.6% (73.1, 78.2)
30.6%	64.2% (61.3, 67.1)
33.0%	58.2% (55.0, 61.4)
36.1%	52.2% (48.9, 55.5)
38.9%	44.9% (41.6, 48.3)
41.7%	35.9% (33.0, 38.8)
44.4%	33.5% (30.5, 36.4)
47.2%	25.1% (22.6, 27.7)
50%	21.0% (18.5, 23.5)
52.8%	17.0% (14.6, 19.5)
55.5%	11.5% (9.2, 13.7)
58.3%	8.9% (7.3, 10.4)
61.1%	6.9% (5.4, 8.3)
63.9%	4.7% (3.5, 5.9)
66.7%	3.6% (2.7, 4.5)

Table 4. Respondent and Household Characteristics by Multidimensional Poverty Status, *Ogumaniha* 2010.

Variables[a]	Non-poor	Poor	Total[d]	P-value[c]
	(n = 1196)	(n = 1682)	(n = 2878)	
Household size (n = 2878)	4 (3–6)	5 (3–6)	4 (3–6)	<0.001
Children under 5 (n = 2878)	1 (0–1)	1 (0–2)	1 (0–2)	<0.001
Age of respondent (n = 2425)	30 (23–40)	32 (25–41)	32 (24–41)	<0.001
Education (n = 2878)	2 (0–4)	0 (0–2)	0 (0–3)	<0.001
*Distance of EA from health facility (km) (n = 2878)	6.8 (3.8–10.8)	7.8 (4.5–12.2)	7.5 (4–11.7)	<0.001
Urban/rural (n = 2878)				<0.001
Rural	40.5%	59.5%	95.7%	
Urban	70.7%	29.3%	4.3%	
Length of residency (years) (n = 2785)	6 (3–18)	6 (3–15)	6 (3–17)	0.997
Primary language of household (n = 2873)				<0.001
Cinyanja	23.2%	76.8%	0.8%	
Cisena	33.7%	66.3%	44.3%	
Echuabo	39.8%	60.2%	25.6%	
Elomwe	55.7%	44.3%	27.6%	
Emakhuwa	45.4%	54.6%	0.3%	
Portuguese	73.5%	26.5%	1.3%	
Respondent understands Portuguese (n = 2876)	54.7%	45.3%	27.5%	<0.001
Marital status (n = 2878)				0.035
Married/Common Law	42.8%	57.2%	72.9%	
Divorced/Separated	29.5%	70.5%	3.4%	
Single	43.0%	57.0%	17.5%	
Widowed	34.0%	66.0%	6.2%	
Religion (n = 2598)				<0.001
Catholic	48.0%	52.0%	45.7%	
Protestant	41.2%	58.8%	10.7%	
Evangelical and Pentecostal	39.6%	60.4%	14.3%	
Other Christian[b]	37.1%	62.9%	4.5%	
Muslim	41.1%	58.9%	8.5%	
Non-Christian Eastern	37.8%	62.2%	4.3%	
Other[b]	34.2%	65.8%	11.9%	
**Monthly household income, Meticais (n = 2691)	150 (0–500)	0 (0–300)	150 (0–500)	<0.001
No household income (n = 2691)	33.4%	66.6%	48.8%	<0.001
Household member has a farm (n = 2856)	41.6%	58.4%	90.7%	0.408
Permanent income (n = 2878)	0.6 (0.3–0.8)	0.3 (0–0.5)	0.4 (0.1–0.7)	<0.001
Ever accessed health facility (n = 2878)	45.4%	54.6%	57.4%	<0.001
Ever accessed pharmacy (n = 2878)	46.5%	53.5%	18.1%	0.004
Ever accessed traditional healer (n = 2878)	43.8%	56.2%	39.7%	0.579
***Ever accessed VCT (n = 2878)	55.1%	44.9%	10.7%	<0.001
****Accessed ANC last pregnancy (n = 2457)	44.7%	55.3%	41.8%	0.001

[a]Continuous variables are reported as weighted estimates of median (interquartile range] and categorical variables are reported as weighted percentages, with each observation being weighted by the inverse of the household sampling probability.
[b]'Other Christian' includes LDS Mormon and Jehovah's Witness. 'Other' includes Spiritual, Traditional Religions, and Agnostic or Atheist.
[c]Tests of associations (continuous) include Wilcoxon rank sum (continuous) and chi-squared test (categorical).
[d]All percentages in the cross tabulations are row percentages. The final column presents column (overall) percentages.
*EA = enumeration area.
**Approximate exchange rate as of October 2013: $1 USD = 30 Meticais.
***VCT = voluntary counseling and testing (for HIV).
****ANC = antenatal clinic.

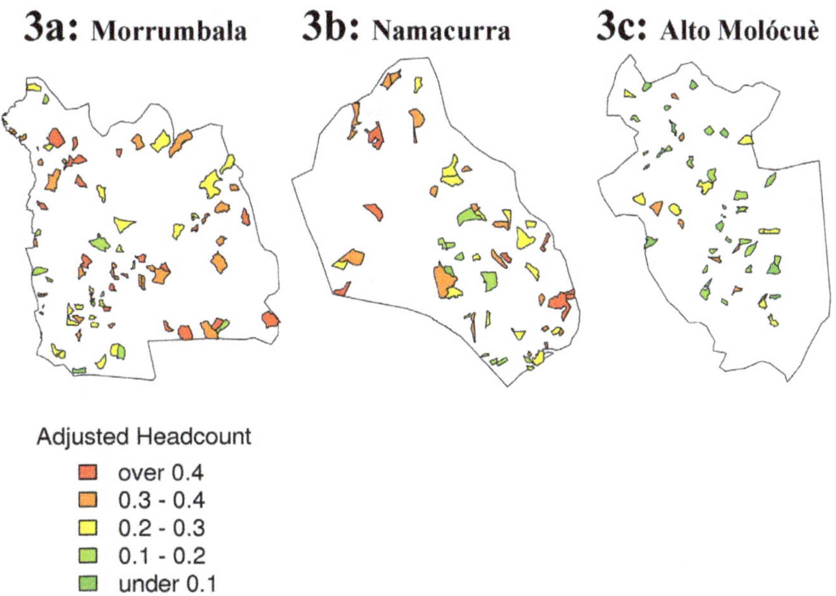

Figure 3. Enumeration Area Distribution in Three Focus District by Adjusted Headcount: Morrumbala, Namacurra and Alto Molócuè. *Enumeration area representations of poverty by adjusted headcount with green being less deprived and red.

1. Creation of a listing of **dimensions** and corresponding **indicators** collected from the household survey. (Table 1, columns 1–2)
2. Setting **poverty lines** at values where a person is identified as deprived or non-deprived for each indicator. (Table 1, column 3)
3. Setting **weights** for contribution of each indicator to the overall metric. (Table 1, column 4)
4. Determining the poverty cut-off for **identification**. (Table 2, row 7)
5. Performing **robustness** checks of the cut-off. (Table 2)
6. Estimating across group or dimension using **aggregation**:

a. Headcount (H): proportion of households that are identified as poor.

b. Average Poverty Gap (A): weighted average deprivation experienced by poor.

c. Adjusted Headcount (called the *Ogumaniha* MPI): multiply headcount by average poverty gap to reflect the breadth of deprivations. Thus, MPI = HxA.

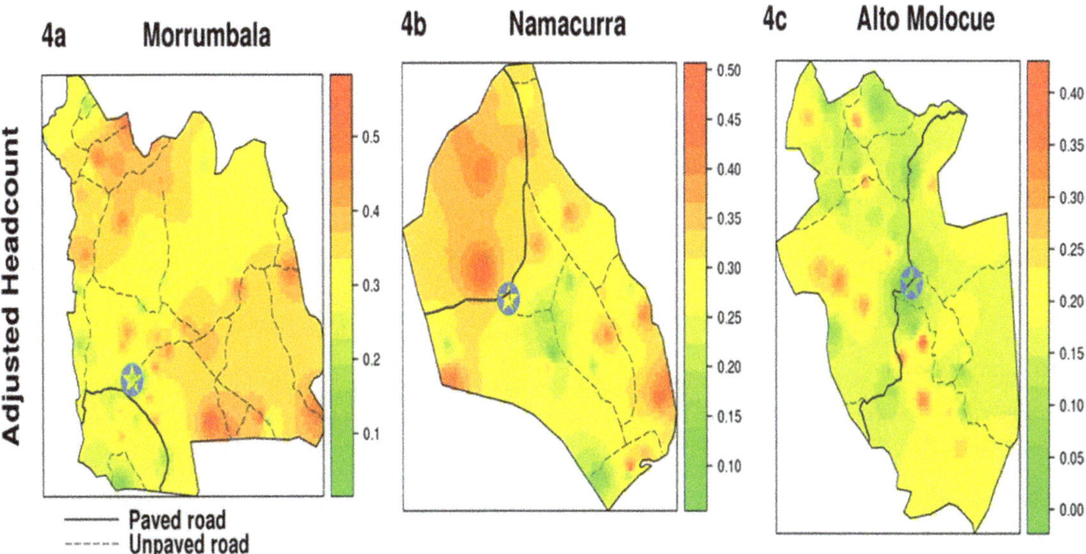

Figure 4. Smoothed Heat Map of Three Focus Districts: Morrumbala, Namacurra, and Alto Molócuè. *Figures 4a, 4b, and 4c show heat map geographical representations of poverty by adjusted headcount with green being less deprived and red most deprived. (Circled Star represents location of district capital).

Proportions include 95% confidence intervals that incorporate the effects of stratification and clustering due to the sample design. [26] Descriptive analysis of continuous variables includes weighted estimates of median, 25th and 75th quantiles (interquartile range). Categorical variables are reported as weighted percentages, with each observation being weighted by the inverse of the household sampling probability. Tests of association by poverty ignore effects of clustering, and they include Wilcoxon rank sum (continuous) and chi-square (categorical) tests.

Map generation

Using Esri shape files provided by INE to identify EA boundaries, a basic heat-map of poverty metrics was generated for the three focus districts. To enhance readability of the maps, ordinary kriging was used to predict poverty metrics for unsampled areas, assuming only spatial correlation. The 'krige' function is in the gstat package of R, which uses generalized least squares prediction with spatial covariances to produce smoothed geospatial representations of poverty. [27] R-software 2.15.1 (www.r-project.org) was employed for all data analyses; analysis scripts are available online at (http://biostat.mc.vanderbilt.edu/ArchivedAnalyses).

Description of permanent income

The measurement of household income is particularly problematic in high poverty areas. [28] In the current sample, 49% report no monetary income whatsoever. Increasingly in economics and development, monetary income is no longer the preferred measure. Instead, a "permanent income", [29] or wealth measure based upon ownership of selected assets is employed. Poverty stemming from lack of resources is associated with low income, but it is perhaps more closely related to low wealth. Low wealth individuals always have low income, but not all low income individuals have low wealth. In that sense, wealth and poverty are more closely related than income and poverty. We applied a measure of permanent income developed by the World Bank. [28] Briefly, a series of 37 asset and other indicator variables were used in a dichotomous hierarchical ordered probit model to derive a latent variable which denotes the permanent income of household to be incorporated into the *Ogumaniha* MPI (Figure 2, orange line) [12].

Ethical Considerations

Participation in the household survey was completely voluntary, no incentive was provided for participation. At enrollment written informed consent was obtained. The protocol for data collection and consent forms were approved by the Mozambican National Bioethics Committee for Health (*Comité Nacional de Bioética em Saúde* [CNBS]) and the Institutional Review Board of Vanderbilt University.

Results and Discussion

Results are presented in two sections. Section 1 describes the methodology we employed to define our metric, the *Ogumaniha* MPI, and demonstrates its usefulness to planning and evaluation of large scale public health and development interventions. Section 2 applies the *Ogumaniha* MPI to households and EAs in the three focus districts by utilizing data collected in the *Ogumaniha* baseline survey, in order to establish baseline multidimensional poverty estimates in Mozambique's Zambézia Province.

Section 1 - Defining the Ogumaniha Multidimensional Poverty Index (MPI)

We employ a method of monitoring and evaluation that looks at the analysis of development interventions in holistic terms, producing an aggregate metric that can be disaggregated by dimension (education, health, and living standard) and further disaggregated by subgroups (e.g., urban/rural, Portuguese proficiency). In the OPHI model, the 3 dimensions were further disaggregated into 10 indicators, weighted evenly within dimension such that each dimension had equal weight, and then a person was defined as poor if they were "deprived" in more than 33% of the indicators (Table 1). We used dimensional weighting similar to the OPHI model that would produce a comparable aggregate metric that could be used to compare across projects while incorporating national norms. Our method allows the isolation of the relative impact of specific inputs on overall well-being, and thus target areas for effective interventions.

This method goes beyond multiple measures and generates a true MPI. Specifically, it 1) uses intentionally selected dimensions of poverty to capture relevant functioning and capability deficits; 2) calculates deficit cut points based on comparative conditions; 3) applies differential weighting of deficits that contribute to poverty level; and 4) combines calculated poverty measures to produce a single metric for comparative purposes (Table 2).

An advantage of the *Ogumaniha* MPI includes its basis on survey data, which takes into account community level impact, perceptions, and buy-in. Additionally, survey data were collected utilizing a low-cost cell phone technology that reduced data entry costs and errors. The *Ogumaniha* MPI may be used for planning purposes to identify areas with high frequency of poor, intense poverty, or both. In being able to isolate not only the direct impact of a particular intervention but also the effect of inputs on other dimensions and overall well-being, this model can also serve as a useful tool in assessing return on investment and cost-benefit analyses.

Section 2 - Identifying Poverty by Household and Enumeration Area

Building upon the OPHI MPI, we maintained the same 3 dimensions (education, health, and living standard), but defined 11 indicators rather than the 10 utilized in the OPHI model. When possible, the same OPHI indicators were used; however, some were adapted for best fit based on the questions asked in the baseline survey. Table 1 shows the OPHI Model in comparison to our adapted *Ogumaniha* MPI with the "weight" column representing the contribution of each indicator to multidimensional poverty. The rightmost column (Table 1) reports the proportion of households that are deprived in each indicator.

Of 2,878 female heads of household interviewed in the three focal districts, the median age was 32 years. The median household size was four persons and the median number of children <5 years old in the home was one. Choosing to maintain the same OPHI poverty definition cut-off, in which the "poor" must be deprived in at least 33% of the indicators, a headcount of 58.2% of our provincially representative sample met that definition and were identified as poor. The highest cut-off would identify 3.6% of households as poor whereas the lowest cut-off would identify 99.2% of households as poor. If the poor were deprived in 50% or more deprivations, then the headcount is 20% (Table 3). Approximately 96% of households lived in an EA designated as rural by INE, of which 59.5% met the criteria for being defined poor, compared to 29.3% of urban households. Looking at the relationship of poverty to the primary language spoken in the household, 26.5% of Portuguese speaking households and 58.6% of households speaking one of the other five local languages were considered poor (Table 4).

Once identified as poor, if the intensity of deprivation increases for a household (say from 33% to 60% of weighted indicators), the headcount remains unchanged. As such, robust models must be able to adjust for changes in both headcount and the average deprivation; this MPI is called adjusted headcount. Using the 33% deprivation cut-off from the OPHI method, we estimated a headcount of 58.2% of the three focal districts sample to be poor; among these, households experienced an average deprivation of 46%; thus the adjusted headcount (= 0.58×0.46) is 0.27 (95% CI: 0.25–0.29). The headcounts for the three focal districts (Morrumbala, Namacurra, Alto Molócuè) plus all three combined are 0.67, 0.60, 0.42, and 0.58, respectively. The average deprivation for the three focal districts, plus all three combined, are 0.48, 0.47, 0.42, and 0.46. Analyzed separately, Morrumbala has the greatest breadth of poverty with an index of 0.32 (0.29–0.34), followed by Namacurra at 0.28 (0.26–0.31), and the least deprived being Alto Molócuè with an index of 0.18 (0.15–0.21). Additionally, the *Ogumaniha* MPI can be further broken down revealing the weight of each dimension's contribution to that index. In all three districts, living standard was the most dominant dimension deprived, followed by health, and then education (Figure 2).

Following calculation of the *Ogumaniha* MPI for each of the 193 EAs in three focal districts, geospatial maps were created that allow for visualization of the dispersion of EAs throughout the three districts (Figure 3) and provide smoothed estimates of poverty at baseline (Figure 4). The mapping of poverty deprivation at baseline provides program implementers a visual needs assessment that characterizes the geographic differences of each target district and aids in prioritizing program planning. Additionally, going forward we can overlay maps depicting the location and intensity of the various *Ogumaniha* sector interventions in the target districts (which were not uniformly implemented) and evaluate the impact of those interventions, or the combination of interventions. This is possible for measured outcomes in the specific individual-level locations in which interventions were implemented and also for a broader area-level evaluation or "neighborhood effect" that interventions may or may not have on nearby locales and/or the district as a whole.

In Morrumbala (Figure 4a), there are two geographic areas of high poverty deprivation, one in the extreme northwest of the district and the other in the southeastern region. Areas of least poverty deprivation, tend to focus around the main transportation corridor in the south, around the district capital and extends to the northeast through the center of the district. The area of high poverty deprivation in the northeast is fairly isolated, and difficult to reach (can take up to 5 hours to reach by car from the district capital). Morrumbala suffers from flooding of the Zambezi and Chire rivers each year. Flood zones are located in the southwest region and extending north along the western border of the district.

In Namacurra (Figure 4b), the largest geographic area of high poverty deprivation is in the northwest side of the district with pockets of high poverty deprivation distributed throughout the southeast. The southern parts of Namacurra can be difficult to reach with roads that flood, cutting them off from the rest of the district during the rainy season. However this area has some of the more fertile farm-land. Furthermore, the southernmost tip of Namacurra is coastal (one of only a handful of natural deep water ports on the eastern African coastline). This port is slated for large investments in infrastructure over the next 5–10 years, and may become an economic hub for the north-central provinces of Mozambique.

Alto Molócuè (Figures 4c) is one of the more economically developed districts with several commercial factories. The national highway cuts across the district and connects Alto Molócuè with commercial centers in the south and Nampula Province to the north. Pockets of high deprivation tend to be located in areas farthest away from transportation corridors.

Conclusions

We seek innovative approaches to conducting evaluation research in public health. [30] Baseline assessments of poverty that are more valid can improve our program planning as well as evaluation of interventions. Advancement in evaluation is increasingly critical due to the pressures created by the burdens of disease in the developing world, and even more so by the increasing complexity of interventions. In developing the measurement and evaluation tools reported here we employ the most current understanding of the crucial interdependency between conditions of poverty and both the need for and effectiveness of public health interventions. However, significant obstacles still limit the potential utility of this new approach to public health program evaluation. While measures taking multidimensionality into account have already been adopted by the Mozambican government, its meaning and use remains relatively unfamiliar. In our sample, relatively few households sampled came from urban areas as the make-up of Zambézia Province is predominantly rural. In our context we feel the MPI measure accurately captures a relevant view of the condition of poverty across the province. However, a limitation to this approach is that if applied to a predominantly urban area, the indicators used to assess poverty may overestimate households as non-deprived based on a lack of dirt floor for example, despite the fact that they may live in a poorly quality structures with crowded conditions and limited space. As a result, analysis must take into account context for what is considered deprived or not. Additionally, the logistics, manpower, and costs of implementing such a large population-based survey at program's beginning and end may limit the accessibility of this approach to only governments, donor agencies, and/or larger multi-sector public health development projects whose outcomes of interest are not isolated to the individual sector specific program indicators.

In this paper, we have reported the estimated baseline MPI for Zambézia Province at initiation of a large scale USAID funded, 5-year multi-sector grant. We believe that our estimates of poverty are a conservative minimum, as our results show that greater than half of our representative sample is poor (based on the 33% deprivation standard), and one-fifth or more are deprived in 50% of indicators. We found that living standard was the dominant dimension of poverty, followed by health and then education. By avoiding a unidimensional income measure, which in the Zambézia context classifies >90% of households as poor based on the generic < $1.25/day standard (Figure 2), the *Ogumaniha* MPI reveals a more nuanced and differentiated view of the conditions of poverty in an area that frequently employs non-monetary economic structures and is reliant on subsistence farming and fishing. This will assist in setting priorities for development in an area of near-universal poverty, as the neediest persons and regions can be differentiated from the less needy.

The implications of this work apply to both program planning and research. The integration of multidimensional poverty measures into planning and implementation design and the use of geospatial visualization of the relationships between interventions and distinct conditions of poverty at baseline have great utility and added value to the field of public health. Geospatial mapping, for instance, can dramatize variations of poverty in microenvironments, helping set program intervention priorities. Key to meeting the twin demands of greater impact and greater efficiency for public health interventions is recognizing and responding to the challenges created by the interdependencies between public health and other dimensions of poverty. Such interdependencies are rarely incorporated into program evaluation, thus leaving public health implementers and researchers struggling to understand both the positive and negative outcomes of interventions.

The MPI technique allows public health professionals and agencies to better target their resources by accounting for variation. With respect to research, we demonstrate how a robust multidimensional measurement can explore the linkages between poverty and health differentials in a population and derive useful inferences for further evidence-based planning. When repeated in Zambézia at the end of the 5-year program, evaluators will be permitted to not only observe the relative impact of *Ogumaniha's* intervention intensity, duration, and composition, but also analyze factors that drive or inhibit direct effectiveness and interaction effects, at both the micro/household level as well as a more macro/provincial level. This work demonstrates the distinctive and highly valuable insights that are created by applying a multidimensional measure of poverty to the evaluation of a complex, large scale public health intervention such as the *Ogumaniha*-SCIP project.

Acknowledgments

We acknowledge the members of the Ogumaniha monitoring and evaluation team including: Jeff Weiser, Lara Vaz, Iranett Manteiga, Ofelia Santiago, Faride Mussagy, Aurélio André Andate, Luciano Bene and Reginaldo Muluco. We give special thanks to the whole OPHI organization for providing excellent instruction to an investigator (MB) at the 2011 OPHI-HDCA Summer School in Delft, Netherlands at Delft University of Technology (course content available online at http://www.ophi.org.uk/resources/online-training-portal). We also thank Spencer James, Post-Bachelor Fellow of University of Washington for sharing his analysis code to estimate permanent income.

Author Contributions

Conceived and designed the experiments: BV MB AG SV AV EF OO TM. Performed the experiments: EN LG AV. Analyzed the data: BV AG MB TM EF OO. Contributed to the writing of the manuscript: BV MB AG SV TM.

References

1. The United Nations Development Agenda: Development for all. Available: http://www.un.org/esa///devagenda/UNDA_BW5_Final.pdf. Accessed 2014 Sep 5.
2. Fanzo JC, Pronyk PM (2011) A review of global progress toward the Millennium Development Goal 1 Hunger Target. Food Nutr Bull, 32: 144–158.
3. Dodd R, Cassels A (2006) Health, development and the Millennium Development Goals. Ann Trop Med Parasitol, 100: 379–387.
4. Gaffikin L, Ashley J, Blumenthal PD (2007) Poverty reduction and Millennium Development Goals: recognizing population, health, and environment linkages in rural Madagascar. Medscape Gen Med, 9: 17.
5. Anand S, Sen A Concepts of human development and poverty: A multidimensional perspective. Available: http://clasarchive.berkeley.edu/Academics/courses/center/fall2007/sehnbruch/UNDP%20Anand%20and%20Sen%20Concepts%20of%20HD%201997.pdf. Accessed 2014 Sep 5.
6. Saith A (2011) Inequality, imbalance, instability: reflections on a structural crisis. Dev Change, 42: 70–86.
7. Sen A (2000) A decade of human development. J Hum Dev, 1: 17–23.
8. International Human Development Indicators - UNDP: Mozambique. Available: http://hdr.undp.org/en/countries/profiles/MOZ. Accessed 2014 Sep 5.
9. Bourguignon F, Chakravarty SR (2003) The measurement of multidimensional poverty. Journal of Economic Inequality, 1: 25–49.
10. Guedes GR, Brondizio ES, Barbieri AF, Anne R, Penna-Firme R, et al (2012) Poverty and inequality in the rural Brazilian Amazon: A multidimensional approach. Hum Ecol, 40: 41–57.
11. Deutsch J, Silber J (2005) Measuring multidimensional poverty: An empirical comparison of various approaches. Rev Income Wealth, 51: 145–174.
12. Victor B, Fischer EF, Cooil B, Vergara A, Mukolo A, et al (2013) Frustrated freedom: The effects of agency and wealth on wellbeing in rural Mozambique. World Dev, 47: 30–41.
13. The multidimensional poverty assessment tool (MPAT): A new approach for measuring rural poverty. Available: http://www.ifad.org/mpat/. Accessed 2014 Sep 5.
14. Alkire S, Santos ME (2011) Acute multidimensional poverty: A new index for developing countries (2011). In Proceedings of the German Development Economics Conference, Berlin, No. 3.
15. Alkire S, Foster J (2011) Counting and multidimensional poverty measurement. J Public Econ, 95: 476–487.
16. Sagar AD, Najam A (1998) The human development index: a critical review. Ecol Econ, 25: 249–264.
17. Country Health Profile of Mozambique - WHO Regional Office for Africa. Available: http://www.afro.who.int/en/mozambique/country-health-profile.html. Accessed 2014 Sep 5.
18. WHO World Health Statistics 2011. Available: http://www.who.int/whosis/whostat/2011/en/index.html. Accessed 2014 Sep 5.
19. INSIDA 2009, Inquérito Nacional de Prevalência, Riscos Comportamentais e Informação sobre o HIV e SIDA em Moçambique. Available: http://www.measuredhs.com/pubs/pdf/AIS8/AIS8.pdf. Accessed 2014 Sep 5.
20. Multiple Indicator Cluster Survey (2008). Available: http://www.unicef.org/mozambique/MICS_Summary_English_201009.pdf. Accessed 2014 Sep 5.
21. Moon TD, Burlison JR, Sidat M, Pires P, Silva W, et al (2010) Lessons learned while implementing an HIV/AIDS care and treatment program in rural Mozambique. Retrovirology: Research and Treatment, 3: 1–14.
22. Moon TD, Burlison JR, Blevins M, Shepherd BE, Baptista A, et al (2011) Enrolment and programmatic trends and predictors of antiretroviral therapy initiation from president's emergency plan for AIDS Relief (PEPFAR)-supported public HIV care and treatment sites in rural Mozambique. Int J STD AIDS, 22: 621–627.
23. Cook RE, Ciampa PJ, Sidat M, Blevins M, Burlison J, et al (2011) Predictors of successful early infant diagnosis of HIV in a rural district hospital in Zambézia, Mozambique. J Acquir Immune Defic Syndr, 56: e104–109.
24. Ciampa PJ, Vaz LME, Blevins M, Sidat M, Rothman RL, et al (2012) The association among literacy, numeracy, HIV knowledge and health-seeking behavior: a population-based survey of women in rural Mozambique. PloS One, 7: e39391.
25. Ministério da Saúde-Moçambique: HIV/SIDA. Available: http://www.misau.gov.mz/index.php/hiv-sida. Accessed 2014 Sep 5.
26. Lumley T (2004) Analysis of complex survey samples. Journal of Statistical Software, 9(1): 1–19.
27. Pebesma EJ (2004) Multivariable geostatistics in S: the gstat package. Comput Geosci, 30: 683–691.
28. Ferguson J (1999) *Expectations of modernity: Myths and meanings of urban life on the Zambian copperbelt*. Berkeley: University of California Press.
29. Friedman M (1957) *A Theory of the Consumption Function*, Princeton: Princeton University Press.
30. Editorial (2010) Evaluation: the top priority for global health. The Lancet, 375: 526.

3

Body Mass Index Development from Birth to Early Adolescence; Effect of Perinatal Characteristics and Maternal Migration Background in a Swedish Cohort

Mohsen Besharat Pour[1]*, Anna Bergström[1], Matteo Bottai[2], Jessica Magnusson[1], Inger Kull[1,3,4], Magnus Wickman[1,4], Tahereh Moradi[1,5]

1 Institute of Environmental Medicine, Division of Epidemiology, Karolinska Institutet, Stockholm, Sweden, 2 Institute of Environmental Medicine, Unit of Biostatistics, Karolinska Institutet, Stockholm, Sweden, 3 Department of Clinical Science and Education, Stockholm South General Hospital, Karolinska Institutet, Stockholm, Sweden, 4 Sachs' Children and Youth Hospital, Stockholm South General Hospital, Stockholm, Sweden, 5 Centre for Epidemiology and Community Medicine, Stockholm County Council, Stockholm, Sweden

Abstract

Background: Well documented diversity in risk of developing overweight and obesity between children of immigrant and of native mothers, might be explained by different body mass index (BMI) development trajectories in relation to maternal and perinatal characteristics of offspring.

Objectives: To assess BMI development trajectories among children born to immigrant and to Swedish mothers from birth to adolescence in relation to perinatal characteristics.

Methods: A cohort of 2517 children born in Stockholm during 1994 to 1996 was followed with repeated measurement of height and weight at eleven time points until age 12 years. We estimated changes over time for BMI in relation to maternal and perinatal characteristics of offspring using mixed linear model analysis for repeated measure data.

Results: We observed a significant BMI change over time in children and time interaction with maternal migration status ($P<0.0001$). Estimated BMI over time adjusted for maternal and perinatal characteristics of offspring, showed slower BMI growth before age of 5, followed by an earlier plateau and steeper BMI growth after 5 years among children of immigrant mothers compared with children of Swedish mothers. These differences in BMI growth were more prominent among children with mothers from outside Europe.

Conclusion: Beside reinforcing early childhood as a crucial period in development of overweight, the observed slower BMI development at early childhood among children of immigrants followed by a steeper increase in BMI compared with children of Swedish mothers is important for further studies and for planning of preventive public health programs.

Editor: Harry Zhang, Old Dominion University, United States of America

Funding: These authors have no support or funding to report.

Competing Interests: The authors have declared that no competing interests exist.

* Email: Mohsen.besharat.pour@ki.se

Introduction

Childhood obesity is a growing epidemic worldwide and recently entitled as a contemporary challenging public health priority by World Health Organization [1]. During the past three decades many western countries including United States have experienced a multiplicative increase in prevalence of childhood obesity [2]. Swedish data shows a similar trend but with a much lower slope as compared with the United States [3]. Despite positive reports indicating flattening childhood obesity trend in Sweden [4], it might be too early to conclude it as in a steady state [5].

The consequences of childhood obesity have a broad spectrum; from psychosocial problems to systemic and metabolic disorders [6,7]. A large proportion of obese children remain overweight or obese through adulthood, and thus are at increased risk of cardiovascular and metabolic morbidity and mortality [7].

Along rising flow of international migration, concerns have been raised about health status among the growing population of immigrants and their offspring [8,9]. The result of previous studies indicates a higher risk of overweight and obesity in children born to immigrant parents compared with the native counterparts [10–15] and even with children in their home countries [10]. Birth weight, as an indicator for prenatal exposures such as maternal

BMI, intrauterine exposure to maternal smoking and maternal diabetes, has been linked to childhood overweight and obesity [16–20]. However, existing studies do not support differences in birth weight, as an indicator for different prenatal exposures and intrauterine growth, between children born to immigrant and to native mothers [21–24]. To explain diversity in risk of developing overweight and obesity thus, we postulate that there are different BMI development trajectories in relation to maternal and perinatal characteristics between children of immigrant and of native Swedish mothers.

In this longitudinal study using an ongoing cohort of children born in Stockholm during 1992 and 1996, we first, assessed BMI development trajectories among children born to immigrant and to Swedish mothers from birth to 12 years of age in relation to perinatal characteristics. Then we investigated critical time points in BMI changes toward development of overweight and obesity among these children.

Material and Methods

Subjects and data collection

A total of 2517 children born in Stockholm were included and followed from birth to the age of 12 years. We retrieved data from the ongoing Swedish prospective birth cohort study BAMSE (Swedish abbreviation for 'Barn/children Allergy Milieu Stockholm Epidemiology'). Initially, 4089 children born in Stockholm between February 1994 and November 1996 were included in the cohort. Inclusion and exclusion criteria as well as the enrolment process have been described in detail elsewhere [25]. Briefly, at baseline, the parents answered a questionnaire when children were at the age of 2 months. Follow-up questionnaires have been sent to the parents when the children were at the ages of 1, 2, 4, 8 and 12 years. The response rates were 96%, 94%, 91%, 84% and 83%, respectively. Information on maternal country of birth, education, smoking habits during pregnancy and breast feeding were elicited from BAMSE cohort.

When the children were on average 12 years old (age range: 11–14 years), 2,887 parents (71% of the original cohort), gave their consent to collect information on their child's weight and height from school health care register which includes data from child health care centers. In Sweden, almost all children below 2 years of age participate in regular physical examinations at child health care centers and at least one additional examination between 2 and 6 years of age [26,27]. In child health care centers children's weight and height are measured by trained nurses according to standard national guidelines [27,28]. When the child starts school, their child health care records are transferred to the school health care. These pre-school health records are then completed with weight and height data routinely measured in 1st, 4th and 7th grade by the school nurses [29].

From the above mentioned sources, available information on weight and height was extracted for 2598 children for 10 predefined ages [6 months (± 2 weeks), 12 months and 18 months (± 4 weeks), 2, 3, 4 and 5 years (±6 months), 7, 10 and 12 years (− 6 to +11 months)]. Then child's BMI was calculated for each predefined ages as weight (kilogram)/height (meter) ^{2}.

Information on birth weight and -height, maternal and prenatal characteristics (i.e. maternal BMI at early pregnancy, age, gestational age) and complications during pregnancy (i.e. pre-eclampsia/eclampsia, diabetes, anemia, placental disease, renal and liver diseases) was obtained from the Swedish Medical Birth Register. The Swedish Medical Birth Register was established 1973 and includes maternal and prenatal information on more than 98% of all infants born in Sweden [30].

The final study population included 2517 children with known maternal country of birth and with information on BMI at least in two time points.

Based on maternal country of birth, children were divided into two groups of immigrant and Swedish mother. We further classified children of immigrant mothers into three sub-groups based on maternal origin: Scandinavian (Finland, Norway, and Denmark), European (excluding Sweden, Finland, Norway, and Denmark) and outside Europe.

Ethics statement

This study was conducted according to the principles of the Declaration of Helsinki and all procedures involving human subjects/patients were approved by the Regional Board of the Ethical Committee in Stockholm (Dnr: 2011/792-32). All parents gave their written informed consent prior to inclusion of their children in the study.

Statistical methods

We used chi-square and t-test for categorical and continuous data, respectively, to examine baseline characteristics among children of immigrant and of Swedish mothers in our study population and also to compare baseline characteristics of our study population with BAMSE cohort.

Mixed linear model analysis for repeated measure data was used to predict changes over time for BMI in relation to maternal and perinatal characteristics of offspring including maternal age (year), maternal education (highest attained level of education ≤12 years and>12 years) early pregnancy BMI (kg/m^2), smoking during pregnancy (at least one cigarette per day any time during pregnancy) (yes/no), pregnancy complications associated with intra uterine growth [31,32] (preeclampsia/eclampsia, diabetes, anemia, placental disease, renal and liver diseases) (yes/no), weight for gestational age, parity and breast feeding (months). Weight for gestational age was divided into 3 categories based on percentiles derived from Swedish reference curves for normal fetal growth [33]: small for gestational age (SGA, birth weight <10th percentile), large for gestational age (LGA, birth weight>90th percentile) and appropriate for gestational age (AGA, 10th ≤ birth weight ≤ 90th percentile) [34].

To find the best fitted model we used residual log likelihood (-2RLL) for comparison of nested models and Akaike's Information Criterion (AIC) for non-nested models. We applied a polynomial transformation to time variable, child's age, to take into account non-linear changes in BMI during the time. The quadratic (age squared) and cubic (age cube) polynomials provided better model fit compared to crude model. Since the model did not describe rapid variation at about 1 year and 5 years, an additional natural log function of child's age added to the model which improved fit of model also better described the functional changes of child's BMI during time [35]. The final model included maternal migration status as exposure, maternal and perinatal characteristics of offspring as covariates, child's age, age squared, age cube and the natural log of age, as time variables, and interaction between time variables and maternal migration status. In the final model effect of child's age and intercept treated as random variables. The same model was used for analysis of different time points if applicable.

We used SAS version 9.3 (SAS Institute, Cary, NC, USA) for analysis and R version 3.0.2 for graphical presentations. P-values <0.05 were considered to be statistically significant.

Results

Demographic characteristics

There were no differences in baseline characteristics between study population and BAMSE cohort with regard to sex, birth weight, gestational age, maternal BMI, maternal smoking during pregnancy, maternal migration status and parity. However, mothers in study population compared with BAMSE cohort had a higher mean age (30.9±4.4 vs. 30.7±4.5 years, $P = 0.02$) as well as higher education (44.1% vs. 41.2% university education, $P = 0.02$) (data not shown).

Table 1 shows maternal and perinatal characteristics of the study population by maternal migration status. In study population 13.3% of the children had foreign born mothers who consist of Scandinavian (30.1%), European (26.8%) and outside Europe (43.1%) origin.

With exception of having higher parity (>2) which was more prevalent among immigrant mothers there were no differences in gestational age, birth weight, or duration of breast feeding between children of immigrant and of Swedish mother. Further stratification by maternal immigration background revealed that immigrant mothers from other European countries had the lowest proportion of low education and immigrant mothers from outside Europe had the highest proportion on no smokers and the longest duration of breast feeding compared with counterpart Swedish mothers (Table 1). Mean BMI among the children by maternal migration status in different ages are presented in Table S1. Using BMI cut points of International Obesity Task Force (IOTF) [36] we observed that at age 2 years higher proportion of children of Swedish mothers are overweight compared with children of immigrant mothers (10.2% vs. 5.8%, $P = 0.046$) while at age 12 years the overweight proportion is higher among children of immigrant mothers compared with counterpart Swedish children (20.9 vs. 13.8, $P =$ 0.001) (data not shown).

Changes in BMI over time

In the final model, we observed a significant BMI change over time, in multivariable mixed linear model analysis adjusted for maternal and perinatal characteristics and time interactions with maternal migration status ($P = <0.0001$) (Table 2). Graphical presentation of these significant observations illustrated in Figure 1&2 which interpreted as significant BMI changes over time by maternal migration background. We further observed that low BMI at birth was associated with female sex ($P = <0.0001$), having older mothers ($P = 0.0352$), low maternal education ($P = 0.0035$), and small for gestational age ($P = <0.0001$). High maternal BMI during early pregnancy ($P = 0.0002$), and being large for gestational age ($P = <0.0001$) were associated with high BMI at birth (Table 2). We found a significant interaction between maternal migration status and BMI development over time ($P = <$ 0.0001) (Table 2). Predicted values for BMI development, adjusted for maternal and perinatal characteristics of offspring, showed that while girls and boys of immigrant mothers had slower BMI growth before age of 5 years, the trajectory reached a plateau earlier among them, and BMI grew at a faster rate after age of 5 years than among children of Swedish mother (Figure 1). Analysis confined to age 10 years showed similar results (results not shown).

Analysis by subgroups of children to immigrant mothers revealed that change in BMI trajectory toward faster BMI development took place earlier among children with mother born outside Europe (after 2 years) and later among children with mothers from other Scandinavian countries (after 5 years) (Figure 2). Children with European mothers continued with a slower BMI growth through early adolescence compared with children of Swedish mother (Figure 2). Similar results were found when we confined the analysis to children with both parents born outside Sweden (results not shown).

We found no interaction between maternal migration status and maternal education, either overall ($P = 0.84$) or in subgroup analysis ($P = 0.20$) (data not presented in table), suggesting similar BMI trajectories for strata of maternal education in relation to migration status.

Discussion

In this population based cohort study with repeated measurements of height and weight among children from birth to 12 years of age, we observed that despite the comparable birth weight and weight for gestational age, the BMI trajectory over time was different between children of immigrant mothers and of Swedish mothers. Up to age 5 years children of immigrant mother experienced slower BMI development compared with children of Swedish mother. The BMI trajectory reversed after age 5 years and became steeper among children of immigrant mother. BMI changes took place earlier (around age 2 years) and steeper among subgroup of children with mother from outside Europe.

This novel observation is important for further studies and for planning of preventive public health programs. To our knowledge, this study is the first conducted in Sweden to explore the BMI development trajectory among offspring of immigrant mothers and of Swedish mothers from birth to late childhood.

Strengths of our study include the cohort design and repeated anthropometric measurements from birth to age 12 years collected by trained nurses in child health care and school health care centers. Linkage to the high quality Swedish Medical Birth register to retrieve maternal and perinatal characteristics is another important merit of our study. Moreover, using linear mixed model analysis for repeated measurements takes into account correlation of different measurements in each subject as well as variation between and within individuals during time. The overlay of crude mean BMI by maternal migration status at each time point on the fitted BMI trajectory line, given perinatal characteristics, provide an overview of goodness of fit for used model.

The observed steeper BMI development toward higher BMI after age of 5 among children of immigrant mother compared with children of Swedish mother is in line with the results of previous studies reporting higher prevalence or risk of overweight and obesity in offspring of immigrants [10–15]. However, to the best of our knowledge, there is no report on slower BMI development before age of 5 years among offspring of immigrants compared with offspring of Swedish mothers. Moreover, most of previous studies among immigrants performed on a cross sectional setting or longitudinal data have been analyzed with conventional methods such as ANOVA or Generalized Estimating Equations assuming constant and equal variation, in other word, an average over time. The few studies that used linear mixed modeling were mostly concerned about difference in generation of immigrants [37], didn't consider early life characteristics [38,39] or had a short follow up period [40]. A longitudinal study of children aged 2–12 years showed that proportion of black ethnicity was higher in both early and late onset overweight trajectories than normal weight trajectory [41]. The privilege of our approach is adding time sequence of events to the whole picture. Moreover, we took into consideration perinatal characteristics which are shown to be involved in BMI programming later in life [17,19,20].

Our results should also be interpreted under the light of some limitations. First, the nature of our exposure, maternal migration status, makes our exposed group a heterogeneous group in respect

Table 1. Maternal and perinatal characteristics of the study population, children born between 1994 and 1996 in Stockholm by maternal migration status.

characteristics		Swedish	Immigrant			
			All immigrant			
				Scandinavian	European	Outside Europe
Number of children		2181	336	101	90	145
Proportion (%)		86.7	13.3	4.0	3.6	5.8
Sex (%)	Girl	49.1	51.8	57.4	55.1	45.8
	Boy	50.9	48.2	42.6	44.9	54.2
Maternal Age in year(±SD[1])		30.9 (±4.4)	31.0 (±4.7)	31.4 (±4.2)	31.2 (±4.7)	30.7 (±5.1)
Maternal Education (%)	≤12 year	55.6	58.1	71.3**	40.5**	59.7
	>12 year	44.4	41.9	28.7	59.6	40.3
Pre-pregnancy BMI[2] (kg/m^2)		22.9 (±3.3)	22.9 (±3.4)	23.4 (±3.5)	22.6 (±3.4)	22.7 (±3.3)
Smoking during pregnancy (%)[3]	Yes	11.9	8.7	13.9	7.9	5.6*
	No	88.1	91.3	86.1	92.1	94.4
Gestational complication (%)	Yes	5.9	3.7	3.0	3.6	4.2
	No	94.1	96.3	97.0	96.4	95.8
Birth weight (gram)		3533 (±572)	3525 (±516.1)	3577 (±484)	3544 (±524)	3476 (±533)
Birth weight (%)[4]	Low BW	3.7	2.5	2	2.3	2.9
	High BW	19.1	17.4	19	17.4	16.6
	Normal BW	77.2	80.1	79	80.2	80.6
Gestational age(week)		39.5 (±1.8)	39.7 (±1.6)	39.8 (±1.5)	39.7 (±1.6)	39.5 (±1.6)
Gestational age (%)[5]	Preterm	9.6	6.4	6.2	9.2	5.0
	Post term	0.5	0.9	2.1	1.2	0.0
	Term	89.9	92.6	91.8	89.7	95
Weight for gestational age[6]	SGA	2.4	1.3	4.2	7.1	10.4
	LGA	4.4	4.7	17.7	11.9	9.6
	AGA	93.2	94.0	78.1	81.0	80.0
Parity (%)	1	55.8	55.4*	52.0	63.2	52.9
	2	33.6	29.1	32.7	20.7	31.4
	>2	10.6	15.6	15.3	16.1	15.7
Breast feeding (months)	Exclusive	5.1 (±2.4)	5.2 (±2.8)	5.1 (±2.6)	4.9 (±2.8)	5.4 (±3.0)
	Total	8.7 (±3.2)	9.1 (±3.7)	9.1 (±3.5)	8.4 (±3.8)	9.5 (±3.8)*

Bolded numbers are statistically significant Comparing immigrant with counterpart Swedish mothers (T-test or chi-square for continuous or categorical variables): * p< 0.05, ** p<0.01, *** p<0.001.
Bolded numbers are statistically significant.
[1]Standard deviation.
[2]Body mass index.
[3]Smoking during pregnancy.
[4]Low BW = BW<2500 gram; High BW = BW≥4000 gram; Normal BW = 2500≤BW<4000 gram.
[5]Preterm = delivery<38 weeks; Post term = delivery> 42 weeks; Term = delivery between 38–42 weeks of gestation.
[6]SGA = small for gestational age; LGA = large for gestational age; AGA = appropriate for gestational age.

to ethnicity, country of birth, genetic and cultural backgrounds and reasons behind migration. We lacked information on genetic and cultural life style factors. Due to lack of statistical power we were not able to perform stratified analysis by specific parental birth country. Nevertheless, we performed analysis in subgroups of children to immigrant mothers based on geographical distance to host country, which might disentangle cultural and lifestyle variations in some degree. This limitation warrants collection of large data with detailed information, specifically on life style factors, in offspring of immigrants.

Furthermore, we defined children of immigrants based on only mother's country of birth due to our concern for perinatal characteristics. It is likely that children with two immigrant parents could differ from children with one immigrant and one Swedish parent in many aspects. The possible misclassification of exposure in our study, however, is probably non-differential which lead to underestimation of the true results, because it is possible for both Swedish and immigrant mothers to have counter-origin husband. Furthermore, this was supported by sensitivity analysis of subgroup of children with both immigrant parents from the same region compared with children of Swedish parents.

We lacked information on child nutrition after weaning until age 5 years; a period were changes in BMI development seem to take place, and could partially explain the observed differences

Table 2. Association between maternal and perinatal characteristics and body mass index (BMI) from birth to 12 years of age in the study population, children born between 1994 and 1996 in Stockholm, using conditional mixed model.

parameter			Estimate	Standard Error	Pr> |t|
Intercept			18.1910	0.2442	<0.0001
Maternal migration status	Swedish		0 (ref)	-	-
	Immigrant	Scandinavia	−0.3094	0.1706	0.0697
		Europe	−0.07528	0.2147	0.7259
		Outside Europe	−0.00275	0.1591	0.9862
Sex	Boys		0 (ref)	-	-
	Girls		−0.1838	0.04563	**<0.0001**
Maternal Age (year)[1]			−0.01221	0.005794	**0.0352**
Maternal Education	> 12 years		0 (ref)	-	-
	≤ 12 years		−0.1443	0.04941	**0.0035**
Pre-pregnancy BMI (kg/m^2)			0.02599	0.007064	**0.0002**
Smoking during pregnancy[2]	No		0 (ref)	-	-
	Yes		0.09235	0.07306	0.2063
Gestational Complication[3]	No		0 (ref)	-	-
	Yes		−0.01182	0.09867	0.9047
Weight for gestational age	AGA[5]		0 (ref)	-	-
	SGA[6]		−0.8891	0.08719	**<0.0001**
	LGA[7]		0.7227	0.06854	**<0.0001**
Parity			0.05863	0.03342	0.0794
Breast feeding (months)[4]			0.009089	0.007266	0.2110
Time [8]					**<0.0001**
Age			−1.5582	0.02657	
Age*Age			0.1874	0.004776	
Age*Age*Age			−0.00577	0.000251	
Age-log			0.7531	0.006858	
Time interaction with Migration Status					**<0.0001**
- Scandinavians					**0.0174**
Migration status(S)* Age			0.001563	0.1189	
Migration status(S)* Age*Age			0.001832	0.02145	
Migration status(S)* Age*Age*Age			0.000188	0.001134	
Migration status(S)* Age-log			−0.07410	0.03098	
- Europeans					**<0.0001**
Migration status(E)* Age			−0.02744	0.1505	
Migration status(E)* Age*Age			−0.00298	0.02688	
Migration status(E)* Age*Age*Age			0.000234	0.001406	
Migration status(E)* Age-log			−0.01387	0.03857	
- Outside Europe					**0.008**
Migration status(O)* Age			−0.0751	0.1115	
Migration status(O)* Age*Age			0.03965	0.0199	
Migration status(O)* Age*Age*Age			−0.0022	0.00104	
Migration status(O)* Age-log			−0.0036	0.02905	

Bold numbers are statistically significant
[1]Age at first antenatal clinic visit, almost around week 12−14 of gestation
[2]Smoking at least one cigarette per day, at any time during pregnancy
[3]Diabetes, preeclampsia and eclampsia, hypertension, anemia, renal disease, liver disease and placental disorders which might affect fetal growth
[4]Total breast feeding: number of months that child has been breastfed, both exclusive and partial
[5]AGA = appropriate for gestational age
[6]SGA = small for gestational age
[7]LGA = large for gestational age
[8]Time variable in this model is 'Age' (year) at weight and height measurement in children. Since the changes in BMI at different ages is not linear or a straight line, different polynomial functions of 'Age' has been used to take into account non-linear changes in BMI in different ages. Then, 'Age' accounts for linear changes, 'Age*Age' accounts for unidirectional curvilinear changes, 'Age*Age*Age' accounts for bi-directional curvilinear changes and 'Age-log' account for sharp changes, either peak or bottom.

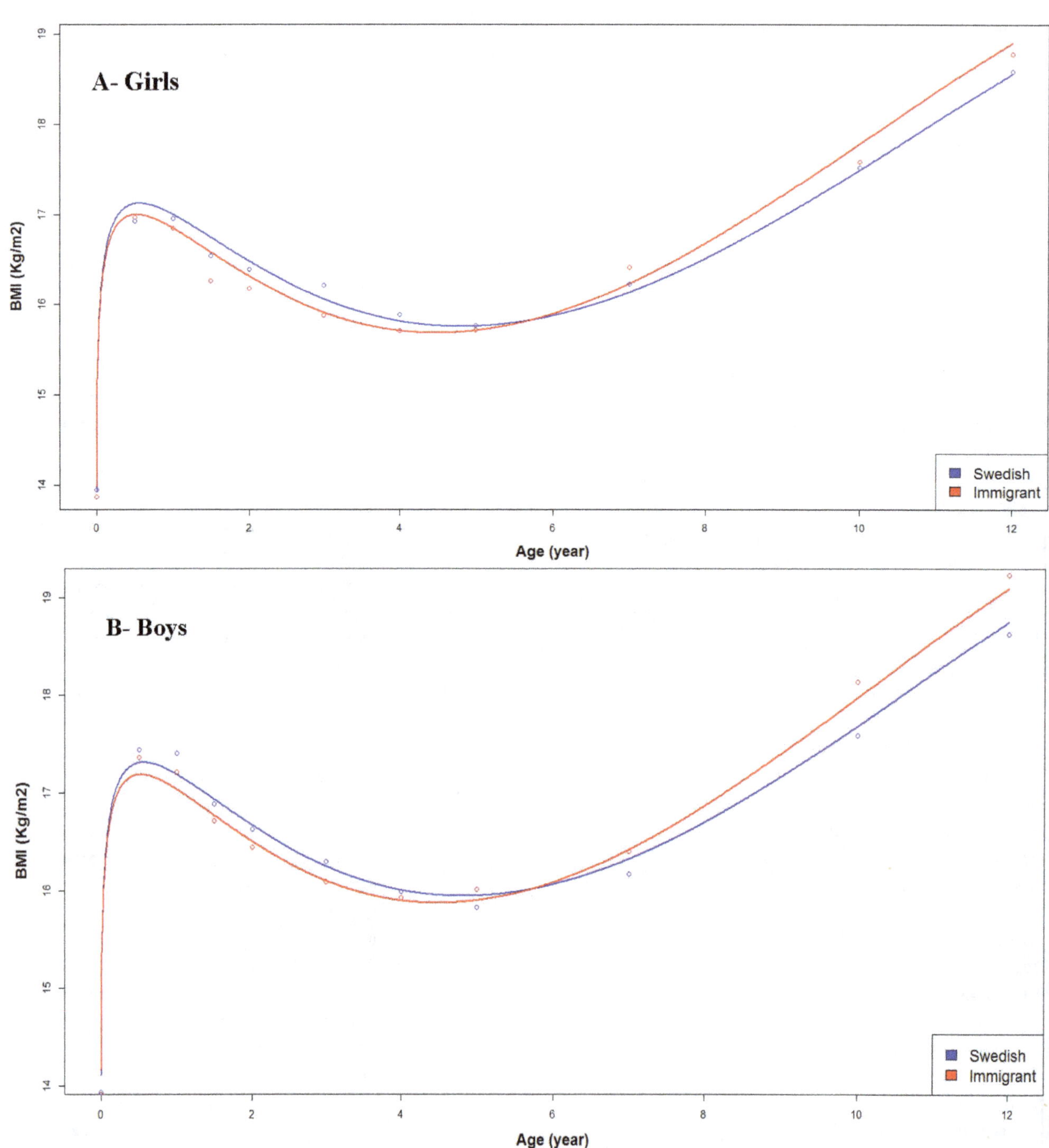

Figure 1. Estimated body mass index (BMI) from birth to 12 years, adjusted for maternal and perinatal characteristics by maternal migration status in girls (A) and boys (B) born between 1994 and 1996 in Stockholm. * Circles represent crude mean BMI.

between offspring of immigrant and of Swedish born mothers. We also lacked accurate time for puberty. However, we conducted a sensitivity analysis excluding data on 12 year time point to confine our results to age periods which are unlikely for puberty in both sexes, and yield similar results.

It might be argued that BMI development is part of normal growth and necessarily doesn't mean overweight or obesity and thus one should use standardized BMI based on age and sex to a reference population. However, direction of BMI changes provides valuable information for preventive purposes and is easy to interpret. In addition it has been shown that BMI changes per se has a better correlation with changes in adiposity especially for assessing adiposity on several time points [42].

Despite the association of perinatal characteristics on programming of BMI development later in life, given controlling for these characteristics, our results suggest that they cannot fully explain the disparity in BMI development in children of immigrant mothers compared with children of Swedish mothers. Neverthe-

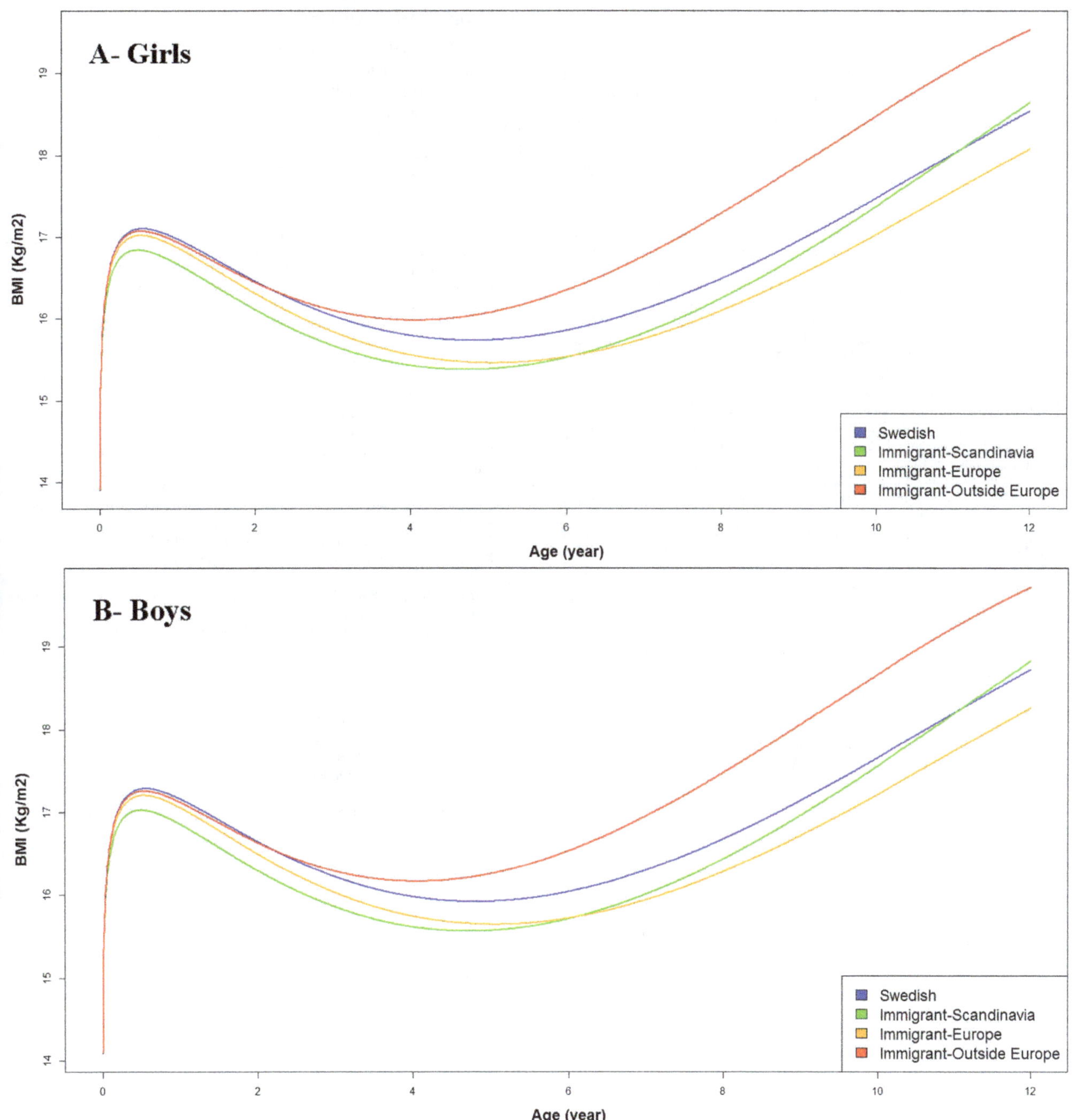

Figure 2. Estimated body mass index (BMI) from birth to 12 years, adjusted for maternal and perinatal characteristics by subgroups of maternal migration status in girls (A) and boys (B) born between 1994 and 1996 in Stockholm.

less, our results reinforce early childhood as a crucial period in development of overweight and obesity later in life, a period which could be influenced mostly by cultural, behavioral and life style factors especially at the family level. This finding is important for public health purpose to plan effective preventive programs with regards to critical period and vulnerable groups to combat childhood overweight and obesity later in life and calls for collection of such data in focused groups of offspring of immigrants.

Supporting Information

Table S1 Mean body mass index (and standard deviation) in the study population, children born between 1994 and 1996 in Stockholm, by maternal migration status and age. Mean body mass index was significantly different in immigrant children compared with Swedish children (t-test): * $p<0.05$, ** $p<0.01$, *** $p<0.001$.

Acknowledgments

We would like to thank all participants in the BAMSE Birth Cohort Study, specially the parents and children, administrative and research team members and also nurses at the child health centers and school nurses who contribute to the data collection. We also appreciate technical and statistical support by Paolo Frumento.

Author Contributions

Conceived and designed the experiments: MBP AB MB TM. Analyzed the data: MBP. Contributed reagents/materials/analysis tools: AB MB JM IK MW. Wrote the paper: MBP. Interpretation of results and critical revision of the manuscript for important intellectual content: MBP AB MB JM IK MW TM. Reading and approve the final sumbited version: MBP AB MB JM IK MW TM.

References

1. WHO (2013) Childhood overweight and obesity. Global strategy on diet, physical activity and health; Available: http://wwwwhoint/dietphysicalactivity/childhood/en/Accessed 2013 July 19.
2. Kosti RI, Panagiotakos DB (2006) The epidemic of obesity in children and adolescents in the world. Cent Eur J Public Health 14: 151–159.
3. Ekblom O, Oddsson K, Ekblom B (2004) Prevalence and regional differences in overweight in 2001 and trends in BMI distribution in Swedish children from 1987 to 2001. Scand J Public Health 32: 257–263.
4. Sundblom E, Petzold M, Rasmussen F, Callmer E, Lissner L (2008) Childhood overweight and obesity prevalences levelling off in Stockholm but socioeconomic differences persist. Int J Obes (Lond) 32: 1525–1530.
5. Kipping RR, Jago R, Lawlor DA (2008) Obesity in children. Part 1: Epidemiology, measurement, risk factors, and screening. BMJ 337: a1824.
6. Kiess W, Galler A, Reich A, Muller G, Kapellen T, et al. (2001) Clinical aspects of obesity in childhood and adolescence. Obes Rev 2: 29–36.
7. Dietz WH (1998) Health consequences of obesity in youth: childhood predictors of adult disease. Pediatrics 101: 518–525.
8. Hjern A (2012) Migration and public health: Health in Sweden: The National Public Health Report 2012. Chapter 13. Scand J Public Health 40: 255–267.
9. Hjern A, Bouvier P (2004) Migrant children–a challenge for European paediatricians. Acta Paediatr 93: 1535–1539.
10. Stillman S, Gibson J, McKenzie D (2012) The impact of immigration on child health: experimental evidence from a migration lottery program. Econ Inq 50: 62–81.
11. Balakrishnan R, Webster P, Sinclair D (2008) Trends in overweight and obesity among 5-7-year-old White and South Asian children born between 1991 and 1999. J Public Health (Oxf) 30: 139–144.
12. Apfelbacher CJ, Loerbroks A, Cairns J, Behrendt H, Ring J, et al. (2008) Predictors of overweight and obesity in five to seven-year-old children in Germany: results from cross-sectional studies. BMC Public Health 8: 171.
13. Fredriks AM, Van Buuren S, Sing RA, Wit JM, Verloove-Vanhorick SP (2005) Alarming prevalences of overweight and obesity for children of Turkish, Moroccan and Dutch origin in The Netherlands according to international standards. Acta Paediatr 94: 496–498.
14. Kirchengast S, Schober E (2006) To be an immigrant: a risk factor for developing overweight and obesity during childhood and adolescence? J Biosoc Sci 38: 695–705.
15. Will B, Zeeb H, Baune BT (2005) Overweight and obesity at school entry among migrant and German children: a cross-sectional study. BMC Public Health 5: 45.
16. Barker DJ (2004) The developmental origins of adult disease. J Am Coll Nutr 23: 588S–595S.
17. Huang JS, Lee TA, Lu MC (2007) Prenatal programming of childhood overweight and obesity. Matern Child Health J 11: 461–473.
18. Eriksson M, Tynelius P, Rasmussen F (2008) Associations of birthweight and infant growth with body composition at age 15–the COMPASS study. Paediatr Perinat Epidemiol 22: 379–388.
19. Rogers I (2003) The influence of birthweight and intrauterine environment on adiposity and fat distribution in later life. Int J Obes Relat Metab Disord 27: 755–777.
20. Oken E, Gillman MW (2003) Fetal origins of obesity. Obes Res 11: 496–506.
21. Alder J, Fink N, Lapaire O, Urech C, Meyer A, et al. (2008) The effect of migration background on obstetric performance in Switzerland. Eur J Contracept Reprod Health Care 13: 103–108.
22. El-Sayed AM, Galea S (2011) Maternal immigrant status and high birth weight: implications for childhood obesity. Ethn Dis 21: 47–51.
23. Forna F, Jamieson DJ, Sanders D, Lindsay MK (2003) Pregnancy outcomes in foreign-born and US-born women. Int J Gynaecol Obstet 83: 257–265.
24. Buekens P, Masuy-Stroobant G, Delvaux T (1998) High birthweights among infants of north African immigrants in Belgium. Am J Public Health 88: 808–811.
25. Wickman M, Kull I, Pershagen G, Nordvall SL (2002) The BAMSE project: presentation of a prospective longitudinal birth cohort study. Pediatr Allergy Immunol 13 Suppl 15: 11–13.
26. Stockholms Läns Landsting (SLL) (2013) Metodbok Barnhälsovården. Bedömning av tillväxt. Stockholm: SLL.
27. Stockholms Läns Landsting (SLL) (2013) Barnhälsovård Årsrapport 2012. Barnhälsovården i Stockholm Län Stockholm: SLL.
28. BarnHälsovård (2012) Mätutrustning och mätteknik. Rikshandboken.
29. Socialstyrelsen (2004) Socialstyrelsens riktlinjer för skolhälsovården. Stockholm: Socialstyrelsen.
30. The Swedish Centre for Epidemiology (2003) The Swedish Medical Birth Register: a summary of content and quality. The National Board of Health & Welfare.
31. Sankaran S, Kyle PM (2009) Aetiology and pathogenesis of IUGR. Best Pract Res Clin Obstet Gynaecol 23: 765–777.
32. Hendrix N, Berghella V (2008) Non-placental causes of intrauterine growth restriction. Semin Perinatol 32: 161–165.
33. Marsal K, Persson PH, Larsen T, Lilja H, Selbing A, et al. (1996) Intrauterine growth curves based on ultrasonically estimated foetal weights. Acta Paediatr 85: 843–848.
34. Battaglia FC, Lubchenco LO (1967) A practical classification of newborn infants by weight and gestational age. J Pediatr 71: 159–163.
35. Chivers P, Hands B, Parker H, Beilin L, Kendall G, et al. (2009) Longitudinal modelling of body mass index from birth to 14 years. Obes Facts 2: 302–310.
36. Cole TJ, Bellizzi MC, Flegal KM, Dietz WH (2000) Establishing a standard definition for child overweight and obesity worldwide: international survey. BMJ 320: 1240–1243.
37. Van Hook J, Balistreri KS (2007) Immigrant generation, socioeconomic status, and economic development of countries of origin: a longitudinal study of body mass index among children. Soc Sci Med 65: 976–989.
38. Balistreri KS, Van Hook J (2009) Socioeconomic status and body mass index among Hispanic children of immigrants and children of natives. Am J Public Health 99: 2238–2246.
39. Wen X, Kleinman K, Gillman MW, Rifas-Shiman SL, Taveras EM (2012) Childhood body mass index trajectories: modeling, characterizing, pairwise correlations and socio-demographic predictors of trajectory characteristics. BMC Med Res Methodol 12: 38.
40. Hof MH, van Dijk AE, van Eijsden M, Vrijkotte TG, Zwinderman AH (2011) Comparison of growth between native and immigrant infants between 0–3 years from the Dutch ABCD cohort. Ann Hum Biol 38: 544–555.
41. Li C, Goran MI, Kaur H, Nollen N, Ahluwalia JS (2007) Developmental trajectories of overweight during childhood: role of early life factors. Obesity (Silver Spring) 15: 760–771.
42. Cole TJ, Faith MS, Pietrobelli A, Heo M (2005) What is the best measure of adiposity change in growing children: BMI, BMI %, BMI z-score or BMI centile? Eur J Clin Nutr 59: 419–425.

4

Modelling Survival and Mortality Risk to 15 Years of Age for a National Cohort of Children with Serious Congenital Heart Defects Diagnosed in Infancy

Rachel L. Knowles[1]*, Catherine Bull[2], Christopher Wren[3], Angela Wade[1], Harvey Goldstein[1], Carol Dezateux[1], on behalf of the UKCSCHD (UK Collaborative Study of Congenital Heart Defects) collaborators¶

1 Population Policy and Practice Programme, Institute of Child Health, University College London, London, United Kingdom, **2** Cardiac Unit, Great Ormond Street Hospital for Children NHS Trust, London, United Kingdom, **3** Department of Paediatric Cardiology, Freeman Hospital, Newcastle-upon-Tyne, United Kingdom

Abstract

Background: Congenital heart defects (CHDs) are a significant cause of death in infancy. Although contemporary management ensures that 80% of affected children reach adulthood, post-infant mortality and factors associated with death during childhood are not well-characterised. Using data from a UK-wide multicentre birth cohort of children with serious CHDs, we observed survival and investigated independent predictors of mortality up to age 15 years.

Methods: Data were extracted retrospectively from hospital records and death certificates of 3,897 children (57% boys) in a prospectively identified cohort, born 1992–1995 with CHDs requiring intervention or resulting in death before age one year. A discrete-time survival model accounted for time-varying predictors; hazards ratios were estimated for mortality. Incomplete data were addressed through multilevel multiple imputation.

Findings: By age 15 years, 932 children had died; 144 died without any procedure. Survival to one year was 79.8% (95% confidence intervals [CI] 78.5, 81.1%) and to 15 years was 71.7% (63.9, 73.4%), with variation by cardiac diagnosis. Importantly, 20% of cohort deaths occurred after age one year. Models using imputed data (including all children from birth) demonstrated higher mortality risk as independently associated with cardiac diagnosis, female sex, preterm birth, having additional cardiac defects or non-cardiac malformations. In models excluding children who had no procedure, additional predictors of higher mortality were younger age at first procedure, lower weight or height, longer cardiopulmonary bypass or circulatory arrest duration, and peri-procedural complications; non-cardiac malformations were no longer significant.

Interpretation: We confirm the high mortality risk associated with CHDs in the first year of life and demonstrate an important persisting risk of death throughout childhood. Late mortality may be underestimated by procedure-based audit focusing on shorter-term surgical outcomes. National monitoring systems should emphasise the importance of routinely capturing longer-term survival and exploring the mechanisms of mortality risk in children with serious CHDs.

Editor: Zaccaria Ricci, Piazza S, Italy

Funding: This work was supported by a British Heart Foundation project grant (reference PG/02/065/13934). RLK was awarded an MRC Special Training Fellowship in Health of the Public and Health Services Research (reference G106/1083). HG and the Centre for Paediatric Epidemiology and Biostatistics benefited from Medical Research Council funding support to the MRC Centre of Epidemiology for Child Health (reference G04005546). Great Ormond St Hospital for Children NHS Trust and the UCL Institute of Child Health receives a proportion of funding from the Department of Health's NIHR Biomedical Research Centres scheme. The funders had no role in the study design, data analysis and interpretation, writing or publication of this paper.

Competing Interests: The authors have declared that no competing interests exist.

* Email: rachel.knowles@ucl.ac.uk

¶ Membership of the UKCSCHD (UK Collaborative Study of Congenital Heart Defects) is provided in the Acknowledgments.

Introduction

Serious congenital heart defects (CHDs), requiring surgery in the first year of life, affect around 1% of births each year in the UK [1–3] and include a broad spectrum of complexity and severity. Without intervention in early life, serious CHDs are often incompatible with long-term survival. Continuous improvement in medical, intensive care and surgical technologies have significantly reduced infant mortality and around 80% of affected babies now survive the first year of life [4–7]. Despite the rising number of paediatric cardiac procedures being undertaken [8], surgical mortality is decreasing and the number of UK adults with CHDs is steadily growing [9]. Nevertheless, long-term survival for individuals within most CHD subgroups remains below that of the unaffected population [10].

Recognising the growing population of adolescents and adults with CHDs, recent research has focused on the epidemiology and health experience of adult survivors. It is generally assumed that

Table 1. Inclusion and exclusion criteria for the UKCSCHD cohort.

Inclusion criteria (for the UKCSCHD and original register). Live born infants:
1) born between 1st January 1992 and 31st December 1995
2) resident in the United Kingdom (UK) at birth
3) with a serious congenital heart defect, defined as a structural malformation of the heart or great vessels, requiring an intervention or resulting in death during the first year of life.
Exclusion criteria (for the UKCSCHD and original register). Live born infants with:
1) isolated cardiovascular defects such as persistent ductus arteriosus, vascular ring or anomalous coronary arteries
2) myocardial dysfunction, arrhythmia or tumours in a structurally normal heart
3) a congenital heart defect that did not require an intervention or result in death during the first year of life.
Excluded from the UKCSCHD but included in the original register:
Babies with a fetal diagnosis of serious congenital heart defect made at prenatal ultrasound but not subsequently live born.

additional mortality between infancy and 15 years of age is extremely low and likely to be related to further surgery, yet observational studies with prospective long-term follow-up of the transition of children with CHDs from infancy through school, adolescence and into adulthood are lacking. While short-term surgical outcome studies provide extensive detail about post-operative survival and mortality, particularly within specific CHD subgroups, the factors associated with mortality risk that are common to all diagnostic subgroups and their significance at different ages are poorly defined [11]. Developing a life course approach [12] to children and adults surviving with CHDs is a vital step in recognising that they experience complex interactions between intrinsic early life factors, cardiac diagnosis and the pressures of the external environment, which have a significant impact on their growth, development and late outcomes. There remains a crucial lack in our understanding of the relevance of different risk factors and exposures at each stage of the lifecourse and how these may modify long-term outcomes, not only when they occur in relation to critical periods but also when experienced as repeated exposures such as multiple surgical interventions. Such information is key to future interventions to improve survival and health outcomes and ensure a smooth transition to adult life for affected children.

The UK Collaborative Study of Congenital Heart Defects (UKCSCHD) was established as a UK-wide multi-centre cohort involving almost 4000 children, diagnosed with serious CHDs during their first year of life, to determine prospectively survival, health, educational and quality of life outcomes. In this paper we examine survival from birth to 15 years of age, characterise the timing and causes of death during childhood and investigate the relative importance of patient-specific and early life factors to mortality risk during childhood for this national cohort that is largely representative of contemporary surgical and medical management.

Materials and Methods

Ethics statement

Ethics approval was granted by Trent Multicentre Research Ethics Committee (MREC 04/4/017). Case notes review was undertaken within collaborating centres under the supervision of the local responsible cardiologist; the names and addresses of the children were not provided to the central study team who carried out analyses on de-identified data.

Methods

The UKCSCHD includes children with serious CHDs born between 1992 and 1995 and prospectively notified to a UK-wide study evaluating fetal diagnosis by paediatric cardiologists (British Congenital Cardiac Association [BCCA] members) in all 17 UK paediatric cardiac surgical centres [13]. Serious CHDs were defined as structural heart malformations requiring intervention or resulting in death during the first year of life [13].

A retrospective hospital records review of 3897 children was co-ordinated by the central research team; 268 children from the original register were excluded as there were insufficient details in the case notes to confirm that all inclusion criteria (Table 1) for the UKCSCHD were met. Local clinicians extracted data and completed a standardised proforma for 3698 (95%) of 3897 children. Record retrieval varied by centre, reflecting local record-keeping, and retrieval was less successful for children who were reported by local clinicians to have died (difference 6% [95% CI 4%, 8%]).

Deaths were traced within hospital systems then validated through the Office for National Statistics (England and Wales) and General Register Office (Scotland). A primary cardiac diagnosis (Table 2) was assigned to every child using a hierarchical classification prioritising the most severe structural defect adapted from Wren et al. [14]; three clinical raters (CB, CW, RK) independently assigned diagnoses (generalised kappa (κ) for rater agreement = 0.83) and the final diagnosis was agreed by consensus. Two cardiologists (CB, CW) designated one procedure for each child as 'definitive', defined as the procedure which would approximate normal anatomy and restore biventricular function or provide long-term palliation without expectation of further surgery during childhood, thus the final stage of a multi-stage repair was considered definitive. The definitive procedure may have taken place at any time during follow-up. Children were assigned to a cardiac prognostic severity (CPS) group, adapted from Lane [15], based on primary diagnosis and whether their definitive procedure was presumed curative, corrective or palliative (Table 2).

Statistical analysis

Descriptive statistics are presented as numbers and percentages, or median and interquartile ranges (IQR), and 95% confidence intervals (CI) were estimated for the difference between two proportions. Table 3 provides information about the numbers of children who died or were censored alive (last seen) during each

Table 2. Cardiac diagnosis and severity for all children in the cohort.

PRIMARY CHD DIAGNOSIS*		Number of children	*Cardiac Prognostic Severity Group*** (% of children within diagnostic group)				
			Curative	*Corrective*	*Palliative*	*No intervention*	*Insufficient information*
HLH/MA	Hypoplastic left heart/mitral atresia	199	*0*	*0*	*65%*	*32%*	*4%*
TA	Tricuspid atresia	67	*0*	*0*	*97%*	*3%*	*0*
DIV	Double inlet ventricle	85	*0*	*0*	*96%*	*4%*	*0*
PA+IVS	Pulmonary atresia with intact ventricular septum	83	*0*	*0*	*99%*	*1%*	*0*
PA+VSD	Pulmonary atresia with ventricular septal defect	151	*0*	*34%*	*62%*	*3%*	*1%*
CAT	Common arterial trunk (Truncus arteriosus)	99	*0*	*89%*	*6%*	*5%*	*0*
CAVSD	Complete atrioventricular septal defect	460	*0*	*74%*	*21%*	*5%*	*0*
TGA	Transposition of the great arteries	597	*0*	*83%*	*17%*	*0%*	*0*
TOF	Tetralogy of Fallot	361	*0*	*81%*	*17%*	*1%*	*1%*
TAPVC	Total anomalous pulmonary venous connection	150	*93%*	*4%*	*1%*	*1%*	*0*
VSD	Ventricular septal defect	760	*63%*	*25%*	*11%*	*2%*	*0*
AS	Aortic stenosis	107	*0*	*92%*	*7%*	*2%*	*0*
PS	Pulmonary stenosis	194	*95%*	*2%*	*2%*	*1%*	*0*
COA	Coarctation of the aorta	395	*0*	*97%*	*1%*	*1%*	*0*
Misc	Miscellaneous	189	*21%*	*25%*	*46%*	*8%*	*1%*
	Total	**3,897**					

Notes:
*adapted from Wren [14];
**adapted from Lane [15].
Assignment of primary CHD diagnosis: The methodology for assigning primary diagnoses to 1,768 children with multiple defects was validated independently by three raters (RK, CB, CW). Based on cardiac diagnoses in medical records, children assigned a primary diagnosis were 1,738 (98%), 1,610 (91%) and 1,146 (65%) for each rater; this increased to 1,761 (99.7%), 1,689 (95.5%) and 1,658 (93.8%) respectively using records of surgical procedures (Interrater agreement: k = 0.83). A 'miscellaneous' category included defects found in fewer than 40 children: congenitally corrected transposition of the great arteries (n = 24), partial atrioventricular septal defect (n = 20), aortopulmonary window (n = 26), atrial septal defect (n = 36) and rarer diagnoses (n = 83).
CPS groups were: *no intervention*-children who received no surgical intervention prior to death during first year of life; *curative*-children who had successful repair of atrial or ventricular septal defect, pulmonary stenosis or total anomalous pulmonary veins and had no additional cardiac defects; *corrective*-children who had a procedure which approximated normal anatomy and restored biventricular function, with no expectation of future surgery during childhood; *palliative*-children whose surgery did not restore biventricular function, including children for whom all stages of multi-stage repair were not achieved, who had a valve replacement which would require later revision, or for whom only a single functional ventricle circulation was possible.

Table 3. Number of children dying or last seen (censored) during each year of follow-up.

Year of follow-up	Number at risk	Deaths	Censored (last seen)
(from birth = 0)	*n*	*n*	*n*
0–1 year	3897	727	681
1–2 years	2489	78	103
2–3 years	2308	35	55
3–4 years	2218	28	46
4–5 years	2144	16	58
5–6 years	2070	11	53
6–7 years	2006	8	48
7–8 years	1950	8	64
8–9 years	1878	3	106
9–10 years	1769	5	168
10–11 years	1596	4	405
11–12 years	1187	4	520
12–13 years*	663	4	424
13–14 years*	235	1	214
14–15 years*	20	0	20

*All children in the cohort were aged 12 years or older at the time of ascertainment of deaths in 2007, thus losses from follow-up at younger ages were due to death or censoring alive on the date last seen (as recorded in hospital case notes). Between 12 and 15 years there are fewer children under follow-up ('at risk') in the older age groups as many children had not reached these ages and this reduced the precision of survival estimates after 12 years.

year of follow-up. The Kaplan-Meier survival function was estimated up to 15 years of age; five children, whose date of death was not known, were censored alive on the date of the last hospital visit.

A multilevel discrete time event history model was developed to investigate the factors influencing survival; this was a binomial logit model with the response variable, death or censoring, coded as a binary variable. The discrete time hazard function represented the conditional probability of an event in each interval given that the event had not occurred in a previous interval: $h(t) = \Pr(T = t \mid T \geq t)$. The period of observation was divided into 24 discrete intervals; 12 intervals of one month duration for the first year of life when the majority of events occurred, then 11 intervals of one year from one to 12 years of age and a final interval of three years duration representing the interval 12 to 15 years of age, in which events were rare. In the final model including multiple predictors, three 'smoothed' categories (representing the first year of life, one to 12 years, and 12 to 15 years of age) were developed by estimating the log-transformed midpoint of each variable and dividing by the number of months within each category. Although the 24 category model had marginally better fit than the 'smoothed' category model (DIC 8887.9 and 8946.8 respectively), the smoothed category model improved model convergence and was therefore used.

Within each interval, it was assumed that the hazards were constant and the binary response variable indicated whether death occurred during the final interval. Covariates specific to the child, such as sex or preterm birth, remained constant whilst factors recorded at each procedure, such as cardiopulmonary bypass duration, were permitted to vary between intervals. Weight and height were converted to age- and sex-standardised z-scores (British 1990 growth reference) [16]. Each predictor was explored in univariable analyses then multivariable models were constructed to determine joint associations.

Missing data were imputed using a hierarchical imputation model developed with MLwiN 2.18–2.20 [17] and Realcom-Impute [18]. The imputation procedure used Markov-chain Monte Carlo (MCMC) procedure to generate 20 imputed datasets during 2500 iterations. Imputation was conditioned on centre availability of records, as this significantly influenced missingness. Imputation excluded 28 children whose date of death or censoring was unknown, and variables with more than 50% missing data; the included variable with the most missing data was clinical status on admission (46%; Table 4). Distributions of continuous variables before and after imputation were compared using density plots (data not shown).

Hierarchical models of mortality risk were developed to take account of the grouping of individual children within cardiac centres and the correlation of procedure-related data within the individual child. For each imputed dataset multilevel discrete-time event models [19,20] were constructed to predict mortality risk from birth to follow-up in 2007, when all surviving children were aged 12 to 15 years. The final results reported are those averaged over these datasets according to 'Rubin's rules'. The results from these analyses using imputed datasets were compared with those using the 'complete case' datasets (including only those children with complete data).

Analyses were undertaken using Stata SE 11 (Timberlake Consulting) and MLwiN 2.18–2.20 [17].

Results

Almost one-quarter of the cohort died (n = 932 deaths) and, of these, 727 (78%) deaths occurred within the first year and 323 (35%) within the first month of life. Although the risk of death was lower after the first year of life, 20% of all cohort deaths occurred after one year of age. Death occurred before intervention, or parents chose palliative care, for 144 (4%) children who died without any procedure; most (n = 63; 44%) of these children had hypoplastic left heart and/or mitral atresia (HLH/MA). The median age at death for children who died without undergoing an

Table 4. Patient-specific characteristics by diagnostic group (n = 3897).

Primary CHD Diagnosis	Boys	Preterm	DS: Down's syndrome	Non-DS non-cardiac malformation	Add. cardiac defects	Unstable clinical status	Age at first intervention*	Death without intervention
	as % of all non-missing values[†]						Median (IQR) days	n
HLH/MA	67%	7%	0	4%	26%	75%	5 (2,14)	63
TA	52%	6%	0	6%	88%	57%	23 (5,83)	2
DIV	71%	4%	0	7%	92%	64%	14 (5,46)	3
PA+IVS	64%	8%	0	5%	29%	82%	3 (2,6)	1
PA+VSD	45%	10%	0	18%	52%	61%	8 (3,81)	5
CAT	52%	10%	0	17%	40%	61%	29 (12,65)	5
CAVSD	47%	8%	43%	5%	43%	42%	103 (55,169)	22
TGA	68%	5%	0	2%	51%	65%	3 (1,14)	1
TOF	59%	10%	3%	12%	29%	33%	133 (42,249)	4
TAPVC	64%	7%	0	6%	19%	76%	16 (3,62)	2
VSD	51%	9%	9%	10%	54%	57%	97 (34,180)	13
AS	70%	2%	2%	5%	44%	60%	15 (3,61)	2
PS	45%	6%	1%	8%	27%	23%	72 (8,71)	2
COA	63%	8%	0	8%	45%	55%	17 (8,71)	4
Misc	52%	9%	7%	7%	63%	65%	81 (14,174)	15
Total	**57%**	**8%**	**8%**	**7%**	**46%**	**55%**	**38 (6,121)**	**144**

Notes:

*excludes 144 children who did not have an intervention;

[†]**Number (%) of children with missing data**: Sex n = 129(3%); Unstable clinical status n = 1784(46%); age at first procedure n = 50(1% of 3753 children who had an intervention); Preterm birth/Down's syndrome (DS)/Non-DS non-cardiac malformations/Additional cardiac defects: no missing data.

Key: **IQR** interquartile range; **preterm** <37 completed weeks gestation at birth; **Add. cardiac defects** - in addition to primary CHD diagnosis; **unstable clinical status** on first admission was defined as unstable if one or more of the following symptoms/signs were present: unwell = significant pallor, breathlessness or sweating, intubated, mechanically ventilated, hypotension = systolic blood pressure [SBP] <50 mmHg, hypertensive = SBP >100 mmHg, cardiac or respiratory arrest, metabolic acidosis, requiring adrenaline or high dose inotropic support; **HLH/MA** hypoplastic left heart and/or mitral atresia; **TA** tricuspid atresia; **DIV** double inlet ventricle; **PA+IVS** pulmonary atresia with intact ventricular septum; **PA+VSD** pulmonary atresia with ventricular septal defect; **CAT** common arterial trunk; **CAVSD** complete atrioventricular septal defect; **TGA** transposition of the great arteries; **TOF** tetralogy of Fallot; **TAPVC** total anomalous pulmonary venous connection; **VSD** ventricular septal defect; **AS** aortic stenosis; **PS** pulmonary stenosis; **COA** coarctation of the aorta; **Misc** miscellaneous cardiac defects (not included within other categories).

Table 5. Characteristics of individuals in the cohort (n = 3897).

Patient-specific factors	N (% of 3897)	Missing N (% of 3897)
Sex		129 (3%)
Boys	2147 (55%)	
Girls	1621 (42%)	
Preterm birth		0
Gestation <37 weeks	296 (8%)	
Gestation ≥37 weeks	3601 (92%)	
Non-cardiac malformations		0
Down's syndrome (DS)	293 (8%)	
Non-DS non-cardiac malformations	290 (7%)	
No non-cardiac malformations	3314 (85%)	
Additional cardiac defects		0
Isolated CHD	1826 (47%)	
Additional cardiac defects	1488 (53%)	
Antenatal diagnosis of CHD		0
Antenatal diagnosis	177 (5%)	
Postnatal diagnosis	3720 (95%)	
Factors related to management		
Clinical status on first admission		1784 (46%)
Stable	953 (24%)	
Unstable	1160 (30%)	
Age at first procedure *(median [IQR])*	38 (6, 121) days	
Weight z-score at first procedure *(median [IQR])*	−1.7 (IQR −2.83, −0.58)	
Height z-score at first procedure *(median [IQR])*	−0.8 (IQR −2.03, 0.42)	
Number of procedures *(median [IQR])*	1 (1, 2)	

Notes:
IQR interquartile range;
Preterm birth - before 37 completed weeks of gestation;
Additional cardiac defects - children who had at least one structural cardiac defect in addition to their primary cardiac diagnosis;
Non-Down's syndrome non-cardiac malformations - a further 290 children had non-cardiac congenital malformations that were not Down's syndrome, including recognised syndromes such as Di George's (n = 61).
Clinical status on first admission was defined as unstable if one or more of the following symptoms/signs were present: unwell = significant pallor, breathlessness or sweating, intubated, mechanically ventilated, hypotension = systolic blood pressure [SBP] <50 mmHg, hypertensive = SBP >100 mmHg, cardiac or respiratory arrest, metabolic acidosis, requiring adrenaline or high dose inotropic support.

intervention was 8.5 days (IQR 3, 75.5 days) and only one-third survived beyond the first month of life. Of 723 children who survived to one year without having undergone a definitive corrective or palliative procedure, 578 (80%) died between age one and 15 years. There was no significant difference in the proportion of girls and boys who died without a procedure. Characteristics of the cohort children and procedure-related factors are presented in Table 5 and Table 6 respectively.

Overall 80% (95% CI 78%–81%) of children were alive at one year and 72% [70%, 73%] at 15 years of age. Survival varied by primary cardiac diagnosis (Figure 1; Table 7). For 2,489 children remaining under follow-up after one year of age, survival between one and 15 years was 90% (95% CI 88%, 91%) overall, however for children within six diagnostic subgroups (HLH/MA, tricuspid atresia [TA], double inlet ventricle [DIV], pulmonary atresia with intact ventricular septum [PA+IVS], PA+VSD and CAVSD), survival post-infancy was lower than 90%.

In univariable models involving *all* children followed from birth, preterm birth (hazard ratio [HR] 1.43 [95% CI: 1.16, 1.77]), non-Down's syndrome non-cardiac malformations (HR 1.56 [1.27, 1.93]), cardiac defects additional to the primary diagnosis (HR 1.24 [1.09, 1.41]) and unstable clinical status on first admission (HR 1.43 [1.07, 1.90]) were statistically significant predictors of higher mortality. Relative to the largest subgroup (ventricular septal defect [VSD]), all primary diagnostic subgroups except pulmonary stenosis (PS) and aortic coarctation (COA) were associated with increased mortality.

In the multivariable model including all children and adjusted for centre effects, higher mortality up to age 15 years was associated with female sex (HR 1.25 [1.06, 1.47]), preterm birth (HR 1.44 [1.15, 1.79]), non-Down's syndrome non-cardiac malformations (HR 1.49 [1.20, 1.86]), additional cardiac defects (HR 1.23 [1.07, 1.42]) and, relative to VSD, all primary diagnoses except for PS and COA (data not shown). When procedure-related risk factors were included in the multivariable model, thus excluding children who died without a procedure, independent predictors of higher mortality risk were female sex, preterm birth, additional cardiac defects, pre-procedure sepsis or hypertension, post-procedure seizures, cardiac arrest, renal failure, stroke, sepsis or disseminated intravascular coagulopathy (DIC), lower weight or

Table 6. Characteristics of procedure-related factors (6351 procedures in 3753 individuals).

Procedure-related factors	Details of procedures	
	N (% of 6351 procedures)	
Pre-procedure variables:		
Any pre-procedure complications/support	786 (12%)*	
Intubated	*590*	
Inotropic support	*252*	
Acidosis	*159*	
Hypotensive (systolic BP <50 mmHg)	*111*	
Sepsis	*93*	
Hypertensive (systolic BP >100 mmHg)	*51*	
Seizures	*46*	
Intra-procedure variables:		
Procedures not requiring bypass‡	2486 (39%)	
Cardiopulmonary bypass (CPB) time†	2346	*median = 87(IQR 60,129) minutes*
Circulatory arrest (CA) time†	1059	*median = 30 (IQR 14,49) minutes*
Aortic cross-clamp (XC) time†	1980	*median = 52 (IQR 32,75) minutes*
Post-procedure variables:		
Any post-procedure complications	816 (13%)*	
Sepsis	*356*	
Re-intubated (after 24 hrs extubation)	*224*	
Renal failure	*202*	
Cardiac arrest	*169*	
Seizures	*113*	
ECMO (extracorporeal membrane oxygenation)	*47*	
DIC (disseminated intravascular coagulopathy)	*31*	
Stroke	*22*	

Notes:
IQR interquartile range; BP blood pressure; hrs hours.
*Procedures at which there was more than one pre-procedure (or post-procedure) complication are only counted once in the totals so the sum of individual complications is greater.
‡Procedures for which cardiopulmonary bypass would not be required, e.g. catheter intervention.
†Excludes procedures in which duration is recorded as 0 minutes.

height z-score, younger age at first procedure, or longer duration of cardiopulmonary bypass or cardiac arrest (Table 8). Non-Down's syndrome non-cardiac malformation and postoperative ECMO were not significant predictors of higher mortality. Mortality risk for children with TGA and COA was similar to VSD, and significantly higher than VSD for all other CHD subgroups.

In sensitivity analyses results from the imputed models were compared with those using complete cases; the imputed data analyses provided greater precision with no significant difference in the magnitude and direction of effect. During stepwise development of the model, the variable representing definitive surgery did not significantly improve the model and was excluded. However in a sensitivity analysis involving only 606 children who had complete data and were alive at age one year, mortality risk was significantly lower for those who had experienced definitive surgery by age one year than for those who did not (HR 0.19, 95%CI 0.05, 0.73; p = 0.015).

Discussion

In this UK-wide cohort involving 3897 children with serious CHDs, mortality was 20% in the first year of life. An additional 8% of the cohort died between one and 15 years of age, thus 20% of all deaths within the cohort occurred after the first year of life. There were 144 children in the cohort who died without any intervention during the first year of life. Overall survival was 79.8% at one year and 71.7% at 15 years of age with variation by primary cardiac diagnosis, thus for children who survived the first year survival into adulthood was generally good. Children with functional single ventricles (HLH/MA, TA and DIV) experienced the highest mortality overall but for children surviving to one year of age, those with PA+VSD and CAVSD had the worst post-infant survival rates.

Primary cardiac diagnosis was an important independent predictor of mortality risk up to 15 years; children with TGA, COA and VSD had the lowest mortality risk. Higher mortality risk regardless of intervention was independently associated with female sex, preterm birth and having a cardiac defect in addition to the primary cardiac diagnosis. For children who had at least one procedure, higher mortality risk was associated with earlier age at

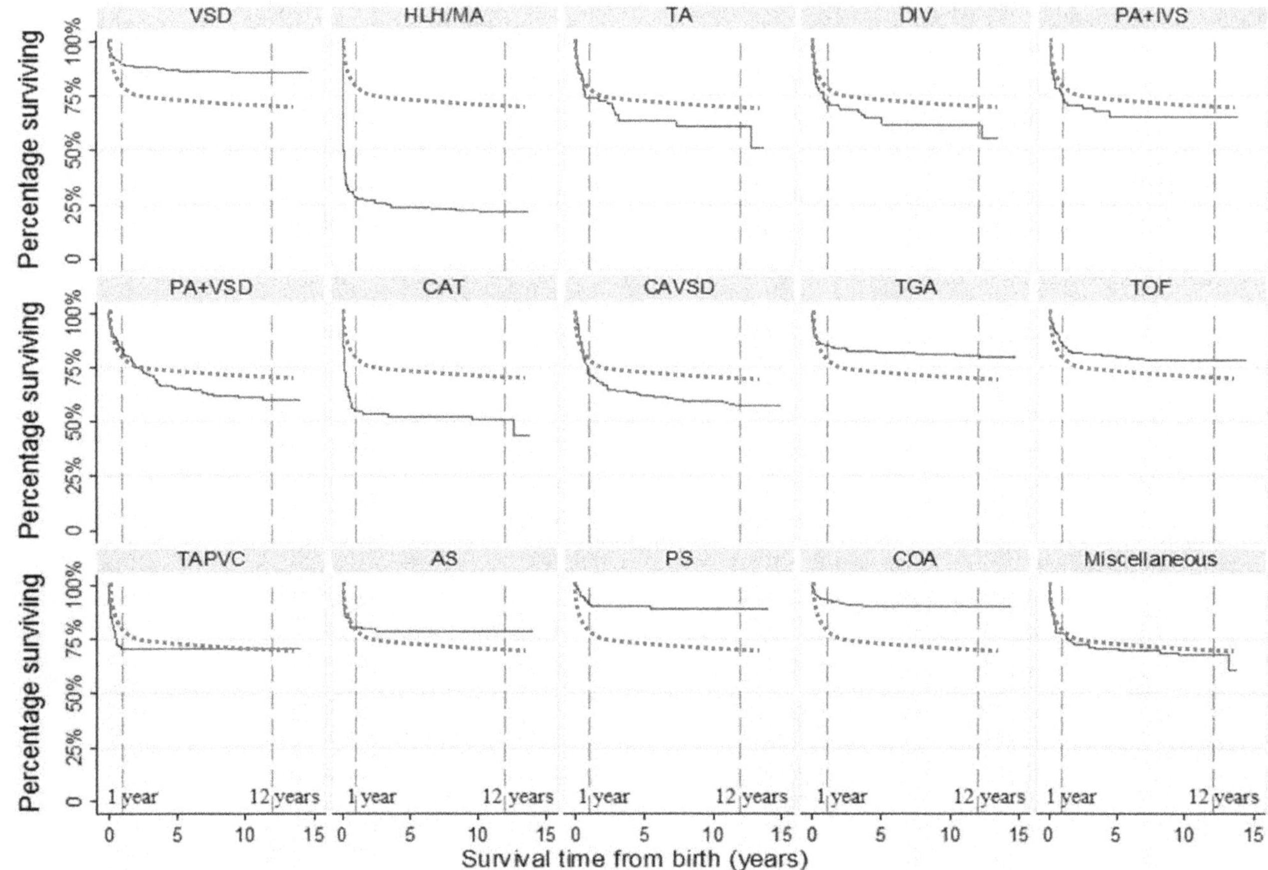

Notes: Interrupted vertical lines represent survival at 1 and 12 years.
The survival curve for all children within the cohort is represented by a **dotted** line.
The survival curve for children with each specific cardiac diagnosis is represented by a **solid** line.

Abbreviations: HLH/MA hypoplastic left heart and/or mitral atresia; **TA** tricuspid atresia; **DIV** double inlet ventricle; **PA+IVS** pulmonary atresia with intact ventricular septum; **PA+VSD** pulmonary atresia with ventricular septal defect; **CAT** common arterial trunk; **CAVSD** complete atrioventricular septal defect; **TGA** transposition of the great arteries; **TOF** tetralogy of Fallot; **TAPVC** total anomalous pulmonary venous connection; **VSD** ventricular septal defect; **AS** aortic stenosis; **PS** pulmonary stenosis; **COA** coarctation of the aorta; **Misc** miscellaneous cardiac defects.

Figure 1. Survival from birth to 15 years by primary diagnosis (for individual diagnoses). Notes: Interrupted vertical lines represent survival at 1 and 12 years. The survival curve for all children within the cohort is represented by a **dotted** line. The survival curve for children with each specific cardiac diagnosis is represented by a **solid** line. **Abbreviations**: **HLH/MA** hypoplastic left heart and/or mitral atresia; **TA** tricuspid atresia; **DIV** double inlet ventricle; **PA+IVS** pulmonary atresia with intact ventricular septum; **PA+VSD** pulmonary atresia with ventricular septal defect; **CAT** common arterial trunk; **CAVSD** complete atrioventricular septal defect; **TGA** transposition of the great arteries; **TOF** tetralogy of Fallot; **TAPVC** total anomalous pulmonary venous connection; **VSD** ventricular septal defect; **AS** aortic stenosis; **PS** pulmonary stenosis; **COA** coarctation of the aorta; **Misc** miscellaneous cardiac defects.

first procedure, pre-procedural sepsis and hypertension (systolic BP>100 mHg), post-procedural complications (including cardiac arrest, stroke, renal failure, seizures and sepsis) and increased duration of cardiopulmonary bypass or cardiac arrest.

Longitudinal cohort studies present important methodological challenges for survival analysis, including the need to model hierarchical data structures, repeated procedures, and to address missing data. An important strength of our study is the development of multilevel models that allowed us to link procedure-related factors across the child's lifecourse and to explicitly order these in time. Children in the cohort underwent varying numbers of procedures, which did not occur at fixed ages, and earlier postoperative experience could influence later management. Despite recognition of the complexity of survival analysis in children with CHDs, for whom both predictors and mortality are time-dependent [11], examples of survival models including time-varying covariates are rare and few previous studies have explicitly stated the temporal ordering of childhood factors and their inter-relationships, directly or through mediating factors, with mortality. We addressed the methodological challenges of repeat observations, and also adjusted for the effects of clustering by cardiac centre, through the development of discrete-time hierarchical survival models [19,20] and multilevel multiple imputation [44,45] of missing values. The use of imputed datasets, by allowing us to include all cohort children and procedures in the analyses, reduced the likelihood of bias that can result from restricting analyses to the small proportion of children with complete data [21]. Our sensitivity analyses evaluating the effect of multiple imputation in comparison with complete-case datasets, demonstrated that imputed data contributed to greater precision in mortality estimates and ensured that the impact of less

Table 7. Data Table for Figure 1.

PRIMARY CARDIAC DIAGNOSIS	Number at birth	Survivor function (95% confidence intervals)	
	n	At 1 year	At 12 years
Hypoplastic left heart/mitral atresia	199	**28%**(22%,35%)	**21%**(15%,27%)
Tricuspid atresia	67	**74%**(62%,83%)	**61%**(48%,72%)
Double inlet ventricle	85	**72%**(61%,80%)	**62%**(50%,71%)
Pulmonary atresia with intact ventricular septum	83	**73%**(62%,82%)	**65%**(53%,74%)
Pulmonary atresia with ventricular septal defect	151	**84%**(77%,89%)	**60%**(51%,68%)
Common arterial trunk (truncus arteriosus)	99	**55%**(44%,64%)	**51%**(40%,61%)
Complete atrioventricular septal defect	460	**71%**(67%,76%)	**57%**(52%,62%)
Transposition of the great arteries	597	**85%**(82%,88%)	**81%**(77%,84%)
Tetralogy of Fallot	361	**85%**(81%,88%)	**79%**(74%,83%)
Total anomalous pulmonary venous connection	150	**71%**(62%,78%)	**71%**(62%,78%)
Ventricular septal defect	760	**90%**(87%,92%)	**86%**(83%,88%)
Aortic stenosis	107	**81%**(72%,87%)	**78%**(69%,85%)
Pulmonary stenosis	194	**91%**(85%,94%)	**89%**(83%,93%)
Coarctation of the aorta	395	**94%**(90%,96%)	**90%**(86%,93%)
Miscellaneous	189	**77%**(70%,83%)	**68%**(60%,75%)

commonly reported factors, such as pre- and post-procedural complications, was quantifiable.

Although we were prevented by our governance permissions [22] from accessing routine mortality data to check for deaths amongst children who clinicians presumed to be surviving, all reported deaths were confirmed against public death registrations. As children with serious CHDs remain under review throughout life, we believe that our ascertainment of deaths through cardiologists, hospital records and GPs was complete.

The heterogeneity of CHDs also presents a significant problem for population-based analyses [23,24] and variability in classification systems often limits comparisons between studies. Our simple hierarchical classification adapted from Wren [14] and validated on data available from medical case notes, ensured that each child was assigned to only one CHD subgroup and avoided double-counting of children with multiple cardiac defects. As similar classifications have been successfully applied in other UK studies [9,25] [26], this provides a sound basis for cross-study comparisons.

Patients do not pay for care within the UK healthcare system, thus there were no financial barrier to accessing surgery and deaths in children who were offered only palliative medical care were related to the inoperability of the defect. As with all long-term follow-up, early management of cohort members who were born in 1992–1995 was determined by clinical era. Although our cohort has its inception after the introduction of neonatal cardiac surgery and key procedures, such as the arterial switch operation, paediatric cardiac surgical and intensive care technologies have continued to advance, notably for children with HLH for whom Norwood-type surgery is now widely available, or with TOF for whom neonatal surgery is now common. Nonetheless, surgical management has not altered markedly for many CHD subgroups. Advances in fetal screening s well as surgery may also alter the proportion of children who would be offered palliative medical care in current practice compared our cohort. Whereas fetal screening detected around 23% of severe CHDs in 1993–94 [13], this has now increased to detection of around one-third of cases [27], which may mean that more children born today would commence specialist care at birth than in our cohort. The findings from our cohort should therefore be interpreted with caution within specific diagnostic subgroups where surgical techniques or screening detection have altered significantly as there may be improved survival for children born today. Nevertheless we believe our results are still likely to remain relevant overall to children born and operated with CHDs today, particularly for diagnostic subgroups in which significant improvements in early postoperative survival have not been seen.

There are relatively few population-based observational cohort studies that describe mortality and survival up to age 12–15 years for children affected by CHDs (Table 9). Although we also present some findings from our model including children who remained unoperated at the time of death, the majority of these children died in the first month after birth, many had HLH and palliative care was chosen by some parents; management of such severe and complex cases has continued to advance in the last decade. Thus our main model excludes these unoperated cases and focuses on survival from birth for the majority of children in the cohort, who did undergo an intervention.

Reviewing all child CHD deaths in Bohemia between 1952 and 1979, Samanek reported that 'natural' survival before the widespread introduction of paediatric cardiac surgery was 67% at 15 years [28]. Three further studies investigated survival in large surgical cohorts [10,29,30], including a Finnish population-based study between 1953 and 1989 in which survival was reported as 78% at 45 years after surgery, significantly lower than for the unaffected population. Only three studies have reported survival after diagnosis in early life, including children who remained unoperated as well as those undergoing surgery, of which two present directly observed survival from diagnosis [31] [32]. These two studies, representing contemporary management, documented better overall survival (Table 10) than we observed but up to 40% of children survived without any interventions suggesting

Table 8. Multivariable survival analysis using multiple imputation (n = 3725*).

Variable	Reference Category	Category	Hazard Ratio	95% CI		P-value
				lower	*upper*	
Sex	*Boys*					
		Girls	1.51	1.24	1.84	<0.0001
Birth gestation	*Term (≥37 weeks)*					
		Preterm (<37 weeks gestation)	1.31	1.01	1.69	0.042
Non-cardiac malformations	*None*					
		Downs Syndrome	0.87	0.62	1.21	0.403
		Non- Downs Syndrome	1.26	0.97	1.64	0.085
Additional cardiac defects	*Isolated CHDs*					
		Additional defects	1.34	1.13	1.57	0.001
Clinical status on admission	*Stable*					
		Unstable	1.17	0.82	1.66	0.383
Primary diagnoses	*VSD*					
		Hypoplastic left heart/mitral atresia	7.58	5.20	11.04	<0.0001
		Tricuspid atresia	4.05	2.45	6.69	<0.0001
		Double inlet ventricle	3.31	2.07	5.29	<0.0001
		Pulmonary atresia with intact ventricular septum	2.98	1.75	5.08	<0.0001
		Pulmonary atresia with ventricular septal defect	2.98	2.01	4.42	<0.0001
		Common arterial trunk (truncus arteriosus)	2.53	1.65	3.89	<0.0001
		Complete atrioventricular septal defect	3.96	2.88	5.42	<0.0001
		Transposition of the great arteries	1.36	0.97	1.90	0.074
		Tetralogy of Fallot	2.55	1.78	3.66	<0.0001
		Total anomalous pulmonary venous connection	2.11	1.35	3.32	0.001
		Aortic stenosis	1.85	1.10	3.13	0.021
		Pulmonary stenosis	1.85	1.06	3.22	0.030
		Coarctation of the aorta	1.11	0.71	1.75	0.645
		Miscellaneous	2.52	1.67	3.80	<0.0001
Procedure- related variables: constant						
Age at first procedure		*per month increase*	0.90	0.86	0.93	<0.0001
Procedure- related variables: time-varying						
Pre-procedure complications	*None*					
		Inotropic support	1.57	0.83	2.97	0.162

Table 8. Cont.

Variable	Reference Category	Category	Hazard Ratio	95% CI		P-value
				lower	*upper*	
		Intubation	0.83	0.48	1.42	0.497
		Seizures	1.38	0.48	4.01	0.551
		Sepsis	2.69	1.27	5.71	0.010
		Metabolic acidosis	0.93	0.43	2.04	0.859
		Hypertension	3.78	1.23	11.60	0.020
		Hypotension	1.84	0.99	3.43	0.053
Post-procedure complications	*None*					
		Seizures	1.54	1.05	2.26	0.027
		Cardiac arrest	4.98	3.78	6.55	<0.0001
		Renal failure	1.78	1.27	2.48	0.001
		Stroke	2.03	1.05	3.90	0.034
		Sepsis	1.46	1.09	1.95	0.010
		Disseminated intravascular coagulopathy (DIC)	6.44	3.78	10.95	<0.0001
		Extra-corporeal membrane oxygenation (ECMO)	1.42	0.83	2.45	0.200
		Re-intubation (after 24 hours extubation)	0.97	0.73	1.30	0.851
Weight and height						
z-score weight		*per one z-score unit increase*	0.92	0.85	1.00	0.048
z-score height		*per one z-score unit increase*	0.87	0.81	0.93	<0.0001
Intra-procedure						
Cardiopulmonary bypass duration		*per 10 min increase*	1.03	1.01	1.05	0.001
Cardiac arrest duration		*per 10 min increase*	1.10	1.08	1.12	<0.0001
Aortic cross-clamping duration		*per 10 min increase*	0.98	0.95	1.01	0.243

*Adjusted for specialist cardiac centre; excludes children who did not have an intervention or who died on same day as birth.

Table 9. Population-based cohort studies reporting mid- and long-term survival for children with congenital heart defects.

Lead author, publication year	Region/State, Country	Period	Study population (n)	Method/Design; Outcome measure	Period of follow-up	Survival/mortality
Morris, 1991 [29]	Oregon, US	Operated 1958–1989	Children aged <18 years (n = 2,701)	Retrospective review of paediatric cardiac procedures (for 8 CHD types); Death after surgery	Up to 25 years after surgery	Varying by CHD: 64% survival at 15 years after surgery (transposition) to 98% survival (atrial septal defect)
Samanek, 1992 [28]	Bohemia, Czech Republic	Diagnosed 1952–1979	Deaths aged ≤15 years (n = 946)	Retrospective review of death registrations; Death ≤15 years old	Up to 16 years of age	71% survival at 1 year of age; 67% survival at 15 years of age
Meberg, 2000 [31]	Vestfold County, Norway	Diagnosed 1982–1996	Children diagnosed clinically or at post-mortem (n = 360)	Prospective follow-up after diagnosis; Death ≤18 years old	Mean 9.5 years (range 3–18 years)	Overall 12% mortality at end of follow-up
Nieminen, 2001 [10]	Finland	Operated 1953–1989	Children aged <15 years old at surgery (n = 6,461)	Retrospective review of paediatric cardiac procedures (all CHDs); Death after surgery	Mean 22 years after surgery (range 9–45 years)	Overall 7% surgical mortality; 78% survival at 45 years after surgery
Wren, 2001 [9]	Northern Region, UK	Born 1985–1994	Children diagnosed clinically or at post-mortem (n = 1,942)	Prospective follow-up from birth/diagnosis; Death ≤15 years old	Up to 16 years of age	82% survival at 1 year of age; *Predicted 78% survival to 16 years of age*
Moons, 2009 [32]	Belgium	Born 2002	Children diagnosed clinically (n = 921)	Prospective follow-up from birth/diagnosis; Death ≤5 years old	Up to 5 years of age	96% survival at 5 years of age
Larsen, 2011 [30]	Western Region, Denmark	Operated 1996–2002	Children operated for CHD (n = 801)	Prospective follow-up after cardiac surgery; Death after surgery	Median 8.2 years after surgery (range 6–12 years)	86% survival at 8.2 years after surgery

Table 10. Childhood survival by primary cardiac diagnosis reported within population-based cohort studies published since 1990.

PRIMARY CARDIAC DIAGNOSIS	UKCSCHD	Samanek, 1992 [28]	Meberg, 2000 [31]	Wren, 2001 [9]
	At age 12 years ('observed')	At age 15 years ('natural')*	At age 9.5 years ('observed')	At age 15 years ('predicted')§
Hypoplastic left heart	21%	11%	22%	0
Pulmonary atresia	60–65%	30%	75%	40%
Common arterial trunk (truncus arteriosus)	51%	11%	50%	31%
Complete atrioventricular septal defect	57%	49%	55%	55%
Transposition of the great arteries	81%	38%	85%	67%
Tetralogy of Fallot	79%	86%	82%	84%
Total anomalous pulmonary venous connection	71%	0	-	70%
Ventricular septal defect	86%	76%	97%	91%
Aortic stenosis	78%	84%	92%	66%
Pulmonary stenosis	89%	94%	93%	92%
Coarctation of the aorta	90%	68%	84%	85%

Notes:
This table compares defect-specific survival reported in childhood within four population-based cohorts that include all children diagnosed in infancy even if no intervention was performed. Most studies present 'observed' cohort survival from diagnosis or first surgery during infancy, with the exception of:
*Samanek presents 'natural' survival in an era prior to widespread surgical correction.
§Wren presents 'predicted' survival up to age 15 years based on observed survival to age 1 year and survival from 1 to 15 years estimated from a review of the published literature.

that, in comparison with the UKCSCHD, they included a higher proportion of mild CHDs that were compatible with survival without intervention.

Surgical case series have highlighted important associations between increased postoperative mortality risk and factors such as low birth weight [33,34], preterm birth [35], sudden clinical deterioration in the neonatal period [36,37], and procedure-associated complications, including sepsis and renal failure [38]. Several studies have demonstrated the detrimental impact of longer intra-procedure duration of cardiopulmonary bypass and cardiac arrest [39–42], also observed in our cohort, although most previous authors estimated the effect at a single procedure only rather than repeated exposure over multiple procedures. Moreover Kang has cautioned that longer duration of cardiopulmonary bypass may only reflect technically more difficult surgery [41].

Although our findings indicate that girls with CHDs are at significantly higher risk of death, published evidence for sex differences in mortality for individuals with CHDs remains inconclusive. Morris [29] demonstrated that girls with COA and TGA had higher mortality prior to intervention, whereas Fyler [43] reported a higher death rate for boys during the first year of life. Other authors have highlighted that girls experience higher perioperative mortality related to paediatric cardiac surgery [44–47]. As the ratio of boys to girls affected varies by specific cardiac defect, these sex differences may be confounded by the severity of cardiac diagnosis. Nevertheless children's cardiac size and function, lung development and immune responses have been shown to vary by sex [47–51], therefore biological differences also provide a plausible explanation for sex differences in mortality risk and would merit further research.

In accordance with previous reports [52,53], we found no independent influence on mortality associated with Down's syndrome. Eskedal [52] has highlighted that children with CHDs who have non-cardiac malformations other than Down's syndrome experience higher mortality than those with isolated cardiac defects. In our cohort, non-Down's non-cardiac malformations were significant predictors of mortality when children who died without intervention were included in the analysis, suggesting that these malformations do contribute to mortality in this subgroup.

It is now over a decade since the Bristol Inquiry addressed concerns about the care of children receiving cardiac surgery at the Bristol Royal Infirmary [54]. Expert evidence presented to the Inquiry emphasised the lack of data on long-term outcomes relevant to children and their families [55]. The Central Cardiac Audit Database (CCAD) now routinely collects national outcome data for cardiac procedures, including survival up to one year after paediatric cardiac intervention; these data are published through the National Institute for Cardiac Outcomes Research (NICOR) Congenital Heart Disease Portal [56].

While routine audit remains essential to monitoring outcomes for children receiving interventions for CHDs in the UK [57], a procedure-based system excludes children who never receive an intervention and often fails to capture late mortality and broader health outcomes, such as educational achievement or quality of life. Improved record linkage between multiple routinely collected data sources, supplemented by focused observational or clinical studies, could enrich current routine data collection and provide more efficient use of existing resources for extended follow-up.

Conclusions

The UKCSCHD has provided a unique opportunity to observe survival and wider health outcomes throughout childhood in a prospectively ascertained UK-wide cohort that is largely representative of contemporary management. We found that infant mortality under age one year for children with serious CHDs was over 30 times greater than for the general population, estimated at six per 1,000 live births [58]. It is also clear from our data that whilst children with CHDs were still most likely to die in infancy in this cohort, over 20% of CHD-related deaths in childhood took place after the first year of life. Surgical management of serious

CHDs carries an initial perioperative risk of death or neurological injury in childhood, but the altered physiology of the operated heart may also result in reduced ability to cope with ageing or cardiac stressors arising in adult life. Long-term survival and health outcomes are influenced by health events across the lifecourse thus optimising the health experience of preschool and school-age children with CHDs is as relevant to future improvements in survival and quality of life of adults with CHDs as successful early surgical repair. Crucially cardiac diagnosis remained an important predictor of outcome particularly as this influenced the type of definitive procedure, whether this was palliative or corrective, and the age at which it was performed. However, we also identified procedure-related predictors of mortality that may be amenable to modification in order to effect further advances in survival or improve health outcomes after surgery. Investigation into the biological mechanisms contributing to higher mortality for girls is warranted to explore the potential for improving future outcomes and reducing health inequalities.

Acknowledgments

We are very grateful to the local cardiologists and members of the British Congenital Cardiac Association (BCCA) within the UKCSCHD collaborating centres without whom this study would not have been possible: We are very grateful to the local cardiologists and members of the British Congenital Cardiac Association (BCCA) in each UKCSCHD collaborating centre, without whom this study would not have been possible: Dr S Adwani, Dr F Bu'Lock, Dr B Craig, Dr P Daubeney, Dr G Derrick, Dr M Elliott, Dr R Franklin, Dr J Gibbs, Dr B Knight, Dr J Lim, Dr A Magee, Dr R Martin, Dr P Miller, Dr S Qureshi, Dr E Rosenthal, Dr A Salmon, Dr I Sullivan, Dr P Thakker, Dr J Thomson, Dr D Wilson, Dr A Wong. UKCSCHD collaborating centres included: Belfast, Birmingham, Bristol, Cardiff, Edinburgh, Glasgow, Leeds, Leicester, Liverpool, London, Manchester, Newcastle, Nottingham, Oxford and Southampton. We would also like to thank Dr Huiqi Pan for her advice and support for the programming of the MLWiN models and the UKCSCHD research assistants (Ms Ugochi Nwulu, Dr Carly Rich and others) for their valuable contribution and hard work. In addition, we appreciate very much the support that we received from Heartline (parent support group).

Author Contributions

Conceived and designed the experiments: RLK CD CB CW. Performed the experiments: RLK CD CB CW. Analyzed the data: RLK AW HG. Contributed reagents/materials/analysis tools: HG. Wrote the paper: RLK. Reviewed and developed the analyses: RLK CD CB CW AW HG. Reviewed and agreed the manuscript: RLK CD CB CW AW HG.

References

1. Dadvand P, Rankin J, Shirley MD, Rushton S, Pless-Mulloli T (2009) Descriptive epidemiology of congenital heart disease in Northern England. Paediatr Perinat Epidemiol 23: 58–65.
2. Lee K, Khoshnood B, Chen L, Wall SN, Cromie WJ, et al. (2001) Infant mortality from congenital malformations in the United States, 1970–1997. Obstet Gynecol 98: 620–627.
3. Khoshnood B, De Vigan C, Vodovar V, Goujard J, Lhomme A, et al. (2005) Trends in prenatal diagnosis, pregnancy termination, and perinatal mortality of newborns with congenital heart disease in France, 1983–2000: a population-based evaluation. Pediatrics 115: 95–101.
4. Samanek M, Voriskova M (1999) Congenital heart disease among 815,569 children born between 1980 and 1990 and their 15-year survival: a prospective Bohemia survival study. Pediatr Cardiol 20: 411–417.
5. Macmahon B, McKeown T, Record RG (1953) The incidence and life expectation of children with congenital heart disease. Br Heart J 15: 121–129.
6. Dastgiri S, Gilmour WH, Stone DH (2003) Survival of children born with congenital anomalies. Arch Dis Child 88: 391–394.
7. Freedom RM, Lock J, Bricker JT (2000) Pediatric cardiology and cardiovascular surgery: 1950–2000. Circulation 102(20 Suppl 4): IV58–68.
8. NHS Information Centre (2009) National Audit of Congenital Heart Disease: Executive Summary 2009. Leeds, UK: NHS Information Centre. Available: http://www.hscic.gov.uk/catalogue/PUB02661/nati-cong-hear-dise-exec-summ-audi-2009-rep.pdf Accessed: 17 July 2014.
9. Wren C, O'Sullivan JJ (2001) Survival with congenital heart disease and need for follow up in adult life. Heart 85: 438–443.
10. Nieminen HP, Jokinen EV, Sairanen HI (2001) Late results of pediatric cardiac surgery in Finland: a population-based study with 96% follow-up. Circulation 104: 570–575.
11. McCrindle BW (2001) Considerations in the appraisal of mortality associated with congenital cardiac lesions. Semin Thorac Cardiovasc Surg Pediatr Card Surg Annu 4: 244–255.
12. Ben-Shlomo Y, Kuh D (2002) A life course approach to chronic disease epidemiology: conceptual models, empirical challenges and interdisciplinary perspectives. Int J Epidemiol 31: 285–293.
13. Bull C (1999) Current and potential impact of fetal diagnosis on prevalence and spectrum of serious congenital heart disease at term in the UK. British Paediatric Cardiac Association. Lancet 354: 1242–1247.
14. Wren C, Richmond S, Donaldson L (2000) Temporal variability in birth prevalence of cardiovascular malformations. Heart 83: 414–419.
15. Lane DA, Lip GY, Millane TA (2002) Quality of life in adults with congenital heart disease. Heart 88: 71–75.
16. Cole TJ, Freeman JV, Preece MA (1998) British 1990 growth reference centiles for weight, height, body mass index and head circumference fitted by maximum penalized likelihood. Stat Med 17: 407–429.
17. Rasbash J, Charlton C, Browne WJ, Healy M, Cameron B (2009) MLwiN version 2.1. University of Bristol, UK: Centre for Multilevel Modelling.
18. Goldstein H (2009) REALCOM-Impute: Multiple Imputation using MLwiN, User Guide. University of Bristol: Centre for Multilevel Modelling.
19. Goldstein H, Browne W, Rasbash J (2002) Multilevel modelling of medical data. Stat Med 21: 3291–3315.
20. Goldstein H (2011) Multilevel Statistical Models. Chichester, UK: John Wiley and Sons.
21. Kenward MG, Carpenter J (2007) Multiple imputation: current perspectives. Stat Methods Med Res 16: 199–218.
22. Knowles RL, Bull C, Wren C, Dezateux C (2011) Ethics, governance and consent in the UK: implications for research into the longer-term outcomes of congenital heart defects. Arch Dis Child 96: 14–20.
23. Brown KL, Crowe S, Pagel C, Bull C, Muthialu N, et al. (2013) Use of diagnostic information submitted to the United Kingdom Central Cardiac Audit Database: development of categorisation and allocation algorithms. Cardiol Young 23: 491–498.
24. Riehle-Colarusso T, Strickland MJ, Reller MD, Mahle WT, Botto LD, et al. (2007) Improving the quality of surveillance data on congenital heart defects in the metropolitan Atlanta congenital defects program. Birth Defects Res A Clin Mol Teratol 79: 743–753.
25. Billett J, Majeed A, Gatzoulis M, Cowie M (2008) Trends in hospital admissions, in-hospital case fatality and population mortality from congenital heart disease in England, 1994 to 2004. Heart 94: 342–348.
26. Crowe S, Brown KL, Pagel C, Muthialu N, Cunningham D, et al. (2013) Development of a diagnosis- and procedure-based risk model for 30-day outcome after pediatric cardiac surgery. J Thorac Cardiovasc Surg 145: 1270–1278.
27. Wren C, Reinhardt Z, Khawaja K (2008) Twenty-year trends in diagnosis of life-threatening neonatal cardiovascular malformations. Arch Dis Child Fetal Neonatal Ed 93: F33–35.
28. Samanek M (1992) Children with congenital heart disease: probability of natural survival. Pediatr Cardiol 13: 152–158.
29. Morris CD, Menashe VD (1991) 25-year mortality after surgical repair of congenital heart defect in childhood. A population-based cohort study. JAMA 266: 3447–3452.
30. Larsen SH, Emmertsen K, Johnsen SP, Pedersen J, Hjortholm K, et al. (2011) Survival and morbidity following congenital heart surgery in a population-based cohort of children–up to 12 years of follow-up. Congenit Heart Dis 6: 322–329.
31. Meberg A, Otterstad JE, Froland G, Lindberg H, Sorland SJ (2000) Outcome of congenital heart defects–a population-based study. Acta Paediatr 89: 1344–1351.
32. Moons P, Sluysmans T, De WD, Massin M, Suys B, et al. (2009) Congenital heart disease in 111 225 births in Belgium: birth prevalence, treatment and survival in the 21st century. Acta Paediatr 98: 472–477.
33. Oppido G, Napoleone CP, Formigari R, Gabbieri D, Pacini D, et al. (2004) Outcome of cardiac surgery in low birth weight and premature infants. Eur J Cardiothorac Surg 26: 44–53.
34. Padley JR, Cole AD, Pye VE, Chard RB, Nicholson IA, et al. (2011) Five-year analysis of operative mortality and neonatal outcomes in congenital heart disease. Heart Lung Circ 20: 460–467.
35. Tanner K, Sabrine N, Wren C (2005) Cardiovascular malformations among preterm infants. Pediatrics 116: e833–e838.
36. Brown KL, Ridout DA, Hoskote A, Verhulst L, Ricci M, et al. (2006) Delayed diagnosis of congenital heart disease worsens pre-operative condition and outcome of surgery in neonates. Heart 92: 1298–1302.

37. Bonnet D, Coltri A, Butera G, Fermont L, Le Bidois J, et al. (1999) Detection of transposition of the great arteries in fetuses reduces neonatal morbidity and mortality. Circulation 99: 916–918.
38. Brown KL, Ridout DA, Goldman AP, Hoskote A, Penny DJ (2003) Risk factors for long intensive care unit stay after cardiopulmonary bypass in children. Crit Care Med 31: 28–33.
39. Vogt PR, Carrel T, Pasic M, Arbenz U, von Segesser LK, et al. (1994) Early and late results after correction for double-outlet right ventricle: uni- and multivariate analysis of risk factors. Eur J Cardiothorac Surg 8: 301–307.
40. Nollert G, Fischlein T, Bouterwek S, Bohmer C, Klinner W, et al. (1997) Long-term survival in patients with repair of tetralogy of Fallot: 36- year follow-up of 490 survivors of the first year after surgical repair. J Am Coll Cardiol 30: 1374–1383.
41. Kang N, Cole T, Tsang V, Elliott M, de Leval M (2004) Risk stratification in paediatric open-heart surgery. Eur J Cardiothorac Surg 26: 3–11.
42. Greeley WJ, Kern FH, Ungerleider RM, Boyd JL, 3rd, Quill T, et al. (1991) The effect of hypothermic cardiopulmonary bypass and total circulatory arrest on cerebral metabolism in neonates, infants, and children. J Thorac Cardiovasc Surg 101: 783–794.
43. Fyler DC (1980) Report of the New England Regional Infant Cardiac Program. Pediatrics 65: 375–461.
44. Chang RK, Chen AY, Klitzner TS (2002) Female sex as a risk factor for in-hospital mortality among children undergoing cardiac surgery. Circulation 106: 1514–1522.
45. Klitzner TS, Lee M, Rodriguez S, Chang RK (2006) Sex-related disparity in surgical mortality among pediatric patients. Congenit Heart Dis 1: 77–88.
46. Seifert HA, Howard DL, Silber JH, Jobes DR (2007) Female gender increases the risk of death during hospitalization for pediatric cardiac surgery. J Thorac Cardiovasc Surg 133: 668–675.
47. Kochilas LK, Vinocur JM, Menk JS (2014) Age-Dependent Sex Effects on Outcomes After Pediatric Cardiac Surgery. J Am Heart Assoc 3: e000608.
48. Sarikouch S, Boethig D, Beerbaum P (2013) Gender-specific algorithms recommended for patients with congenital heart defects: review of the literature. Thorac Cardiovasc Surg 61: 79–84.
49. Dezateux C, Stocks J (1997) Lung development and early origins of childhood respiratory illness. Br Med Bull 53: 40–57.
50. Postma DS (2007) Gender differences in asthma development and progression. Gend Med 4 Suppl B: S133–146.
51. Falagas ME, Mourtzoukou EG, Vardakas KZ (2007) Sex differences in the incidence and severity of respiratory tract infections. Respir Med 101: 1845–1863.
52. Eskedal L, Hagemo P, Eskild A, Aamodt G, Seiler KS, et al. (2004) A population-based study of extra-cardiac anomalies in children with congenital cardiac malformations. Cardiol Young 14: 600–607.
53. Frid C, Bjorkhem G, Jonzon A, Sunnegardh J, Anneren G, et al. (2004) Long-term survival in children with atrioventricular septal defect and common atrioventricular valvar orifice in Sweden. Cardiol Young 14: 24–31.
54. Bristol Royal Infirmary Inquiry (2001) Learning from Bristol: the report of the public inquiry into children's heart surgery at the Bristol Royal Infirmary 1984 - 1995. Norwich, UK: The Stationery Office Ltd.
55. Bull C (2001) Key Issues in Retrospective Evaluation of Morbidity Outcomes Following Paediatric Cardiac Surgery. Final Report of the Bristol Royal Infirmary Inquiry (CM 5207). Norwich, UK: The Stationery Office Ltd.
56. NICOR (2012) National Institute for Cardiovascular Outcomes Research: Congenital Heart Disease Website. London, UK: University College London. Available: https://nicor4.nicor.org.uk/CHD/an_paeds.nsf/vwContent/home?Opendocument Accessed: 17 July 2014.
57. Gibbs JL, Monro JL, Cunningham D, Rickards A (2004) Survival after surgery or therapeutic catheterisation for congenital heart disease in children in the United Kingdom: analysis of the central cardiac audit database for 2000-1. BMJ 328: 611.
58. Office for National Statistics (2010) Infant and perinatal mortality by health areas in England and Wales, 2009. Office for National Statistics Statistical Bulletin. Newport, UK: Office for National Statistics.

5

Ethnicity and Child Health in Northern Tanzania: Maasai Pastoralists Are Disadvantaged Compared to Neighbouring Ethnic Groups

David W. Lawson[1]*, Monique Borgerhoff Mulder[2,3], Margherita E. Ghiselli[4], Esther Ngadaya[5], Bernard Ngowi[5], Sayoki G. M. Mfinanga[5], Kari Hartwig[6], Susan James[3]

1 Department of Population Health, London School of Hygiene and Tropical Medicine, London, England, United Kingdom, **2** Department of Anthropology, University of California Davis, Davis, California, United States of America, **3** Savannas Forever Tanzania, Arusha, Tanzania, **4** University of Minnesota, Minneapolis, Minnesota, United States of America, **5** National Institute for Medical Research, Muhimbili Medical Research Centre, Dar es Salaam, Tanzania, **6** St. Catherine University, Minneapolis, Minnesota, United States of America

Abstract

The Maasai of northern Tanzania, a semi-nomadic ethnic group predominantly reliant on pastoralism, face a number of challenges anticipated to have negative impacts on child health, including marginalisation, vulnerabilities to drought, substandard service provision and on-going land grabbing conflicts. Yet, stemming from a lack of appropriate national survey data, no large-scale comparative study of Maasai child health has been conducted. Savannas Forever Tanzania surveyed the health of over 3500 children from 56 villages in northern Tanzania between 2009 and 2011. The major ethnic groups sampled were the Maasai, Sukuma, Rangi, and the Meru. Using multilevel regression we compare each ethnic group on the basis of (i) measurements of child health, including anthropometric indicators of nutritional status and self-reported incidence of disease; and (ii) important proximate determinants of child health, including food insecurity, diet, breastfeeding behaviour and vaccination coverage. We then (iii) contrast households among the Maasai by the extent to which subsistence is reliant on livestock herding. Measures of both child nutritional status and disease confirm that the Maasai are substantially disadvantaged compared to neighbouring ethnic groups, Meru are relatively advantaged, and Rangi and Sukuma intermediate in most comparisons. However, Maasai children were less likely to report malaria and worm infections. Food insecurity was high throughout the study site, but particularly severe for the Maasai, and reflected in lower dietary intake of carbohydrate-rich staple foods, and fruits and vegetables. Breastfeeding was extended in the Maasai, despite higher reported consumption of cow's milk, a potential weaning food. Vaccination coverage was lowest in Maasai and Sukuma. Maasai who rely primarily on livestock herding showed signs of further disadvantage compared to Maasai relying primarily on agriculture. We discuss the potential ecological, socioeconomic, demographic and cultural factors responsible for these differences and the implications for population health research and policy.

Editor: Andrea S. Wiley, Indiana University, United States of America

Funding: Data analysis and the production of this manuscript were funded by a UK Medical Research Council (MRC) Fellowship Award to DWL (grant number: MR/K021672/1). This fellowship is jointly funded by the MRC and the UK Department for International Development (DFID) under the MRC/DFID Concordat agreement. All data come from the Whole Village Project (WVP). The WVP was generously funded by the United States Agency for International Development (www.usaid.gov), Partners for Development (www.pfd.org), the University of Minnesota, including the Institute on the Environment (environment.umn.edu), and the Canadian Foodgrains Bank (www.foodgrainsbank.ca). The funders had no role in study design, data collection and analysis, decision to publish, or preparation of the manuscript.

Competing Interests: The authors have declared that no competing interests exist.

* Email: David.Lawson@lshtm.ac.uk

Introduction

As we approach their 2015 target, there has been mounting criticism of the strong emphasis the Millennium Development Goals, and related development objectives, have placed on national averages, because such estimates dangerously obscure considerable and often rising inequality in health within developing countries [1–3]. Most scholarship focuses on socioeconomic dimensions of health (e.g. [4]), but, in some contexts, ethnic disparities can be of equal or greater importance [5,1]. A particular concern is the status of minority populations, or of "indigenous" ethnic groups, which systematically fail to benefit from wider improvements in health experienced by the general population. This is especially true when such groups are geographically or linguistically remote, or when they rely on alternative modes of production to agriculture, which benefits selectively from national and international investments and technological innovation [6,7,8]. In this paper we investigate ethnic variation in child health in Northern Tanzania, focusing on the comparison of the Maasai to neighbouring ethnic groups, and furthermore between farming and pastoralist households among the Maasai.

Many researchers have emphasised the numerous difficulties faced by the Maasai, and by pastoralists more generally [9–13]. A number of Tanzanian non-governmental organisations (NGOs) also specifically address development issues in the Maasai, many of which are included in the Pastoralists and Indigenous NGOs Forum (www.pingosforum.or.tz), an advocacy coalition of over 50 NGOs. However, due to the lack of national data disaggregating health outcomes by ethnicity or livelihood, there has so far been no large-sample comparative assessment of the true extent to which the health of the Maasai can be considered disadvantaged relative to the wider population [12]. This lack of data is an important concern since such invisibility in aggregate datasets represents a crucial barrier to motivating both productive discourse and support for initiatives addressing the specific needs of disadvantaged and/or marginalised ethnic groups [7].

The Maasai people inhabit Tanzania and Kenya, and are often characterised as archetypal pastoralists i.e. subsistence is based primary or exclusively on livestock herding. However, specialised pastoralism, traditionally the core of Maasai cultural identity, declined throughout the twentieth century and today livelihoods are increasingly diversifying towards agro-pastoralism and off-farm activities [14,15]. Owing to their proximity to the major East African game parks and their distinctive customs and dress, the Maasai have become perhaps the most globally recognizable ethnic group in sub-Saharan Africa [15]. Indeed they are commonly (mis)represented in advertisements and tourist commercials for both Kenya and Tanzania, and in recent years have become the focus of a burgeoning cultural tourism economy [16,17].

There are a number of reasons to suspect that the fame of the Maasai is not matched with good fortune with respect to child health. First, the Maasai reside in a semi-arid ecology prone to erratic rainfall and periodic drought. The year we initiated data collection (2009) witnessed a particularly devastating drought leading to high levels of pasture depletion, which by some reports the Maasai describe as the worst drought in living memory [18]. Such vulnerability is likely to be reflected in high food insecurity and poor health outcomes. Second, Maasai communities tend to be relatively remote, and livestock herding requires most household units to be at least semi-nomadic. In contrast to other ethnic groups, they also have a relatively poor command of Swahili, the national language. These factors reduce opportunities for both health service provision and educational attainment [12]. Third, these disadvantages have been exacerbated by on-going land ownership conflicts, fuelled in large part by the expansion of parks and protected areas for the profitable ecotourism industry, causing the Maasai to be displaced from historical and often the most fertile rangelands [19,20]. Such conflicts are anticipated to have both direct and indirect negative trickle-down consequences for child well being.

The question of ethnic variation in child health is also particularly interesting in Tanzania because, with an estimated 120 distinct ethnicities inhabiting its borders, it combines the highest level of ethnic diversity in Sub-Saharan Africa [21], with a tradition of downplaying ethnic differences in order to emphasize collective national identity. This stems from the socialist ideology that characterized the emergence of an independent Tanzania, and contrasts with Kenya, where ethnicity is highly politicized [22,23]. While playing a relatively modest role in national politics, ethnic identity (locally referred to as "tribe" or "kabila" in Kiswahili) is widely recognised and remains closely associated with region of residence, and linguistic and cultural distinctions, see Spear and Waller [15] for a specific discussion of the construction and expression of Maasai ethnic identity. Despite this diversity, ethnicity data are not routinely collected in national surveys. Five Tanzanian Demographic and Health Surveys (DHS), the only source of nationally representative data on child health, have so far been conducted (1991/2, 1996, 1999, 2004/5, 2010). To our knowledge, only the 1991/2 and 1996 DHS provide ethnicity data and such information has never been used to consider ethnic variation in child health.

We are aware of only a handful of previous studies that explicitly address ethnic variation in child health in Tanzania [24–27]. Hadley [26], for example, in a sample of several hundred children living in the Rukwa valley, reports that Sukuma children had significantly lower mortality and superior nutritional status compared to the Pimbwe. Unable to account for these differences in terms of (measured) variation in wealth or seasonal food insecurity, Hadley speculates that different infant feeding practices accounted for observed differences, see also [28,29]. In a large sample, Kruger et al. [27] reported that Datoga pastoralists had significantly lower child immunisation coverage compared to other ethnicities resident in the Mbulu area of northern Tanzania, a pattern they attribute to the relatively remote Datoga being both less accessible to and less trusting of health services. Numerous small-scale studies have also measured child survival and health within specific ethnic groups (e.g. Datoga: [30,31]; Pwimbwe and Sukuma: [26,32]; Maasai: [33]; Hadza: [34]). However, comparing estimates across studies is problematic due to differences in sampling methodology, timing, statistical methodology, and health measures considered.

In this study we conduct a systematic analysis of ethnic variation in child health using data collected by Savannas Forever Tanzania (SFTZ), an NGO specialising in the evaluation of rural development projects. SFTZ surveyed 56 villages spanning seven administrative regions in northern Tanzania between 2009 and 2011 as part of the Whole Village Project (WVP). Substantial sampling in the Arusha region and surrounding area lead to the inclusion of large number of Maasai households, making the collected data a uniquely valuable resource for the study of the Maasai relative to neighbouring ethnic groups. For comparison, in the 1996 Tanzanian DHS only 2% (n = 195/8120) of sampled women identified as Maasai [35]: p77–78, compared to 21% (n = 735/3584) of SFTZ sampled households. The main other ethnic groups sampled by SFTZ were the Sukuma, Rangi and Meru. All of these ethnicities are Bantu ethno-linguistic groups and, in contrast to the predominantly pastoralist and Nilotic-speaking Maasai, their livelihoods are typically based on agro-pastoralism or small-scale agriculture. The Sukuma are the largest ethnic group in Tanzania by a clear margin, estimated to represent 16% of the national population, while no other ethnicity comprises more than 5% [35]: p77–78.

Following the literature described above, we hypothesize that child health will be poorest in Maasai communities relative to neighbouring ethnic groups, and particularly for those Maasai who rely primarily on livestock herding. We contextualize our analyses by presenting descriptive data on household socioeconomic, demographic and cultural characteristics by ethnicity, but do not attempt to isolate the role of these more distal factors via multivariate analysis. Instead our focus here is on establishing a systematic and detailed characterisation of the nature of ethnic disparities in health across a large range of measures. Such information is valuable to the design and implementation of health policies and initiatives that typically focus on specific health risks and proximate determinants (e.g. nutrition, breastfeeding, vaccination), but rarely consider ethnic variation. Furthermore, since a number of development organisations in Tanzania focus specifically on Maasai communities or on pastoralists more generally, our data provide a much-needed clarification of the extent to which such groups can be meaningfully understood to be disadvantaged with regard to child health.

In the analyses that follow, we compare each ethnic group on the basis of (**i**) measures of child health, including anthropometric indicators for nutritional status, subjective health ratings and the self-reported incidence of specific illnesses. We also compare these groups on (**ii**) several important proximate determinants of child health, including food insecurity, diet, breastfeeding and vaccination coverage. We then (**iii**) further contrast households among the Maasai by the extent to which they rely on livestock herding as their primary livelihood. For the purposes of the present study, we do not conceptualize ethnicity as a causal determinant of child health, nor do we attempt to analytically isolate ethnic differences that are independent from socioeconomic or demographic variation. Our objective is simply to quantify disparities in child health on the basis of self-reported ethnicity (see below); disparities that may ultimately originate from a complex suite of interrelated determinants. We do however include a supplementary analysis of the contribution of a limited number of ecological factors (village rainfall, distance to district capital and presence/absence of health clinics/dispensaries) to village-level differences in child anthropometric indicators. The implications of our results for both policy makers and population health scientists are discussed.

Materials and Methods

The Whole Village Project

All data come from the WVP, a project run by SFTZ and the University of Minnesota, and in collaboration with the National Institute for Medical Research (NIMR), Muhimbili Medical Research Centre in Tanzania. The purpose of the WVP is to provide baseline data for evaluating rural development projects in the region, as well as a general source of information on Tanzanian villages. Overall, 56 villages were sampled, between mid 2009 and mid 2011, across the northern and central regions of Arusha (19 villages), Manyara (11 villages), Dodoma (7 villages), Singida (5 villages), Shinyanga (8 villages), Mwanza (3 villages), and Mara (3 villages). The sampling of villages was based in part on the priorities of development agency partners and the permission of government leaders, although effort was made to randomize village sampling where possible and to ensure a wide geographic spread. SFTZ and WVP have no agenda with regard to Maasai settlement or pastoralist rights, and village sampling was not influenced by the ethnicity or livelihood of residents. **Figure 1** shows the location of each village in relation to major settlements, main roads, national parks and game reserves.

The WVP collected quantitative and qualitative data at the level of village, household and child. This study primarily utilises quantitative data from the household and child level. Within each village between 60–75 households were randomly selected for participation from a list provided by village administrators, leading to a total of 3584 surveyed households. Household heads responded to questionnaire modules surveying their demographic, cultural and socioeconomic characteristics. Within each household, a child health module was administered collecting anthropometric and questionnaire data for all eligible children under the age of five years. More information on the WVP, including descriptive statistics on village characteristics by district, is available on the SFTZ website (sftz.org) or by request to the first author. All data utilized in this study are available from SFTZ to interested researchers upon request, and following approval from the SFTZ board of directors (see sftz.org).

Ethics Statement

Informed oral consent was obtained from participants and all individual data were anonymized before analysis. Consent was oral rather than written because this format is most appropriate in rural Tanzanian communities with limited literacy skills, and where many individuals harbour mistrust of written communication. Participant consent was recorded in separate documentation. The WVP, including consent procedures, received ethical approval from the University of Minnesota (Institutional Review Board code number: 0905S65241) and from the National Health Research Ethics Review Committee, at NIMR.

Ethnicity and Livelihoods

The study area is ethnically diverse, but four main ethnicities, the Maasai, Sukuma, Rangi and Meru, make up 60% of the households sampled and 65% of the households contributing child health data. Maasai (21% of households) were primarily sampled in the Arusha and Manyara regions. Sukuma (20% of households) were primarily sampled in the Mwanza and Shinyanga regions. Rangi (12% of households) were primarily sampled in the Dodoma region. Meru (8% of households) were primarily sampled in the Arusha region. Ethnicity was self-reported by the household head as a freeform response to the question "What is your tribe?" ("kabila" in Kiswahili). Most villages tended to be largely ethnically homogenous i.e. most households sampled stated the same tribal identity, particularly for villages in which the Maasai or Sukuma were most common (typically 85%+) and to a lesser extent for Meru and Rangi villages. However, many Maasai (12%) and Sukuma households (10%) were located in villages where they were not the majority ethnic group. Supporting information in **File S1** provides further details of the sampling by ethnicity, village, district and region. **File S2** and **File S3** provide supporting information on household and village-level data.

For the purpose of this study, livelihood categorization was based on self-reported primary livelihood strategy rather than a quantified behavioural measure. Around two-thirds of Maasai (68%) stated livestock herding as their "primary occupation", while a quarter stated farming, the most common occupation for all other ethnicities. A small percentage of households stated their occupation as business, most commonly in the Meru (11%). We make the assumption that stated occupation serves as an effective proxy for primary mode of subsistence. We note however that many households identifying their primary livelihood as "farming" also kept livestock (i.e. agro-pastoralists), and that with recent trends in pastoralist livelihood diversification, some Maasai may still identify themselves as livestock herders despite considerable reliance on farming or wage-labour. Indeed, around half of Maasai households who identified their primary occupation as livestock herding reported cultivating at least some land.

Child Health Data

Out of 3584 sampled households, 2268 (63%) contributed data on child health for children under five years of age, and just under half of those households provided data on more than one child (2 children: 35%; 3+ children: 10%), leading to a total of 3586 surveyed children. The mean age of sampling was 28.9 months, with roughly even sampling across the age range of zero to 60 months (**SI4**). An ANOVA showed a significant difference in mean ages of sampled children by ethnicity ($F(4,3581) = 3.09$, $p < 0.05$). The largest difference was very small in magnitude with Sukuma children sampled at a mean age of 27.8 months compared

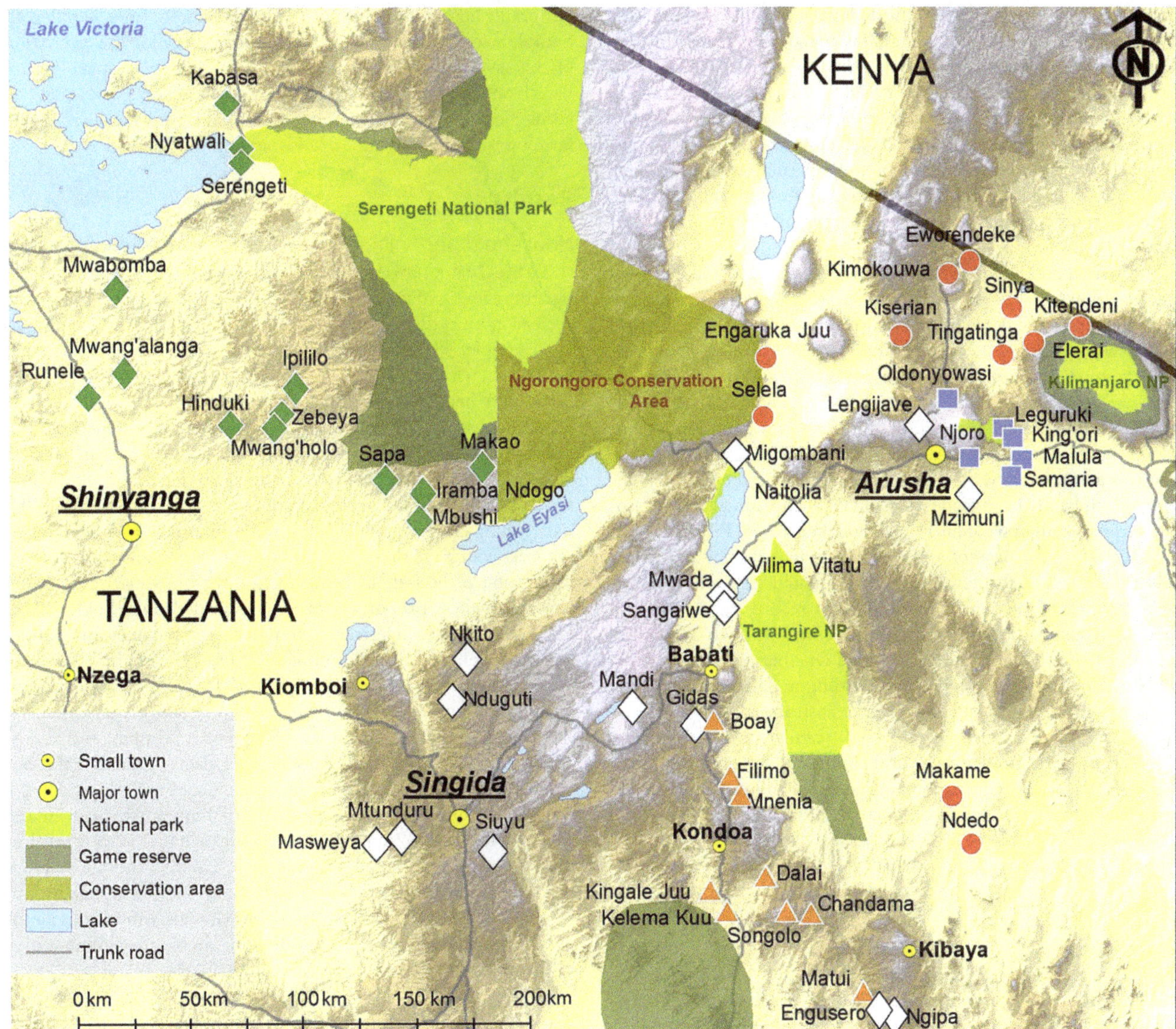

Figure1. Location of the 56 Study Villages Included in the Whole Village Project. Ethnicity is coded as the most common ethnicity in each village (**File S1** for details). Red circle = Maasai village; orange triangle = Rangi village; green diamond = Sukuma village; blue square = Meru village; white diamond = Other ethnicity village. Figure adapted from Aichele et al. [76] and initially published under an open-access license (CC-BY).

to the Rangi at 31.3 months. There was no statistically significant difference in the sampling of boys vs. girls (51% female) across ethnicities (chi-squared $(4,3586) = 0.50$, $p>0.05$).

Child weight was measured to the nearest 100 g using a Salter-type spring hanging scale for infants, and electronic scales for children able to stand. Child height was measured to the nearest millimetre using a measuring board for young children, and using a stadiometer for children of two years or older. All measurements were made once and immediately entered into a database. Children were measured by different field staff depending on the village sampled, but training of enumerators by UNICEF staff and oversight of anthropometric sessions by NIMR personnel ensured high levels of inter-rater reliability prior to data collection.

Three anthropometric indicators were derived using World Health Organisation (WHO) age and sex-specific growth standards [36] Height-for-age Z-scores (HAZ) serves as an indicator of long-term effects of malnutrition. A child with a HAZ of <-2 standard deviations from the WHO reference is considered "stunted" i.e. chronically malnourished, which reflects failure to receive adequate nutrition over a long period of time and is influenced by recurrent and chronic illness. Weight-for-height Z-scores (WHZ) measure body mass in relation to body height/length and describes current nutritional status. A child with a WHZ <-2 standard deviations is considered acutely malnourished (i.e. "wasted"), which represents the failure to achieve adequate nutrition in the period immediately preceding measurement and may result from inadequate food intake or illness. Weight-for-age Z-scores (WAZ) can be considered as a composite index, taking into account both chronic and acute malnutrition. Children with WAZ <-2 standard deviations are classified as "underweight". Following WHO guidelines (**File S4**), extreme values, potentially resulting from measurement error, were removed leading to 3411, 3426 and 3507 valid HAZ, WHZ and WAZ scores respectively.

In all villages, carers were asked to categorize the health of each child as either "good" or "frequently sick", and whether or not the child had *ever* suffered from the following illnesses/symptoms: fever, diarrhoea, pneumonia, cough/flu, malaria or worms. In 37/56 villages an additional question asked whether each illness/symptom had been experienced *in the last 3 months*. Recognizing the potential for recall bias when reporting childhood symptoms over a long period, particularly in older children, priority is given to the latter short-term version of this question in the present analysis. Locally recognisable terms for each illness/symptom were used following consultation with medical practitioners and NIMR staff.

Household and child-level surveys carried out in all villages also asked a number of questions relating to important proximate determinants of child health. First, the Household Food Insecurity Access Scale (HFIAS), was used to assess the extent to which households experienced problems assessing food during the last 30 days [37]. The HFIAS has previously been validated as a useful survey tool in rural Tanzania [38] and is described in more detail in the supplementary material (**File S2**). Second, food consumption was also measured by a diet survey recording the foods eaten by each child in the previous day divided into nine food group categories for analysis. The list of food items (see **File S4**) was constructed on the basis of a review of previous studies and prior field experience by the authors, and was piloted successfully as an inclusive dietary measure. Surveys did not record the amount of each food eaten, only whether or not some of each food was consumed. Third, enumerators recorded whether or not the carer stated the child was currently breastfeeding and/or eating solids, and whether the child had consumed colostrum in early infancy. Finally, survey respondents were asked whether or not the child had received recommended vaccinations (BCG (tuberculosis), Polio, DPT and Measles) and vitamin A supplementation. **File S4** provides further information on child-level data.

Data Analysis

To address ethnic variation in child health we use multilevel linear and logistic regression models for continuous and dichotomous dependent variables respectively, accounting for the clustering of child-level data (level 1, n = 3568) within villages (level 2, n = 56) using random intercepts. Comparisons on the HFIAS are made at the household (n = 2268) rather than child-level, with multilevel logistic regression predicting whether or not a household is categorized as "severely food insecure". Multilevel modelling is the appropriate statistical technique because failure to adjust estimates for non-independent sampling inflates the risk of Type 1 error. Furthermore, multilevel analysis quantifies unexplained variance at each hierarchical level, thus enabling us to assess the extent to which ethnicity accounts for variance in child health within and between villages. The average village provides data on 64 children from 41 households. In our child health analyses we do not include an intermediate hierarchical level for household because the mean number of children per household was only 1.58 and Clarke [39] has demonstrated that when clusters are unbalanced and sparsely populated (i.e. $\leq$2 cases per level) both fixed and random effects may be overestimated. All models were fit using maximum likelihood estimation in Stata version 13 using the "xtmixed" and "xtmelogit" commands [40]

For each outcome, we first contrast the four main ethnic groups, and then contrast households *among the Maasai* that self report as either farmers or livestock herders. All analyses adjust for effects of child age, child age-squared and child sex. We also adjust all analyses for the timing of village surveys in order to take into account whether or not the village was sampled in the hunger season (see **File S2**). Note that livelihood comparisons are derived from separate models with cases restricted to Maasai farming and pastoralist households only (715 Maasai children, from 21 villages). Sample size was also reduced for models estimating the estimation of child symptoms over the past 3 months. These comparisons are based on 2496 children from 37 villages when contrasting all ethnicities, and on 282 children from 8 villages when contrasting farming vs. pastoralist households among the Maasai.

Results

Household and village characteristics by ethnic group

Table 1 summarises household and village level characteristics by ethnicity, and by livelihood among the Maasai. Dramatic socioeconomic differences between ethnic groups are apparent. For example, 68% of Maasai male household heads had no formal education whatsoever; while among the Meru 84% of male household heads had completed at least primary education. A wealth index, based on non-livestock asset ownership (**File S2**) indicates the Maasai had on average the lowest material wealth, while the Meru are the wealthiest. With regard to household structure, Sukuma households were the largest, and contained the most young children, while Meru were the smallest and contained the least young children. Maasai households contained the highest proportion of household heads in a polygynous marriage (40%), and the highest proportion of female-headed households (39%). Polygyny was also relatively common in the Sukuma and Rangi, but almost entirely absent among the Meru. Christianity (Catholic or Protestant) was the stated religion of two-thirds of Maasai, and around one half of Sukuma, who otherwise stated they practiced "traditional" religions. Almost all Rangi were Muslim, and almost all Meru were Protestant. Village-level data (see also **File S3**) confirm that Maasai pastoralists were resident in the driest villages overall (625 mm per year), while Meru households lived in the wettest villages (982 mm per year). Meru households were less remote compared to all other ethnic groups, and most often resided in villages with a health dispensary or clinic, compared to all other ethnic groups. Two-thirds of Maasai farmer households lived in a village with a health clinic or dispensary compared to just over half of Maasai pastoralist households.

Are there ethnic differences in child health?

Tables 2–6 present unadjusted descriptive statistics for each dependent variable by ethnicity, and by livelihood among the Maasai, along with fixed effects coefficients from corresponding multivariate multilevel regression models, which are adjusted for village-level clustering (i.e. using random intercepts), along with fixed effects of child age, child age squared, child sex and season of data collection. **File S5** reports the fixed effects for all covariates in each model, along with random effects estimating the unexplained variance within and between villages before and after models have been adjusted for ethnicity.

There are striking ethnic differences in child nutritional status as indicated by anthropometric measurements (**Table 2**). Maasai children are at a considerable disadvantage, while Meru children are at a relative advantage. Nearly three times as many Maasai children are stunted (57%) compared to Meru children (21%), and almost double as many when compared to Sukuma children (32%). Rangi children had a level of stunting intermediate between the Sukuma and Maasai (44%). In terms of adjusted HAZ values, the contrast between Maasai and Meru children corresponds to almost a full standard deviation (B = 0.92, 95% Confidence Interval (CI) = 0.60–1.25, $p<0.001$). Wasting showed a similar pattern, with more than three times as many Maasai children recorded as wasted (10%) compared to any other ethnic group (2–3%). Adjusted WHZ scores show these differences correspond to

Table 1. Descriptive Statistics for Households Contributing Child Health Data by Ethnicity.

		MAASAI						
			Primary occupation					
		All	*Livestock*	*Farming*	**SUKUMA**	**RANGI**	**MERU**	**OTHER**
No. of villages where ethnic group is the majority (n = 56)		11	-	-	14	9	6	16
No. of households contributing child health data (n = 2268)		542	366	124	517	240	165	804
No. of children sampled (n = 3586)		788	523	192	1025	354	213	1206
Household-Level								
Primary occupation of household head	Livestock Herding (%)	68	100	-	<1	<1	3	5
	Farming (%)	23	-	100	92	95	73	82
	Business (%)	3	-	-	4	3	11	7
	Other (%)	6	-	-	4	2	13	6
Education level (male household heads only)	None (%)	68	70	61	27	19	4	21
	<Standard 7 (%)	6	5	8	18	18	11	14
	Standard 7+ (%)	26.4	25	31	55	64	84	65
Mean wealth index		1.8 *[1.5]*[a]	1.6 *[1.4]*	2.2 *[1.5]*	3.0 *[1.5]*	3.3 *[1.6]*	5.6 *[2.5]*	3.4 *[2.1]*
Mean household size		5.8 *[2.3]*	5.7 *[4.2]*	6.3 *[2.4]*	8.4 *[3.9]*	6.2 *[2.1]*	5.6 *[1.7]*	6.3 *[2.3]*
Mean no. of children per household		1.5 *[0.8]*	1.5 *[0.8]*	1.5 *[0.8]*	2.0 *[1.1]*	1.4 *[0.7]*	1.2 *[0.5]*	1.5 *[0.7]*
Household type	Polygynously Married Household Head (%)	40	44	34	26	16	2	16
	Female-Headed Household (%)	39	42	31	18	16	10	16
Religion	Protestant (%)	48	44	52	24	<1	98	44
	Catholic (%)	21	23	21	22	3	1	22
	Muslim (%)	<1	<1	<1	3	97	<1	22
	Traditional/Other (%)	30	32	27	52	<1	<1	12
Village-Level								
Mean Village Annual Rainfall (mm)		653 *[132]*	625 *[64]*	727 *[213]*	841 *[68]*	688 *[39]*	982 *[121]*	779 *[187]*
Mean Village Distance from district capital (km)		32.1 *[18.9]*	30.7 *[18.1]*	36.1 *[21.2]*	34.3 *[17.7]*	33.2 *[13.8]*	21.3 *[17.5]*	33.0 *[17.0]*
Village has own health dispensary/clinic? (% yes)		54	53	66	56	52	70	59

[a]Numbers in square brackets are standard deviations.

Table 2. Multilevel Linear Regressions Predicting Child Anthropometric Status.

		Height for Age Z Score (n = 3411)			Weight for Height Z Score (n = 3426)			Weight for Age Z Score (n = 3507)		
		Mean (SD)	% stunted	Adjusted B coefficient (95% CI)	Mean (SD)	% wasted	Adjusted B coefficient (95% CI)	Mean SD	% underweight	Adjusted B coefficient (95% CI)
Ethnicity	Maasai	−2.13 (1.78)	57	0.00	−0.20 (1.60)	10	0.00	−1.38 (1.48)	33	0.00
	Sukuma	−1.34 (1.41)	32	**0.59***** *(0.36–0.82)*	0.40 (1.20)	2	**0.44***** *(0.26–0.63)*	−0.47 (1.15)	7	**0.72***** *(0.55–0.89)*
	Rangi	−1.83 (1.34)	44	0.22 *(−0.05–0.49)*	−0.07 (1.12)	3	0.04 *(−0.18–0.27)*	−1.06 (1.07)	17	**0.27*** *(0.06–0.47)*
	Meru	−0.93 (1.37)	21	**0.92***** *(0.60–1.25)*	0.38 (1.36)	3	**0.43**** *(0.16–0.70)*	−0.26 (1.17)	5	**0.87***** *(0.62–1.12)*
	Other	−1.69 (1.56)	43	**0.32**** *(0.13–0.51)*	0.18 (1.26)	3	**0.26**** *(0.10–0.41)*	−0.80 (1.20)	13	**0.46***** *(0.31–0.60)*
Livelihood [a] (*Maasai only*)	Livestock	−2.21 (1.75)	59	0.00	−0.25 (1.62)	12	0.00	−1.44 (1.46)	35	0.00
	Farmer	−1.84 (1.84)	51	**0.39*** *(0.06–0.71)*	−0.02 (1.63)	6	0.20 *(−0.09–0.48)*	−1.12 (1.55)	27	**0.39**** *(0.13–0.65)*

Adjusted B coefficients are adjusted for child age, child sex, hunger season and a random intercept for village.
*p<0.05,
**p<0.01,
***p<0.001,
[a]Livelihood parameters are derived from separate models including only Maasai households.

around half a standard deviation when contrasting the Maasai to the Sukuma or Meru (B = 0.44, 95%CI = 0.26–0.63, p<0.001; and B = 0.43, 95%CI = 0.16–0.70, p<0.001 respectively), but the comparison did not reach statistical significance when contrasting the Maasai to the Rangi. WAZ similarly places Maasai children as having the worst, and Meru the best, nutritional status compared to other ethnic groups. Random effects indicate that 5–10% of variance in child anthropometric status is between rather than within villages, and that adding ethnicity into each model greatly reduces the amount of unexplained between-village variance (**File S5**). **Figure2** illustrates the substantial village and ethnic variation in anthropometric status, displaying the means of HAZ for each village coded by the most common resident ethnicity.

There are also ethnic differences in subjective health and self-reported incidence of symptoms/illnesses in the three months prior to the survey (**Table 3**). Overall 17% of children were described as frequently sick by their carers. Compared to the Maasai, Rangi children were not significantly different on this measure. However the odds of being described as frequently ill was 42% lower for the Sukuma (Odds Ratio (OR) = 0.58, 95%CI = 0.40–0.84, p<0.01), and 76% lower for the Meru (OR = 0.24, 95%CI = 0.12–0.48, p<0.001). Symptoms of diarrhoea and fever were significantly more common in the Maasai compared to the Meru. Maasai children were also more often reported to have recently had pneumonia, with 12% of Maasai children reported to have had pneumonia compared to only 3–4% in all other ethnicities.

Maasai children were not at a disadvantage for all forms of illness. Reported incidence of malaria was significantly more common among the Rangi compared to the Maasai. Furthermore, Meru children, who otherwise appear to be relatively advantaged on most measures, had considerably elevated odds of stating the child had suffered from a worm infection, with 17% of children reported to have had worms in the Meru compared to 5–7% for other ethnic groups. **File S5** also reports ethnic comparisons when carers were asked whether the child had *ever had* each symptom/illness. This analysis produces a similar picture. Notably the odds of having *ever had* malaria are substantially higher for both the Sukuma (OR = 1.58, 95%CI = 0.94–2.65, p<0.1) and Rangi (OR = 2.08, 95%CI = 1.15–3.37, p<0.05) compared to the Maasai. Unexplained between-village variance in child symptoms/illness ranged between 1% (cough/flu) to 14% (pneumonia) of total variance without ethnicity, but reduced substantially after adding ethnicity into each model (**File S5**).

Supplementary analyses confirm that rainfall is a strong correlate of village differences in child health (**File S5**). For example, a child living in a village in the wettest quartile for annual rainfall had both substantially higher HAZ (B = 0.40, 95%CI = 0.09–0.71, p<0.001) and WHZ scores (B = 0.41, 95%CI = 0.19–0.65, p<0.001). Including this effect in our multivariate analyses also reduces the magnitude of ethnic comparisons, particularly when comparing Maasai and Meru children, and particularly for WHZ scores (i.e. acute malnutrition), although most comparisons remain statistically significant. This attenuation suggests that rainfall at least part mediates the ethnic differences reported here. Presence of a health clinic/dispensary and distance from district capital however were not clearly associated with child health, at least with regard to anthropometric indicators (**File S5**).

Are there ethnic differences in the proximate determinants of child health?

Food insecurity was high across the study villages. Only 9% of households were categorized as "*food secure*", and 6% as

Table 3. Multilevel Logistic Regressions Predicting Subjective Health and Self-Reported Incidence of Specific Illnesses/Symptoms.

		Subjective Health (n = 3585)		*"Has the Child Had X in the Past Three Months?" (n = 2496)*											
		"Good" vs. "Frequently Sick"		Fever		Diarrhoea		Pneumonia		Cough/Flu		Malaria		Worms	
		% sick	Adjusted Odds Ratio (95% CI)	% yes	Adjusted Odds Ratio (95% CI)	% yes	Adjusted Odds Ratio (95% CI)	% yes	Adjusted Odds Ratio (95% CI)	% yes	Adjusted Odds Ratio (95% CI)	% yes	Adjusted Odds Ratio (95% CI)	% yes	Adjusted Odds Ratio (95% CI)
Ethnicity	Maasai	22	1.00	55	1.00	30	1.00	12	1.00	53	1.00	18	1.00	5	1.00
	Sukuma	13	**0.58**** *(0.40–0.84)*	58	1.12 *(0.82–1.52)*	32	1.00 *(0.67–1.50)*	4	0.48 *(0.18–1.28)*	58	1.32 *(0.94–1.87)*	24	1.26 *(0.79–2.03)*	6	1.37 *(0.62–3.01)*
	Rangi	19	0.90 *(0.58–1.38)*	46	0.70 *(0.48–1.03)*	27	0.93 *(0.56–1.52)*	3	**0.31*** *(0.10–0.96)*	63	1.40 *(0.92–2.11)*	33	**1.77*** *(1.03–3.07)*	6	1.05 *(0.41–2.71)*
	Meru	6	**0.24***** *(0.12–0.48)*	37	**0.48**** *(0.30–0.77)*	10	**0.28**** *(0.13–0.60)*	3	0.37 *(0.10–1.39)*	56	1.17 *(0.71–1.93)*	22	1.06 *(0.54–2.05)*	17	**3.27*** *(1.24–8.6)*
	Other	17	0.78 *(0.57–1.06)*	46	**0.70*** *(0.51–0.94)*	25	0.76 *(0.51–1.14)*	4	**0.43+** *(0.18–1.02)*	54	1.05 *(0.75–1.45)*	27	1.43 *(0.91–2.27)*	7	1.24 *(0.57–2.69)*
Livelihood [a] *(Maasai only)*	Livestock	23	1.00	52	1.00	33	1.00	12	1.00	52	1.00	16	1.00	2	1.00
	Farmer	18	0.71 *(0.44–1.15)*	63	**1.74*** *(1.04–2.91)*	24	0.63 *(0.36–1.12)*	11	1.00 *(0.45–2.23)*	59	1.20 *(1.45–3.21)*	20	1.51 *(0.78–2.89)*	9	**4.91*** *(1.41–17.04)*

Adjusted odds ratios are adjusted for child age, child sex, hunger season and a random intercept for village.+ $p<0.1$,
* $p<0.05$,
**$p<0.01$,
***$p<0.001$,
[a]Livelihood parameters are derived from separate models including only Maasai households.

Table 4. Multilevel Logistic Regression Predicting Household Food Insecurity (n = 2208).

		% Food Secure	% Mildly Food Insecure	% Moderately Food Insecure	% Severely Food Insecure	Adjusted Odds Ratio Predicting Severe Food Insecurity (95% CI)
Ethnicity	Maasai	4.7	2.1	15	78	1.00
	Sukuma	8	4.9	55	32	**0.18***** *(0.12–0.28)*
	Rangi	6	6	41	47	**0.32***** *(0.20–0.51)*
	Meru	12	12	53	24	**0.13***** *(0.07–0.24)*
	Other	11	7	46	36	**0.20***** *(0.14–0.29)*
Livelihood [a] (*Maasai only*)	Livestock	3.9	1.7	14	81	1.00
	Farmer	5	4.0	19	72	0.78 *(0.41–1.49)*

Adjusted odds ratios are adjusted for hunger season and a random intercept for village. See File SI2 for details on the Household Food Insecurity Access Scale.
***p<0.001,
[a]Livelihood parameters are derived from separate models including only Maasai households.

experiencing "*mild food insecurity*". The majority of households were either categorised as "*moderately food insecure*" (39%); meaning food quality was sacrificed frequently, by eating a monotonous diet or undesirable foods sometimes or often, and/or cutting back on quantity by reducing the size of meals or number of meals, rarely or sometimes; or "*severely food insecure*" (46%); meaning they cut back on meal size or number of meals often, and/or experienced any of the three most severe conditions (running out of food, going to bed hungry, or going a whole day and night without eating) at least once a month [37]. **Table 4** shows the percentage of households in each food insecurity category and the results of logistic regression analyses predicting the odds of being severely food insecure by ethnic group. Maasai were substantially more likely to be categorized as severely food insecure compared to any other ethnic group. At the most extreme comparison, four out of five of Maasai households were classified as "severely food insecure", compared to only one in four Meru households, representing a 87% reduction in the adjusted odds of severe food insecurity when comparing Meru to Maasai (OR = 0.13, 95%CI = 0.07–0.24, $p<0.001$). As anticipated food insecurity was significantly higher during hunger season months (OR = 1.41, 95%CI = 1.04–1.92, $p<0.05$, SI5).

There are large differences between ethnic groups in the specific food items consumed in the previous day. These differences are illustrated in **Figure3**, which plots ethnic differences in child diet, by food category and child age (see **File S5** and text below for adjusted odds ratios from multivariate analyses including all villages). Consumption of carbohydrate-rich staple foods, such as ugali, was substantially lower among the Maasai compared to all other ethnic groups, where such foods were eaten almost universally by all children between the ages of one and five years. At the largest comparison, the age-adjusted odds of consuming carbohydrate-rich foods was almost six times higher for the Meru compared to the Maasai (OR = 5.92, 95%CI = 2.69–13.05, $p<0.001$). Maasai children were also the least likely to have eaten beans, legumes or peanuts, and leafy green vegetables compared to other ethnic groups, but there was no significant difference in the odds of consuming tomatoes, carrots or other vegetables. Fruit consumption was significantly lower in the Maasai compared to all other ethnic groups, but particularly compared to the Meru, where around 30–40% of children ate fruit in the previous day, compared to around 5–10% of Maasai children (OR = 2.59, 95%CI = 1.25–4.69, $p<0.01$).

Meat consumption occurred at low frequency for Maasai, Rangi and Meru children (around 10%). However, the odds of meat consumption was significantly higher for the agro-pastoralist Sukuma (OR = 1.98, 95%CI = 1.09–3.59, $p<0.05$). Fish consumption was also low for most ethnic groups, but particularly low for Maasai children (2% ate fish on the previous day), and considerably more common in the Sukuma (53% ate fish on the previous day). This difference is likely attributable to the proximity of many Sukuma villages to Lake Victoria (**Figure1**), with ethnic differences attenuated in adjusted analyses including a random intercept for village (**File S5**). Egg consumption was low for all ethnic groups, with borderline significantly lower consumption for Maasai compared to Sukuma and Meru children. Cow's milk was the only food category consumed significantly more often in the Maasai, and was consumed by around 90% of the children in previous day during non-hunger season months, compared to around 30–70% among other ethnic groups (**Figure3**). At the largest comparison, the odds of milk consumption was 77% lower in the Sukuma compared to the Maasai (OR = 0.23, 95% 0.15–0.35, $p<0.001$).

Breastfeeding behaviour varied by ethnic group (**Table 5**). In all ethnicities, over 90% of children were reported to have been fed colostrum in early infancy, although this was significantly less common among the Sukuma (91% vs. 96% or more for all other ethnic groups). Most notably Maasai children were more likely to be currently breastfeeding compared to children of any other ethnicity, even adjusting for child age. This implies a relatively late age at weaning (see **Figure4**, which plots the percentage of children currently breastfeeding by age and ethnic group). There was also an indication that Maasai and Meru children under the age of one were less likely to be currently eating solids; suggestive of relatively low levels of complementary feeding (**Figure4**). However this difference was not significant in multivariate models (**Table 5**). Unexplained village-level variance in food insecurity, child diet and breastfeeding analyses ranged between 15–49% without ethnicity, but reduced substantially in most cases after adding ethnicity into each model (**File S5**)

Vaccination coverage was high for all ethnicities, with over 90% of all children reporting to have had recommended vaccinations for BCG, Polio and DPT (**Table 6**). However, Maasai children

Table 5. Multilevel Logistic Regressions Predicting Breastfeeding Behaviour.

		Baby Had Colostrum		Currently Breastfeeding		Currently Eating Solids	
		(n = 3530)		(n = 3195)		(n = 3586)	
		% yes	Adjusted Odds Ratio	% yes	Adjusted Odds Ratio	% yes	Adjusted Odds Ratio
			(95% CI)		(95% CI)		(95% CI)
Ethnicity	Maasai	98	1.00	44	1.00	85	1.00
	Sukuma	91	**0.22***** *(0.10–0.48)*	30	**0.15***** *(0.09–0.25)*	90	1.76 *(0.81–3.85)*
	Rangi	96	0.73 *(0.27–1.99)*	29	**0.27***** *(0.14–0.51)*	95	2.07 *(0.78–5.47)*
	Meru	99	2.53 *(0.49–13.11)*	31	**0.41*** *(0.20–0.84)*	84	0.77 *(0.26–2.25)*
	Other	97	0.58 *(0.28–1.22)*	32	**0.27***** *(0.18–0.41)*	88	1.45 *(0.78–2.69)*
Livelihood [a]	Livestock	99	1.00	45	1.00	84	1.00
(Maasai only)	Farmer	97	0.50 *(0.14–1.70)*	37	0.77 *(0.46–1.30)*	85	1.43 *(0.70–2.92)*

Adjusted odds ratios are adjusted for child age, child sex, hunger season and a random intercept for village.
*p<0.05,
**p<0.01,
***p<0.001,
[a]Livelihood parameters are derived from separate models including only Maasai households.

Table 6. Multilevel Logistic Regressions Predicting Vaccination Coverage and Vitamin A Supplementation.

		BCG Vaccination (n = 3586)		Polio Vaccination (n = 3586)		DPT Vaccination (n = 3586)		Measles Vaccination (n = 3586)		Vitamin A Supplementation (n = 3586)	
		%	Adjusted Odds	%	Adjusted Odds Ratio	%	Adjusted Odds Ratio	%	Adjusted	%	Adjusted Odds Ratio
		yes	Ratio	yes		yes		yes	Odds Ratio	yes	
Ethnicity	Maasai	95	1.00	95	1.00	93	1.00	76	1.00	77	1.00
	Sukuma	94	1.38 *(0.64–2.99)*	94	1.49 *(0.73–3.03)*	92	1.34 *(0.70–2.62)*	67	0.84 *(0.50–1.40)*	60	0.75 *(0.44–1.25)*
	Rangi	97	1.94 *(0.68–5.54)*	97	2.54 *(0.94–6.89)*	96	**2.56*** *(1.03–6.35)*	82	**2.02*** *(1.08–3.80)*	76	1.03 *(0.58–1.83)*
	Meru	98	2.01 *(0.49–8.27)*	99	**4.50*** *(1.07–18.81)*	96	1.93 *(0.69–5.32)*	86	**2.66*** *(1.22–5.83)*	89	**2.43*** *(1.15–5.13)*
	Other	95	1.25 *(0.66–2.37)*	96	1.43 *(0.79–2.59)*	95	1.49 *(0.87–2.56)*	78	**1.58*** *(1.03–2.41)*	76	1.26 *(0.84–1.90)*
Livelihood [a] *(Maasai only)*	Livestock	96	1.00	95	1.00	94	1.00	77	1.00	78	1.00
	Farmer	92	*0.50 (0.22–1.15)*	94	0.85 *(0.39–1.86)*	92	0.76 *(0.36–1.62)*	76	1.17 *(0.66–2.07)*	76	1.24 *(0.68–2.26)*

Adjusted odds ratios are adjusted for child age, child sex, hunger season and a random intercept for village.
*p<0.05,
[a]Livelihood parameters are derived from separate models including only Maasai households.

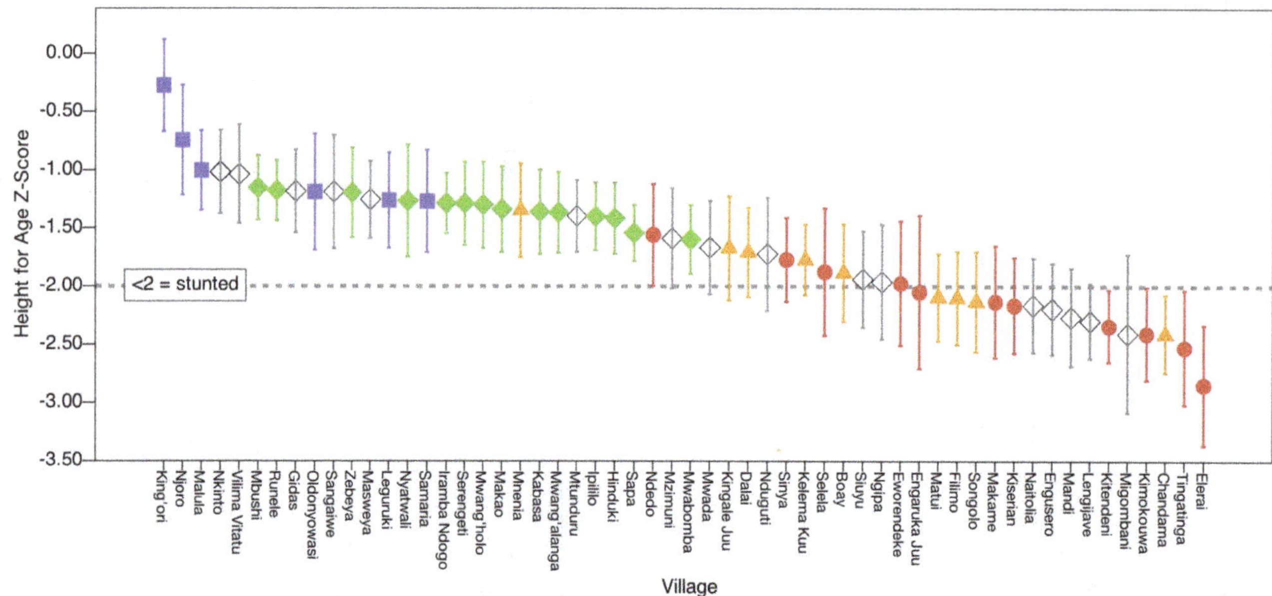

Figure2. Mean Height for Age Z-Score (HAZ) by Village and Ethnicity. Village means arranged in descending order, with 95% confidence intervals. Ethnicity is coded as the most common ethnicity in each village (see **File S1** for details). Children in Maasai majority villages tend to have relatively low HAZ scores and children in Meru majority villages tend to have relatively high HAZ scores, with Sukuma and Rangi majority villages intermediate between these extremes. Red circle = Maasai village; orange triangle = Rangi village; green diamond = Sukuma village; blue square = Meru village; white diamond = Other ethnicity village. HAZ scores falling below <2 are categorized as "stunted" by the World Health Organization.

were less likely to have received a measles vaccination compared to the Rangi, Meru and "Other Ethnicity" categories. In addition the Meru were more likely to have reported their children had received a Polio vaccination than the Maasai, and the Rangi were more likely to report children had received a DPT vaccination than the Maasai. Reported levels of Vitamin A supplementation varied between 60% among the Sukuma to 89% among the Meru. Vitamin A supplementation was significantly more common in the Meru than in the Maasai (**Table 6**). Between 10–20% of unexplained variance in vaccination and vitamin supplementation was between villages, but this was not notably reduced by the inclusion of ethnicity into each model.

How do Maasai households that rely on livestock herding compare to those that rely on farming?

We examined associations between primary occupation and child health outcomes among the Maasai adjusting for the same set of covariates, and found that Maasai pastoralists appear to be at a relative disadvantage when compared to Maasai farmers (see the "livelihood" row in Tables 2–6). With regard to anthropometric measurements, adjusted estimates place farmers as 0.39 Z-scores in height-for-age (B = 0.39, 95%CI = 0.06–0.71, $p<0.05$), and 0.39 Z-scores in terms of weight for age (B = 0.39, 95%CI = 0.13–0.65, $p<0.05$) above pastoralists. For the most part, reported occurrence of specific illnesses/symptoms did not differ between Maasai farmers and pastoralists. However, Maasai farmers more commonly stated that their children had worms in the past 3 months compared to Maasai pastoralists (OR = 4.91, 95CI% = 1.41–17.04).

Pastoralists were more often categorized as severely food insecure (81%) compared to farmers (72%), however this difference was not statistically significant in adjusted analyses. Dietary analyses confirm a number of differences between Maasai farmer and pastoralist food intake (**Figure5**; see also **FileS5** for adjusted odds ratios). The children of Maasai farmers had a significantly higher odds of eating leafy greens (OR = 3.11, 95%CI = 1.72–5.61, $p<0.001$) and fruit (OR = 2.95, 95%CI = 1.44–6.02, $p<0.001$), and were borderline significantly more likely to have recently eaten carbohydrate-rich staple foods (OR = 1.76, 95%CI = 0.99–1.42, $p<0.01$), tomatoes, carrots or other vegetables (OR = 1.82, 95%CI = 0.97–3.40, $p<0.1$) and eggs (OR = 2.40, 95%CI = 0.95–6.07, $p<0.1$). There was no significant difference in the recent consumption of milk, meat or fish between farmers and pastoralists. Multilevel regression models also estimated no overall significant difference in the consumption of beans, legumes and peanuts. However analysing these data by child age indicates more common intake of these foods among the children of farmers above the age of three years (**Figure5**). Breastfeeding behaviour and vaccination coverage did not differ between the children of Maasai pastoralists and those of Maasai farmers.

Discussion

Ethnic Differences in Child Health in Northern Tanzania

We demonstrate the existence of strong ethnic differences in child health. Maasai children are substantially disadvantaged compared to neighbouring ethnic groups and this disadvantage is concentrated in the majority of Maasai who record livestock herding as their primary livelihood. Many authors have emphasised the numerous difficulties faced by the Maasai, and by pastoralist populations more generally, [9–13], leading us to the strong expectation that the health of Maasai children would be relatively poor. However, this is the first study to quantitatively contrast child health and its proximate determinants between the Maasai and neighbouring ethnic groups using large sample data. Differences in chronic malnutrition are particularly striking. The most recent Tanzanian DHS (2010) states that 45% of children resident in rural areas are stunted [41], while we place 59% of

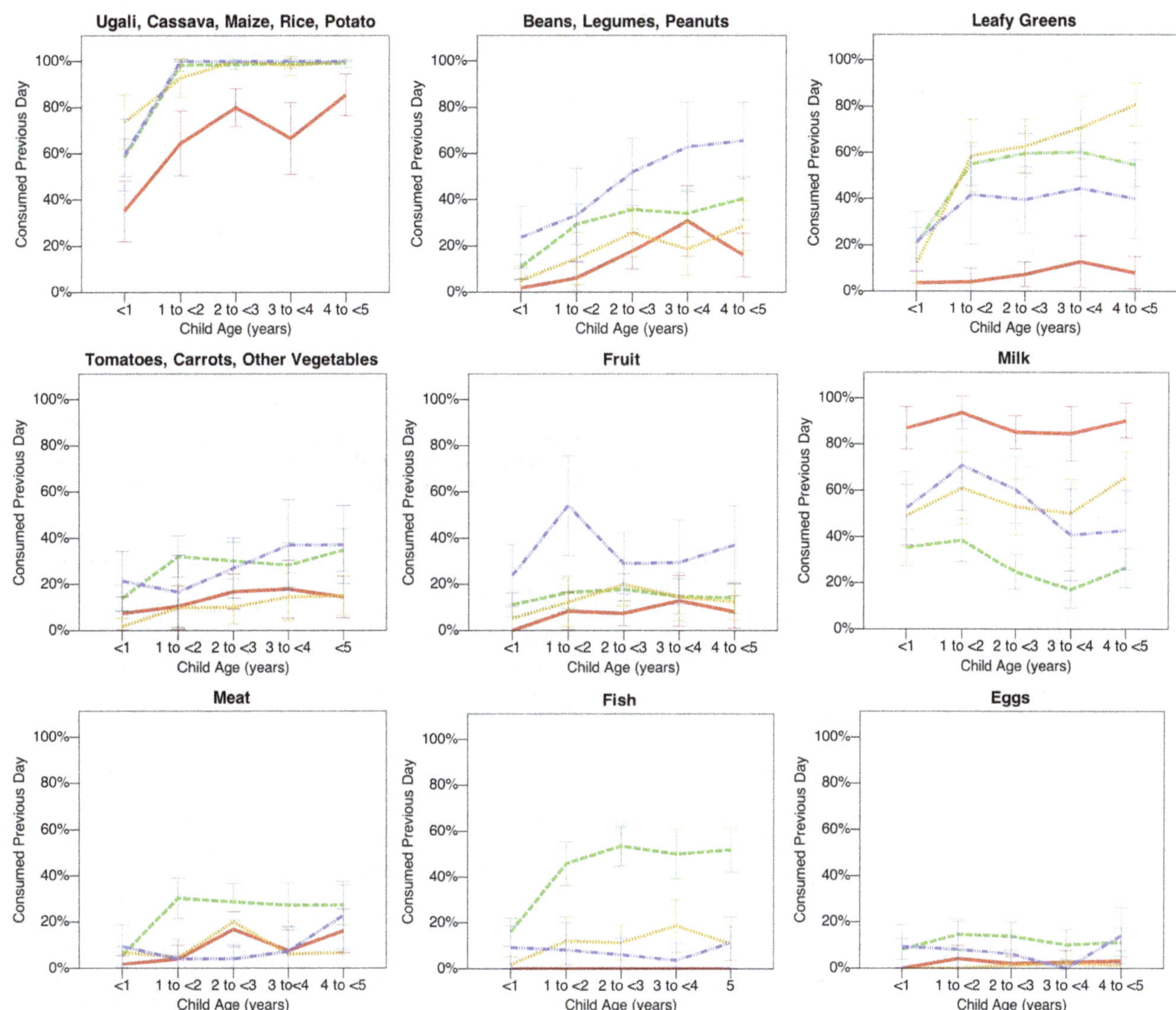

Figure3. Child Diet by Age and Ethnicity. Dietary analyses reveal substantial ethnic variation in reported child diet. Red solid line = Maasai children; orange dotted line = Rangi children; green dashed line = Sukuma children; blue dotted and dashed line = Meru children. Data plotted only for the 31 villages sampled outside of the hunger season (n = 1903 children), to avoid confounding between ethnicity and season of sampling. 95% confidence intervals calculated using normal approximation. See **File S5** for multilevel logistic regression models predicting food consumption for all children and villages adjusted for child age, child sex, hunger season and a random effect for village.

Maasai pastoralist children, but only 21% of Meru children, in the same category. Self-report data further suggest that the Maasai are at an elevated risk of certain illnesses/symptoms, including pneumonia, which is closely linked to poverty and malnutrition [1], but also fever and diarrhoea. Food insecurity, a well-substantiated cause of poor child health in low-income settings [42], presents a strong candidate proximate determinant behind these differences. Maasai were considerably more likely to be categorised as severely food insecure compared to all other ethnic groups (78% vs. 24–47% respectively). Maasai children also had a lower intake of carbohydrate-rich staple foods, nutritious leafy green vegetables and fruit, and important non-milk sources of protein (beans, legumes and peanuts, fish, eggs). As has been reported for other pastoralist populations in Tanzania [27], the Maasai also had lower vaccination coverage, consistent with relatively low engagement with/availability of health services.

Maasai children are unmistakeably at an overall disadvantage, but by considering a broader range of health measures beyond anthropometric status, our study also indicates that they experience a reduced vulnerability to at least some pathogens. Maasai children had a lower self-reported incidence of malaria than the Sukuma and Rangi. In addition, Maasai households reported the lowest incidence of worm infections, which was markedly more common in otherwise relatively advantaged Meru children. Maasai farmers also reported more worm infections compared to pastoralist households. Previous studies of pastoralist populations have recorded similar patterns; with both Kenyan Turkana and Malian Tuareg reported to have lower levels of intestinal parasites compared to agriculturalists, see [43,44] cited in [45]: p505. One potential explanation is that the low rainfall environment of the Maasai, particularly in pastoralist villages, reduces opportunities for pathogen transmission. Corbett et al. [46], p.208, for example, suggest that the relative lack of standing

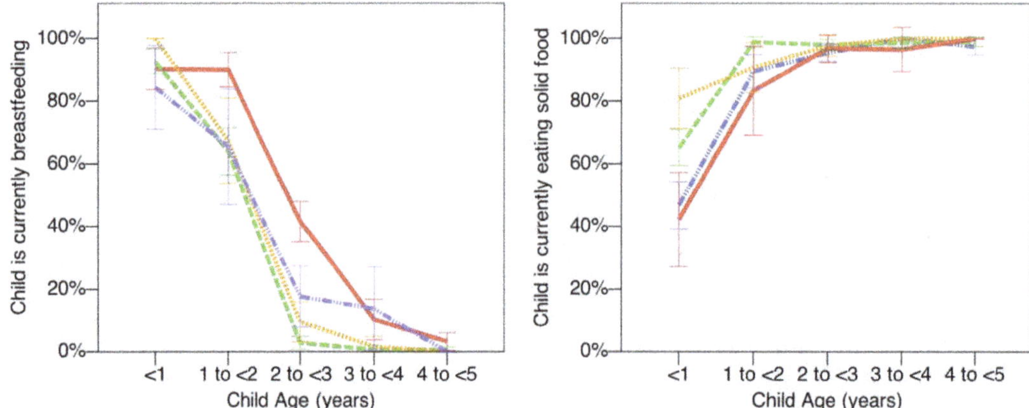

Figure4. Breastfeeding Behaviour by Child Age and Ethnicity. Current patterns indicate relatively delayed weaning in the Maasai compared to other ethnic groups. Red solid line = Maasai children; Orange dotted line = Rangi children; green dashed line = Sukuma children; blue dotted and dashed line = Meru children. Data plotted for all 56 villages. 95% confidence intervals calculated using normal approximation.

water in semi-arid areas occupied by Turkana pastoralists lowers mosquito frequency and consequently malaria exposure compared to neighbouring wetter areas inhabited by farmers.

Maasai children were also more likely to have recently consumed milk than other ethnic groups, consistent with previous research reporting high milk consumption for pastoralists, e.g. [33,44,47]. A considerable body of research has emphasised the benefits of milk consumption for child health and growth [48–51], and milk consumption has been proposed to account for the relatively tall adult height of east African pastoralist populations, including the Maasai (e.g. [52,53]). Our study suggests that, at least with regard to early childhood health and growth, potential benefits of higher milk consumption do not offset the challenges of severe food insecurity and a greater burden of illness faced by the Maasai. Milk consumption may however be an important contributing factor to continued growth into and during adolescence; the period of growth responsible for the relatively tall attained adult height for African pastoralists like the Maasai and Turkana [53,54]. In this context, we caution that population-level comparisons in adult height should not be interpreted as evidence of health disparities. Indeed, adult height is positively correlated with child mortality when comparing African nations [55], a trend that may be partly accounted for by mortality selection, i.e. early death of those children that would otherwise have grown up to be short adults [55], and the evolved adaptation of later growth patterns to related features of the ecology [56].

It is also interesting that, despite the apparent availability of cow's milk, breastfeeding was relatively prolonged in the Maasai compared to neighbouring ethnic groups. This finding is consistent with Sellen and Smay [57] who conclude that weaning food availability is poorly predictive of weaning age, at least when making population-level comparisons. Wander and Mattison [58] also report that cattle-holding households did not wean children earlier than households without cattle in the Chagga ethnic group in the Kilimanjaro region.

A comparison of household characteristics (**Table 1**) and a review of the relevant literature suggest that a combination of factors may be ultimately responsible for marked ethnic differences in child health we observe. Unsurprisingly, socioeconomic variation runs parallel to differences in child health and food insecurity, with Maasai households being relatively poor and undereducated. Furthermore as anticipated, sampled Maasai households were resident in villages with lower annual rainfall, which makes both productive pastoralism and farming more difficult. In contrast, the Meru, who generally had the best child health outcomes, occupy the relatively high rainfall, fertile slopes of mount Meru in close proximity to Arusha city, benefiting from increased health care and education infrastructure, along with opportunities for beneficial forms of livelihood diversification. Supplementary analyses (**File S5**) confirm that annual rainfall is a strong correlate of village-level differences in child health, and contributes to the ethnic differences documented here. Interestingly, however, distance to district capital and presence of a health clinic/dispensary were not predictive of child health, at least with regard to anthropometric indicators. Yet, we caution these measures may be only weakly informative of the quality of services provided. Indeed, many rural health clinics are poorly stocked and understaffed. Previous research has also emphasized the Maasai suffer from relatively ineffective interaction with health services, even when health services are available, due to language differences, distrust and potentially culturally inappropriate services [7,12].

The objective of the present study is to provide a systematic comparison of ethnic differences in child health across a broad range of measures. Further analysis, guided by the patterns established here, would be instructive in quantifying the relative contribution of alternative explanatory factors to the ethnic differences observed, unpicking the causal chain from distal to more proximate health determinants. Such analyses should include a consideration of notable ethnic differences in household structure (**Table 1**), including a particularly high frequency of female-headed and polygynous households among the Maasai [59,60], but see [61]. Differences in ratio of dependent children to productive adults may also be important [62]. Furthermore, as has been emphasised in prior literature [28,63] ethnic differences in child health may be partly attributable to cultural norms more or less independently of ecological, socioeconomic or demographic pathways. For example, the Maasai are notable for practicing dietary restrictions during pregnancy [64], which could have negative consequences for children.

Limitations

Household sampling was random within villages, but villages were not randomly sampled from the districts and regions of northern Tanzania included in the study site (see *Methods*). With the absence of alternative forms of representative data, we caution

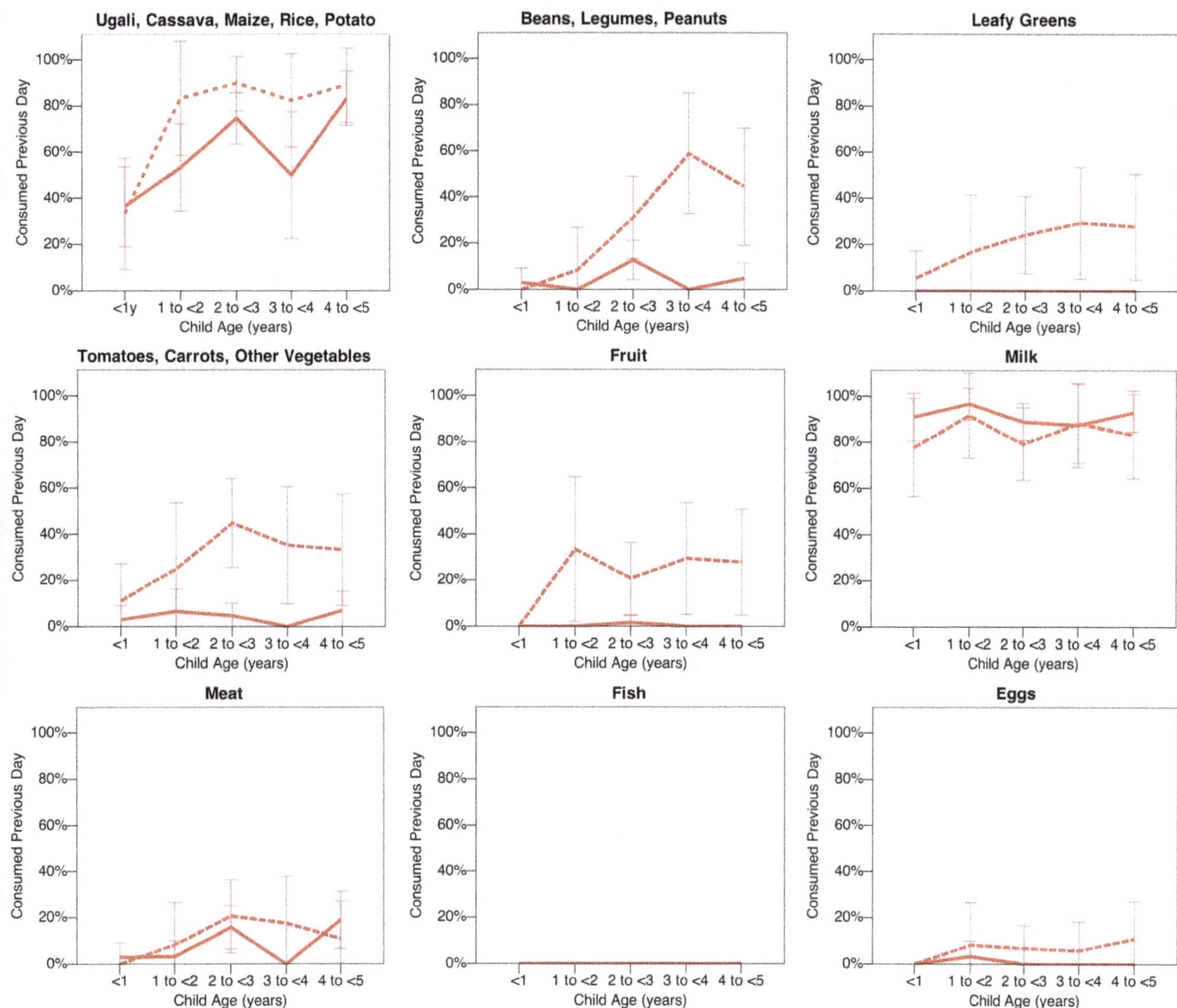

Figure5. Child Diet by Age for Pastoralist and Farming Maasai Households. Maasai child diets differ depending on livelihood. Red solid line = Maasai pastoralist children; red dashed line = Maasai farming children. Data plotted only for the 7 villages containing Maasai households sampled outside of the hunger season (n = 298 children). 95% confidence intervals calculated using normal approximation. See **File S5** for multilevel logistic regression models predicting food consumption for all Maasai children adjusted for child age, child sex, hunger season and a random effect for village.

against extrapolating observed patterns outside their context of measurement. Nonetheless, given the large geographic spread of villages, and large sample sizes achieved, we believe our findings broadly approximate wider trends, and we are certainly not aware of any comparable datasets of this size enabling ethnic comparisons. All analyses adjust for hunger season and include random-effects for village in attempt to control for potential confounding effects of temporal variation in child health across the two-year study period. Such controls are unavoidably imperfect and so we acknowledge that variation in the timing of household surveys represents a limitation of our analyses. It is also possible that we overestimate the disadvantages of the Maasai that might be observed in a more typical year because our surveys were conducted during and immediately following the 2009 drought, which is believed to have been particularly devastating for Maasai pastoralists [18]. However, droughts are a periodic occurrence, and some of the largest ethnic differences we observe are in height-for-age, a measure reflecting chronic nutritional stress, suggesting our conclusions reflect longer-term trends of Maasai disadvantage.

We recognize that several health measures, including measures of disease incidence, vaccination and diet, rely on self-report, and as such may be subject to recall issues and other forms of respondent bias e.g. familiarity and conceptual recognition of health conditions. For example, there may be much ambiguity in the parental categorisation of child respiratory illness as cough/flu vs. pneumonia (although our analysis indicates these outcomes have a distinct distribution). In the absence of comparable large-sample data from other sources, we believe our use of self-report data is justified for the purpose of this study; establishing important sources of ethnic variation, which through directed further study may inform future interventions aiming to improve child health and reduce inequality. More detailed comparative analysis of ethnic variation in diet, going beyond the crude food group categories and recall method used here, would also be valuable.

This would, for example, enable a fuller consideration of the impact of animal sourced foods and milk consumption [51,65], and the role of "indigenous knowledge" regarding food preparation and use, as emphasized by Oiye et al. [66] in a detailed dietary study of a Kenyan Maasai community.

Implications and Conclusion

Our conclusions echo wider international findings that marginalised ethnic groups that rely on alternative modes of production to agriculture are disadvantaged in terms of health outcomes and access to health services [6–8]. There are a large number of organisations that seek to improve the situation of the Maasai [67]. Our results reinforce support for these initiatives, particularly those combating issues of food insecurity and child nutrition, along with a greater emphasis on the specific needs of pastoralists in Tanzanian health policy [12]. We also emphasize that the situation of the Maasai is perhaps particularly troubling given on-going "land grabbing" conflicts (reviewed in [19]), and the widespread commodification of their culture for profit, both inside and outside of Tanzania. Studies of the impact of cultural tourism attractions, such as so-called "cultural bomas", where Maasai pose for photographs, sing, dance and sell handmade products to tourists in an artificial settlement, indicate a complex mix of benefits and costs to local communities [16,17,68]. Moreover, it has been estimated that many foreign companies made multi-million dollar profits in the last decade from Maasai-themed products, ranging from clothing and bed covers, to car accessories and stationary, capitalising on the exotic image of the Maasai to a western audience [69]. In recognition that these profits rarely find their way to the Maasai people, efforts are being made to enforce intellectual property rights, including the recent formation of a Maasai Intellectual Property Initiative (maasaiip.org).

Our results caution against a simple narrative that numerical minority status alone necessitates disparities in health. The Maasai are one of many ethnic groups in Tanzania that make up only a very small fraction of its total population, and, in the area covered by SFTZ, outnumber the Meru who had the best child health outcomes in this study. Likewise, the Sukuma, by far the most common ethnic group in Tanzania, were not the most advantaged. Indeed the Maasai can only be viewed a marginalised "minority" when we consider broader distinctions of ecology, livelihood, and wider ethnic and cultural distinctions in Tanzania (e.g. Nilotic vs. Bantu). Furthermore the usage of the term "indigenous" in Africa, and its specific and popular application to the Maasai, is not without controversy [70,71] Maasai-focused organisations have been instrumental in their use of the indigenous label [67], but they cannot be considered "first peoples" in the region, having migrated into Kenya and Tanzania only in last several hundred years, nor are they the only non-agriculturalists in Tanzania. Indeed there exist many other ethnic groups in Tanzania who antedate the Maasai, and/or share similar issues of cultural and economic marginalisation, but are rarely included in the indigenous rights movement [70,71]. Whatever the case, irrespective of both minority and indigeneity, contrasting welfare indicators between ethnic groups is an important endeavour because it identifies vulnerable communities in need and, through directed further analysis, can improve our understanding of the structural and cultural factors underlying health inequality amendable to change, e.g. [5,28].

Much has been written about the health consequences pastoralists face when transitioning to agriculture and/or permanent settlement. Previous research has largely relied on small opportunistic samples and produced conflicting conclusions [43,46,72–74], most likely reflecting differences among sites in agricultural productivity, compatibility with continued pastoralist production and exposure to diseases in more permanent homesteads, and the varying existence of economic alternatives contingent on settlement. In this study, we found that Maasai who identify as farmers experience lower food insecurity (although this difference was not statistically significant), and report their children have less restricted diets (e.g. higher reported consumption of carbohydrate-rich food, fruit and certain vegetables) and better nutritional status as indicated by anthropometric measures. It is tempting to see this as evidence of positive effects of farming on child health, with the implication farming should be encouraged. However, such an interpretation cannot be inferred from the current analysis. Farming households were also resident in higher rainfall villages, and were more often resident in villages with a health clinic or dispensary (**Table 1**). These differences highlight that cultivation is unlikely to be ecologically or economically feasible in all contexts, and that service provision may also vary with livelihood shifts. Consequently cross-sectional analyses may be vulnerable to false comparisons. Previous research has also emphasized that wealthy pastoralists diversify as a risk avoidance strategy, while poorer households may do so out of necessity [73], and our study can not distinguish between these alternatives. Clearly, longitudinal studies are needed to better understand the health consequences of subsistence transitions.

We conclude by emphasizing the value of disaggregated data by ethnicity and livelihood in the measurement of population health. Given the lack of ethnicity data in recent national surveys in Tanzania, there has been unsurprisingly little discussion of the role of ethnicity in structuring inequalities in health and progress towards development targets (e.g. [2,75]). Previous research has also specifically lamented the lack of data available for monitoring the health of Tanzania's pastoralists and their contribution to social and economic disparities within the nation [12]. Without such data, important dimensions of inequality are likely to go underestimated and unaddressed [7]. Furthermore, as we demonstrate, ethnicity and livelihood type are related not only to child health, but also a range of other ecological, socioeconomic, demographic and cultural variables. We also demonstrate high levels of clustering in child health outcomes and determinants at the village-level. Naïve analysts of aggregate data may therefore easily confound such parameters and draw erroneous conclusions regarding health determinants. We encourage future DHS in Tanzania to reincorporate the collection and dissemination of ethnicity data, and, where such data remain absent, we urge analysts to be vigilant of the limitations to ignoring ethnic and spatial variation (see also [61]). Finally, we hope that this study contributes to an increased recognition of the disadvantages currently experienced by the Maasai, and the support and development of initiatives targeting their specific needs.

Supporting Information

File S1 Ethnicity and Sampling by Village, District and Region.

File S2 Supporting Information on Household-Level Data.

File S3 Supporting Information on Village-Level Data.

File S4 Supporting Information on Child-Level Data.

Acknowledgments

We thank the village residents for taking part in this study, Craig Packer and Deborah Levison (University of Minnesota) for their contributions to the success of the WVP, and also the WVP field team leaders: Majory Kaziya, Fenella Rabison Msangi, Jovit Felix, and Edward Sandet. We thank Andrew Ferdinands and Asma Mohseni for the contribution of village location and rainfall data, and Jonathan Salerno, Cristina Moya, Rebecca Sear, Andrea Wiley, Alyson Young, Jed Stevenson and an anonymous reviewer for insightful comments and constructive critique on the manuscript.

Author Contributions

Analyzed the data: DWL. Contributed reagents/materials/analysis tools: MBM MEG EN BN SGMM KH SJ. Wrote the paper: DWL MBM.

References

1. Mulholland EK, Smith L, Carneiro I, Becher H, Lehmann D (2008) Equity and child-survival strategies. Bull World Health Organ 86: 399–407.
2. Ruhago GM, Ngalesoni FN, Norheim OF (2012) Addressing inequity to achieve the maternal and child health millennium development goals: looking beyond averages. BMC Public Health 12: 1119.
3. Wirth ME, Balk D, Delamonica E, Storeygard A, Sacks E, et al. (2006) Setting the stage for equity-sensitive monitoring of the maternal and child health Millennium Development Goals. Bull World Health Organ 84: 519–27.
4. Moradi A, Baten J (2005) Inequality in Sub-Saharan Africa: New Data and New Insights from Anthropometric Estimates. World Development 33: 1233–1265.
5. Brockerhoff M, Hewett P (2000) Inequality of child mortality among ethnic groups in sub-Saharan Africa. Bull World Health Organ 78: 30–41.
6. Crawhall N (2006) MDGs, Globalisation and Indigenous Peoples in Africa. Indigenous Affairs 1: 6–13.
7. Walker B (2013) State of the World's Minorities and Indigenous Peoples 2013. London: Minority Rights Group International.
8. Ohenjo N, Willis R, Jackson D, Nettleton C, Good K, et al. (2006) Health of Indigenous people in Africa. The Lancet 367: 1937–1946.
9. Catley A, Lind J, Scoones I (2013) Pastoralism and Development in Africa: Dynamic Change at the Margins. New York: Routledge.
10. Hampshire K (2002) Networks of nomads: negotiating access to health resources among pastoralist women in Chad. Soc Sci Med 54: 1025–1037.
11. Sellen DW (1996) Nutritional status of African pastoralists: a review of the literature. Nomad People 39: 107–134.
12. Sika NK, Hodgson DL (2006) In the shadow of the MDGs: pastoralist women and children in Tanzania. Indigenous Affairs 1: 30–37.
13. Zinsstag J, Ould Taleb M, Craig PS (2006) Health of nomadic pastoralists: new approaches towards equity effectiveness. Trop Med Int Health 11: 565–8.
14. Homewood K, Kristjanson P, Trench P (2010) Staying Maasai: Livelihoods, Conservation and Development in East African Rangelands. New York: Springer.
15. Spear T, Waller R (1993) Being Maasai: ethnicity and identity in East Africa. James Currey.
16. Buzinde CN, Kalavar JM, Melubo K (2013) Tourism and community well-being: The case of the Maasai in Tanzania. Annals of Tourism Research 44: 20–35
17. Kalavar JM, Buzinde CN, Melubo K, Simon J (2014) Intergenerational Differences in Perceptions of Heritage Tourism Among the Maasai of Tanzania. J Cross Cult Gerontol 29: 53–67.
18. Goldman MJ, Riosmena F (2013) Adaptive capacity in Tanzanian Maasailand: Changing strategies to cope with drought in fragmented landscapes. Glob Environ Change 23: 588–597.
19. Galaty JG (2013) Land grabbing in the east African rangelands. In Catley A, Lind J, Scooness I, editors. Pastoralism and Development in Africa: Dynamic Change at the Margins. New York: Routledge. pp. 131–142.
20. Ngoitiko M, Sinandei M, Meitaya P, Nelson F (2010) Pastoral Activists: Negotiating Power Imbalances in the Tanzanian Serengeti. In Nelson F, editor. Community rights, conservation and contested land: the politics of natural resource governance in Africa. London: Earthscan. pp. 269–289
21. Fearon JD (2003) Ethnic and Cultural Diversity by Country. Economic Growth 8: 195–222.
22. Campbell J (1999) Nationalism, ethnicity and religion: fundamental conflicts and the politics of identity in Tanzania. Nations and Nationalism 5: 105–125.
23. Weber A (2009) The Causes of Politicization of Ethnicity: A Comparative Case Study of Kenya and Tanzania. Centre for Comparative and International Studies, University of Zurich and ETH Zurich.
24. Armstrong Schellenberg JRM, Mrisho M, Manzi F, Shirima K, Mbuya C, et al. (2008) Health and survival of young children in southern Tanzania. BMC Public Health 8: 194.
25. Batura N (2013) The determinatns and impact of long-term child undernutrition: Evidence from rural Tanzania. PhD thesis. SOAS, University of London.
26. Hadley C (2005) Ethnic expansions and between-group differences in children's health: a case study from the Rukwa Valley, Tanzania. Am J Phys Anthropol 128: 682–92.
27. Kruger C, Olsen OE, Mighay E, Ali M (2013) Immunisation coverage and its associations in rural Tanzanian infants. Rural Remote Health 13: 2457.
28. Hadley C, Patil CL, Gulas C (2010) Social Learning and Infant and Young Child Feeding Practices. Curr Anthropol 51: 551–560.
29. Hadley C, Mulder MB, Fitzherbert E (2007) Seasonal food insecurity and perceived social support in rural Tanzania. Pub Health Nutr 10: 544–551.
30. Sellen DW (1999) Growth patterns among seminomadic pastoralists (Datoga) of Tanzania. Am J Phys Anth 2: 187–209.
31. Sellen DW (2000) Age, sex and anthropometric status of children in an African pastoral community. Ann J Hum Biol 27: 345–65.
32. Borgerhoff Mulder M, Beheim BA (2011) Understanding the nature of wealth and its effects on human fitness. Philos Trans R Soc Lond B Biol Sci 366: 344–56.
33. Homewood KM (1992) Development and the ecology of Maasai pastoralist food and nutrition. Ecol Food Nutr 29: 61–80.
34. Hawkes K, Connell JFO, Jones NGB (1997) Hadza Women' s Time Allocation, Offspring Provisioning, and the Evolution of Long Postmenopausal Life Spans. Curr Anthropol 38: 551–577.
35. Garenne M, Zwang J (2006) Premarital Fertility and Ethinicity in Africa. DHS Comparative Reports No.13.
36. De Onis M, Onyango A, Borghi E, Siyam A, Blössner M, et al. (2012) Worldwide implementation of the WHO Child Growth Standards. Public Health Nutrition 15: 1603–1610.
37. Coates J, Swindale A, Bilinsky P (2007) Household Food Insecurity Access Scale (HFIAS) for Measurement of Food Access: Indicator Guide (v.3) Washington DC: Food and Nutrition Technical Assistance Project, Academy for Educational Development, August 2007.
38. Knueppel D, Demment M, Kaiser L (2010) Validation of the Household Food Insecurity Access Scale in rural Tanzania. Public Health Nutrition 13: 360–7.
39. Clarke P (2008) When can group level clustering be ignored? Multilevel models versus single-level models with sparse data. J Epidemiol Community Health 62: 752–8.
40. StataCorp (2013) Stata statistical software: release 13. College Station, TX: StataCorp LP.
41. National Bureau of Statistics (NBS) [Tanzania] and ICF Macro (2011) Tanzania Demographic and Health Survey 2010. Dar es Salaam, Tanzania: NBS and ICF Macro.
42. Hadley C, Crooks DL (2012) Coping and the biosocial consequences of food insecurity in the 21st century. Am J Phys Anthropol 149: 72–94.
43. Hill AG (1985) Population, Health and Nutrition in the Sahel. London: Routledge and Kegan Paul.
44. Little MA, Galvin KA, Leslie PW (1988) Health and energy requirements of nomadic Turkana pastoralists. In Coping with Uncertainty in Food Supply. London: Oxford University Press. pp. 288–315.
45. Nathan MA, Fratkin EM, Roth ER (1996) Sedentism and Child Health Among Rendille Pastoralists of Northern Kenya. Soc Sci Med 43: 503–515.
46. Corbett S, Gray S, Campbell B, Leslie PW (2003) Comparison of body composition among settled and nomadic Turkana of Kenya. Ecol Food Nutr 42: 193–212.
47. Nestel PS (1989) Food intake and growth in the Maasai. Ecol Food Nutr 23: 17–30.
48. Hoppe C, Mølgaard C, Michaelsen KF (2006) Cow's milk and linear growth in industrialized and developing countries. An Rev Nutr 26: 131–73.
49. Wiley AS (2011) Cow milk consumption, insulin-like growth factor-I, and human biology: a life history approach. Am J Hum Biol 24: 130–8.
50. de Beer H (2012) Dairy products and physical stature: a systematic review and meta-analysis of controlled trials. Econ Hum Biol 10: 299–309.
51. Iannotti LL, Dulience SJL, Green J, Joseph S, François J, et al. (2014) Linear growth increased in young children in an urban slum of Haiti: a randomized controlled trial of a lipid-based nutrient supplement. Am J Clin Nutr 99: 198–208.
52. Little MA, Johnson BR (1987) Mixed-longitudinal growth of nomadic Turkana pastoralists. Hum Biol 59: 695–707.
53. Galvin KA (1991) Nutritional Ecology of Pastoralists in Dry Tropical Africa. Am J Hum Biol 4: 209–221.
54. Migliano AB, Vinicius L, Mirazo M (2007) Life history trade-offs explain the evolution of human pygmies. PNAS 104: 18–21.
55. Deaton A (2007) Height, health, and development. PNAS 104: 13232–7.
56. Walker R, Gurven M, Hill K, Migliano A, Chagnon N, et al. (2006) Growth rates and life histories in twenty-two small-scale societies. Am J Hum Biol 18: 295–311.
57. Sellen D, Smay D (2001) Relationship between subsistence and age at weaning in "preindustrial" societies. Human Nature 12: 47–87.

58. Wander K, Mattison SM (2013) The evolutionary ecology of early weaning in Kilimanjaro.
59. Omariba D, Boyle M (2007) Family Structure and Child Mortality in Sub-Saharan Africa: Cross-National Effects of Polygyny. J Marriage Fam 69: 528–543.
60. Strassmann BI (1997) Polygyny as a Risk Factor for Child Mortality Among the Dogon. Curr Anthropol 38: 688–695.
61. Lawson DW, Uggla C (2014) Family Structure and Health in the Developing World: What Can Evolutionary Anthropology Contribute to Population Health Science? In Applied Evolutionary Anthropology: Darwinian Approaches to Contemporary World Issues pp. 85–118.
62. Lawson DW, Mace R (2011) Parental investment and the optimization of human family size. Phil Trans Roy Soc B: Biol Sci 366: 333–343.
63. Hadley C, Borgerohoff Mulder M, Fitzherbert E (2007) Seasonal food insecurity and perceived social support in rural Tanzania. Pub Health Nutr 10: 544–51.
64. Coast E (2001) Maasai demography. University College London. PhD thesis. University of London.
65. Wiley AS (2009) Consumption of milk, but not other dairy products, is associated with height among U.S. preschool children in NHANES 1999–2002. Ann Hum Biol 36: 125–138
66. Oiye S, Simel JO, Oniang'o R, Johns T (2009) The Maasai food system and food and nutrition security. In Kuhnlein HV, Erasmus B & Spigelski D. (Eds) Indigenous Peoples' Food Systems: The many dimensions of culture, diversity and environment for nutrition and health. FAO Food and Agriculture Organization of the United Nations. Centre for Indigenous Peoples' Nutrition and Environment, Rome, Italy pp. 231–249
67. Hodgson DL (2011) Being Maasai, Becoming Indigenous: Postcolonial Politics in a Neoliberal World. Indiana University Press.
68. Azarya V (2004) Globalization and international tourism in developing countries: marginality as a commercial commodity. Curr Sociol 52: 949–967.
69. Faris S (24 Oct 2013) Can a tribe sue for copyright? The Maasai want royalties for use of their name. Bloomberg Buisnessweek. Available: http://www.businessweek.com/articles/2013-10-24/africas-maasai-tribe-seek-royalties-for-commercial-use-of-their-name. Accessed: 2014 Sep 26.
70. Hodgson DL (2002) Precarious Alliances: The Cultural Politics and Structural Predicaments of the Indigenous Rights Movement in Tanzania. Am Anthropol 104: 1086–1097.
71. Levi JM, Maybury-Lewis B (2012) Becoming Indigenous: Identity and Heterogeneity in a Global Movement. In Hall GH, Anthony Patrinos, H, editors. Indigenous Peoples, Poverty and Development. Cambridge University Press. pp. 73–117.
72. Fratkin EM (2013) Seeking alternative livelihoods in pastoral areas. In Catley A, Lind J, Scoones I, editors. Pastoralism and Development in Africa: Dynamic Change at the Margins New York: Routledge. pp. 197–205.
73. McCabe JT, Leslie PW, Deluca L (2010) Adopting Cultivation to Remain Pastoralists: The Diversification of Maasai Livelihoods in Northern Tanzania. Hum Ecol 38: 321–334.
74. Brainard JM (1991) Health and development in a rural Kenyan community. Peter Lang.
75. Masanja H, de Savigny D, Smithson P, Schellenberg J, John T, et al. (2008) Child survival gains in Tanzania: analysis of data from Demographic and Health Surveys. Lancet 371: 1276–1283
76. Aichele SR, Borgerhoff Mulder M, James S, Grimm K (2014) Attitudinal and Behavioral Characteristics Predict High Risk Sexual Activity in Rural Tanzanian Youth. PLoS ONE 9(6): e99987. doi: 10.1371/journal.pone.0099987.

6

A Genome-Wide Association Study Identifies Potential Susceptibility Loci for Hirschsprung Disease

Jeong-Hyun Kim[1,2], Hyun Sub Cheong[3], Jae Hoon Sul[4], Jeong-Meen Seo[5], Dae-Yeon Kim[6], Jung-Tak Oh[7], Kwi-Won Park[8], Hyun-Young Kim[8], Soo-Min Jung[5], Kyuwhan Jung[9], Min Jeng Cho[10], Joon Seol Bae[11], Hyoung Doo Shin[1,2,3]*

1 Research Institute for Basic Science, Sogang University, Seoul, Republic of Korea, **2** Department of Life Science, Sogang University, Seoul, Republic of Korea, **3** Department of Genetic Epidemiology, SNP Genetics, Inc., Seoul, Republic of Korea, **4** Department of Computer Science, University of California Los Angeles, Los Angeles, California, United States of America, **5** Division of Pediatric Surgery, Department of Surgery, Samsung Medical Center, Sungkyunkwan University School of Medicine, Seoul, Republic of Korea, **6** Department of Pediatric Surgery, Asan Medical Center, University of Ulsan College of Medicine, Seoul, Republic of Korea, **7** Department of Pediatric Surgery, Severance Children's Hospital, Yonsei University College of Medicine, Seoul, Republic of Korea, **8** Department of Pediatric Surgery, Seoul National University Children's Hospital, Seoul, Republic of Korea, **9** Department of Surgery, Seoul National University Bundang Hospital, Seongnam, Gyeonggi, Republic of Korea, **10** Department of Surgery, Konkuk University Medical Center, Seoul, Republic of Korea, **11** Laboratory of Translational Genomics, Samsung Genome Institute, Samsung Medical Center, Seoul, Republic of Korea

Abstract

Hirschsprung disease (HSCR) is a congenital and heterogeneous disorder characterized by the absence of intramural nervous plexuses along variable lengths of the hindgut. Although *RET* is a well-established risk factor, a recent genome-wide association study (GWAS) of HSCR has identified *NRG1* as an additional susceptibility locus. To discover additional risk loci, we performed a GWAS of 123 sporadic HSCR patients and 432 unaffected controls using a large-scale platform with coverage of over 1 million polymorphic markers. The result was that our study replicated the findings of *RET-CSGALNACT2-RASGEF1A* genomic region (${}_{raw}P=5.69\times10^{-19}$ before a Bonferroni correction; ${}_{corr}P=4.31\times10^{-13}$ after a Bonferroni correction) and *NRG1* as susceptibility loci. In addition, this study identified *SLC6A20* (${}_{adj}P=2.71\times10^{-6}$), *RORA* (${}_{adj}P=1.26\times10^{-5}$), and *ABCC9* (${}_{adj}P=1.86\times10^{-5}$) as new potential susceptibility loci under adjusting the already known loci on the *RET-CSGALNACT2-RASGEF1A* and *NRG1* regions, although none of the SNPs in these genes passed the Bonferroni correction. In further subgroup analysis, the *RET-CSGALNACT2-RASGEF1A* genomic region was observed to have different significance levels among subgroups: short-segment (S-HSCR, ${}_{corr}P=1.71\times10^{-5}$), long-segment (L-HSCR, ${}_{corr}P=6.66\times10^{-4}$), and total colonic aganglionosis (TCA, ${}_{corr}P>0.05$). This differential pattern in the significance level suggests that other genomic loci or mechanisms may affect the length of aganglionosis in HSCR subgroups during enteric nervous system (ENS) development. Although functional evaluations are needed, our findings might facilitate improved understanding of the mechanisms of HSCR pathogenesis.

Editor: Stacey Cherny, University of Hong Kong, Hong Kong

Funding: This work was supported by grants from the Basic Science Research Program through the National Research Foundation of Korea (NRF) funded by the Ministry of Education, Science and Technology (2010-0007857 and 2012-0006690) and the Ministry of Education (2013R1A1A2008335). The funders had no role in study design, data collection and analysis, decision to publish, or preparation of the manuscript.

Competing Interests: The authors of this manuscript have read the journal's policy and have the following competing interests: SNP Genetics, Inc. provided the iScan scanner instrument and GenomeStudio software used in the research. Authors employed in the company also were involved in the study design, data collection and analysis, decision to publish and preparation of the manuscript. Jeong-Meen Seo is employed by Division of Pediatric Surgery, Department of Surgery, Samsung Medical Center, Sungkyunkwan University School of Medicine, Seoul, 135-710, Republic of Korea and Joon Seol Bae is employed by Laboratory of Translational Genomics, Samsung Genome Institute, Samsung Medical Center, Seoul 135-710, Republic of Korea.

* Email: hdshin@sogang.ac.kr

Introduction

Hirschsprung disease (HSCR, or aganglionic megacolon) is a rare congenital disease (1 in 5000 live births) that leads to intestinal obstruction or chronic constipation. HSCR manifests a sex-dependent penetrance (male:female ratio of ~4:1) and involves mostly sporadic cases; however, 5–20% are familial forms. Based on the length of aganglionosis, patients can be further classified into three groups as follows: (1) short-segment (S-HSCR, ~80% of cases) with aganglionosis affecting the rectum and not extending beyond the upper sigmoid, (2) long-segment (L-HSCR, ~15%) with aganglionosis affecting longer tracts of the colon, and (3) total colonic aganglionosis (TCA, ~5%) [1,2]. Genetic variations in eight genes, including *RET*, have been implicated in less than 30% of HSCR development, indicating the need to identify additional HSCR-causing variations.

The *RET* proto-oncogene, encoding a tyrosine-kinase receptor, has been identified as the major HSCR gene. In particular, a common variant rs2435357 (also known as RET+3) within a conserved enhancer-like sequence in intron 1 of *RET* showed a significant association with HSCR susceptibility, with different genetic effects between male and female patients [3]. Since this variant is located in an enhancer-like sequence, it was further speculated that additional factors might interact with this variant to affect *RET* expression. Two downstream genes that are near *RET*, *CSGALNACT2* and *RASGEF1A*, are differentially expressed between the colon and small intestine [3], although the functions of these genes have not been adequately characterized.

Mutations in other genes (*EDNRB*, *GDNF*, *NRTN*, *SOX10*, etc.) have also been identified as contributing to HSCR development [1,2,4,5]. Recently, the first genome-wide association study (GWAS) of HSCR has additionally identified *neuregulin 1* (*NRG1*), one of the molecular regulators in the development and maintenance of the enteric nervous system (ENS), as a susceptibility locus for HSCR [6]. Follow-up studies have also evaluated the potential effects of NRG1 on HSCR, including aberrant *NRG1* expression [7,8]; however, results from these studies suggest that other alleles or epigenetic factors might affect *NRG1* expression. Moreover, still other factors (for instance, *APOB*, *RELN*, *GAL*, etc.) have been proposed that may be associated with HSCR development [9,10].

Given that HSCR is a heterogeneous disorder, new confounders with small-to-modest effects on HSCR development have yet to be discovered. *RET* coding sequence mutations account for about 50% in familial HSCR and 15–20% in sporadic HSCR [1]. In this study, we have performed GWAS using sporadic HSCR to discover additional risk loci and to validate previous discoveries using a larger number of single nucleotide polymorphism (SNP) markers.

Subjects and Methods

Study subjects

Study subjects were collected from Samsung Medical Center, Asan Medical Center, Severance Children's Hospital, and Seoul National University Children's Hospital in Korea. The study protocol was approved by the Institutional Review Board of each hospital (IRB No. SMC_2010-02-028-003 of Samsung Medical Center; 2010-0395 of Asan Medical Center; 4-2010-0436 of Severance Children's Hospital; 1006-129-322 of Seoul National University Children's Hospital), and guardians of all subjects provided written informed consent. All subjects were of Korean ethnicity. A total of 124 sporadic HSCR patients (102 males and 22 females) were recruited, and their biopsy specimens or surgical materials were used to make the diagnosis of HSCR by histological examination based on the absence of the enteric ganglia. Patients were composed of 76 S-HSCR, 31 L-HSCR, and 17 TCA. For the controls, 450 unaffected subjects (250 males and 200 females) with no history of HSCR based on the questionnaire information about concomitant disease, but without exclusion criteria for other neurological diseases or gastroenterological diseases, were included from Ansan cohort provided by Korea BioBank, Center for Genome Science, National Institute of Health, Korea Centers for Disease Control and Prevention. However, 19 subjects (1 S-HSCR patient and 18 controls) were excluded from all analyses because they were detected as outliers based on the principal component analysis (PCA) and revealed as mixed-bloods.

Genome-wide genotyping

Genomic DNAs were extracted from the peripheral blood lymphocytes of the patients and unaffected controls, using the Wizard Genomic DNA Purification Kit (Promega, WI, USA), according to the manufacturer's protocol. A whole-genome genotype scan was performed using about 200 ng of the genomic DNAs on Illumina's HumanOmni1-Quad BeadChip (Illumina, San Diego, USA), according to the manufacturer's protocol. All samples were scanned using the Illumina iScan system (Illumina), and the normalized bead intensity data were loaded into the GenomeStudio software (Illumina). Considering a potential association between rare variants and rare diseases such as HSCR, this study included all polymorphic markers for association analysis. For 1,140,419 markers on the chip, SNP marker quality control (QC) was applied as follows: (1) only SNP with call rate (> 98%, 995,666 markers) in both cases and controls was included, (2) 221,556 monomorphic markers were excluded, and (3) visual inspection of the genotype cluster image was performed for the SNPs with deviation from Hardy-Weinberg equilibrium (HWE, $P<0.0001$), and 16,850 SNPs deviating from HWE were excluded from the analysis. The 757,260 markers that remained after QC were ultimately used for further association analysis.

Statistics

Associations of genotype distributions were calculated by logistic regression analysis using HelixTree software (Golden Helix, Bozeman, MT, USA). The possible population stratification was examined by PCA using HelixTree software. A Bonferroni correction applied by the number of independent SNPs (757,260), which resulted in the threshold of GWAS significance ($_{corr}P = 6.6 \times 10^{-8}$), was calculated. In order to remove the effects of primary top signals from the known *RET-CSGALNACT2-RASGEF1A* genomic region on chromosome 10q11.2 and the effect of the first GWAS-discovered *NRG1* on chromosome 8p12, four SNPs, including rs2435357, rs1800860, and rs7078220 on *RET-CSGALNACT2-RASGEF1A* region and rs16879552 on *NRG1*, were adjusted as covariates. In the case of the three SNPs on *RET-CSGALNACT2-RASGEF1A* region, they were likely to make a major contribution to the strongest signal according to our GWAS results. Therefore, *P*-values were defined as follows: $_{raw}P$ for raw *P*-value before a Bonferroni correction, $_{corr}P$ after a Bonferroni correction, and $_{adj}P$ under adjusting the known *RET-CSGALNACT2-RASGEF1A* and *NRG1* loci. The FaST-LMM (Factored Spectrally Transformed Linear Mixed Models) program was applied to correct for hidden relatedness [11]. Statistical power of the sample size was calculated using the Power for Genetic Association Analyses (PGA) software [12], with false positive rate of 5%, disease prevalence of 0.02% (1 in 5000 live births) [1], given minor allele frequencies of the most significant allele and sample sizes of case (n = 123) and control (n = 432), and assuming a relative risk of 1.5, resulting in the statistical power = 58.5%. Analysis of linkage disequilibrium (LD) among the SNPs was performed using the Haploview v4.2 software downloaded from the Broad Institute (http://www.broadinstitute.org/mpg/haploview) based on LD coefficients ($|D'|$ and r^2) between all pairs of biallelic loci.

Results

Characteristics of study subjects

After excluding outliers based on the PCA (Figure S1), a total of 555 subjects (123 sporadic HSCR patients and 432 unaffected controls) were involved in the GWAS. Although our study subjects showed genomic control inflation factor (λ) of 1.077, this inflation factor was reduced to 1.015 after correcting for hidden relatedness using FaST-LMM. Male:female ratio was ~4.9:1, as was expected based on general sex differences in HSCR. Patients were classified into groups of 75 S-HSCR (60.1% of cases; 65 male, 10 female), 31 L-HSCR (25.2% of cases; 24 male, 7 female), and 17 TCA (13.8% of cases; 13 male, 4 female), indicating that the proportion of patients with L-HSCR and TCA in this study was slightly higher than the expected prevalence of each subgroup.

Association analysis and identification of new susceptibility locus

A quantile-quantile (Q-Q) plot for the association test with HSCR showed a significant deviation of measures at the tail (Figure 1A), even after excluding SNPs in the *RET-CSGALNACT2-RASGEF1A* region on chromosome 10q11.2 (Figure S2), indicating potentially true associations between the SNPs and HSCR. Our GWAS confirmed two facts previously reported. First, the strongest significant association was observed at the *RET-CSGALNACT2-RASGEF1A* genomic region (Figure 1B), with top signal at kgp4676284 (rs1864400, $_{raw}P = 5.69 \times 10^{-19}$ before a Bonferroni correction; $_{corr}P = 4.31 \times 10^{-13}$ after a Bonferroni correction, Table S1). Second, *NRG1* also showed association signals (Table S2).

No other individual SNPs reached a genome-wide significance (Bonferroni-corrected significance) level, except for five SNPs (two intronic rs12739262 and rs35198051; three intergenic rs12752277, rs2809867, and rs36019094; Figure 1B and Table S3). To identify additional signals under exclusion of effects from the *RET-CSGALNACT2-RASGEF1A* region and from the first GWAS-discovered *NRG1*, further analysis was employed by adjusting for four SNPs, rs2435357, rs1800860, and rs7078220 on the *RET-CSGALNACT2-RASGEF1A* region (these three SNPs were confirmed to sufficiently represent the region) and rs16879552 on *NRG1*. The strongest association was detected at *SLC6A20* encoding solute carrier family 6, proline IMINO transporter, member 20 (rs4299518, $_{adj}P = 2.71 \times 10^{-6}$; rs2159272, $_{adj}P = 2.66 \times 10^{-5}$; Table 1 and Figure 2). In the regional association of 400 kb around *SLC6A20* on chromosome 3p21.3 (Figure 3A), seven SNPs of *SLC6A20* showed relatively robust association signals (minimum $_{adj}P = 2.71 \times 10^{-6}$, Table S4). LD analysis revealed that *SLC6A20* SNPs showing potential associations with HSCR were likely to not be in LD with nearby genes (Figure 3A). In addition, *RORA* (minimum $_{adj}P = 1.26 \times 10^{-5}$) and *ABCC9* (minimum $_{adj}P = 1.86 \times 10^{-5}$), along with relatively strong regional associations (Figure 3B and 3C), were detected as potential risk loci for HSCR (Table 1 and Table S4).

In the further analysis under adjusting the known *RET-CSGALNACT2-RASGEF1A* and *NRG1* loci, other genes including *CDKAL1* ($_{adj}P = 1.96 \times 10^{-5}$), *ACCSL* ($_{adj}P = 1.13 \times 10^{-5}$), and *ASTN1* ($_{adj}P = 7.63 \times 10^{-5}$) also showed potential associations with HSCR (Table 1 and Table S5).

Analysis of HSCR subgroups

In addition to *RET*, two of its downstream genes, *CSGALNACT2* and *RASGEF1A*, showed similar levels of significance regarding HSCR susceptibility and were in tight LD (Figure S3). In our further analysis among subgroups, this *RET-CSGALNACT2-RASGEF1A* genomic region showed different significance levels among subgroups ($_{corr}P = 1.71 \times 10^{-5}$ in S-HSCR; $_{corr}P = 6.66 \times 10^{-4}$ in L-HSCR; $_{corr}P > 0.05$ in TCA; Table S6 and Figure 4).

Discussion

HSCR is a complex and heterogeneous disease. In addition, the incidence of HSCR is much higher in males, and a higher maternal inheritance than paternal (largely transmitted to the son) is observed in *RET* coding sequence mutations, based on the assumption of parent-of-origin effect [13]. Although mutations in *RET* (in particular, a common variant rs2435357 within a conserved enhancer-like sequence) and other genes (such as *GDNF*, *SOX10*, and endothelin-related genes) have partially accounted for HSCR development [3–5,14], comprehensive genetic implications for HSCR and ENS development are still not fully understood. Inspired by the discovery of *NRG1* as an additional susceptibility locus from GWAS of HSCR, we performed another GWAS using a large-scale platform with coverage of over 1 million markers to identify additional risk factors and to investigate potential genetic effects among HSCR subgroups. As a result, this study identified *SLC6A20* and *ABCC9* as potential susceptibility loci and the possible reduced effects of the *RET-CSGALNACT2-RASGEF1A* genomic region according to length of aganglionosis.

Consistent with results of the first GWAS [6], we also replicated the finding that *NRG1* on chromosome 8 might be a susceptibility locus for HSCR (Figure 1B and Table S2). Due to the different GWAS array platforms, only *NRG1* rs16879552 in our GWAS was matched and could be compared to that of the previous GWAS. This study showed a nominal relevance at rs16879552 (Table S2), whereas the first GWAS revealed a higher association signal [6]. Since this study included no hereditary HSCR cases,

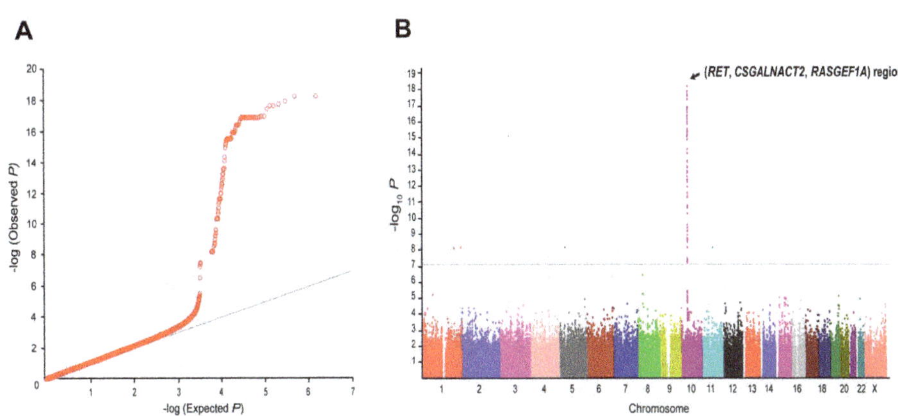

Figure 1. Overview of genome-wide association results. (A) Q-Q plot. The observed *P*-value (y-axis) is compared with the expected $_{raw}P$-value (x-axis, under null distribution) before a Bonferroni correction. (B) Graphical summary (Manhattan plot) presenting $_{raw}P$-values for the association with HSCR in 123 sporadic HSCR patients and 432 unaffected controls. The $-\log_{10}P$ (logistic regression analysis) is plotted against its physical position on successive chromosomes. Gray line represents the threshold for GWAS significance after a Bonferroni correction.

Table 1. Top 20 SNPs under analysis adjusted by SNPs of *RET* region on chr. 10 and *NRG1* on chr. 8.

SNP	Chr.	Position	Minor allele	Location	(Closest) gene	MAF		$_{adj}P$-value* (Adjusted analysis)	$_{corr}P$-value**
						Case (n = 123)	Control (n = 432)		
rs11725593	4	27066038	A	Intergenic	(*STIM2*)	0.317	0.204	1.80×10^{-6}	NS
rs4299518	3	45809273	C	Intron	*SLC6A20*	0.004	0.053	2.71×10^{-6}	NS
rs6074578	20	191797	T	Intergenic	(*DEFB129*)	0.549	0.389	3.71×10^{-6}	NS
rs12639288	3	167661136	A	Intergenic	(*LOC100509398*)	0.085	0.036	5.11×10^{-6}	NS
rs13069589	3	167680850	A	Intergenic	(*LOC100509398*)	0.081	0.035	6.66×10^{-6}	NS
rs12284962	11	44077227	A	Intron	*ACCSL*	0.041	0.121	1.13×10^{-5}	NS
rs1351544	15	61042867	T	Intron	*RORA*	0.354	0.213	1.26×10^{-5}	NS
rs8025324	15	61043378	A	Intron	*RORA*	0.354	0.213	1.26×10^{-5}	NS
rs704192	12	22015114	T	Intron	*ABCC9*	0.390	0.251	1.86×10^{-5}	NS
rs6078500	20	182013	C	Intergenic	(*DEFB128*)	0.549	0.398	1.86×10^{-5}	NS
rs9348455	6	21043852	T	Intron	*CDKAL1*	0.362	0.249	1.96×10^{-5}	NS
rs704191	12	22015022	A	Intron	*ABCC9*	0.390	0.253	2.16×10^{-5}	NS
rs9920560	15	61047930	A	Intron	*RORA*	0.358	0.219	2.37×10^{-5}	NS
rs4148669	12	22024093	C	Intron	*ABCC9*	0.386	0.253	2.60×10^{-5}	NS
rs2159272	3	45829995	T	Intron	*SLC6A20*	0.472	0.360	2.66×10^{-5}	NS
rs6033398	20	183222	T	Intergenic	(*DEFB128*)	0.541	0.391	2.70×10^{-5}	NS
rs12466120	2	53587240	A	Intergenic	(*GPR75-ABS3*)	0.524	0.396	2.82×10^{-5}	NS
rs8050612	16	51025933	A	Intergenic	(*LOC100652974*)	0.159	0.081	3.03×10^{-5}	NS
rs7183955	15	61049569	C	Intron	*RORA*	0.358	0.220	3.09×10^{-5}	NS
rs704190	12	22014473	C	Intron	*ABCC9*	0.362	0.249	3.74×10^{-5}	NS

**P*-value after adjustment by sex and 4 SNPs (rs2435357, rs1800860, and rs7078220 on/nearby *RET* and rs16879552 on *NRG1*) as covariates.
***P*-value after the Bonferroni correction.
Chr., chromosome; MAF, minor allele frequency; NS, not significant.

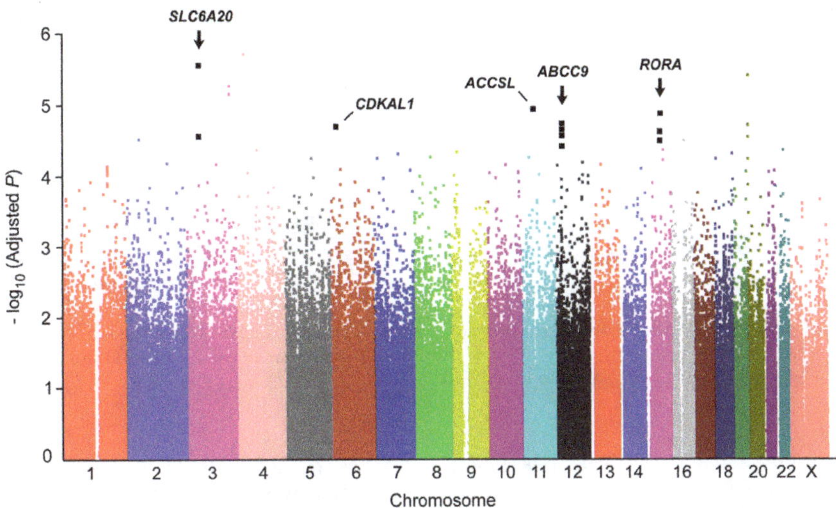

Figure 2. Result of the analysis adjusted by *RET-CSGALNACT2-RASGEF1A* and *NRG1* and top SNPs within the gene region. The $_{adj}P$-value (y-axis) after adjustment by rs2435357, rs1800860, and rs7078220 on *RET-CSGALNACT2-RASGEF1A* region and rs16879552 on *NRG1* is plotted against its physical position on successive chromosomes.

this discrepancy between the Chinese and Korean studies might be due to ethnic differences among Asian populations or different inclusion ratios of the subgroups. However, among 41 *NRG1* SNP markers in our GWAS, several variants (for instance, rs7005606, rs4733130, and rs6996957) also showed increased association signals for HSCR (Table S2).

Five SNPs (rs12739262, rs12752277, rs2809867 on chromosome 1; rs36019094 on chromosome 5; rs35198051 on chromosome 11) showed genome-wide significance levels (Table S3). Among these SNPs, *PPP1R12B* rs12739262 and *SHANK2* rs35198051 ($_{corr}P = 0.005$ for both SNPs) are positioned at the intron of the genes, whereas others are in intergenic or gene desert regions. However, despite potential associations of *SHANK2* with the nervous system and neurodevelopmental diseases [15,16], no observation of additionally significant associations of *SHANK2* and *PPP1R12B* SNPs in our regional association results suggests that these loci with genome-wide significance might be false-positive findings. This study identified *SLC6A20*, *RORA*, and *ABCC9* as new potential susceptibility loci for HSCR. Four, nine, and nineteen SNPs of *SLC6A20*, *RORA*, and *ABCC9*, respectively, showed relatively robust association signals ($_{adj}P<0.001$, Table S4), suggesting that these genes might play a role in HSCR susceptibility without the effects of the *RET-CSGALNACT2-RASGEF1A* and *NRG1* regions.

Although the functions of *SLC6A20* and its gene product are poorly understood, there are a few intriguing clues to the relationship between *SLC6A20* and HSCR. The human *SLC6A20* that is abundantly expressed in much of the gastrointestinal tract has been suggested as a target gene for a renal tubular disorder of iminoaciduria [17,18]. Also, the combined mutations in *SLC6A20* and other genes have been observed to affect its related human phenotypes [19], suggesting that genetic variations

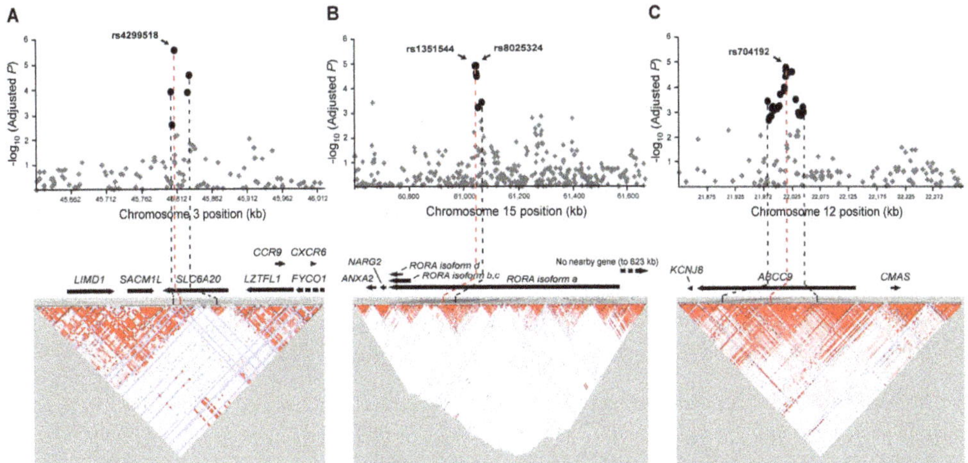

Figure 3. Regional association and LD plots of *SLC6A20, RORA*, and *ABCC9* SNPs for HSCR. Associations of SNPs across approximately (A) a 400 kb region around *SLC6A20* on chromosome 3p21.3, (B) a 1,065 kb region around *RORA* on chromosome 15q22.2, and (C) a 500 kb region around *ABCC9* on chromosome 12p12.1, under analysis adjusted by *RET-CSGALNACT2-RASGEF1A* and *NRG1*, are shown. In the upper panel of each regional association, strong associations are shown as large black circles; relatively weak associations are shown as small gray diamonds. In the lower panel, LDs are indicated with LD coefficient (r^2) between all pairs of biallelic loci.

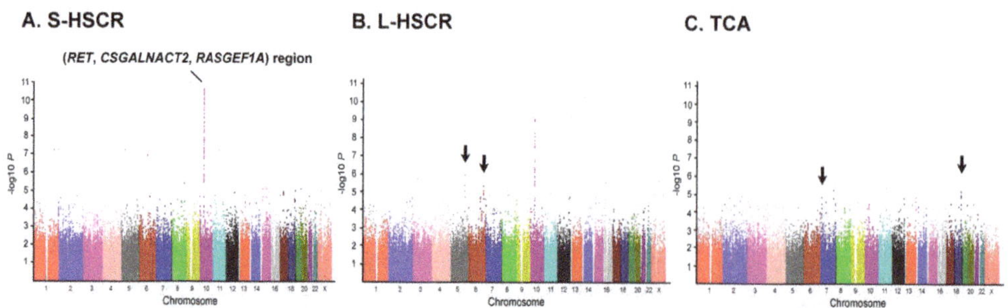

Figure 4. Manhattan plots of HSCR subgroup analysis. The strongest association *RET-CSGALNACT2-RASGEF1A* genomic region is observed at chromosome 10. Other potential loci are indicated by arrows. *P*-value indicates the significance before a Bonferroni correction. (A) short-segment (S-HSCR); (B) long-segment (L-HSCR); (C) total colonic aganglionosis (TCA).

of *SLC6A20* may also contribute to the development of the enteric system when combined with other risk factors. On the other hand, since *LIMD1*, a nearby gene of *SCL6A20*, has been shown to affect cell migration that is essential during development [20], we also analyzed LD between the seven *SLC6A20* SNPs ($_{adj}P<0.01$) and two nearby genes (*LIMD1* and *SACM1L*) that were most likely to be in LD with *SLC6A20*. However, *SLC6A20* showed no LD with the nearby genes (Table S7), indicating that *SLC6A20* may have roles without correlation to nearby genes, but may interact with other regulators [21]. For other potential genes of *RORA* and *ABCC9*, no literature clues related to HSCR or ENS development could be found.

This study confirmed strong associations of SNPs on *CSGALNACT2* and *RASGEF1A* as nearby genes of *RET* and being in tight LD with one another. However, the functions of CSGALNACT2 and RASGEF1A are little understood. Only differential expressions of these three genes have been previously observed in human tissues: for instance, higher expression of *RASGEF1A* in the colon but lower in the small intestine, when compared to *RET* expressions [3]. Despite the insufficient sample size (in particular, the low number of L-HSCR and TCA cases), our results also identified other potential loci (Figure 4) that might contribute to the phenotypes, such as length of aganglionosis, of the L-HSCR and TCA subgroups. This evidence suggests that other regulators, including distant-acting factors or chromosomal abnormalities, may affect the development of ENS as well as HSCR [22,23]. Therefore, further studies, including replications in large cohorts and deep sequencing of the *RET-CSGALNACT2-RASGEF1A* region in HSCR patients, are needed.

Notably, there are additional observations from this study. First, although the common *RET* rs2435357 within a conserved enhancer-like sequence has been evaluated to be associated with HSCR, possibly by affecting *RET* expression [3,24], this study has found more significant associations at the top three intronic SNPs, kgp4676284 (rs1864400, $_{corr}P=4.31\times10^{-13}$, Table S1), kgp3302846 (rs741968, $_{corr}P=4.31\times10^{-13}$), and kgp11922846 (rs2742233, $_{corr}P=9.54\times10^{-13}$), which are in tight LD with each other but not in LD with rs2435357 (Figure S4). However, in our further in silico prediction analysis of potential branch point (BP) sites for alternative splicing using the Human Splicing Finder (http://www.umd.be/HSF/), these top three intronic SNPs did not emerge as potential BP sites. Second, in the case of *DSCAM* as a candidate gene in this study (Table S5), a most recent study has reported that this gene may be a predisposing locus in HSCR [25]. Therefore, further functional evaluations of these new observations may also be required.

To date, the association between *RET* genetic variations and HSCR has been identified in less than 30% of sporadic HSCR cases [1]. To investigate the genetic heterogeneity for genomic regions that showed the Bonferroni-corrected significances for HSCR, SNPs across approximately a 196 kb region around the *RET-CSGALNACT2-RASGEF1A* on chromosome 10 were further analyzed. As a result, this genomic region showed a relatively strong LD block (Figure S3). In addition, when a multidimensional scaling (MDS) of the *RET-CSGALNACT2-RASGEF1A* region for genetic heterogeneity was plotted, patients were not divided into subgroups with specific genotypes, showing a single cluster (Figure S5). Therefore, it is suggested that there may be no genetic heterogeneity in these *RET-CSGALNACT2-RASGEF1A* genomic regions showing significant associations with HSCR.

Finally, several well-known HSCR- and/or enteric development-related genes (*EDNRB*, *GDNF*, *NRTN*, *SOX10*, *PHOX2B*, etc.) [1,2,26] showed no significant association signals in this study ($_{corr}P>0.05$, Table S8). Only, SNPs of *EDNRB* and *ECE1* revealed nominal associations. The lack of associations in *NRTN* and *SOX10* is consistent with reports that have conflicting results [27,28]. For *EDN3* and *ZFHX1B*, the genetic diversity or the complex phenotypes of patients with combined clinical features might affect no replication of associations in this study [1,29,30].

This study found a small amount of inflation of test statistics as the genomic control inflation factor is around 1.07. We applied the linear mixed models (FaST-LMM) to correct for hidden relatedness and found that inflation factor becomes 1.015. This indicates that the linear mixed models successfully removed effects of hidden relatedness as our inflation factor is close to 1. It was also found that *P*-values of most of significant associations detected before correcting for relatedness were consistent with *P*-values after applying the linear mixed models.

In conclusion, our preliminary findings suggest that new potential susceptibility loci, including *SLC6A20*, *RORA*, and *ABCC9* under adjusting the *RET-CSGALNACT2-RASGEF1A* and *NRG1* regions, may be related to the development of HSCR or ENS-related disorders. However, there are several limitations of this study, such as insufficient sample size and lack of replication. In the case of statistical power of the sample size, it was calculated as 58.5% due to the low numbers of subjects (in particular, L-HSCR and TCA cases due to the rareness of the conditions). Therefore, further replication study with independent samples and functional evaluations of candidate genes are required. In order to share data for further meta-analysis elsewhere, the summary statistics (SNP ID, chromosome, position, allele variation, MAF, OR with 95% CI, and *P*-value) for SNPs with association signals (42,447 SNPs, $_{raw}P<0.05$) were summarized in Table S9. In addition, further observation on differential expressions of *RET*, *CSGALNACT2*, and *RASGEF1A* among HSCR subgroups may help our understanding of HSCR pathogenesis and/or ENS development.

Supporting Information

Figure S1 The result of principal component analysis.

Figure S2 Q-Q plot after excluding SNPs in the *RET-CSGALNACT2-RASGEF1A* region on chromosome 10q11.2.

Figure S3 Regional and LDs of SNPs on *RET*, *CSGALNACT2* and *RASGEF1A* region on chromosome 10.

Figure S4 LDs of top three SNPs (kgp4676284, kgp3302846, kgp11922846) and major known risk allele rs2435357 of *RET*.

Figure S5 MDS plot of the *RET-CSGALNACT2-RASGEF1A* region on chromosome 10 that shows Bonferroni-corrected significances for the HSCR association.

Table S1 Top 100 SNPs from association in GWAS analysis.

Table S2 *NRG1* SNPs with significance (GWAS Raw P<0.05 in this study.

Table S3 SNPs with genome-wide significance except for *RET-CSGALNACT2-RASGEF1A* genomic region.

Table S4 List of all SNPs of *SLC6A20*, *RORA*, and *ABCC9* in this GWAS.

Table S5 Potential genes showing significant associations ($_{adj}P<10^{-4}$) with HSCR under adjusted analysis (only SNPs with P<0.05 shown).

Table S6 Top 10 SNPs of *RET-CSGALNACT2-RASGEF1A* region in each subgroup.

Table S7 LD of *SLC6A20* SNPs with significant associations ($_{adj}P<0.01$) with SNPs of *LIMD1* and *SACM1L*.

Table S8 SNPs (in this GWAS) of previously known HSCR-related genes.

Table S9 Summary statistics for SNPs with association signals (42,447 SNPs, $_{raw}P<0.05$).

Acknowledgments

The authors thank the patients and their parents without whom this study would not have been possible.

Author Contributions

Conceived and designed the experiments: JHK HDS. Performed the experiments: JHK JSB. Analyzed the data: JHK HSC JHS JSB. Contributed reagents/materials/analysis tools: JMS DYK JTO KWP HYK SMJ KJ MJC. Contributed to the writing of the manuscript: JHK HDS.

References

1. Amiel J, Sproat-Emison E, Garcia-Barcelo M, Lantieri F, Burzynski G, et al. (2008) Hirschsprung disease, associated syndromes and genetics: a review. J Med Genet 45: 1–14.
2. Heanue TA, Pachnis V (2007) Enteric nervous system development and Hirschsprung's disease: advances in genetic and stem cell studies. Nat Rev Neurosci 8: 466–79.
3. Emison ES, McCallion AS, Kashuk CS, Bush RT, Grice E, et al. (2005) A common sex-dependent mutation in a RET enhancer underlies Hirschsprung disease risk. Nature 434: 857–63.
4. Carrasquillo MM, McCallion AS, Puffenberger EG, Kashuk CS, Nouri N, et al. (2002) Genome-wide association study and mouse model identify interaction between RET and EDNRB pathways in Hirschsprung disease. Nat Genet 32: 237–44.
5. Shen L, Pichel JG, Mayeli T, Sariola H, Lu B, et al. (2002) Gdnf haploinsufficiency causes Hirschsprung-like intestinal obstruction and early-onset lethality in mice. Am J Hum Genet 70: 435–47.
6. Garcia-Barcelo MM, Tang CS, Ngan ES, Lui VC, Chen Y, et al. (2009) Genome-wide association study identifies NRG1 as a susceptibility locus for Hirschsprung's disease. Proc Natl Acad Sci U S A 106: 2694–9.
7. Tang CS, Tang WK, So MT, Miao XP, Leung BM, et al. (2011) Fine mapping of the NRG1 Hirschsprung's disease locus. PLoS One 6: e16181.
8. Tang W, Li B, Xu X, Zhou Z, Wu W, et al. (2012) Aberrant high expression of NRG1 gene in Hirschsprung disease. J Pediatr Surg 47: 1694–8.
9. Evangelisti C, Bianco F, Pradella LM, Puliti A, Goldoni A, et al. (2012) Apolipoprotein B is a new target of the GDNF/RET and ET-3/EDNRB signalling pathways. Neurogastroenterol Motil 24: e497–508.
10. Saeed A, Barreto L, Neogii SG, Loos A, McFarlane I, et al. (2012) Identification of novel genes in Hirschsprung disease pathway using whole genome expression study. J Pediatr Surg 47: 303–7.
11. Lippert C, Listgarten J, Liu Y, Kadie CM, Davidson RI, et al. (2011) FaST linear mixed models for genome-wide association studies. Nat Methods 8: 833–5.
12. Menashe I, Rosenberg PS, Chen BE (2008) PGA: power calculator for case-control genetic association analyses. BMC Genet 9: 36.
13. Jannot AS, Amiel J, Pelet A, Lantieri F, Fernandez RM, et al. (2012) Male and female differential reproductive rate could explain parental transmission asymmetry of mutation origin in Hirschsprung disease. Eur J Hum Genet 20: 917–20.
14. Sham MH, Lui VC, Fu M, Chen B, Tam PK (2001) SOX10 is abnormally expressed in aganglionic bowel of Hirschsprung's disease infants. Gut 49: 220–6.
15. Raab M, Boeckers TM, Neuhuber WL (2010) Proline-rich synapse-associated protein-1 and 2 (ProSAP1/Shank2 and ProSAP2/Shank3)-scaffolding proteins are also present in postsynaptic specializations of the peripheral nervous system. Neuroscience 171: 421–33.
16. Tse MT (2012) Neurodevelopmental disorders: exploring the links between SHANK2 and autism. Nat Rev Drug Discov 11: 518.
17. Procopis PG, Turner B (1971) Iminoaciduria: a benign renal tubular defect. J Pediatr 79: 419–22.
18. Takanaga H, Mackenzie B, Suzuki Y, Hediger MA (2005) Identification of mammalian proline transporter SIT1 (SLC6A20) with characteristics of classical system imino. J Biol Chem 280: 8974–84.
19. Broer S, Bailey CG, Kowalczuk S, Ng C, Vanslambrouck JM, et al. (2008) Iminoglycinuria and hyperglycinuria are discrete human phenotypes resulting from complex mutations in proline and glycine transporters. J Clin Invest 118: 3881–92.
20. Bai SW, Herrera-Abreu MT, Rohn JL, Racine V, Tajadura V, et al. (2011) Identification and characterization of a set of conserved and new regulators of cytoskeletal organization, cell morphology and migration. BMC Biol 9: 54.
21. Dierking K, Polanowska J, Omi S, Engelmann I, Gut M, et al. (2011) Unusual regulation of a STAT protein by an SLC6 family transporter in C. elegans epidermal innate immunity. Cell Host Microbe 9: 425–35.
22. Panza E, Knowles CH, Graziano C, Thapar N, Burns AJ, et al. (2012) Genetics of human enteric neuropathies. Prog Neurobiol 96: 176–89.
23. Tang CS, Cheng G, So MT, Yip BH, Miao XP, et al. (2012) Genome-wide copy number analysis uncovers a new HSCR gene: NRG3. PLoS Genet 8: e1002687.
24. Miao X, Leon TY, Ngan ES, So MT, Yuan ZW, et al. (2010) Reduced RET expression in gut tissue of individuals carrying risk alleles of Hirschsprung's disease. Hum Mol Genet 19: 1461–7.
25. Jannot AS, Pelet A, Henrion-Caude A, Chaoui A, Masse-Morel M, et al. (2013) Chromosome 21 scan in Down syndrome reveals DSCAM as a predisposing locus in Hirschsprung disease. PLoS One 8: e62519.

26. Garcia-Barcelo M, Sham MH, Lui VC, Chen BL, Ott J, et al. (2003) Association study of PHOX2B as a candidate gene for Hirschsprung's disease. Gut 52: 563–7.
27. Fernandez RM, Ruiz-Ferrer M, Lopez-Alonso M, Antinolo G, Borrego S (2008) Polymorphisms in the genes encoding the 4 RET ligands, GDNF, NTN, ARTN, PSPN, and susceptibility to Hirschsprung disease. J Pediatr Surg 43: 2042–7.
28. Pan ZW, Lou J, Luo C, Yu L, Li JC (2011) Association analysis of the SOX10 polymorphism with Hirschsprung disease in the Han Chinese population. J Pediatr Surg 46: 1930–4.
29. Edery P, Attie T, Amiel J, Pelet A, Eng C, et al. (1996) Mutation of the endothelin-3 gene in the Waardenburg-Hirschsprung disease (Shah-Waardenburg syndrome). Nat Genet 12: 442–4.
30. Yamada K, Yamada Y, Nomura N, Miura K, Wakako R, et al. (2001) Nonsense and frameshift mutations in ZFHX1B, encoding Smad-interacting protein 1, cause a complex developmental disorder with a great variety of clinical features. Am J Hum Genet 69: 1178–85.

7

The Impact of Prior Tonsillitis and Treatment Modality on the Recurrence of Peritonsillar Abscess: A Nationwide Cohort Study

Ying-Piao Wang[1,2,3], Mao-Che Wang[2,4], Hung-Ching Lin[1,3], Pesus Chou[2]*

1 Department of Otolaryngology, Head and Neck Surgery, Mackay Memorial Hospital, Taipei, Taiwan, **2** Institute of Public Health and Community Medicine Research Center, National Yang-Ming University, Taipei, Taiwan, **3** Department of Audiology and Speech Language Pathology and School of Medicine, Mackay Medical College, New Taipei City, Taiwan, **4** Department of Otolaryngology, Head and Neck Surgery, Taipei Veterans General Hospital and School of Medicine, National Yang-Ming University, Taipei, Taiwan

Abstract

Background: Studies suggest an increased risk of peritonsillar abscess (PTA) recurrence in patients with prior tonsillitis. However, this association is inconsistent and could be confounded by different treatment modalities. This study aimed to assess the risk of recurrence among PTA patients with different degrees of prior tonsillitis and treatment modalities, and the role of tonsillectomy in current practice.

Methods: All in-patients with peritonsillar abscess between January 2001 and December 2009 were identified in a nationwide, retrospective cohort study. Recurrence was defined as the first occurrence of PTA ≥30 days from the initial PTA. Factors independently associated with recurrence were analyzed using Cox proportional hazard model after adjusting for demographic and clinical data.

Results: There were 28,837 patients, with a 5.15% recurrence rate and 4.74 years of follow-up. The recurrence rates were significantly higher among subjects with more than five prior tonsillitis or 1–4 prior tonsillitis compared to those without prior tonsillitis (adjusted hazard ratio, 2.82 [95% confidence interval, 2.39–3.33] and 1.59 [95% CI: 1.38–1.82]). The adjusted HR in patients treated with needle aspiration was 1.08 compared to those treated with incision & drainage (95% CI: 0.85–1.38). After age stratification, the adjusted HRs of more than five prior tonsillitis increased to 2.92 and 3.50 in patients aged ≦18 and 19–29 years respectively. The adjusted HR ofneedle aspiration only increased in patients ≦18 years old (aHR: 1.98 [95% CI: 0.99–3.97]). The overall tonsillectomy rate was 1.48% during our study period.

Conclusions: The risk of PTA recurrence increases with higher degrees of prior tonsillitis in all age groups and management by needle aspiration only in the pediatric population. Patients younger than 30 years old with PTA and more than five prior tonsillitis have the greatest risk of recurrence.

Editor: Salomon Amar, Boston University, United States of America

Funding: This study was funded by the Mackay Memorial Hospital (MMH-100-063), and no additional external funding was received for this work. The funders had no role in study design, data collection and analysis, decision to publish, or preparation of the manuscript.

Competing Interests: The authors have declared that no competing interests exist.

* Email: pschou@ym.edu.tw

Introduction

Deep neck infection is one of the most lethal infectious diseases in the complex framework formed by the three layers of the deep cervical fascia, with potential morbidity and mortality ranging from 1.6% to 40% [1–4]. Peritonsillar abscess (PTA) is the most common type of deep neck infection, colloquially referred to as "Quinsy", and accounts for approximately 30% of head and neck abscesses [5–7]. Even in the antibiotic era, PTA remains a common condition, with an incidence that has increased by 18% in the United Kingdom over the last 10 years [8,9]. Appropriate management has been debated for more than two decades. In a National Audit of PTA treatment in the UK, the main strategies are needle aspiration along with antibiotics (60%), incision and drainage (25%), intravenous antibiotics only (5%), and abscess tonsillectomy (1%) [8,10,11].

Although all treatments are initially effective, a substantial proportion of PTA tend to recur [12]. The recurrence rate of PTA is poorly defined in the literature, ranging from 5% to 22%, with variability in age, sex, duration of follow-up, and different managements [8,13–19]. To date, there is no direct estimate of the frequency of PTA recurrence in a nationwide study in the world. The higher PTA recurrence rates reported in some observational studies are associated with recurrent tonsillitis prior to the development of PTA [8,13,20–22]. Conversely, two retrospective studies indicated no significant difference in recurrence rates between patients with and those without prior tonsillitis [14,19].

The mode of treatment may influence the recurrence rates of PTA. In descriptive studies, patients treated with needle aspiration have a higher incidence of residual and recurrent PTA compared to incision and drainage (I&D) patients [14,21]. In contrast, a retrospective study of 38 pediatric PTA patients has revealed no difference in different treatment modalities [19]. Data from current literature are inconclusive regarding factors associated with PTA recurrence. Most observational studies are small-sized, unable to analyze recurrent tonsillitis and treatment modalities simultaneously, unable to adjust for important covariates like demographic factors and co-morbidities, have relatively short follow-up periods, and not population-based.

Under the hypothesis that prior tonsillitis and treatment modality are independently associated with increased risk of PTA recurrence, this retrospective nationwide study assessed how recurrent tonsillitis and mode of treatment affected the risk of PTA recurrence. The role of tonsillectomy as PTA treatment remains controversial, as quinsy or interval tonsillectomy is reported in 10–20% of patients after PTA episodes [16,23–25]. This study also provided tonsillectomy data on PTA patients that had not been addressed in a nationwide setting.

Materials and Methods

Study design and data source

A retrospective, nationwide cohort study was conducted to determine the recurrence rate of PTA with a specific follow-up period and to investigate the influence of prior tonsillitis and treatment mode on the risk of PTA recurrence. Data were obtained from the National Health Insurance Claims database. The National Health Insurance (NHI) program was launched in March 1995 and covers over 98% residents and medical utilities in Taiwan [26]. The electronic files contained details of health care services for every patient, including demographic characteristics, complete out-patient visits, hospital admissions, diagnoses, prescriptions, clinical orders of participants. The Institutional Review Board of Mackay Memorial Hospital approved this study (12MMHIS129). Because the personal information and identification numbers of the subjects included in this study were de-identified in the Claims database, the review board stated that the written informed consent from patients was not required.

Study population

All the PTA patients in Taiwan between 2001 to 2009 were identified from the entire population in the NHI program. Claims data from both the out-patient and in-patient database were studied. All subjects with claims data with the in-patient codes relevant to PTA (ICD-9-CM 475) between 2001 to 2009 were enrolled as target subjects. All ambulatory and in-patient claims data, details of in-patient, and ambulatory orders and registry files from 2000 to 2009 were used in the research. The index date was defined as the date of the first PTA episode.

Patients with abnormal or inconsequent registry data, or missing data; those with tonsillectomy before censoring or PTA occurrence; and those with a PTA episode in the year 2000 were excluded (Fig. 1).

Outcome definition

The primary study outcome was the first occurrence of any PTA ≥30 days from the index date of the initial PTA [14]. Censor days were determined from the date when the patient had the initial PTA until the date when he or she was defined as having recurrent PTA, death, or the last day he or she was covered by the NHI program for those who did not have recurrent PTA.

Independent variables

Information regarding demographics, prior tonsillitis, treatment modalities, and co-morbidities were obtained from the claims data of each individual. Age was categorized into three groups for further analysis: ≦18 years, 19–29 and ≥30 years. The patients were also stratified by sex.

To determine a history of prior tonsillitis, the number of outpatient visits for acute tonsillitis in the preceding year before subject's index date was categorized into mutually exclusive categories: 0, 1–4, and ≥5 visits. The diagnosis of tonsillitis was dependent on the ICD-9 codes in the administrative claims data. Treatment modalities included needle aspiration, incision and drainage, and intravenous antibiotics only. All of the patients included in this study were treated as inpatient and intravenous antibiotics were given regardless of the use of drainage procedures. The overall mean time for inpatient antibiotics were 4.5±4.4 days. The mean time for inpatient antibiotics were 4.4±3.2 days for the patients received needle aspiration, 4.2±2.7 days for incision & drainage and 4.8±5.8 days for antibiotics only.

Ambulatory and in-patient claims data will be searched for the subject's co-morbidities. Each co-morbidity was defined as positive if the patient had more than three outpatient visits or one hospitalization claim for the specific disease a year before the index date. Co-morbidities include diabetes mellitus (ICD-9-CM codes 250.00–250.90), hypertension (ICD-9-CM codes 401–405), cardiovascular disorder (ICD-9-CM codes 410–414), chronic kidney disease (ICD-9-CM codes 581–583, 585,586), chronic liver disease (ICD-9-CM codes 571), and cancer (ICD-9-CM codes (140–203). Each co-morbidity was analyzed as a binominal variable.

Statistical analyses

The SAS statistical package version 9.3 was used for all analysis. Cox proportional hazard model was used to estimate the independent association between prior tonsillitis and recurrent PTA after adjustments for numerous confounding factors, including treatment modalities, co-morbidities, and demographic factors. The 95% confidence intervals (CIs) of the adjusted hazard ratios (aHRs) were calculated. Significance was set at a two-sided $p<0.05$.

Results

Patient Characteristics

This study included 28,837 patients with initial episode of PTA between 2001 and 2009 in Taiwan. The mean age was 25.5±18.9 years for the entire PTA cohort and 13.8±15.6 years for the recurrent PTA patients. Overall, 19083 (66.2%) were males, 18907 (65.6%) were younger than 30 years old, 20150 (69.9%) had prior tonsillitis, and 14726 (51.1%) were treated with needle aspiration. There were 1486 (5.15%) patients experienced PTA recurrence during a 4.74-year follow-up. The recurrence rate was 6.7% in patients aged <30 years and 2.1% to those aged ≥30 years ($p<0.0001$). The mean time to recurrence was 1.16±1.28 years after initial PTA. Recurrence rates also differed significantly in different degrees of prior tonsillitis, treatment modality and co-morbidities including diabetes, hypertension, cardiovascular disease, renal disease, chronic liver disease and cancer. However, the recurrence rates in females and males did not differ significantly (5.4% and 5.0%, respectively) (Table 1).

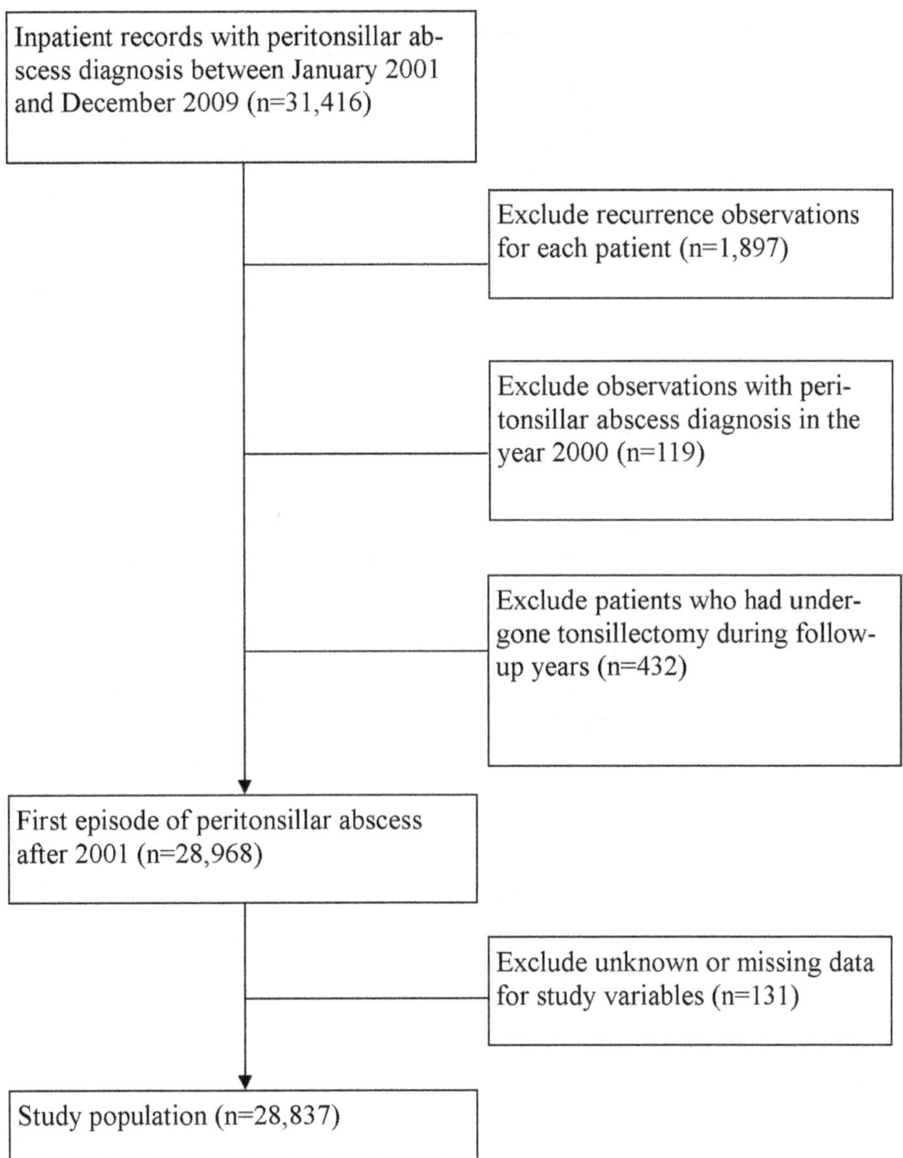

Figure 1. Assembly of PTA cohort.

Prior tonsillitis, treatment modalities and recurrent PTA

Among the 1486 recurrent PTA patients, 82.6% had prior tonsillitis compared to 69.2% in the 27351 non-recurrent cohort ($p<0.0001$). Patients with a history of prior tonsillitis ≥5 visits had a 2.82 fold increased risk of PTA recurrence (aHR: 2.82; 95% CI: 2.39–3.33). The risk of recurrent PTA among patients with 1–4 prior tonsillitis was also significantly different from those without prior tonsillitis (aHR: 1.59; 95% CI: 1.38–1.82) (Table 2).

Among 28,837 PTA patients, 14,726 (51.1%) were treated with needle aspiration, 2357 (8.2%) by incision and drainage, and 11,754 (40.8%) by intravenous antibiotics only. The aHR in patients treated with needle aspiration was 1.08 compared to those treated with incision & drainage (95% CI: 0.85–1.38) (Table 2).

Age stratification

Results of stratified analysis were presented in Table 3. Stratified by age, the risk of PTA recurrence increased significantly in patients aged ≦18 years (aHR: 2.92; 95% CI: 2.37–3.61) and 19 to 29 years (aHR: 3.50; 95% CI: 2.27–5.38) among patients with a prior history of tonsillitis ≥5 visits. The risk of recurrent PTA among patients with a prior history of 1–4 tonsillitis was significantly different from those without prior tonsillitis (aHR: 1.67; 95% CI: 1.37–2.03 in patients aged ≦18 years and aHR: 2.04; 95% CI: 1.54–2.70 in patients aged 19–29 years). In contrast, the impact of prior tonsillitis on the risk of PTA recurrence decreased among patients aged ≥30 years old (aHR: 1.76; 95% CI: 1.02–3.03 for ≥5 prior tonsillitis)and subsequently became statistically insignificant in patients with a prior history of 1–4 tonsillitis (aHR: 1.01; 95% CI: 0.75–1.36). In terms of treatment modalities, the aHR of patients treated with needle aspiration only increased in patients ≦18 years old (aHR: 1.98 [95% CI: 0.99–3.97]); however, no association was found between PTA recurrence and treatment modalities in patients older than 18 years old (Table 3). Overall, the recurrence rate in the high risk group aged under 30 years with ≥5 prior tonsillitis was 13.70%

Table 1. Characteristics of patients with peritonsillar abscess (PTA).

	Peri-tonsillar abscess			
	Total (n = 28,837)	Recurrence (n = 1,486)		
Characteristics	**No.(%)**	**No.**	**Rate (%)**	***p* value**
Age, mean (SD)	25.5(18.9)	13.8(15.6)		<0.001
Age stratification				<0.001
≥30 years	9,930(34.4)	211	2.1	
19–29 years	8,883(30.8)	296	3.3	
≦18 years	10024(34.8)	979	9.8	
Sex				0.12
Female	9,754(33.8)	530	5.4	
Male	19,083(66.2)	956	5.0	
Frequency of tonsillitis (1Y)				<0.001
0 times	8,687(30.1)	258	3.0	
1–4 times	17,324(60.1)	887	5.1	
≥5 times	2,826(9.8)	341	12.1	
Treatment				<0.001
Incision & drainage	2,357(8.2)	76	3.2	
Antibiotics only	11,754(40.8)	530	4.5	
Needle aspiration	14,726(51.1)	880	6.0	
Co-morbidity				
Diabetes	1,005(3.5)	15	1.5	<0.001
Hypertension	1,817(6.3)	35	2.0	<0.001
Cardiovascular disease	766(2.7)	17	2.2	<0.001
Renal disease	272(0.9)	6	2.2	0.03
Chronic liver disease	1,432(5.0)	35	2.4	<0.001
Cancer	259(0.9)	5	1.9	0.03

Abbreviations: SD, standard deviation.

(325/2373) compared to 4.39% (1161/26464) in the others ($p<0.001$).

Tonsillectomy performed in PTA patients in Taiwan

Tonsillectomy patients were included and the data was re-analyzed in terms of tonsillectomy rate. The overall tonsillectomy rate was 1.48% (432/29269) during our study period. In 1486 patients with PTA recurrence, tonsillectomy rate after PTA recurrence was 3.84% (57/1486).

Discussion

The present study is the first nationwide report of PTA recurrence that includes all PTA patients in the NHI dataset from 2001 to 2009. Overall, the recurrence rate is 5.15% during a 4.74-year follow-up, which is lower than most of the rates reported in other studies [8,13–19]. The reason for this may be that all of the patients with recurrence within one month from the initial episode are considered as residual diseases instead of PTA recurrence and have been excluded from our study. The residual diseases account for up to 40–47% of cases of PTA recurrence in a previous study [14,27]. The data here also show that 20.5% are residual diseases, accounting for 1.33% of all PTA subjects.

With a large, nationwide cohort, the results here confirm the association that prior tonsillitis increases the risk of PTA recurrence. There is a 2.82-fold relative increase in the risk of recurrent PTA in patients with ≥5 prior tonsillitis during the year preceding the initial abscess compared to patients who did not suffer from prior tonsillitis. The aHR is 1.59-fold higher in patients with 1–4 prior tonsillitis in the preceding year. The risk varied according to the different degrees of prior tonsillitis, and the dose response effect is statistically significant.

Before this study, results have been inconsistent in the literature. Kronenberg conducted a retrospective study and found the patients with previous history of recurrent tonsillitis had four times higher incidence of developing PTA recurrence than those without prior history (40% vs. 9.6%) [20]. However, previous episodes of tonsillitis was not clearly defined by time period and frequency. Savolainen found that patients with more than three episodes of previous tonsillitis had a significantly higher recurrence rate compared to those with three or less episodes of previous tonsillitis. Of note, most of the recurrence (17/19) happened within two months after the initial PTA diagnosis. They might contaminate the residual PTA cases and prevent the establishment of a reliable association between recurrent tonsillitis and PTA recurrence [13]. In contrast, Wolf's study demonstrated a history of recurrent tonsillitis before PTA did not have a significant increase on the recurrence rate of PTA [14]. A small retrospective cohort study was done in children under 15 years old (n = 38), but did not find any significant difference between the groups with or without a previous history of recurrent tonsillitis [19]. Again, these

Table 2. Adjusted hazard ratios for the risk of PTA recurrence.

Variable	aHR	95% CI
Age		
≥30 years	1.00	
19–29 years	1.48	1.23–1.79
≦18 years	3.92	3.31–4.64
Sex		
Female	1.00	
Male	1.13	1.01–1.26
Frequency of tonsillitis (1Y)		
0 times	1.00	
1–4 times	1.59	1.38–1.82
≥5 times	2.82	2.39–3.33
Treatment		
Incision & drainage	1.00	
Antibiotics only	0.88	0.69–1.13
Needle aspiration	1.08	0.85–1.38
Co-morbidity		
Diabetes	0.70	0.40–1.21
Hypertension	0.95	0.64–1.43
Cardiovascular disease	1.24	0.72–2.13
Renal disease	1.00	0.44–2.26
Chronic liver disease	1.10	0.77–1.56
Cancer	0.89	0.37–2.17

Abbreviations: aHR, adjusted hazard ratio; CI, confidence interval.

studies did not define the frequency of recurrent tonsillitis and might have included residual infections instead of PTA recurrence.

The most appropriate treatment of PTA has been debated for more than two decades, with lack of evidence-based studies focusing on the issues of efficacy, patient discomfort, and PTA recurrence [7,8,10]. Although most studies indicate that needle aspiration and incision and drainage provide similar efficacy for the initial PTA treatments [7,8,10,12,28,29], little evidence has been noted addressing PTA recurrence among different treatment modalities. In a retrospective study with 160 admitted patients, patients treated with needle aspiration are associated with higher PTA recurrence rate compared to those who underwent incision

Table 3. Risk of PTA recurrence stratified by age.

	≦18 years of age (n = 10,024)		19–29 years of age (n = 8,883)		≥30 years of age (n = 9,930)	
Variables	aHR	95% CI	aHR	95% CI	aHR	95% CI
Sex						
Female	1.00		1.00		1.00	
Male	1.12	0.99–1.27	1.21	0.91–1.60	1.15	0.86–1.54
Frequency of tonsillitis (1Y)						
0 times	1.00		1.00		1.00	
1–4 times	1.67	1.37–2.03	2.04	1.54–2.70	1.01	0.75–1.36
≥5 times	2.92	2.37–3.61	3.50	2.27–5.38	1.76	1.02–3.03
Treatment						
Incision & drainage	1.00		1.00		1.00	
Antibiotics only	1.54	0.76–3.10	0.89	0.55–1.23	0.93	0.61–1.44
Needle aspiration	1.98	0.99–3.97	0.94	0.66–1.33	0.97	0.57–1.44

Abbreviations: aHR, adjusted hazard ratio; CI, confidence interval.
Note: Adjusted for diabetes, hypertension, cardiovascular disease, renal disease, chronic liver disease, and cancer.

and drainage [14]. The other study revealed no differences in different modes of treatment in 38 children [19]. However, there are some flaws in these studies. First, they used phone interviews and questionnaire to obtain the final recurrence data and might be affected by recall bias. Second, they did not analyze the history of prior tonsillitis simultaneously which was considered an independent risk factor for PTA recurrence. Third, the second study had a very small case number and found no significant difference. This might be a type II error, which represented the case numbers not large enough to detect a significant difference that actually existed. To date, the present study is the most comprehensive evaluation of the treatment modality and prior tonsillitis associated with PTA recurrence accounting for confounding factors such as demographic factors and co-morbidities. The study design here can address some limitations of the previous studies [13,14,19–21]. Furthermore, the treatment modalities differ greatly between the pediatric and adult populations. In this study, we noted I&D accounted for only 1.55% in the pediatric group, compared to more than 11% in the adult population. Thus, we stratified the PTA cohorts into 3 categories, ≦18 years old, 19–29 years old and ≥30 years old, which was not done in previous studies. The aHR of needle aspiration only increased in the pediatric group (aHR: 1.98 [95% CI: 0.99–3.97]). The possible explainations for this finding may be that I&D was performed only in cooperative child or child under general anesthesia, and it would be easier to drain the abscess completely in this setting than in child underwent needle aspiration. I&D also prolonged the duration of drainage and led to less repeated drainage procedure. On the other hand, repeated drainage procedures are common in PTA patients treated with needle aspiration before the abscess resolved. However, repeated needle aspirations are often difficult to perform in children. Thus, the risk of PTA recurrence increased in pediatric patients treated with needle aspiration compared to I&D patients, but this association was not found in patients aged 19–29 and ≥30 years.

The role of tonsillectomy in the treatment of PTA remains controversial and varies widely among different countries and even within countries [12,23]. A PTA review mentions that tonsillectomy is indicated in patients with high risk of PTA recurrence, such as a prior history of tonsillitis and <40 years of age [8]. In 2000, 83% of head and neck surgeons in the UK advised interval tonsillectomy in PTA patients with a prior history of tonsillitis [17]. Recent tonsillectomy guidelines for children from the American Academy of Otolaryngology-Head and Neck Surgery (AAO-HNS) suggest that clinicians should assess the need for tonsillectomy in children with recurrent throat infections associated with peritonsillar abscess [24,25,30]. In Finland, Wiksten reported the tonsillectomy rate after peritonsillar abscess or peritonsillar cellulitis in patients aged over 6 years. Quinsy or planned interval tonsillectomy was performed on 19.9% (159/798) of patients during a 5-year follow-up period. Delayed tonsillectomy was performed on 25.5% (163/639) of those who were not initially treated with Quinsy or interval tonsillectomy [16]. On the other hand, Mak conducted a small study and observed only 2.9% (2/67) of PTA patients eventually underwent tonsillectomy in a two-year follow-up in the UK [15].

Results of our study shows that the tonsillectomy has been performed in only 432 patients (1.48%) during a 4.74-year follow-up. Furthermore, the tonsillectomy rate after PTA recurrence is 3.84% in 1486 patients with PTA recurrence. These indicate that most of the patients with initial PTA or PTA recurrence in Taiwan are treated successfully with repetition of aspiration or incision and drainage and/or antibiotics. There is no clinical practice guideline existed, and PTA treatment varies widely among different countries. To the best of our knowledge, this is the first study providing nationwide data regarding treatment modalities in PTA patients, including tonsillectomy.

The strength of this study is the use of a nationwide database in Taiwan, which provides all the PTA subjects covered by the national health insurance program (>98%) and enables a comprehensive investigation of the association between prior tonsillitis, treatment modality, and PTA recurrence. The high insurance-covered dataset also minimizes the possibility for selection bias due to loss to follow-up of the PTA subjects. Nonetheless, some limitations of this study should be addressed. First, the diagnoses of PTA, acute tonsillitis, and medical co-morbidities are completely dependent on ICD-9 codes in the administrative database that includes both in-patients and out-patients. Regarding the definition of tonsillitis, there was no clinical data like fever, cervical adenopathy, tonsillar exudate or a positive culture for group A β-hemolytic Streptococcus. Thus, validation of accuracy of diagnoses is not possible by individual medical record review. This is the limitation of administrative data analysis studies. Second, admitted patients with a principal diagnosis of peritonsillar abscess have been chosen to reduce misdiagnosis. However, this may cause selection bias that will limit the application of the findings to all PTA patients. Fortunately, the vast majority (90%) of PTA patients are treated as inpatients in Taiwan, very similar to the report from a national audit in the UK (94% of patients are managed as inpatients) whilst in some other countries such as the USA, outpatient management is preferred for the majority of patients. [11,23,28]. Since the majority of the patients are included, this study has produced relatively generalizable results. Overall, given the robust magnitude of the effects with statistical significance in this study, the limitations are unlikely to compromise the results.

In conclusion, this study confirms the associations regarding increased risk of PTA recurrence among patients with a history of prior tonsillitis in all age groups and managed by needle aspiration in pediatric subgroup. Patients younger than 30 years old with more than five prior tonsillitis episodes have the greatest risk of PTA recurrence.

Author Contributions

Conceived and designed the experiments: YPW PC. Performed the experiments: YPW MCW PC. Analyzed the data: YPW MCW. Contributed reagents/materials/analysis tools: YPW HCL PC. Contributed to the writing of the manuscript: YPW HCL PC.

References

1. Rana RS, Moonis G (2011) Head and neck infection and inflammation. Radiol Clin North Am 49: 165–182.
2. Ridder GJ, Technau-Ihling K, Sander A, Boedeker CC (2005) Spectrum and management of deep neck space infections: an 8-year experience of 234 cases. Otolaryngol Head Neck Surg 133: 709–714.
3. Huang TT, Liu TC, Chen PR, Tseng FY, Yeh TH, et al. (2004) Deep neck infection: analysis of 185 cases. Head Neck 26: 854–860.
4. Bottin R, Marioni G, Rinaldi R, Boninsegna M, Salvadori L, et al. (2003) Deep neck infection: a present-day complication. A retrospective review of 83 cases (1998–2001). Eur Arch Otorhinolaryngol 260: 576–579.
5. Epperly TD, Wood TC (1990) New trends in the management of peritonsillar abscess. Am Fam Physician 42: 102–112.
6. Steyer TE (2002) Peritonsillar abscess: diagnosis and treatment. Am Fam Physician 65: 93–96.
7. Johnson RF, Stewart MG, Wright CC (2003) An evidence-based review of the treatment of peritonsillar abscess. Otolaryngol Head Neck Surg 128: 332–343.
8. Powell J, Wilson JA (2012) An evidence-based review of peritonsillar abscess. Clin Otolaryngol 37: 136–145.

9. Al-Hussaini A, Owens D, Tomkinson A (2013) Health costs and consequences: have UK national guidelines had any effect on tonsillectomy rates and hospital admissions for tonsillitis? Eur Arch Otorhinolaryngol 270: 1959–1965.
10. Khayr W, Taepke J (2005) Management of peritonsillar abscess: needle aspiration versus incision and drainage versus tonsillectomy. Am J Ther 12: 344–350.
11. Mehanna HM, Al-Bahnasawi L, White A (2002) National audit of the management of peritonsillar abscess. Postgrad Med J 78: 545–548.
12. Johnson RF, Stewart MG (2005) The contemporary approach to diagnosis and management of peritonsillar abscess. Curr Opin Otolaryngol Head Neck Surg 13: 157–160.
13. Savolainen S, Jousimies-Somer HR, Makitie AA, Ylikoski JS (1993) Peritonsillar abscess. Clinical and microbiologic aspects and treatment regimens. Arch Otolaryngol Head Neck Surg 119: 521–524.
14. Wolf M, Even-Chen I, Kronenberg J (1994) Peritonsillar abscess: repeated needle aspiration versus incision and drainage. Ann Otol Rhinol Laryngol 103: 554–557.
15. Mak CC, Spielmann PM, Hussain SS (2012) Recurrence of peritonsillar abscess: a 2-year follow-up. Clin Otolaryngol 37: 87–88.
16. Wiksten J, Hytonen M, Pitkaranta A, Blomgren K (2012) Who ends up having tonsillectomy after peritonsillar infection? Eur Arch Otorhinolaryngol 269: 1281–1284.
17. Raut VV, Yung MW (2000) Peritonsillar abscess: the rationale for interval tonsillectomy. Ear Nose Throat J 79: 206–209.
18. Herbild O, Bonding P (1981) Peritonsillar abscess. Arch Otolaryngol 107: 540–542.
19. Wolf M, Kronenberg J, Kessler A, Modan M, Leventon G (1988) Peritonsillar abscess in children and its indication for tonsillectomy. Int J Pediatr Otorhinolaryngol 16: 113–117.
20. Kronenberg J, Wolf M, Leventon G (1987) Peritonsillar abscess: recurrence rate and the indication for tonsillectomy. Am J Otolaryngol 8: 82–84.
21. Szuhay G, Tewfik TL (1998) Peritonsillar abscess or cellulitis? A clinical comparative paediatric study. J Otolaryngol 27: 206–212.
22. Harris WE (1991) Is a single quinsy an indication for tonsillectomy? Clin Otolaryngol Allied Sci 16: 271–273.
23. Herzon FS (1995) Harris P. Mosher Award thesis. Peritonsillar abscess: incidence, current management practices, and a proposal for treatment guidelines. Laryngoscope 105: 1–17.
24. Schraff S, McGinn JD, Derkay CS (2001) Peritonsillar abscess in children: a 10-year review of diagnosis and management. Int J Pediatr Otorhinolaryngol 57: 213–218.
25. Baugh RF, Archer SM, Mitchell RB, Rosenfeld RM, Amin R, et al. (2011) Clinical practice guideline: tonsillectomy in children. Otolaryngol Head Neck Surg 144: S1–30.
26. Wen CP, Tsai SP, Chung WS (2008) A 10-year experience with universal health insurance in Taiwan: measuring changes in health and health disparity. Ann Intern Med 148: 258–267.
27. Apostolopoulos NJ, Nikolopoulos TP, Bairamis TN (1995) Peritonsillar abscess in children. Is incision and drainage an effective management? Int J Pediatr Otorhinolaryngol 31: 129–135.
28. Stringer SP, Schaefer SD, Close LG (1988) A randomized trial for outpatient management of peritonsillar abscess. Arch Otolaryngol Head Neck Surg 114: 296–298.
29. Maharaj D, Rajah V, Hemsley S (1991) Management of peritonsillar abscess. J Laryngol Otol 105: 743–745.
30. Randel A (2011) AAO-HNS Guidelines for Tonsillectomy in Children and Adolescents. Am Fam Physician 84: 566–573.

8

Factors Likely to Affect Community Acceptance of a Malaria Vaccine in Two Districts of Ghana: A Qualitative Study

Arantza Meñaca[1]*, Harry Tagbor[2], Rose Adjei[2], Constance Bart-Plange[3], Yvette Collymore[4], Antoinette Ba-Nguz[5], Kelsey Mertes[4], Allison Bingham[6]

1 Departmento de Antropología Social, Universidad Complutense de Madrid, Madrid, Spain, **2** Malaria in Pregnancy Group, Department of Community Health, School of Medical Sciences, Kwame Nkrumah University of Science and Technology, Kumasi, Ghana, **3** National Malaria Control Programme, Ghana Health Service, Accra, Ghana, **4** PATH Malaria Vaccine Initiative, Washington DC, United States of America, **5** PATH Malaria Vaccine Initiative, Nairobi, Kenya, **6** PATH Kenya, Kisumu, Kenya

Abstract

Malaria is a leading cause of morbidity and mortality among children in Ghana. As part of the effort to inform local and national decision-making in preparation for possible malaria vaccine introduction, this qualitative study explored community-level factors that could affect vaccine acceptance in Ghana and provides recommendations for a health communications strategy. The study was conducted in two purposively selected districts: the Ashanti and Upper East Regions. A total of 25 focus group discussions, 107 in-depth interviews, and 21 semi-structured observations at Child Welfare Clinics were conducted. Malaria was acknowledged to be one of the most common health problems among children. While mosquitoes were linked to the cause and bed nets were considered to be the main preventive method, participants acknowledged that no single measure prevented malaria. The communities highly valued vaccines and cited vaccination as the main motivation for taking children to Child Welfare Clinics. Nevertheless, knowledge of specific vaccines and what they do was limited. While communities accepted the idea of minor vaccine side effects, other side effects perceived to be more serious could deter families from taking children for vaccination, especially during vaccination campaigns. Attendance at Child Welfare Clinics after age nine months was limited. Observations at clinics revealed that while two different opportunities for counseling were offered, little attention was given to addressing mothers' specific concerns and to answering questions related to child immunization. Positive community attitudes toward vaccines and the understanding that malaria prevention requires a comprehensive approach would support the introduction of a malaria vaccine. These attitudes are bolstered by a well-established child welfare program and the availability in Ghana of active, flexible structures for conveying health information to communities. At the same time, it would be important to improve the quality of Child Welfare Clinic services, particularly in relation to communication around vaccination.

Editor: David J. Diemert, The George Washington University Medical Center, United States of America

Funding: This work was funded by the PATH Malaria Vaccine Initiative (MVI), Washington, DC, with support from the Bill & Melinda Gates Foundation and the ExxonMobil Foundation. MVI had a role in overall project management and in writing of the manuscript and decision to publish. The views expressed herein do not necessarily reflect the views of PATH or its funders.

Competing Interests: The authors have declared that no competing interests exist.

* Email: arantzamenaca@gmail.com

Introduction

Malaria is one of the main causes of mortality among children younger than five years in Africa, where approximately half a million children died from malaria in 2010 [1]. The disease also has severe effects on pregnant women [2] and people living with HIV [3]. The Ghana Ministry of Health describes the disease as the leading cause of morbidity and mortality in the country, accounting for more than one-third of all outpatient cases reported each year, 20 percent to 30 percent of deaths in children younger than five, and 11 percent of maternal deaths [4]. While no malaria vaccine has ever been licensed for use, the global health community is working toward a 2015 time frame for a policy recommendation for a first-generation product that could be deployed for use with existing interventions to help protect young children against the deadly *Plasmodium falciparum* malaria parasite [5].

In order to ensure timely access to such a vaccine, some African countries have begun to build a base of evidence that can help to accelerate national decision-making, so that when a malaria vaccine is recommended for use, countries are also prepared to make decisions on whether to introduce a particular vaccine to complement the existing arsenal of malaria control tools [5,6]. African policymakers and their international partners have identified the need for a range of data to inform the decision-making process, including data on perceptions of vaccines and malaria [7]. Data on community perceptions would also inform the development of a communications strategy to help ensure that the introduction of a partially efficacious malaria vaccine [8] does not jeopardize continued use of current malaria control measures or reduce confidence in vaccines for other diseases currently in use. Other qualitative studies on community perceptions of malaria and vaccines have been conducted, including in Kenya [9,10], Mozambique [11], Burkina Faso [12], and in a malaria vaccine trial setting in Ghana, Kintampo [13]. This article provides further data from two non-trial settings in different provinces of Ghana. The study was guided by the following research questions:

1. How is malaria prevention (and treatment) understood and undertaken in the communities?
2. What is the knowledge and acceptance of existing vaccines in the study communities? How do they affect vaccination practices?
3. What are the characteristics of the discourse in the communities about the possibility of a malaria vaccine?
4. What is the decision-making process with regard to child health within families in the study?
5. What audiences and communication channels have been used in previous health information campaigns? Which were the most successful campaigns?

Ghana malaria and immunization context

Ghana is among the ten countries in the world with the highest malaria morbidity rates and among the 15 with the highest malaria mortality rates [1]. Since the 1950s, the Ministry of Health and the Ghana Health Service have adopted various strategies to control malaria in the population, with special emphasis on children younger than five and pregnant women. These strategies include the distribution of insecticide-treated bed nets door to door (including hanging of the nets), and through schools, antenatal care, child welfare clinics, and public health institutions. Strategies also include the adoption of the Home Management of Malaria program for children younger than five and the use of intermittent preventive treatment of malaria in pregnancy (IPTp) [4]. According to the 2011 Multiple Indicator Cluster Survey, only 51 percent of households owned a mosquito net (whether treated or untreated), and only 39 percent of children younger than five and 33 percent of pregnant women slept under a treated mosquito net the night before the survey [14].

The Expanded Programme on Immunization (EPI) was introduced in Ghana in 1978. In accordance with the World Health Organization and United Nations Children's Fund guidelines for vaccinating children, the Ghana EPI calendar includes seven types of vaccines for 11 diseases (Table 1). Of these, vaccines for rotavirus and pneumococcal disease and a booster for measles were introduced in 2012. Vaccine coverage in Ghana is among the highest in sub-Saharan Africa. The percentage of children ages 12 months to 23 months who are fully vaccinated (against tuberculosis [with Bacillus Calmette-Guérin], diphtheria-tetanus-pertussis, polio, and measles) increased in the past 20 years in Ghana from 47 percent in 1988 to 84 percent in 2011 [14,15]. EPI is conducted mainly through programs of the Child Welfare Clinic (CWCs), which are operated at established health centers or hospitals and at outreach clinics. Intensive campaigns are also organized to improve immunization rates and to respond to disease outbreaks. Two immunization campaigns were held in 2012, prior to the start of data collection for this study: the national immunization days for polio in March and May [16] and emergency vaccination in the Upper East Region during the same period, following a cerebrospinal meningitis (CSM) outbreak that caused 23 deaths in the first two months of the year [17]. A CSM mass vaccination campaign for meningococcal meningitis in the three northern regions in October followed the first phase of data collection for this study [18].

Ghana is one of a few countries in Africa that has successfully implemented a health insurance system. The National Health Insurance Scheme (NHIS), which covers primary care services and the cost of a range of basic drugs, has intentionally low fees, including a yearly registration fee of two USD for individuals younger than 18 years (if both parents are subscribed), people older than 70 years, and the needy. Pregnant women are exempt from any financial contribution to the NHIS [19]. CWC visits, including routine vaccines, are free for all children, even if they are not registered in the NHIS.

Methods

Sites

Two districts were purposively selected for this study. The selection took into account the important ethnic, religious, geographic, climatic, and malaria transmission heterogeneity of Ghana.

In the district selected for the Ashanti Region, located in a southern area of tropical forest, the majority of the population is Asante (Akan), the country's main ethnic group [20]. They are also Christian and year-round subsistence farmers. In the district selected for the Upper East Region–a savannah area at the border with Burkina Faso–the predominant ethnic group is Frafra (Mole Dagbon), the country's second main ethnic group [20]. In contrast to the Ashanti district, this area has a more heterogeneous religious profile, including Christianity (mainly Catholicism), Islam, and Animism. As opposed to year-round farming, the single farming season coincides with the rainy season from March/April to September/October. The rest of the year, part of the population migrates to other regions.

In general, malaria in Ghana is hyperendemic, with year-round transmission. However, there is a pronounced seasonal variation in the northern part of the country, where the typical duration of the intense malaria transmission season is about seven months, coinciding with the rainy season [21]. Malaria transmission is therefore more seasonal in the Upper East Region site than in the Ashanti Region site.

Noteworthy public health interventions in the Upper East Region referenced by study participants included the vaccination campaigns for CSM held in 2012 [17,18]; the filariasis eradication project held between 2001 and 2011 [22]; and the pilot introduction of intermittent preventive treatment of malaria in infants (IPTi) that began with implementation studies in 2007 and continued during data collection for this study [23]. No specific health program of relevance for this research was found in the Ashanti Region.

Within the two districts studied, four urban and rural communities were selected to enhance the diversity of the samples, and the public health facilities that served those communities were also identified. Three hospitals in the Ashanti Region and one hospital and three health centers in the Upper East Region were selected. Semi-structured observations were conducted at the hospitals and CWCs.

Participant selection and data collection

The qualitative methodology used in this study has its roots in anthropological research. Given the important differences that are known to exist between people's normative discourses, their actual practices, and their assessment of these practices and knowledge [24], researchers used a diversity of tools to focus both on discourse and behavior:

- **Focus group discussions** permitted a rapid assessment of the normative discourse in the communities regarding malaria and vaccine perceptions. In order to promote practical

Table 1. Ghana vaccination calendar 2013.

Month	0	1	2	3	9	18
Visit to CWC	1st visit	2nd visit	3rd visit	4th visit	10th visit	19th visit
BCG	♦[1]					
Polio	●[1]	●	●	●		
Pentavalent[2]		■	■	■		
Pneumococcal		■[3]	■[3]	■[3]		
Rotavirus		●[3]	●[3]			
Measles					■	■[3]
Yellow fever					■	

BCG: Bacillus Calmette-Guérin for tuberculosis; CWC: Child Welfare Clinic.
Administration path: ♦ Intradermic, ● Oral, ■ Intramuscular.
[1]If the baby was delivered in a hospital/health center, it is given at birth.
[2]Pentavalent includes diphtheria-tetanus-pertussis (DTP), hepatitis B, and *Haemophilus influenzae* type b. It was introduced in 2002 as a substitute to DTP.
[3]Introduced in February 2012 (second dose of measles) and May 2012 (rotavirus and pneumococcal disease).

participatory debate, discussion around vignettes or stories and free-listing and sorting techniques were included in their design (Tables S1, S2).

- **In-depth interviews** allowed researchers to gain deeper insight into the attitudes, knowledge, contradictions, and gaps in information of different participants. These interviews also provided preliminary data on malaria and vaccination practices within the community (Tables S3, S4, S5, S6).
- **Semi-structured observations** added data on practical matters that did not surface in interviews or discussions, perhaps because they were considered too obvious for discussion or seemed to contradict the normative views. Research assistants observed the interactions during the provision of routine childhood immunization services and wrote ethnographic notes on previously defined themes (Table S7).

The triangulation of data from interviews, group discussions, and observations allowed for deeper insight into community members' perceptions related to vaccinations and their actual practices and experiences at immunization clinics. This approach also permitted the analysis of provider-client communication practices within the context of vaccination services–an important perspective given that community confidence in the quality of vaccine delivery has been shown to influence use of immunization services [25,26,27,28].

A purposive sample (Table S8) was designed for the selection of study participants, using the following criteria: those who make decisions on whether or not to vaccinate young children (parents and other caregivers), and those within communities who influence childhood vaccination decisions (health administrators, health system workers involved in infant and child care, and relevant community members, including teachers, religious leaders, political and traditional authorities, and traditional healers). Mothers of small children were recruited at vaccination clinics and directly in the communities, and some fathers were also selected through previously interviewed mothers (Table 2).

Data were collected between May 2012 and mid-January 2013 by four research assistants with experience in qualitative data collection and knowledge of the local languages (Twi and Gruni). Prior to data collection, research assistants were trained, data collection tools piloted, and community stakeholders informed about the research. The translation/transcription of the data collected was completed by the research assistants and double-checked by the site coordinators.

The final sample size across both regions was 286 participants, including 107 in-depth interviewees and 179 in group discussions. This number does not include the semi-structured observations at vaccination clinics, where the number of participants was difficult to determine (Table 2). In the Ashanti Region, all planned collection events were completed. In the Upper East Region, unforeseen delays in the field limited the number of collection events in the scheduled phase (between May and October 2012). In order to achieve conclusive results, preliminary data analysis was conducted in November 2012 to assess the quality and main gaps of the data collected so far, and a short, intensive phase of data collection was held in early January 2013 to ensure the saturation of data for the key points of the research.

Analysis and interpretation were an iterative and flexible part of the anthropological data collection process [29]. Regular meetings occurred throughout the process between those in charge of data collection and those in charge of analysis. These meetings allowed the discussion of perceived relevant themes at the different sites, the development of new questions based on the interpretation of previous data, and the debate of team preconceptions, unexpected findings, contradictions, and doubts. Using Atlas.ti 7, a theme-based, iterative approach was employed to analyze the data. A preliminary list of codes was created based on the topics of the research, and the list was enriched with new categories during analysis. At different stages during the analysis, the research team held discussions in order to clarify and arrive at a consensus on coding, merging categories, and the final comparative analysis and narrative of the findings.

Ethics statement

Ethical approvals were obtained from the Committee on Human Research, Publication and Ethics of the School of Medical Sciences KNUST, Kumasi, Ghana. 'Exempt' approval status was also obtained from the PATH Research Ethics Committee in Seattle, Washington, USA. This meant that the research was deemed exempt from a full research ethics committee review because it fell into a low-risk category, as defined in the US federal

Table 2. Study groups and number of collection events.

Tool	Study group	Ashanti Region	Upper East Region	Total
Group discussions	Mothers	8	6	**14**
	Men/Relevant community members	8	3	**11**
In-depth interviews	Health administrators	4	4	**8**
	Health professionals	12	6	**18**
	Formal and informal leaders	16	6	**22**
	Mothers	24	15	**39**
	Fathers	12	8	**20**
Semi-structured observations in vaccination clinics		12	9	**21**

regulations. As approved by both ethics committees, participants provided verbal informed consent. Interviewers obtained verbal consent by reading aloud a written script that had been approved by both ethics committees. Verbal rather than written informed consent was preferred in order to avoid the possible negative influence of a written consent on rapport between research assistants and participants. After the agreement of respondents, verbal consent was voice recorded prior to each in-depth interview or focus group discussion.

Results

Malaria perceptions

In both regions, study participants considered malaria to be one of the most common health problems among children. Participants differentiated between mild and severe episodes of malaria and described malaria as a very serious disease that could lead to death. Children, followed by pregnant women and the elderly, were considered to be the groups most at risk of contracting malaria.

Study participants used multiple terms to refer to malaria, some of them related to specific symptoms of the disease (Table 3). In the Ashanti Region, the preferred terms were *malaria* and *fever*. While most study participants considered *malaria* and *fever* to be terms for the same condition, they recognized differences between the two. Three contrasting but overlapping meanings were found for *fever*. In some cases, *fever* was associated with a rise in temperature, whereas *malaria* was associated with other perceived symptoms, such as paleness, yellowish eyes, and green vomit. In other cases, *fever* was linked to mild malaria, whereas *malaria* was linked to severe cases. Other participants associated *fever* with yellowness in the eyes and urine. In the Upper East Region, the preferred terms were the local ones that emphasized high temperature (*entolegaban*) and feeling cold from fever (*ooro*).

Local terminology and its use revealed that malaria overlapped with different locally recognized conditions in each of the districts. In the Ashanti Region, the main overlap was between malaria, as referred to when talking of *fever* and *atiridee* (yellowish eyes), and yellow fever (commonly called *jaundice*). Both diseases shared descriptions of yellowish eyes and urine. On the other hand, in the Upper East Region, the main overlap was between malaria and pneumonia, as they shared key symptoms used in local terminologies and the cold weather as a cause.

Mosquitoes were considered to be the main cause of malaria, with dirt and stagnant water–associated with mosquito breeding–seen as indirect causes. These two ideas were generally shared with health professionals and conveyed during health talks. In most cases, though, people from the communities did not strictly separate causes of malaria from causes of disease in general. They also did not isolate malaria-specific preventive practices from general hygiene and healthy practices. In this regard, other causes mentioned were the presence of houseflies around food and, in some cases, the eating of very cold food. Participants from the Upper East Region said that wet weather–particularly linked to *ooro*–contributed to malaria. In the Ashanti Region, *malaria*, and especially *fever*, was occasionally associated with the consumption of unripe fruits and oily food.

There was consensus that no one preventive measure stopped malaria transmission completely. At both sites, bed nets were the most cited preventive tool, but certain factors were seen to limit

Table 3. Malaria terms.

	Ashanti Region	Upper East Region
Most frequent	*Malaria*	*Ooro* (feeling cold from fever)
	Fever	*Entolegaban* (high temperature)
	Whuraye (paleness)	*Zuwaka* (headache)
	Atiridee (yellowish eyes)	*Malaria*
	Ebunu (green vomit)	*Fever*
Least frequent		*Duusi Ban* (mosquito sickness)

their use. Participants said they were not distributed for free as frequently as they would have liked and in some houses, three or more people shared the same net, making it very hot inside. Participants also cited general hygienic measures, whether indirectly associated with mosquito breeding or not, illustrating the wide range of measures taken for general sickness prevention. While participants occasionally mentioned other malaria prevention strategies such as the use of sprays and coils, price limited the use of sprays, while coils were seen as a fire hazard and linked to some discomfort. In most interviews, it was only when prompted (and not in all cases) that people remembered the preventive use of the drug sulfadoxine-pyrimethamine in pregnant women and the programs in trial areas for IPTi and IPTc (intermittent preventive treatment of malaria in children).

I(interviewer): Are all (preventive) measures effective? (...)
R(respondent)6: It does not matter whether we use these measures we can still get sick because mosquitoes bite us outside even before we sleep so all that we have to do is protect ourselves. (...)
R5: When you do all of them, they are effective.
R2: When you do them, the malaria can still come but will not be severe. (...)
R8: I use both bed net and coil but mosquitoes still bit us.
R6: The net is effective but the mosquitoes can still bite us.
(Ashanti Region, group discussion with relevant women)

Vaccine perceptions

Study participants universally acknowledged vaccination as the main activity conducted within the health system to promote child health. However, the perception of vaccination was closely related to two other concepts: injections and the package of activities at CWCs. The issue was especially evident when people talked about malaria, as treatment in hospitals for severe malaria often includes injections highly valued by community participants. *Pania* in Gruni (Upper East Region) and *panie* in Twi (Ashanti Region) were the words for both vaccine and injection. In order to specify that the conversation was only about vaccines, it was necessary to add the notion of protection in Gruni (*adin gu pania*); whereas, in the Ashanti Region, vaccines were referred to as injections for children (*nkora panie*). The perception was that both vaccines and injections fought children's diseases–that injections fought diseases that were already "visible," while vaccines either fought diseases that were "hidden," or prepared the body to fight in case the disease was coming.

I: What is your general perception about nkora panie?
R: It is good because, when a child has a sickness, the panie is able to take it away...it helps the child to become healthy. (...)
I: And what benefits do you get from the nkora paine?
R: Nkora panie... the benefit I get is, when the child is sick you will not know, so the vaccines are able to cure the child of the sickness...
(Ashanti Region, interview with a mother)
I: when the drugs (vaccine) enter into the body, how does it protect the child?
R: the drugs poisons the blood so when the virus or the bacteria come, it cannot affect the child.
(Ashanti Region, interview with a political leader)

The understanding of what vaccines do ranged from "fighting diseases" in general to partial knowledge of the diseases they protected against. When discussing the concept of 'efficacy', some participants understood that vaccines had helped to eliminate some diseases from the community, whereas other participants saw vaccines as diminishing the severity of the disease.

R: (...) the kasua (measles) that could have attacked the child and you will lose the child when it is serious, if the child is given this vaccine, this time even if it attacks the child, it cannot get to the state where you lose the child.
(Upper East Region, interview with a mother)

While health professionals directly involved in vaccination programscould name the required vaccines for children in Ghana, this was not the case for other study participants. Some community members could specify a number of them, while others recognized that there were many vaccines. The most common response was somewhere in the middle: while most mothers did not know the specific illnesses the vaccines were for, they could distinguish them through the mode of administration, injection site, or the age of the child at vaccination. As such, differences were seen if the vaccines were given orally or by injection, if they were given in the arm or the leg, or if they were given at one, two, three, or nine months of age.

In naming vaccines against common childhood diseases, the measles vaccine was the most widely known, followed by polio and tetanus. Few study participants mentioned hepatitis B or *Haemophilus* vaccines. Knowledge of vaccines introduced a few months before was slightly higher and was associated with information provided on the radio and at CWCs.

R3: I took my child to the clinic recently and they injected both left and right thighs that pneumonia and diarrhea. They used to inject only one leg and then, the following month we go back. But they have realized that the diarrhea is disturbing the children a lot that is why they inject the two thighs. That is what they told me before injecting my child.
(Upper East Region, group discussion with mothers)

Participants could also distinguish between vaccines based on whether they were administered at CWCs or through campaigns, as would be the case with polio, CSM, and yellow fever vaccines. When prompted, participants also mentioned vaccines for pregnant women (tetanus) and for adults (campaigns included H1N1 in 2010). In the Upper East Region, participants referred to other non-vaccine prevention activities, such as IPTi and the filariasis eradication program. Vitamin A supplementation was not mentioned.

All study participants acknowledged that vaccines had minor side effects and that these side effects were a negative aspect of an intervention that otherwise had important benefits. Minor side effects were seen to include general discomfort, high body temperature, and swelling. Mothers talked or complained openly about these side effects during semi-structured observations. In addition, health professionals sometimes told mothers what to do in case they occurred, and mothers consulted providers on ways to alleviate them. For the majority of our study participants, these minor side effects were not seen as a reason to stop vaccinating children.

Narratives also suggest that when families associate a vaccine with the occurrence of a serious health problem, they may choose not to have their children vaccinated. In some cases, families seemed to link more serious side effects with questions about the expertise of nurses. For example, in the Ashanti Region, many community members associated vaccines–especially the perceived failure of health professionals to properly administer vaccines–with paralysis. This was evident in the Upper East Region with regard to the CSM vaccine. Participants also linked drugs distributed for filariasis to unspecific, "very serious negative effects" and even deaths. In one example, an Upper East father spoke of "the drug they brought to vaccinate people against elephantiasis".

I: Can you mention the vaccine that has these negative effects?
R: I have never experienced it in my children but what I have witnessed before is the drug they brought to vaccine people against elephantiasis. For that one, the side effects are nothing to talk about. In fact, I insulted the nurses and prevented my mother from taking it.
I: Are some vaccines better than others?
R: Yes most vaccines are better than the vaccine for elephantiasis because it disturbed a lot of people. But for the chills and fever in children after vaccinations, it is normal.
(Upper East Region, father)

Rumors were said to have influenced community members' perceptions of vaccination. However, rumors had been associated mostly with vaccines administered during vaccination campaigns as opposed to vaccines administered as part of established services at CWCs. More specifically, study participants spoke of rumors of deaths related to the H1N1 campaign, a school vaccination campaign for polio in the Ashanti Region, and filariasis drug distribution in the Upper East Region. The radio was one of the main sources for the rumors the participants had heard.

Child Welfare Clinics

Child Welfare Clinics offer a well-established package of activities for children that includes registration for clinic services, vaccination, the administration of other preventive drugs, weighing, and health talks (Table 4). On occasions mainly related to droughts in the north of the country, CWCs have also been a point for distribution of nutritious food for children. Women are expected to bring their children to the CWC monthly up to the age of five, and the services are free of charge. Perceptions, evaluation, and acceptance of vaccines are strongly linked to experiences at CWCs.

Motivation to attend the clinics was said to include overall appreciation for the value of vaccination and weighing. This appreciation was mixed with a sense of obligation that was reinforced every time women were asked at the CWC to give reasons for missing visits. In addition to the sense of appreciation and obligation, community members stressed that they were motivated by the fact that food was sometimes distributed, especially in the Upper East Region.

CWCs also provided opportunities to socialize and do business. Women dressed in fine clothes and brought money with them, and various businesses were evident. Some people took photos and others sold food and items for babies, including clothes, weighing pants (designed to attach the baby to the scale), baby powder, napkins, and baby bottles. In addition, some people offered pomades, health cards, and protectors for the cards. Nurses at both sites participated in the trading, even though there were references to the fact that they were forbidden from doing business at the CWC.

Most of the costs incurred by mothers during CWC visits were related to socializing. In the Upper East Region and in the urban health centers in the Ashanti Region, some women spent money only on the things they bought around the CWC and in preparing themselves for the visit (e.g., buying clothes and having their hair braided). Some also spent money on transportation, though most women walked to the clinics. Though services were generally supposed to be free, women visiting rural outreach clinics in the Ashanti Region were charged 0.1 USD. The money was provided as an incentive to the Community-Based Agents (CBAs)–volunteers trained by the health system who helped to organize the clinics and who were generally responsible for weighing. In some cases, the money was collected to pay town criers or information centers that helped to mobilize the mothers. All the costs, whether related to socializing or for health services, were seen in the communities as constraints to full CWC attendance.

Time spent at the clinics was another cost considered by mothers. While nurses preferred that women arrive early in the morning, they usually made the first arrivals wait until there were enough women to start the activities. From the structured observations, it was calculated that women who arrived early generally spent between one and two hours at the clinic. When logistical issues claimed the health workers' attention, some women spent even more time at the CWC.

While women were supposed to go monthly to the CWC for the first five years of the child's life, most did not go for that long. Significantly, as community members and health professionals noted, parents generally stopped bringing their children to the CWC after the perceived end of the vaccination schedule at nine months. After that, time and cost were given as reasons not to continue with the other CWC activities, which were less valued than vaccines. It was exceptional to find a woman who had continued to bring her child to the CWC for five years.

I: so at what age are vaccines when given is better off?
R: just as you are here talking but usually, from birth, up to nine months. It is usually the last time of giving the children pania. We are supposed to continue sending the children there but I do not do it because of time.

(Upper East Region, in-depth interview with a mother)

CWC settings offered two opportunities for counseling and providing vaccine information. Nurses delivered a health talk at the beginning of the session or when they considered there were enough women gathered, and an opportunity for more personal counseling came during vaccination. During the semi-structured observations, health talks were given at almost every session in the Ashanti Region, but they occurred in fewer than half of the observations in the Upper East Region. The main topic for health education was child nutrition–exclusive breastfeeding in the first six months and nutritious foods afterward. Other health talks focused on health programs that were being established. For example, pneumococcal and rotavirus vaccines, introduced in May, were topics of some of the health talks observed in June-July. In these talks, nurses explained the conditions vaccines prevented–pneumonia and diarrhea–and their seriousness, and the number of doses and path of administration of the vaccines. They also encouraged women to "take these new vaccines seriously".

Direct counseling for mothers was brief and irregular, and women tended not to ask many questions. In some cases, the lack of interaction was associated with the heavy workload of nurses

Table 4. Child Welfare Clinic structure.

	Waiting area	Registering	Weighing	Vaccination
Average time spent at station.	Most of the total 1–2 hours.	Less than 5 minutes.	Less than 5 minutes.	Less than 5 minutes.
	Health talk lasted 10–20 minutes.			
What happened at the station?	1. Health talk at some centers.	1. Information was registered in Registration Books and Child Welfare Booklets.	All the children were weighed. (In outreach clinics, this activity is organized by CBAs.)	Administration of vaccines, vitamin A supplementation, IPTi (only in Upper East Region).
	2. Waiting before the activities began and between activities.	2. Mothers were directed to vaccination area if necessary.		
What health information was given?	Health talks about breastfeeding/new health programs.	N/A	Comments on whether the child is growing properly/advice on breastfeeding (though not given to every mother).	Partial information on vaccines and side effects (though not given to every mother).
What discussion occurred?	1. Nurses asked mothers if they had questions/doubts.	Discussion centered on missed sessions, delayed visits, and premature visits.	Discussion centered on missed sessions, delayed visits, and premature visits.	Discussion centered on missed sessions, delayed visits, and premature visits.
	2. Mothers generally did not ask many questions.			
What comments did mothers have about the services at the station?	Mothers saw it as a place for social gathering and trading things for babies.	Mothers had no comments on this area.	Weighing appreciated by some mothers. CWCs are informally called "weighing."	Mothers said that vaccination was the main reason for the clinic visit.
What comments did providers have about mothers who were at this station?	Complaints when patients did not respond when called.	Complaints about missed visits and people using different CWCs.	No comments.	No comments.
Average time spent discussing immunization/child vaccine issues.	Irregular: information was only given in the months around the implementation of a new vaccine (full health talk).	N/A	N/A	Brief and irregular (less than 5 minutes).

CBA: Community-Based Agent; CWC: Child Welfare Clinic; IPTi: intermittent preventive treatment of malaria in infants.

who were feeling the pressure to get everything done, and information was generally incomplete. Nurses prioritized instructions on what to do in case side effects occurred. Information on the diseases the vaccines targeted and on the remaining vaccines in the schedule was provided less often. During a majority of the observed vaccinations in the Ashanti Region, the nurses did not provide information on the vaccines they were giving. In the Upper East Region, some women received information on the vaccines, whereas others were only told where on the child's body the vaccine was to be administered.

During the semi-structured observations, observers noted that nurses often reprimanded mothers for a variety of reasons. Nurses would scold mothers for skipping one or more clinic visits or for giving water to the children when they had been told to breastfeed exclusively. In other situations, nurses would castigate women whom they thought were being impolite. At the same time, none of the mothers complained about nurses being disrespectful. Only some Upper East opinion leaders and Ashanti nurses said the quality of health professionals' attitudes toward community members deterred women from going to the CWC.

Malaria vaccine

Even as community members and health professionals agreed that it would be important to have a vaccine against malaria, some participants had the perception that a malaria vaccine already existed. This confusion was associated with limited knowledge of specific vaccines: the perception that vaccines as a whole fought against childhood diseases in general; the perception that there were no clear differences between vaccines and injections, and between vaccines and other preventive strategies such as IPT; and the overlap between malaria and other diseases with fever as a symptom for which there are vaccines available (e.g., yellow fever in the Ashanti Region and pneumonia in the Upper East Region).

R4: because malaria is rampant, they vaccinate the child the first day you give birth to the child. (...)
I: ok. who should be given vaccines?
R4: as for vaccination, everybody can be given injection. For example, if I am sick of malaria and goes to the hospital, they give me injection.
I: I am talking about injection they give during vaccination period.
R4: they normally give those injections to the children.
I: what about adults?
R4: they don't give some to adult but they give to the pregnant women. When you go for antenatal they give you malaria vaccination and yellow fever and tetanus.
(Ashanti Region, group discussion with relevant women)

When discussing the possibility of a malaria vaccine with partial efficacy, there was consensus among study participants that people were unlikely to stop using other preventive measures. Data presented so far suggest three reasons for this consensus. Firstly, many participants saw vaccines as only reducing the severity of disease and never providing complete protection. Secondly, community members were already combining different preventive methods–mainly bed nets and hygienic measures–because no single measure was seen as totally efficacious. These factors suggest that community members are open to the use of a combination of methods. Moreover, bed nets and hygienic measures were considered to be good not only for malaria but also to prevent the nuisance of mosquito bites (bed nets) and to prevent many other diseases (hygiene). The prevalent holistic understanding of prevention associated with these two measures suggests communities will continue with them even if there is a malaria vaccine.

R: the pania is to prevent my child from malaria so it does not mean that I should allow dirt to take over my entire house. So I will continue to clean my home, sleep in the nets with my children and all the rest to prevent other diseases.
(Upper East Region, in-depth interview with a mother)

When discussing the possible mode of administration for a future malaria vaccine, community members indicated that they generally look to health professionals and vaccine developers to decide how vaccines are to be administered. However, when asked about their preferred route of administration, opinion was divided. Some considered injections painful and said that too many vaccines were administered this way. These study participants, most of them in the Ashanti Region, generally preferred the oral method of delivery. Others, including traditional leaders in the Upper East Region, saw injections to be more efficacious, as they go "straight to the blood" and cannot be vomited up, as sometimes happened with "malaria drugs" and the rotavirus vaccine.

Finally, many people asked if a malaria vaccine would be available for adults in addition to children, as is the case with other preventive medicine campaigns. They wondered whether a future malaria vaccine would be introduced in CWCs and only given to children, or if, following the CSM model in the Upper East Region, it would be available for adults as well through campaigns in the communities.

Communication preferences

Community members highlighted four main avenues for receiving health information: via radio, information vans, health talks, and trusted relevant people in the community. The communication tools least mentioned were posters and television. In urban areas, people preferred radio and information vans, whereas in rural areas, people preferred community durbars (gatherings of chiefs and people of the community), and they trusted their leaders and community health volunteers to provide the relevant information.

Each community described different formal community processes for disseminating health information. In some places, the health system contacted traditional leaders directly, whereas in others, health volunteers (including CBAs) were the ones to deliver the message. Village Health Committees were active in some places but not in others. And while some villages used local information centers to transmit messages, in others, leaders preferred to use the town crier or gong beater. Coordination with the health professionals involved in community sensitization was seen to be necessary in order to determine the best information channel in a given area.

In addition to formal processes, certain informal information networks existed. When deciding on vaccine use, different women stressed that they valued the opinions of other women who had previous experience with the vaccine. Women also said they valued advice on health issues when it came from people involved in the health field, including CBAs, volunteers of previous programs, and traditional birth attendants.

Health administrators and health professionals described the actual strategy of the Ghana Health Service to transfer communication from its headquarters to districts and communities. The picture portrayed seemed to clearly address participants' preferences: to allow the flexibility needed at the community level; to include communication both with the relevant leaders and, through them, with male heads of households, who had the ultimate responsibility to make decisions; and with mothers, who made the day-to-day decisions, especially those regarding routine trips to the CWC (Table 5).

Discussion

The study identified a number of factors that could facilitate the introduction of a licensed malaria vaccine. They include the need to build on the generally positive attitude toward vaccines in the communities, an understanding that malaria prevention requires a comprehensive approach, the availability of well-established programs to deliver new vaccines, the need to increase and improve communication around childhood vaccination, and the identification of flexible, active health communication structures and processes to disseminate information.

Building on positive attitudes toward vaccines

The findings suggest that communities placed a high value on vaccines in general and were positive about the idea of a malaria vaccine. This positive attitude is the general trend seen in other studies conducted in other districts in Ghana [13] and in other African countries [9–12]. Community members acknowledged that malaria was one of the most common and serious diseases,

Table 5. Information channels and activities.

Channel	Source	Target audience	Activities
Formal structures	Ghana Health	Local health	Letters
	Service	professionals	Workshops
		General population	Television
			Radio
			Posters
	Local health	General population	Local radio stations
	professionals	(urban)	Vans
		Communities (rural)	Workshops for relevant people (e.g., CBAs and local authorities)
		Mothers (urban and rural)	CWCs: health talks and direct interaction
Community channels	Local authorities, CBAs, etc.	Communities (men and women)	Durbars Community meetings
	CBAs, other relevant health-related people	Mothers	Informal interactions

CBA: Community-Based Agent; CWC: Child Welfare Clinic.

especially among children, and they showed a positive attitude toward new interventions that might help in the control of the disease, as had been previously reported for IPTi in Ghana and other African countries [30] and IPTc [31]. Significantly, study participants considered vaccination the most important activity at the CWCs.

Understanding that malaria prevention requires a comprehensive approach

Findings suggest that a malaria vaccine would not affect the use of other preventive measures. Firstly, current practices reflect a holistic approach to household health and disease prevention [30,32,33] that includes the use of bed nets as well as general hygiene practices, not only for malaria prevention but also to address other health-related concerns–bed nets to address the nuisance of mosquito bites and hygiene practices to prevent multiple diseases. Communities also acknowledged that none of the methods used is totally effective and understood the value of employing different preventive methods at the same time.

Findings also suggest that community members would not see the concept of partial efficacy as new or exclusive to a possible malaria vaccine. While for some, vaccines had been effective in eradicating certain diseases from their communities, for others a disease could be contracted even if a person was vaccinated against it. Community perceptions of vaccines as giving just partial protection were already reported in the 1980s and 1990s in many different countries of Africa and Asia [34]. Findings in this study suggest that this way of understanding the role of vaccines is facilitating more recent community acceptance of new vaccines such as those for pneumococcal disease and rotavirus, and could also facilitate the acceptance of a partially efficacious malaria vaccine in the future.

Taking advantage of well-established and packaged child welfare programs

The package of services offered at the CWCs appears to provide the best context within which to implement a new vaccine strategy. CWCs are a well-established program that is widely known and respected in communities and regularly attended by mothers and children–at least during the first nine months of a child's life. On the other hand, rumors were found to influence attendance at vaccination campaigns. The introduction in the last few years of new vaccines and malaria control strategies and the limited number of concerns generated prior to this study could be regarded as an example of how well-established routines and the use of a trusted program considered beneficial by the community can help to ensure the acceptance of new practices [35,36]. Further, a new intervention would be more likely to be accepted if its administration path, its delivery calendar, and its side effects are similar to those of existing interventions.

Improving the quality of service and communication around vaccination

Even though CWCs provide a good setting in which to deliver a new vaccine, some limits were observed. Findings in this study show that with most children's visits ending after the age of nine months, the administration of additional vaccine doses past this time period could pose challenges. Thus, the introduction of the measles booster at 18 months may need to be monitored. The high rates of attendance at CWCs both for antenatal care during pregnancy and during the first nine months of a child's life show that a monthly routine for pregnant women and newborns could be successful for a limited time before [37] and after birth (Ghana's EPI coverage is among the highest in Africa [38,39]). At the same time, a different strategy may need to be found in order to achieve effective attendance after the child's ninth month.

Even though communities were concerned about side effects and would like full information about the implementation of a new vaccine, data from clinic observations showed that little information was actually provided to caregivers on existing vaccines as part of the routine at the CWCs. Effective communication can close this gap at CWCs, where health professionals have two opportunities to engage with mothers.

The health talk at the beginning of CWC sessions is an opportunity for health workers to provide general information and for mothers, fathers, and other caregivers to share their concerns and ask questions. At this time, vaccine information could be included as one of the regular topics–along with nutrition and breastfeeding–rather than only addressed when a new vaccine has been included on the calendar. Health professionals could also be trained to adjust their communication model. A friendly and dynamic model that community members do not perceive as punitive could be helpful. Strategies could be incorporated to involve mothers in the conversation and to motivate them to express their concerns and ask questions. In regions such as the Upper East, where health talks are not held regularly, it would be important to increase the frequency of these talks.

The personal counseling that takes place while a child is being vaccinated provides another key opportunity for nurse-mother interactions. Observations during this study showed that the workload of the nurses is an important structural factor that has the potential to limit both the quality and length of such interactions. As with the health talks, the focus could be on addressing the specific concerns and questions mothers have rather than on controlling attendance and reprimanding women.

Identifying a flexible, active health communication structure

A well-established, formal health communications process facilitates the flow of information for a particular strategy from the central offices of the Ghana Health Service to relevant regions and districts, to health professionals involved in direct implementation, and finally to the general public, communities, and caregivers (in the case of an intervention for children). The structure is flexible and allows different approaches in urban and rural areas and is complemented by other community channels that may vary locally. Given the local variability in the community actors involved in distributing health information, the final design of information flows would best be completed in specific local settings, with close attention paid to integrating the views and experiences of health professionals working in the area.

The communication network identified would involve the relevant actors within the context of a vaccination campaign, particularly during the months following the introduction of a new vaccine. However, while CWCs allow for regular direct interaction and communication with mothers, there are no regular activities that target fathers and community leaders, who also play a key role in decision-making related to child health [40,41]. Regular direct contact between health professionals and community leaders and men that is not limited to specific campaigns could be helpful. Such interactions could help in detecting doubts and rumors and in engaging community discussions related to national decision-making processes, as well as offset the role of radio in the spread of rumors.

Addressing messaging challenges

In addition to considering all of these factors within the context of vaccine introduction, an effective communications strategy for a future malaria vaccine would take into account certain challenges that relate directly to perceptions of malaria and vaccines. They include:

- **The variety of terms used to refer to malaria and their overlap with other biomedical conditions** [42,43]. Similar symptoms are used to identify malaria and yellow fever in the Ashanti Region and malaria and pneumonia in the Upper East Region. Moreover, in the Upper East Region, important differences are evident in the terminology and understanding of malaria even in neighboring areas. Examples can be found in Gruni and neighboring Nankani, where the languages are so closely related that people using one language can perfectly communicate with people using the other. In Gruni, malaria is referred to as *entolegaban* and *ooro*, while Nankani residents mainly use the word *poa*, which refers to a traditional disease in Gruni [43]. Given this variability and overlap, local health workers could be trained to actively include their local knowledge and experience in the final steps of the design of health messages so that they are prepared to communicate with the communities where they work.
- **Partial knowledge of vaccines.** Results have shown that with the exception of a limited number of health workers, study participants could not name the different vaccines given to children. This finding is in line with those presented in previous studies in the Upper East [30] and Ashanti Regions [44], and in Kintampo [13]. These studies also showed that the lack of knowledge is not incompatible with high coverage both of routine vaccines and vaccines given during national immunization days. They also highlighted an expressed interest in vaccinating children against all important childhood diseases, including malaria. Nevertheless, other authors have argued that accurate knowledge and expectations of vaccines and what they do increases the active demand of vaccines. This can be defined as adherence to programs by an informed public who perceives the benefits and need for specific vaccinations, as opposed to passive acceptance or compliance, dependent on authoritative or even coercive recommendations and social pressure [34].
- **Perception that a malaria vaccine already exists.** This understanding is closely related to the two previous points discussed, to the weak distinction between injections and vaccines, and to the use of the malaria preventive measures (e.g., IPTp, IPTi, and IPTc) that are given within antenatal care and with routine childhood vaccines at CWCs. In the design of the health education strategy for a future malaria vaccine, it would be helpful to address the existence of this perception directly, or messages stating its relevance could be easily misunderstood.

Understanding the overall context for vaccine acceptance

Finally, understanding the context within which communities accept health interventions is also important. In line with previous studies, the results of this study show that final acceptance of new health strategies is more related to the perceived general good and routine acceptance of a package of health activities–such as the CWC and antenatal care–than to the specific knowledge of each intervention [30,35,37]. Moreover, there is a general trust in the competence and knowledge of health professionals and health decision-makers [35,45]. A discussion on the risks of manipulation and misuse of that trust and on the value of full engagement between community members and community-level institutions could be extremely useful.

Strengths and limitations

Given that qualitative data are always influenced by the interaction between researchers and participants, the study employed both discursive and observational methods in an effort to control and understand these influences. The methods allowed for triangulation and in-depth insight into the relationship between community perceptions of vaccines and community experiences and communication at CWCs. Researchers also used team meetings to discuss linguistic ambiguities and interactions that occurred during field work in order to attune data analysis and interpretation. A different purposive sample design could have allowed find differences in discourse and practices depending on educational level and socioeconomic status The regional differences found in the study highlight two critical points: the importance of careful local planning of communications strategies [46] and the impossibility of generalizing data from two study settings to the whole country.

Conclusion

This study has identified several factors that may facilitate the introduction of a malaria vaccine. These factors include the highly accepted and well-established routines of the CWCs, the high value placed on vaccination by communities despite their limited knowledge of vaccines, and the shared understanding that malaria prevention requires a comprehensive approach. The finding that communities appeared to be open to using a combination of methods to fight diseases suggests that a partially efficacious malaria vaccine could be part of a tool kit of malaria control strategies. The study has also confirmed the existence of an active and flexible national health communication structure and processes that allow for dissemination and local coordination of messages and activities.

A number of challenges could be addressed through a well-planned communications strategy and well-designed messages. A key challenge to be taken into account is the perception by some community members that a malaria vaccine already exists. This perception is associated with the vague knowledge of vaccines and other preventive strategies. Another challenge is the variety of terms used to refer to malaria and their overlap with other conditions, such as yellow fever and pneumonia. This lack of clarity regarding malaria and its symptoms could have implications for the perceived efficacy of an eventual malaria vaccine. Finally, there is space for reviewing the communications aspects of CWC service delivery to allow for an increase in vaccine information and the use of a dynamic communication model that seeks to engage caregivers of vaccinated children and that community members do not perceive as being punitive. Communicating with mothers about the need to continue CWC visits past the nine-month mark would also be important to ensure administration of any additional vaccination, including the measles booster, which is administered at 18 months.

Supporting Information

Table S1 Group discussion guide. Malaria.

Table S2 Group discussion guide. Vaccines.

Table S3 In-depth interview guide. Health administrators.

Table S4 In-depth interview guide. Health professionals.

Table S5 In-depth interview guide. Formal and informal leaders.

Table S6 In-depth interview guide. Mothers and fathers.

Table S7 Semi-structured observation guide.

Table S8 Purposive sample per site.

Acknowledgments

The authors would like to thank the participants in the study who took the time to share their experiences and opinions with members of the research team. We would also like to express our gratitude to Agnes Ataa Amofa Snr., Ernest Ekutor, Charles Atakbire Ateem, and Helen Azupogo, the research assistants who collected the data. Support for this project was provided by the PATH Malaria Vaccine Initiative. The views expressed by the authors do not necessarily reflect the views of PATH.

Author Contributions

Conceived and designed the experiments: AM HT CB-P YC AB-N KM AB. Performed the experiments: HT RA. Analyzed the data: AM RA. Contributed reagents/materials/analysis tools: AM HT YC AB-N KM AB. Wrote the paper: AM HT RA CB-P YC AB-N KM AB.

References

1. World Health Organization (WHO) (2012) World Malaria Report 2012. Geneva: WHO.
2. Desai M, ter Kuile FO, Nosten F, McGready R, Asamoa K, et al. (2007) Epidemiology and burden of malaria in pregnancy. Lancet Infect Dis 7: 93–104.
3. Flateau C, LeLoup G, Pialoux G (2011) Consequences of HIV infection on malaria and therapeutic implications: a systematic review. Lancet Infect Dis 11: 541–556.
4. Ghana Ministry of Health (2007) Strategic Plan for Malaria Control in Ghana 2008–2015. Accra: Ghana Ministry of Health.
5. Malaria Vaccine Funders Group (2013) Malaria Vaccine Technology Roadmap. Available: http://www.who.int/immunization/topics/malaria/vaccine_roadmap/TRM_update_nov13.pdf. Accessed 18 November 2013.
6. Malaria Vaccine Decision-Making Framework (2012). Available: http://malvacdecision.net. Accessed 18 November 2013.
7. World Health Organization (WHO) (2005) Vaccine Introduction Guidelines. Geneva: WHO.
8. Agnandji ST, Lell B, Soulanoudjingar SS, Fernandes JF, Abossolo BP, et al. (2011) First results of Phase 3 trial of RTS, S/AS01 malaria vaccine in African children. N Engl J Med 365: 1863–1875.
9. Ojakaa DI, Ofware P, Machira YW, Yamo E, Collymore Y, et al. (2011) Community perceptions of malaria and vaccines in the South Coast and Busia Regions of Kenya. Malar J 10: 147. doi:10.1186/1475-2875-10-147.
10. Ojakaa D, Yamo E, Collymore Y, Ba-Nguz A, Bingham A (2011) Perceptions of malaria and vaccines in Kenya. Hum Vaccin 7: 1096–1099.
11. Bingham A, Gaspar F, Lancaster K, Conjera J, Collymore Y, et al. (2012) Community perceptions of malaria and vaccines in two districts of Mozambique. Malar J 11: 394. doi:10.1186/1475-2875-11-394.
12. Yaya Bocoum F, Kouanda S, Hinson L, Ba-Nguz A, Collymore Y, et al. (2014) Perceptions des communautés sur le paludisme et les vaccins: étude qualitative réalisée dans les districts sanitaires de Kaya et Houndé au Burkina Faso. Glob Health Promot 21: In press.
13. Febir LG, Asante KP, Dzorgbo DBS, Senah KA, Letsa T, et al. (2013) Community perceptions of a malaria vaccine in the Kintampo districts of Ghana. Malar J 12: 156. doi:10.1186/1475-2875-12-156.
14. Ghana Statistical Service (GSS) (2011) Ghana Multiple Indicator Cluster Survey with an Enhanced Malaria Module and Biomarker, 2011, Final Report. Accra: GSS.
15. Ghana Statistical Service (GSS), Ghana Health Service (GHS), ICF Macro (2009) Ghana Demographic and Health Survey 2008. Accra: GSS, GHS, ICF Macro.
16. Ghana Health Service (2012) Expanded Programme on Immunization. Upcoming Events. Available: http://www.ghanahealthservice.org/epi_events.php. Accessed 18 November 2013.

17. International Federation of Red Cross and Red Crescent (IFRC) (2012) Disaster Relief Emergency Fund (DREF) final report. Ghana: Meningitis. Available: http://ifrc.org/docs/Appeals/12/MDRGH006dfr.pdf. Accessed 18 November 2013.
18. World Health Organization Regional Office for Africa (2012) A mass campaign to vaccinate nearly 3 million people against meningitis "A" starts today in Ghana. Press materials. Available: http://www.afro.who.int/en/ghana/press-materials/item/5013-a-mass-campaign-to-vaccinate-nearly-3-million-people-against-meningitis-%E2%80%9Ca%E2%80%9D-starts-today-in-ghana.html. Accessed 18 November 2013.
19. Sarapong N, Loag W, Fobil J, Meyer CG, Adu-Sarkodie Y, et al. (2010) National health insurance coverage and socio-economic status in a rural district of Ghana. Trop Med Int Health 15: 191–197.
20. Service GS (2008) Ghana Population and Housing Census 2000. Accra: Office of the President.
21. Mara Arma (2000) Mapping Malaria Risk in Africa. Ghana: Duration of the Malaria Transmission Season. Available: www.mara.org.za. Accessed 18 November 2013.
22. World Health Organization Regional Office for Africa. Ghana Publications (2008) Lymphatic Filariasis elimination (LFE). Available: http://www.afro.who.int/en/ghana/ghana-publications/1728-lymphatic-filariasis-elimination-lfe.html. Accessed 18 November 2013.
23. Abotsi AK, Inkoom E, Ribaira E, Le Mentec R, Levy P, et al. (2012) Cost effectiveness of intermittent preventive treatment of malaria in infants in Ghana. International Journal of Tropical Disease & Health 2: 1–15.
24. Pool R, Geissler W (2005) Medical Anthropology: Understanding Public Health. London: Open University Press.
25. Streefland PH, Chowdhury AMR, Ramos-Jimenez P (1999) Quality of vaccination services and social demand for vaccinations in Africa and Asia. Bull World Health Organ 77: 722–730.
26. Jheeta M, Newell J (2008) Childhood vaccination in Africa and Asia: the effects of parents' knowledge and attitudes. Bull World Health Organ 86: 419–420.
27. Andrus JK, Lewis MJ, Goldie SJ, García PJ, Winkler JL, et al. (2008) Human papillomavirus vaccine policy and delivery in Latin America and the Caribbean. Vaccine 26: L80–L87. doi:10.1016/j.vaccine.2008.05.040.
28. Stanton BF (2004) Assessment of relevant cultural considerations is essential for the success of a vaccine. J Health Popul Nutr 22: 286–292.
29. Bernard HR (2011) Research Methods in Anthropology. Plymouth: AltaMira Press.
30. Gysels M, Pell C, Mathanga DP, Adongo P, Odhiambo F, et al. (2009) Community response to intermittent preventive treatment of malaria in infants (IPTi) delivered through the expanded programme of immunization in five African settings. Malar J 8: 191. doi:10.1186/1475-2875-8-191.
31. Pitt C, Diawara H, Ouédraogo DJ, Diarra S, Kaboré H, et al. (2012) Intermittent preventive treatment of malaria in children: a qualitative study of community perceptions and recommendations in Burkina Faso and Mali. PLOS ONE 7: e32900. doi:10.1371/journal.pone.0032900.
32. Hausmann Muela S, Muela Ribera J, Mushi AK, Tanner M (2002) Medical syncretism with reference to malaria in a Tanzanian community. Soc Sci Med 55: 403–413.
33. Musoke D, Karani G, Ssempebwa JC, Musoke MB (2013) Integrated approach to malaria prevention at household level in rural communities in Uganda: experiences from a pilot project. Malar J 12: 327. doi:10.1186/1475-2875-12-327.
34. Nichter M (1995) Vaccinations in the Third World: a consideration of community demand. Soc Sci Med 41: 617–632.
35. Streefland P, Chowdhury AMR, Ramos-Jimenez P (1999) Patterns of vaccination acceptance. Soc Sci Med 49: 1705–1716.
36. Pool R, Munguambe K, Macete E, Aide P, Juma G, et al. (2006) Community response to intermittent preventive treatment delivered to infants (IPTi) through the EPI system in Manhiça, Mozambique. Trop Med Int Health 11: 1670–1678.
37. Pell C, Meñaca A, Were F, Afrah NA, Chatio S, et al. (2013) Factors affecting antenatal care attendance: results from qualitative studies in Ghana, Kenya and Malawi. PLOS ONE 8: e53747. doi:10.1371/journal.pone.0053747.
38. Chandramohan D, Webster J, Smith L, Awine T, Owusu-Agyei S, et al. (2007) Is the Expanded Programme on Immunisation the most appropriate delivery system for intermittent preventive treatment of malaria in West Africa? Trop Med Int Health 12: 743–750.
39. Webster J, Lines J, Bruce J, Armstrong Schellenberg JRM, Hanson K (2005) Which delivery systems reach the poor? A review of equity of coverage of ever-treated nets, never-treated nets and immunization to reduce child mortality in Africa. Lancet Infect Dis 5: 709–717.
40. Tolhurst R, Nyonator FK (2006) Looking within the household: gender roles and responses to malaria in Ghana. Trans R Soc Trop Med Hyg 100: 321–326.
41. Tolhurst R, Amekudzi YP, Nyonator FK, Bertel Squire S, Theobald S (2008) "He will ask why the child gets sick so often": the gendered dynamics of intra-household bargaining over healthcare for children with fever in the Volta Region of Ghana. Soc Sci Med 66: 1106–1117.
42. Ahorlu C, Koram K, Ahorlu C, de Savigny D, Weiss M (2005) Community concepts of malaria-related illness with and without convulsions in Ghana. Malar J 4: 47. doi:10.1186/1475-2875-4-47.
43. Meñaca A, Pell C, Manda-Taylor L, Chatio S, Afrah NA, et al. (2013) Local illness concepts and their relevance for the prevention and control of malaria during pregnancy in Ghana, Kenya and Malawi: findings from a comparative qualitative study. Malar J 12: 257. doi:10.1186/1475-2875-12-257.
44. Browne EN, Bonney AA, Agyapong FA, Essegbey IT (2002) Factors influencing participation in national immunization days in Kumasi, Ghana. Ann Trop Med Parasitol 96: 93–104.
45. Smith L, Jones C, Adjei R, Antwi G, Afrah N, et al. (2010) Intermittent screening and treatment versus intermittent preventive treatment of malaria in pregnancy: user acceptability. Malar J 9: 18. doi:10.1186/1475-2875-9-18.
46. Cockcroft A, Andersson N, Omer K, Ansari NM, Khan A, et al. (2009) One size does not fit all: local determinants of measles vaccination in four districts of Pakistan. BMC Int Health Hum Rights 9: S4.

Impact of a Participatory Intervention with Women's Groups on Psychological Distress among Mothers in Rural Bangladesh: Secondary Analysis of a Cluster-Randomised Controlled Trial

Kelly Clarke[1]*, Kishwar Azad[2], Abdul Kuddus[2], Sanjit Shaha[2], Tasmin Nahar[2], Bedowra Haq Aumon[2], Mohammed Munir Hossen[2], James Beard[1], Anthony Costello[1], Tanja A. J. Houweling[1,3], Audrey Prost[1], Edward Fottrell[1]

1 Institute for Global Health, University College London, London, United Kingdom, **2** Perinatal Care Project, Diabetic Association of Bangladesh, Dhaka, Bangladesh, **3** Department of Public Health, Erasmus MC University Medical Center Rotterdam, Rotterdam, The Netherlands

Abstract

Background: Perinatal common mental disorders (PCMDs) are a major cause of disability among women and disproportionately affect lower income countries. Interventions to address PCMDs are urgently needed in these settings, and group-based and peer-led approaches are potential strategies to increase access to mental health interventions. Participatory women's health groups led by local women previously reduced postpartum psychological distress in eastern India. We assessed the effect of a similar intervention on postpartum psychological distress in rural Bangladesh.

Method: We conducted a secondary analysis of data from a cluster-randomised controlled trial with 18 clusters and an estimated population of 532,996. Nine clusters received an intervention comprising monthly meetings during which women's groups worked through a participatory learning and action cycle to develop strategies for improving women's and children's health. There was one group for every 309 individuals in the population, 810 groups in total. Mothers in nine control clusters had access to usual perinatal care. Postpartum psychological distress was measured with the 20-item Self Reporting Questionnaire (SRQ-20) between six and 52 weeks after delivery, during the months of January to April, in 2010 and 2011.

Results: We analysed outcomes for 6275 mothers. Although the cluster mean SRQ-20 score was lower in the intervention arm (mean 5.2, standard deviation 1.8) compared to control (5.3, 1.2), the difference was not significant (β 1.44, 95% CI 0.28, 3.08).

Conclusions: Despite promising results in India, participatory women's groups focused on women's and children's health had no significant effect on postpartum psychological distress in rural Bangladesh.

Editor: Gabriele Fischer, Medical University of Vienna, Austria

Funding: A Big Lottery Fund International Strategic Grant (IS/2/010281409) funded the implementation and evaluation of the women's groups. The study was also supported by funds from a Wellcome Trust Strategic Award (085417ma/Z/08/Z). The funders had no role in study design, data collection and analysis, decision to publish, or preparation of the manuscript.

Competing Interests: The authors have declared that no competing interests exist.

* Email: k.clarke.09@ucl.ac.uk

Introduction

Perinatal common mental disorders (PCMDs) are defined as depressive, anxiety, panic and somatic disorders occurring in pregnancy or the postpartum period [1]. PCMDs are a major cause of disability among women, and depression is a strong predictor of suicide [2–5]. PCMDs also have adverse consequences for children's growth and development, and disrupt the mother-infant bond [6–8]. Women in low and lower middle-income countries are disproportionately affected, with 16% (95% Confidence Interval [CI] 15.0–16.8%) experiencing a PCMD during pregnancy and 20% (95% CI 19.2–20.6%) in the postpartum period [9]. However, to date there are few trials of interventions for PCMDs in these countries [10,11]. Interventions delivered by non-mental health specialists and integrated into existing maternal and child health programmes are needed [10–12].

Women's groups practising participatory learning and action to address women's, newborn and child health problems have been implemented in several African and south Asian settings [13]. Groups are facilitated by lay women or community health volunteers and are open to all community members, though they target women of reproductive age. Although groups do not explicitly address PCMDs, a recent meta-analysis showed that exposure to groups is associated with a 37% reduction in neonatal mortality (Odds Ratio [OR] 0.63 95% Confidence Interval [CI] 0.32, 0.94) a key predictor of PCMDs [13]. Groups may also reduce maternal complications during the perinatal period and neonatal deaths, improve social support and problem-solving skills, and are therefore a potential strategy to improve maternal mental health [14,15]. In rural eastern India exposure to groups reduced moderate postpartum psychological distress, a proxy for PCMDs, by 57% (OR 0.43 95% CI 0.23, 0.80) within geographical clusters that had received the intervention, albeit only in the third year of the trial [15].

Population coverage, as well as the proportion of pregnant women attending groups, predict the effect size of women's groups on neonatal and maternal mortality [13]. In rural eastern India, population coverage was 468 per group and the proportion of pregnant women attending at least one group meeting was 55% in the final year of intervention, during which time the reduction in moderate postpartum psychological distress was detected [14]. In rural Bangladesh women's groups have been evaluated in two trials. In the first trial (2005–2007) coverage was 1414 per group, only 3% of pregnant women attended groups (477/15,695) and there was no impact on neonatal mortality [16]. In the second trial (2009–2011) coverage increased to 309 per group, attendance among pregnant women increased to 36% (3326/9109) and neonatal mortality was reduced by 38% (Risk Ratio [RR] 0.62 95% CI 0.43, 0.89) [17]. In Bangladesh there is a high prevalence of PCMDs ranging from 22 to 52%, and a lack of mental health resources in rural areas [18–20]. In light of proven mental health benefits of women's groups in rural eastern India, and using data from the second Bangladeshi trial, we aimed to assess the impact of groups on postpartum psychological distress in rural Bangladesh.

Methods

Ethics statement

The trial was approved by the Ethical Review Committee of the Diabetic Association of Bangladesh and by University College London Research Ethics Committee (ID number: 1488/001), and registered as ISRCTN01805825. Permission for the trial was obtained from community leaders. The consent process, approved by the ethics committees, involved briefing respondents about the trial aims, the interview process and data storage and usage, and respondents were free to decline participation. We sought verbal, as opposed to written, consent from respondents because many of them were illiterate. Consent was documented by the interviewer at the time of interview and subsequently entered into the trial database. Respondents were made aware of appropriate health-care facilities if they or their children were ill.

Study setting and design

We conducted a secondary analysis of a cluster-randomised controlled trial of participatory women's groups to address women's, newborn and child health problems in rural Bangladesh. Neonatal mortality was the primary outcome and postpartum psychological distress, a proxy for PCMDs, was an additional outcome. The full design of the trial has been reported elsewhere [17,21]. Briefly, January to December 2008 was the baseline period and the trial ran from 1st January 2009 to 30th June 2011. The trial was located in Moulvibazar, Faridpur and Bogra districts, which were purposively selected because of the presence of Diabetic Association of Bangladesh (BADAS) programmes, and to represent the geographically diversity of rural Bangladesh. In each district two upazillas (sub-districts) and three unions per upazilla were sampled on the basis of being accessible from BADAS district headquarters but having limited access to perinatal health care facilities. Unions comprise a group of adjacent villages, are the lowest administrative unit in Bangladesh and were the unit of clustering in the trial.

The six unions in each district (18 unions in total) were randomly allocated to both intervention and control arms by drawing folded papers from a bottle using a pre-specified allocation sequence. The estimated population size in the study unions was 532,996 people, in 117,914 households [17]. Around 80% of the population is Muslim, and the rest are mainly Hindu. Around half of the women who recently delivered never went to school or only attended primary education. Baseline neonatal (38/1000) and pregnancy-related (188/100000) mortality rates in the study districts were high [17]. In Moulvibazar there are several tea garden estates. Workers on these estates (tea garden residents) are mainly of Indian descent and Hindu, since their ancestors were brought from India by former British rulers [22,23]. They tend to be socioeconomically disadvantaged compared to non-tea garden residents.

Intervention and control arm activities

Women's groups comprised 162 'old groups' from the first trial (2005–2007) plus 648 'new groups' implemented during the second trial (2009–2011). Groups convened monthly and worked through a learning and action cycle that involved group members identifying and prioritising issues affecting the health of mothers and newborns (Cycle 1) or women and children (Cycle 2) in their communities, and developing and implementing strategies to address these issues. New groups worked through Cycle 1, whereas old groups who had previously completed Cycle 1 during the first trial worked through Cycle 2. Groups were participatory, rather than prescriptive, ensuring strategies were culturally appropriate. Strategies differed across groups and included home visits, using social dramas and picture card games to raise awareness of common health problems, prevention and treatment strategies, and collecting voluntary donations to community funds to facilitate care seeking. Mental health issues were not explicitly addressed during either cycle. Local women of reproductive age with at least some high school education were recruited to facilitate group meetings, and groups held community meetings to encourage the wider community to engage with their strategies. Groups took approximately 20 months to work through the cycles. Both intervention and control clusters received health strengthening activities, including training of traditional birth attendants in essential newborn and maternal care, essential obstetrics and neonatology education sessions for doctors and provision of health equipment for community clinics.

Target group and respondents

Women's groups were open to all community members, however the target group was women of reproductive age, especially pregnant and newly married women. The women's group intervention was expected to have effects reaching beyond group members to non-attenders. We therefore collected data at a population level from all women permanently residing in the study districts who gave birth during the trial period. We excluded women who were not permanently residing in the study area, as it was unlikely they were exposed to the women's group intervention.

Data collection and measurement of postpartum psychological distress

Traditional birth attendants identified all deaths and births in the study districts and received a financial incentive for reporting each event. Monitors visited the households to verify the birth or

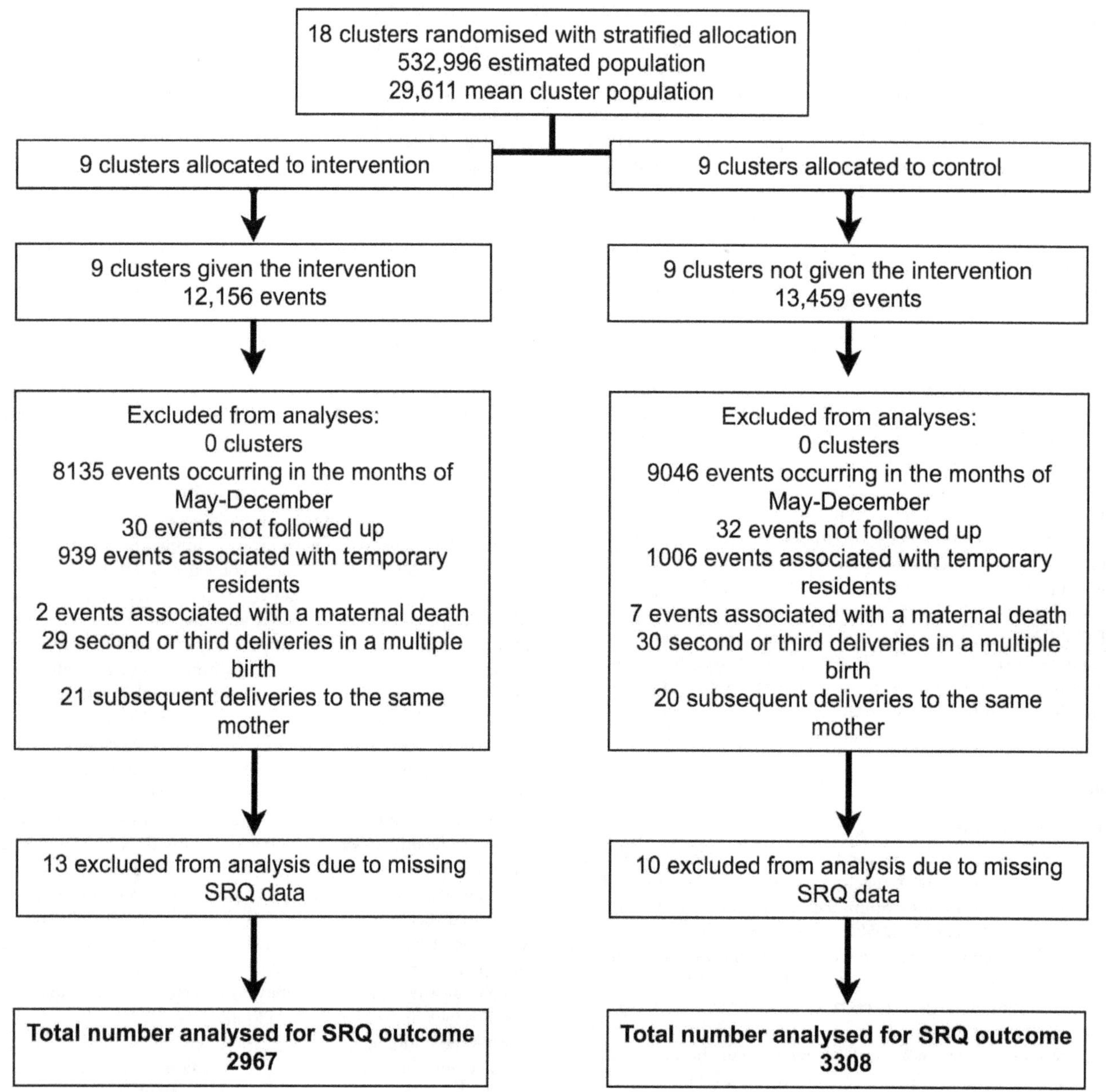

Figure 1. Sample selection procedure for evaluation of the effect of women's groups on postpartum psychological distress. From 25,615 births and deaths ('events') over the 24 study months in 2010 and 2011 we excluded data from: 17,181 events that did not occur within the SRQ-20 data collection periods; 62 events where it was not possible to conduct an interview due to migration or refusal; 1945 events associated with mothers who were temporary residents in the study area; nine events associated with a maternal death; 100 events associated with mothers who had previously delivered during the SRQ-20 data collection periods, either because of multiple births or through repeated births; 23 mothers due to missing SRQ-20 data. In total, 6275 mothers were included in the final sample.

death. After a birth an interview was conducted between a minimum of six weeks and a maximum of 52 weeks postpartum. The interview included questions about healthcare, socioeconomic status and postpartum psychological distress. As in several community-based randomised controlled trials of participatory interventions, monitors and respondents were aware of allocation, however there were no incentives or disincentives for over- or under-reporting births, deaths or postpartum psychological distress. Furthermore, mechanisms existed to identify any inaccuracies, such as monitoring process data on a monthly basis and cross-checking a sample of data through re-interview [21].

Postpartum psychological distress was measured using the 20-item Self Reporting Questionnaire (SRQ-20) [24]. This tool has been used to screen for common mental disorders, including PCMDs, in a variety of low-income settings [25]. The tool comprises 20 yes/no questions about symptoms of depression and anxiety experienced in the past 30 days. Responses were summed to produce a total score ranging from 0 to 20.

The main trial sample size calculations were carried out for neonatal mortality. We also sought to estimate the power of the study to detect changes in postpartum psychological distress among mothers. We carried out power calculations using a cut-off SRQ score ≥6 to indicate the presence of distress for baseline

Table 1. Respondent characteristics for intervention and control areas (with and without tea garden residents) at baseline and during the SRQ-20 data collection period.

	BASELINE (JANUARY–DECEMBER 2008)			SRQ-20 DATA COLLECTION (JAN–APRIL 2010 & 2011)		
	Intervention	Control	Control	Intervention	Control	Control
	(N = 5027)	Excluding tea-garden residents (N = 5013)	Including tea-garden residents (N = 5571)	(N = 2967)	Excluding tea garden residents (N = 2823)	Including tea garden residents (N = 3308)
Age (years)						
Mean (SD)	24.7 (5.6)	24.6 (5.5)	24.6 (5.4)	24.5 (5.3)	24.8 (5.4)	24.8 (5.4)
Age at first pregnancy (years)						
Mean (SD)	18.4 (2.8)	18.5 (2.7)	18.6 (2.6)	18.4 (2.6)	18.6 (2.6)	18.7 (2.6)
Gravidity						
Mean (SD)	2.7 (1.7)	2.5 (1.6)	2.5 (1.6)	2.5 (1.6)	2.5 (1.6)	2.5 (1.6)
Religion						
Islam (%)	4539 (90.3)	4523 (90.2)	4605 (82.7)	2626 (88.5)	2551 (90.4)	2594 (78.5)
Hindu (%)	479 (9.5)	487 (9.7)	959 (17.2)	341 (11.5)	270 (9.6)	708 (21.4)
Other (%)	9 (0.2)	3 (0.1)	7 (0.1)	0 (0)	1 (0.0)	1 (0.0)
Education						
Never went to school (%)	1261 (25.1)	1091 (21.8)	1437 (25.8)	617 (20.8)	529 (18.7)	810 (24.5)
Primary education (%)	1795 (35.7)	1609 (32.1)	1727 (31.0)	1129 (38.1)	942 (33.4)	1059 (32.0)
Secondary or above (%)	1971 (39.2)	2313 (46.1)	2407 (43.2)	1221 (41.2)	1352 (47.9)	1439 (43.5)
Household assets**						
None (%)	1840 (36.6)	1635 (32.6)	1939 (34.8)	630 (21.2)	534 (18.9)	737 (22.3)
One (%)	1056 (21.0)	1017 (20.3)	1087 (19.5)	802 (27.0)	708 (25.1)	801 (24.1)
Two (%)	722 (14.4)	636 (12.7)	697 (12.5)	438 (14.8)	449 (15.9)	511 (15.5)
Three or more (%)	1409 (28.0)	1723 (34.4)	1846 (33.1)	1097 (37.0)	1132 (40.1)	1259 (38.1)
Perinatal health care utilization						
Facility deliveries (%)	943 (18.8)	1065 (21.3)	1114 (20.0)	820 (27.6)	796 (28.2)	862 (26.1)
4 or more ANC check-ups by formal provider (%)	546 (10.9)	648 (12.9)	676 (12.1)	541 (18.2)	386 (13.7)	398 (12.0)
Counts of births and deaths						
Number of births	4965	4930	5485	2876	2749	3216
Neonatal mortality rate per 1000 livebirths	38.3	35.3	37.2	14.6	28.0	28.3

**Assets included in the variable: radio, electric fan, television, fridge, mobile phone, bicycle, generator and electricity.

prevalences ranging between 10–20%, with an estimated k value of 0.3 [26,27]. Assuming 500 births per year per cluster, if the baseline prevalence of postpartum psychological distress was 10%, collecting data over 12 months would allow us to detect a 35% reduction in distress with 64.4–70.2% power at the 95% confidence level, and between 69 and 75% power if the baseline prevalence was 20%. Collecting data for 24 months would only yield a marginal increase in power (68.7–74.4%). In order not to impose a burden of continuous data collection on the monitoring team, we therefore planned to collect data on postpartum psychological distress for four months (January to April) per year over three years. We screened each mother for postpartum psychological distress once per birth: data are therefore cross-sectional. We did not exclude any mothers for mental ill-health reasons. Some mothers delivered more than once in the study period, because of multiple births (twins or triplets) or through repeated pregnancies. To avoid duplicating cases we therefore only used data associated with the firstborn infant of a multiple birth, or the first birth during the SRQ-20 data collection period.

Statistical analysis

A researcher who was not involved in the design or management of the trial (KC) carried out the analysis independently. We assigned mothers to the cluster in which their delivery was registered, and estimated the intra-cluster correlation coefficient (ICC) for postpartum psychological distress using a large one-way ANOVA to assess how symptoms clustered. We used an SRQ-20 score ≥6 to report the prevalence of psychological distress because a previous study in urban Bangladesh found that this score discriminated best for psychiatric disorders, though the

Table 2. Women's group participation rates among respondents screened with the SRQ-20.

	Proportion of women in intervention clusters (%) N = 2967	Proportion of women in intervention clusters that attended groups (%) N = 1037
Age group		
<20 years	505 (17.0)	137 (13.2)
20–29 years	1889 (63.7)	676 (65.2)
30–39 years	549 (18.5)	220 (21.2)
40 years or older	24 (0.8)	4 (0.4)
Religion		
Muslim	2626 (88.5)	933 (90.0)
Hindu	341 (11.5)	104 (10.0)
Other	0 (0)	0 (0)
Maternal education		
Never went to school/less than 1 year	617 (20.8)	231 (22.3)
Primary education/non-formal	1129 (38.1)	441 (42.5)
Secondary or above	1221 (41.2)	365 (35.2)
Household		
None (%)	630 (21.2)	381 (19.7)
One (%)	802 (27.0)	537 (27.8)
Two (%)	438 (14.8)	267 (13.8)
Three or more (%)	1097 (37.0)	745 (38.6)
Primigravid	996 (32.6)	253 (24.0)
Experienced a neonatal death or stillbirth	133 (4.5)	53 (5.1)
SRQ-20 score >6	1028 (34.7)	351 (33.9)

sensitivity (62%) and specificity (69%) were quite low [28]. In order to avoid over-reliance on this cut-off score, we therefore evaluated the impact of women's groups using the SRQ-20 data as a continuous outcome, through a t-test of cluster means weighted by inverse variance, accounting for clustering at the union and district level [27]. We log transformed SRQ-20 data, adding 0.1 to each value to account for scores of zero. The results are reported on the original scale, interpreted as the ratio of the geometric mean SRQ-20 score in the intervention arm over the geometric mean score in the control arm. Analyses were not adjusted for confounders such as age, education or asset ownership, since these factors were relatively balanced across trial arms at baseline. We excluded a small number of cases with missing SRQ-20 data (0.4% 23/6275). We decided a priori to conduct analyses with and without tea garden residents. The trial in eastern India only reported a significant effect of women's groups on distress in its final year [15]. We therefore planned to stratify our analyses by year of birth. Our main analyses used data collected during the trial period in 2010 and 2011. After the trial, groups carried on meeting and surveillance and data collection continued. Systematic differences in neonatal mortality rates between control and intervention arms were only evident from April 2011. If an intervention effect of women's groups on postpartum psychological distress was dependent on a reduction in neonatal mortality, we would have been unable to detect it using data from the trial period only, since SRQ-20 data were collected only during the months of January to April. We therefore conducted a post-hoc sensitivity analysis including further SRQ-20 data collected between 1 January and 30 April 2012. All analyses were carried out in Stata version 12 [29]. We will make an anonymised version of the dataset used for the analyses in this article available to researchers upon completion of a simple data request form, which can be obtained from Dr Audrey Prost (Audrey.Prost@ucl.ac.uk).

Results

Figure 1 shows the selection process of data included in the trial analysis for the postpartum psychological distress outcome. In total, data were available for 25,615 births and deaths over the 24 study months in 2010 and 2011. After excluding data from events that did not occur within the SRQ-20 data collection periods (January to April inclusive, 2010 and 2011), there were 4021 and 4413 events in intervention and control clusters, respectively. Of these we excluded 62 events where it was not possible to conduct an interview due to migration or refusal. Although the exact number or mothers who refused interview is not known it is believed to be extremely low (<1%). We excluded data from 1945 events associated with mothers who were temporary residents in the study area and nine events associated with a maternal death. In order to remove data from duplicate interviews associated with the same mother, we excluded data from 100 events associated with mothers who had previously delivered during the SRQ-20 data collection period, either because of multiple births or through repeated births. At this stage the denominator for analyses was mothers rather than events and we excluded 23 mothers due to missing SRQ-20 data. In total, 6275 mothers were included in the final sample. The median interval between childbirth and interview was 70 days (interquartile range: 52–102) and it was similar in control and intervention areas.

Table 3. Summary measures of postpartum psychological distress (SRQ-20 score ≥6) in intervention and control areas (with and without tea garden residents), by year.

	Mothers (N)	Overall prevalence	District prevalence			Mean cluster score	Mean cluster prevalence	Mean (SD)	Median (IQR)
			Bogra	Faridpur	Moulvibazar				
2010 and 2011									
Intervention	2967	1028 (34.7)	320 (34.7)	296 (27.9)	412 (41.9)	5.2 (1.8)	34.8 (16.8)	5.2 (4.3)	4 (2–8)
Control excluding tea garden residents	2823	1014 (35.9)	286 (30.2)	381 (34.3)	347 (45.4)	5.3 (1.4)	33.7 (14.0)	5.5 (4.5)	4 (2–9)
Control including tea garden residents	3308	1180 (35.7)	286 (30.2)	381 (34.3)	513 (41.1)	5.3 (1.2)	34.3 (12.2)	5.4 (4.6)	4 (2–8)
2010, 2011 and 2012									
Intervention	4260	1354 (31.8)	437 (32.8)	378 (25.4)	539 (37.5)	4.9 (1.7)	32.1 (16.3)	4.9 (4.1)	4 (2–8)
Control excluding tea garden residents	4072	1420 (34.9)	464 (33.5)	484 (30.5)	472 (42.8)	5.2 (1.4)	33.1 (15.0)	5.4 (4.5)	4 (2–8)
Control including tea garden residents	4760	1631 (34.3)	464 (33.5)	484 (30.5)	683 (38.1)	5.2 (1.3)	33.4 (13.1)	5.3 (4.5)	4 (2–8)
2010									
Intervention	1507	624 (41.4)	178 (39.7)	183 (33.7)	263 (51.0)	5.9 (1.8)	41.3 (15.7)	5.9 (4.6)	5 (2–9)
Control excluding tea garden residents	1389	566 (40.8)	143 (32.2)	219 (39.8)	204 (51.7)	5.7 (1.5)	38.5 (15.2)	5.9 (4.6)	5 (2–9)
Control including tea garden residents	1644	647 (39.4)	143 (32.2)	219 (39.8)	285 (43.9)	5.7 (1.3)	38.0 (12.7)	5.8 (4.7)	5 (2–9)
2011									
Intervention	1460	404 (27.7)	142 (30.0)	113 (21.8)	149 (31.8)	4.5 (2.2)	28.1 (21.4)	4.5 (3.9)	4 (1–7)
Control excluding tea garden residents	1434	448 (31.2)	143 (28.4)	162 (28.8)	143 (38.8)	4.8 (1.5)	30.3 (14.4)	5.1 (4.4)	4 (2–8)
Control including tea garden residents	1664	533 (32.0)	143 (28.4)	162 (28.8)	228 (38.1)	4.9 (1.3)	30.3 (14.4)	5.1 (4.4)	4 (1.5, 8)
2012									
Intervention	1293	326 (25.2)	117 (28.5)	82 (19.1)	127 (28.1)	4.3 (1.7)	25.6 (16.3)	4.2 (3.6)	3 (1–7)
Control excluding tea garden residents	1249	406 (32.5)	178 (40.7)	103 (21.8)	125 (36.9)	5.1 (2.0)	31.7 (20.8)	5.2 (4.2)	4 (2–8)
Control including tea garden residents	1452	451 (31.1)	178 (40.7)	103 (21.8)	170 (31.4)	5.0 (1.9)	31.2 (19.8)	5.0 (4.3)	4 (2–8)

Table 4. Evaluation of the effect of participatory women's groups on postpartum psychological distress.

	Including tea garden residents			Excluding tea garden residents		
	Ratio of means	95% CI	P-value	Ratio of means	95% CI	P-value
2010	1.41	0.39, 3.53	0.509	1.14	0.35, 3.20	0.801
2011	1.78	0.17, 3.18	0.391	1.89	0.18, 3.37	0.350
2012	0.74	0.15, 2.94	0.662	0.70	0.14, 2.83	0.617
2010 and 2011	1.44	0.28, 3.08	0.524	1.38	0.28, 3.02	0.586
2010, 2011 and 2012	1.28	0.24, 2.91	0.680	1.23	0.23, 2.86	0.735

Mothers' characteristics and women's group participation

Table 1 shows that mothers in intervention and control arms were similar with respect to baseline characteristics. Overall, the average age of mothers was 25 years. Most were Muslim and a quarter had never been to school. Around a third had three or more household assets such as a radio, television, bicycle or mobile phone. Only a fifth delivered in facilities and most did not receive adequate antenatal healthcare. The socioeconomic status of respondents excluding the tea garden residents was higher.

Table 1 also shows that the sample of mothers screened with the SRQ-20 was similar to the full baseline sample in terms of socioeconomic characteristics. During the trial period, among the sample screened with the SRQ-20, more mothers received antenatal care in the intervention arm compared to the control arm and the neonatal mortality rate was lower in the intervention arm. These effects were probably due to the women's group intervention. Otherwise, characteristics were balanced across trial arms. Table 2 shows rates of participation in women's group activities for different subgroups of the study sample in intervention clusters. Participation was marginally lower among mothers living in the poorest households, as well as those who were primigravid, younger, or had a secondary education or above. The percentage of respondents who attended at least one group meeting was 33% (490/1507) in 2010, rising to 37% (547/1460) in 2011. Among mothers who had attended meetings, 83% (860/1037) attended on a monthly basis.

Impact of the women's groups on postpartum psychological distress

Using a cut-off score of ≥6, the overall prevalence of postpartum psychological distress was 35% (2208/6275) (Table 3). Prevalence and mean SRQ-20 score were lower in the intervention arm, and between 2010 and 2011 there were substantial reductions in prevalence and mean SRQ-20 score in both intervention and control arms. Prevalence was highest in Moulvibazar, especially in 2010. The ICC for SRQ-20 scores was 0.10 (95% CI 0.04, 0.17), suggesting that mothers' SRQ-20 scores within the same cluster were more similar to mothers' scores across clusters. A weighted t-test of log transformed cluster mean SRQ-20 scores showed that overall there was no significant difference in mean SRQ-20 scores between intervention and control arms (β 1.44 95% CI 0.28, 3.08) (Table 4). Similarly we found no effect of the intervention by year, or when we excluded tea garden residents. We conducted a sensitivity analysis using data from January to April 2012 in order to assess the impact of women's groups on postpartum psychological distress after a difference in neonatal mortality rates between trial arms had become apparent. We found no significant impact of the groups when these data were included in the analysis (including tea garden residents: β 1.28 95% CI 0.24, 2.91 P = 0.680; excluding tea garden residents: β 1.23 95% CI 0.23, 2.86 P = 0.735) or analysed separately (including tea garden residents: β 0.74 95% CI 0.15, 2.94 P = 0.662; excluding tea garden residents: β 0.70 95% CI 0.14, 2.83 P = 0.617).

Discussion

Consistent with previous studies, we report a high prevalence of postpartum psychological distress among mothers in rural Bangladesh [18,19]. However, in contrast to our expectations, a participatory intervention with women's groups did not significantly reduce postpartum psychological distress in this setting This is surprising given that the intervention substantially reduced neonatal mortality, a risk factor for distress, and that a similar intervention in rural eastern India significantly reduced postpartum psychological distress. Furthermore, coverage of groups and participation among pregnant women in Bangladeshi groups was relatively high, and these factors have been shown to predict effectiveness, at least for neonatal and maternal mortality outcomes [13].

One possible explanation for the absence of a mental health effect is that neonatal mortality was less important as a predictor of postpartum psychological distress in Bangladesh compared to eastern India because the baseline neonatal mortality rate was lower and/or because factors not addressed by the women's groups were more important for maternal mental health. For example, communities in rural Bangladesh are strongly patriarchal and factors associated with gender-based victimization, including domestic violence, marital relationship problems and lack of education, are known to be associated with PCMDs in this setting [19,30,31]. Also, communities in rural Bangladesh are exposed to flooding, storms and epidemics. These environmental stressors possibly contribute to psychological distress through effects on income and physical health [32]. The increased prevalence of postpartum psychological distress in Moulvibazar during 2010 may have been due to severe flooding in the district at this time.

Another possible explanation for the null result is that mechanisms other than a reduction in neonatal mortality account for the mental health benefits of women's groups in eastern India, and these mechanisms were not fully realised in Bangladesh. Contextual factors, including gender and social equality, are likely to influence the way in which women's groups engage with non-group members in their communities. In rural Bangladesh women are secluded and confined to the house, and although group members disseminated health information among non-group members, with benefits for maternal and child health, social barriers may have prevented them from engaging with women in a way that empowered them more generally, and reduced psychological distress. Further investigation is needed to understand how contextual factors influence strategies used by women's groups, as is research to establish mechanisms for their effects on postpartum psychological distress in eastern India. In India it took until the third year for these effects to be detected. It remains possible that the small differences we observed between trial arms in Bangladesh would increase over time, with the benefits of group participation in reducing distress emerging later.

Our study suggests that women's groups practising participatory learning and action focused on women's, newborn and child health are not universally effective to improve maternal mental health. Evaluations of alternative approaches are urgently needed in Bangladesh and other low-income countries in order to address the lack of evidence-based interventions for PCMDs in these settings. Women's groups are a cost-effective method to engage with disadvantaged women. One approach could therefore be to adapt existing groups by integrating mental health content into participatory learning and action cycles in order to improve awareness of the consequences and causes of PCMDs, and to develop appropriate strategies to address them. Content on context-specific predictors of PCMDs, such as domestic violence and environmental resilience could also be included. Another approach would be to deliver psychological therapy through women's groups. In Uganda, Chile and China, trials of interventions involving group-based cognitive behaviour and interpersonal therapy reported benefits for general and postpartum depression [33–38]. Formative work is needed to assess the cultural acceptability and feasibility of this approach in other settings.

Alternatively interventions could be delivered individually. Evidence from middle-income countries suggests that preventive and treatment programmes for PCMDs delivered during home visits can be effective. For example, a cognitive behaviour intervention delivered by lady health workers in Pakistan and an intervention to improve the quality of the mother infant relationship in South Africa showed promising results for postpartum depression [39,40]. However, individually delivered interventions may be more resource-intensive than group approaches and data are needed to assess the cost-effectiveness of these interventions.

Study limitations

Our analysis has three main limitations. First, we only collected data between January and April in 2010, 2011 and 2012. The confidence intervals associated with results in Table 4 are wide, and collecting more data would have enabled greater precision. Also, in March and April, farm labourers may be unemployed after the *boro* crop has been planted and households may therefore be at risk of financial hardship and food insecurity [41]. During these months benefits of the women's groups for maternal mental health may have been masked. Second, we did not assess inter-rater reliability for the SRQ-20, and therefore differences in mean cluster SRQ-20 scores could be related to inconsistencies between assessors. However, this is unlikely to have resulted in systematic bias since there were many assessors working in multiple unions, in both control and intervention arms. Intervention and surveillance teams were aware of cluster allocation, though there were no incentives for under or over reporting psychological distress. Finally, although we screened most mothers for distress in the first few weeks after childbirth, some were screened up to a year after delivery and we were unable to investigate differential effects of the intervention on early versus late postpartum psychological distress. Because the women's group intervention was designed to benefit individuals beyond those attending groups, we assessed its impact at the population level and did not conduct subanalyses of individuals in the intervention arm.

Conclusions

Participatory women's groups in rural Bangladesh did not reduce postpartum psychological distress, possibly due to contextual factors and the relative importance of neonatal mortality as a population-level predictor of distress in this setting. An investigation of how contextual factors affect the mechanisms of women's groups across settings is needed, as is local, formative research to identify ways of adapting group-based or individually delivered interventions for maternal mental health.

Acknowledgments

We are grateful to the women and families who took part in the trial. We thank the Diabetic Association of Bangladesh for supporting the work and Badrun Nahar Bithi for managing the data.

Author Contributions

Conceived and designed the experiments: KA AK SS TN BHA MMH JB AC TH AP EF. Analyzed the data: KC. Wrote the paper: KC. Commented on the draft: KA AK SS TN BHA MMH JB AC TH AP EF. Approved the final version: KC KA AK SS TN BHA MMH JB AC TH AP EF.

References

1. Goldberg D, Huxley P (1992) Common mental disorders: a biosocial model. London, UK: Tavistock/Routledge.
2. Harris EC, Barraclough B (1997) Suicide as an outcome for mental disorders: a meta-analysis. British Journal of Psychiatry 170: 205–228.
3. Prince M, Patel V, Saxena S, Maj M, Maselko J, et al. (2007) No health without mental health. Lancet 370: 859–877.
4. Rahman A, Iqbal Z, Bunn J, Lovel H, Harrington R (2004) Impact of maternal depression on infant nutritional status and illness: a cohort study. Archives of General Psychiatry 61: 946–952.
5. Senturk V, Hanlon C, Medhin G, Dewey M, Araya M, et al. (2012) Impact of perinatal somatic and common mental disorder symptoms on functioning in Ethiopian women: The P-MaMiE population-based cohort study. Journal of Affective Disorders 136: 340–349.
6. Cooper PJ, Tomlinson M, Swartz L, Woolgar M, Murray L, et al. (1999) Postpartum depression and the mother-infant relationship in a South African peri-urban settlement. British Journal of Psychiatry 175: 554–548.
7. Parsons CE, Young KS, Rochat TJ, Kringelbach ML, Stein A (2012) Postnatal depression and its effects on child development: a review of evidence from low- and middle-income countries. British Medical Bulletin 101: 57–79.
8. Surkan PJ, Kennedy CE, Hurley KM, Black MM (2011) Maternal depression and early childhood growth in developing countries: systematic review and meta-analysis. Bulletin of the World Health Organization 89.
9. Fisher J, Mello CD, Patel V, Rahman A, Tran T, et al. (2012) Prevalence and determinants of common perinatal mental disorders in women in low- and lower-middle- income countries: a systematic review. Bulletin of the World Health Organisation 90: 139–149.
10. Clarke K, King M, Prost A (2013) Psychosocial Interventions for Perinatal Common Mental Disorders Delivered by Non-Mental Health Specialists in Low and Middle-Income Countries: A Systematic Review and Meta-Analysis. PLoS Medicine 10: e100154.
11. Rahman A, Fisher J, Bower P, Luchters S, Tran T, et al. (2013) Interventions for common perinatal mental disorders in women in low- and middle-income countries: a systematic review and meta-analysis. Bulletin of the World Health Organization.
12. Hanlon C (2012) Maternal depression in low- and middle- income countries. International Health 5: 4–5.
13. Prost A, Colbourn T, Seward N, Azad K, Coomarasamy A, et al. (2013) Women's groups practising participatory learning and action to improve maternal and newborn health in low-resource settings: a systematic review and meta-analysis. Lancet 381: 1736–1746.

14. Rath S, Nair N, Tripathy P, Barnett S, Rath S, et al. (2010) Explaining the impact of a women's group led community mobilisation intervention on maternal and newborn health outcomes: the Ekjut trial process evaluation. BMC Health and Human Rights 10.
15. Tripathy P, Nair N, Barnett S, Mahapatra R, Borghi J, et al. (2010) Effect of a participatory intervention with women's groups on birth outcomes and maternal depression in Jharkhand and Orissa, India: a cluster-randomised controlled trial. Lancet 375: 1182–1192.
16. Azad K, Barnett S, Banerjee B, Shaha S, Khan K, et al. (2010) Effect of scaling up women's groups on birth outcomes in three rural districts in Bangladesh: a cluster-randomised controlled trial. Lancet 375: 1193–1202.
17. Fottrell E, Azad K, Kuddus A, Younes L, Shaha S, et al. (2013) The effect of increased coverage of participatory women's groups on neonatal mortality in Bangladesh: a cluster randomized trial. JAMA Pediatrics 20: 1–9.
18. Black MM, Baqui AH, Zaman K, McNary SW, Le K, et al. (2007) Depressive symptoms among rural Bangladeshi mothers: implications for infant development. Journal of Child Psychology and Psychiatry 48: 764–772.
19. Gausia K, Fisher C, Ali M, Oosthuizen J (2009) Magnitude and contributory factors of postnatal depression: a community-based cohort study from a rural subdistrict of Bangladesh. Psychological Medicine 39: 999–1007.
20. World Health Organisation (2007) WHO-AIMS report on mental health system in Bangladesh. Dhaka.
21. Houweling TA, Azad K, Younes L, Kuddus A, Shaha S, et al. (2011) The effect of participatory women's groups on birth outcomes in Bangladesh: does coverage matter? Study protocol for a randomized controlled trial. Trials 12: 208.
22. Chowdhury M, Hasan G, Karim M (2011) A study on existing WATSAN condition in two twa gardens in Maulvibazar. Journal of Environmental Science and Natural Resources 4: 13–18.
23. Ahmed M, Begum A, Chowdhury M (2010) Social constraints before sanitation improvement in tea gardens of Sylhet, Bangladesh. Environmental Monitoring and Assessment 164: 263–271.
24. World Health Organization (1994) A user's guide to self-reporting questionnaires. Geneva.
25. Harpham T, Reichenheim M, Oser R, Thomas E, Hamid N, et al. (2003) Measuring mental health in a cost-effective manner. Health Policy and Planning 18: 344–349.
26. Hayes RJ, Bennett S (1999) Simple sample size calculation for cluster-randomised trials. International Epidemiological Association 28: 319–326.
27. Hayes RJ, Moulton LH (2009) Cluster randomised trials: Chapman & Hall/ CRC Interdisciplinary Statistics.
28. Islam MM, Ali M, Ferroni P, Underwood P, Alam MF (2000) Validity of a self reporting questionnaire (SRQ) in detecting psychiatric illnesses in an Uraban [sic] community in Bangladesh. Bangladesh Journal of Psychiatry 14: 31–43.
29. StataCorp (2011) Stata Statistical Software: Release 12. In: College Station, editor. TX. StataCorp LP,.
30. Gausia K, Fisher C, Ali M, Oosthuizen J (2009) Antenatal depression and suicidal ideation among rural Bangladeshi women: a community-based study. Archives of Women's Mental Health 12: 351–358.
31. Nasreen HE, Kabir ZN, Forsell Y, Edhborg M (2011) Prevalence and associated factors of depressive and anxiety symptoms during pregnancy: a population based study in rural Bangladesh. BMC Women's Health 11.
32. Choudhury WA, Quraishi FA, Haque Z (2006) Mental health and psychosocial aspects of disaster preparedness in Bangladesh. International Review of Psychiatry 18: 529–535.
33. Araya R, Rojas G, Fritsch R, Gaete J, Rojas M, et al. (2003) Treating depression in primary care in low-income women in Santiago, Chile: a randomised controlled trial. Lancet 361: 995–1000.
34. Bolton P, Bass J, Betancourt T, Speelman L, Onyango G, et al. (2007) Interventions for depression symptoms among adolescent survivors of war and displacement in northern Uganda. Journal of the American Medical Association 298: 519–527.
35. Bolton P, Bass J, Neugebauer R, Verdeli H, Clougherty KF, et al. (2003) Group interpersonal psychotherapy for depression in rural Uganda: a randomized controlled trial. Journal of the American Medical Association 289: 3117–3124.
36. Gao L, Chan SW, Li X, Chen S, Hao Y (2010) Evaluation of an interpersonal psychotherapy-oriented childbirth education programme for Chinese first-time childbearing women: a randomised controlled trial. International Journal of Nursing Studies 47: 1208–1216.
37. Mao H-J, Li H-J, Chiu H, Chan W-C, Chen S-L (2012) Effectiveness of antenatal emotional self-management training program in prevention of postnatal depression in Chinese women. Perspectives in Psychiatric Care 48: 218–224.
38. Rojas G, Fritsch R, Solis J, Jadresic E, Castillo C, et al. (2007) Treatment of postnatal depression in low-income mothers in primary-care clinics in Santiago, Chile: a randomised controlled trial. Lancet 370: 1629–1637.
39. Cooper PJ, Tomlinson M, Swartz L, Landman M, Molteno C, et al. (2009) Improving quality of mother-infant relationship and infant attachment in socioeconomically deprived community in South Africa: randomised controlled trial. British Medical Journal 338: 997.
40. Rahman A, Malik A, Sikander S, Roberts C, Creed F (2008) Cognitive behaviour therapy-based intervention by community health workers for mothers with depression and their infants in rural Pakistan: a cluster-randomised controlled trial. Lancet 372: 902–909.
41. Zug S (2006) Monga - Seasonal food insecurity in Bangladesh - Bringing the information together. Journal of Social Studies 11.

10

Viral Etiology of Respiratory Tract Infections in Children at the Pediatric Hospital in Ouagadougou (Burkina Faso)

Solange Ouédraogo[1], Blaise Traoré[1], Zah Ange Brice Nene Bi[1], Firmin Tiandama Yonli[1], Donatien Kima[1], Pierre Bonané[1], Lassané Congo[1], Rasmata Ouédraogo Traoré[1], Diarra Yé[1], Christophe Marguet[2], Jean-Christophe Plantier[3], Astrid Vabret[4], Marie Gueudin[3]*

1 Charles de Gaulle Pediatric University Hospital, Ouagadougou, Burkina Faso, **2** Respiratory Diseases, Allergy and CF Unit, Paediatric Department, Rouen University Hospital Charles Nicolle, EA3830, Inserm CIC204, Rouen, France, **3** Laboratory of Virology, GRAM EA 2656 Rouen University Hospital Charles Nicolle, Rouen, France, **4** Laboratory of Human and Molecular Virology, Caen University Hospital Clemenceau, Caen, France

Abstract

Background: Acute respiratory infections (ARIs) are a major cause of morbidity and mortality in children in Africa. The circulation of viruses classically implicated in ARIs is poorly known in Burkina Faso. The aim of this study was to identify the respiratory viruses present in children admitted to or consulting at the pediatric hospital in Ouagadougou.

Methods: From July 2010 to July 2011, we tested nasal aspirates of 209 children with upper or lower respiratory infection for main respiratory viruses (respiratory syncytial virus (RSV), metapneumovirus, adenovirus, parainfluenza viruses 1, 2 and 3, influenza A, B and C, rhinovirus/enterovirus), by immunofluorescence locally in Ouagadougou, and by PCR in France. Bacteria have also been investigated in 97 samples.

Results: 153 children (73.2%) carried at least one virus and 175 viruses were detected. Rhinoviruses/enteroviruses were most frequently detected (rhinovirus n = 88; enterovirus n = 38) and were found to circulate throughout the year. An epidemic of RSV infections (n = 25) was identified in September/October, followed by an epidemic of influenza virus (n = 13), mostly H1N1pdm09. This epidemic occurred during the period of the year in which nighttime temperatures and humidity were at their lowest. Other viruses tested were detected only sporadically. Twenty-two viral co-infections were observed. Bacteria were detected in 29/97 samples with 22 viral/bacterial co-infections.

Conclusions: This study, the first of its type in Burkina Faso, warrants further investigation to confirm the seasonality of RSV infection and to improve local diagnosis of influenza. The long-term objective is to optimize therapeutic management of infected children.

Editor: Pierre Roques, CEA, France

Funding: Sanofi Pasteur funded this study in its entirety. The funder approved the study design but had no role in data collection and analysis, decision to publish, or preparation of the manuscript.

Competing Interests: This study was funded by Sanofi Pasteur. An agreement was signed with the university hospital of Rouen which managed the funds.

* Email: Marie.Gueudin@chu-rouen.fr

Introduction

Respiratory viruses are ubiquitous, but most epidemiological knowledge relates to developed countries. In contrast, the burden of acute respiratory infections (ARIs) is particularly heavy among children in developing countries, with high mortality and hospital admission rates. The number of deaths related to ARIs has been estimated at 1.9 million children aged less than 5 years, 70% of whom live in Africa or South-East Asia [1]. In Burkina Faso (West Africa), ARIs are also a major cause of child admissions to hospital [2] with a 17.6% mortality rate in children aged under 5 years [3]. For a long time now, *Streptococcus pneumonia*, *Haemophilus influenza* and *Staphylococcus aureus* have been considered as the sole causal agents of severe ARIs in developing countries, and guidelines recommend prescribing antibiotics. Conversely, detection of viruses by molecular methods has provided evidence that a growing number of respiratory viruses are potent pathogenic agents for the respiratory tract. Thus, respiratory syncytial virus (RSV), human metapneumovirus (hMPV), rhinoviruses, parainfluenza (PIVs) and influenza viruses are currently recognized as common ARI etiologies in young children in developed countries [4,5]. The etiology of ARI is complex and emphasized by the demonstration of viral, bacterial or mixed co-infections in the respiratory tracts [5,6,7].

However, in developing countries and especially in Africa, studies on virus-related ARIs are limited to very few countries. Nevertheless, the results of these studies confirm epidemiological data reported in developed countries and underline the fact that viruses also cause frequent upper or lower airway infections. Early diagnosis facilitates early management and is recognized as one way to combat ARIs [8]. In fact, lack of sensitivity and specificity of symptoms prevents differentiation between influenza or any other viral infection and malaria [9,10]. The recommended early and easy use of antibiotics is not effective in viral ARIs, and can only prevent occurrence of bacterial super infection. In this context, viral diagnosis can prevent use of unnecessary costly antibiotics or antimalarial treatments.

To our knowledge, no specific data concerning the circulation of these viruses is currently available for Burkina Faso, even for influenza virus, which is the most documented virus internationally [11].

We carried out a prospective study, over a period of one year at Charles de Gaulle pediatric University Hospital in Ouagadougou (Burkina Faso). The aim was to determine the microbiological agents of these respiratory diseases using rapid detection of antigens by immunofluorescence, multiplex molecular tests, and bacterial cultures on nasopharyngeal samples. We aimed to improve our knowledge on the circulation of viruses and the type of ARIs that they cause.

Materials and Methods

Patients

This prospective study was conducted at Charles de Gaulle pediatric hospital in Ouagadougou, between July 1st 2010 and June 30th 2011. Inclusion criteria were as follows: Children aged under three years attending or hospitalized with an upper or lower airway infection. Upper respiratory infections were defined as congestive otitis, rhinitis associated with fever, and a hoarse cough suggesting tracheitis or laryngitis. Lower respiratory infection were defined as acute febrile respiratory distress, acute bronchiolitis, acute coughing or wheezing, febrile chest sounds suggesting pneumonia, bronchiolitis, asthma exacerbation. Oral parental consent was obtained to use a part of the nasopharyngeal aspiration for PCRs and clinical data were collected. In French law, the right to use the end of the samples is written in the code of public health: Code de la santé publique - Article L1211-2. The ethics committee in Burkina Faso was not consulted as it was recent when the study started.

Detection of viruses

At the hospital laboratory in Ouagadougou, antigens for RSV, hMPV, influenza virus A and B, parainfluenza type 1, 2, and 3, and adenovirus were detected by direct immunofluorescence assay (DFA) from nasopharyngeal aspiration (NPA) samples, employing commercial monoclonal antibodies conjugated with fluorescein isothiocyanate (Imagen, Oxoid, UK). A positive result was indicated by DFA, if a technician noted presence of at least one cell showing a typical fluorescence pattern, provided that at least 20 respiratory cells were available in the sample. All the samples were frozen at −80°C and further analyzed by molecular methods at the virology laboratory of Caen University Hospital. Nucleic acids were extracted with a Qiasymphony kit (Qiasymphony Virus/Bacteria Minikit, Qiagen, Courtaboeuf, France), and RT-PCR was carried out for detection of RSV, hMPV, influenza A and B viruses (RSV/hMPV r-gene, Influenza A/B r-gene, Argène Biomérieux) and rhinovirus/enterovirus and influenza C virus (in-house multiplex RT-PCR) [12]. Viral subtyping was carried out according to the National Reference Center for Influenza techniques (Institut Pasteur, Paris, France).

Bacterial growths

Bacteriological examinations were carried out only on 97 samples collected between the end of March and end of June 2011. NPA cultures were performed for growth of common and potentially pathogenic aerobic bacteria: *Streptococcus pneumoniae, Haemophilus influenzae, Moraxella catharralis, Staphylococcus aureus*, and *Klebsiella pneumonia*.

Climatic data

Burkina Faso has a tropical Sudanian-Sahelian climate with two opposite seasons: a rainy season, with 300 to 1200 mm of precipitation, and a dry season characterized by the Harmattan, a hot dry wind loaded with dust and originating in the Sahara Desert. The data used were obtained from the meteorological archives of Ouagadougou Airport *(source http://rp5.ru/archive.php?wmo_id = 65503&lang = fr)*. From daily data available, we calculated mean monthly values for temperature and humidity at 6 AM and 12 noon.

Statistical analysis

MedCalc software was used for the comparison of rates realized in Table 1. A P value of 0.05 was considered statistically significant. For the climatic data, mean monthly values for humidity and temperature for the months with or without detection of RSV or influenza A virus were compared using t-test after verification of the equality of variances by a F-test.

Results

Two hundred and nine children (boys: 58.4%) were included in this study. They were all aged less than three years, and 60.8% of them were less than 1 year old. Seventy-three children (34.9%) attended outpatient consultation, and 136 (65.1%) were admitted to hospital. Respiratory symptoms are described in Table 1.

One hundred and fifty-three children (73.2%) carried at least one virus (table 1). Children with positive results were mostly identified by RT-PCR (n = 149, 71.3%), and only 21 (10%) were detected by DFA. Positive results by DFA were as follows: adenovirus ($n = 3$), parainfluenza virus 1 ($n = 2$), parainfluenza virus 2 ($n = 1$), parainfluenza virus 3 ($n = 5$), and RSV ($n = 10$). RT-PCR detected: rhinovirus (n = 88; 59.1%), enterovirus (n = 38; 25.5%), RSV (n = 24; 16.1%), influenza (n = 13, including one case of influenza C; 8.7%), and one case of hMPV. Co-infections were detected in 14 samples (9.4%). Only one discordant result was observed for one sample, which was positive for RSV by DFA and negative by PCR. Among the viruses tested, only influenza B was never detected. Twenty-two (14.4%) viral co-infections were observed involving mainly rhinovirus or enteroviruses. Ninety eight (72.1%) of the inpatients carried at least one virus and 55 (75.3%) of the outpatients.

Bacterial cultures were carried out for 97 samples. Eighteen (18.6%) were negative for Bacteria and Viruses, 50 (51.5%) were positive for one or more viruses, 7 (7.2%) were positive for one or more bacteria and 22 (22.7%) were positive with a viral/bacterial co-infection. *Staphylococcus aureus, Klebsiella pneumonia*, and *Streptococcus pneumonia* were isolated in 14 cases (42.4%), 10 cases (30.3%), and 9 cases (27.7%) respectively.

Twenty-two viral/bacterial co-infections were diagnosed, 20 of which involved an enterovirus and/or a rhinovirus. The remaining two viral/bacterial co-infections associated *Staphylococcus aureus*/PIV-3 and *Staphylococcus aureus*/adenovirus. Four bacterial co-infections were detected: *Staphylococcus aureus/Klebsiella pneumoniae* ($n = 2$) and *Staphylococcus aureus/Streptococcus pneumoniae* ($n = 2$). Rhinovirus was also detected in three of these four cases. 76 of the 97 children (78.4%) were hospitalized and 26 (34.2%) of them were infected with a Bacteria.

Table 1. Respiratory viruses detected either by direct immunofluorescence or RT-PCR and the associated final diagnosis (in some cases, more than one), * significant difference (p = 0.0006) with the group where no virus was detected.

Virus and viral co-infection	N (%) results		Children under 1 year old	Children admitted to hospital	Pneumonia	Bronchiolitis	Bronchitis/Asthma	Laryngitis	Nasopharyngitis/Otitis
None	56	26.8%	37	38	8	6	26	3	28
Adenovirus only	2	1.0%	1	2		1	2		1
Adenovirus + Rhinovirus	1	0.5%	1	1					1
Influenza A only	8	3.8%	4	3	2		3	1	4
Influenza A + Enterovirus	1	0.5%	0	0					1
Influenza A + Rhinovirus	2	1.0%	2	2		2	1		1
Influenza A + Rhinovirus + Enterovirus	1	0.5%	0	0					1
Influenza C + Rhinovirus	1	0.5%	1	1		1			
Parainfluenza 1 + Rhinovirus	1	0.5%	0	0					1
Parainfluenza 1 + RSV	1	0.5%	1	0			1		1
Parainfluenza 2	1	0.5%	1	1			1		
Parainfluenza 3 + Enterovirus	4	1.9%	2	3	1	1	3		2
Parainfluenza 3 + Rhinovirus	1	0.5%	0	1		1			
RSV only	19	9.1%	14	14	6	10*	8		5
RSV + Rhinovirus	3	1.4%	2	3	1	2	1		
RSV + Enterovirus	2	1.0%	2	2		2	2		
Metapneumovirus	1	0.5%	1	0		1	1		
Enterovirus only	26	12.4%	12	18	3	2	11	1	18
Rhinovirus only	74	35.4%	43	44	8	11	35	3	37
Rhinovirus + Enterovirus	4	1.9%	3	3	1	2	1		3
Total	**209**	**100.0%**	**127**	**136**	**30**	**42**	**96**	**8**	**104**

Monthly distribution and weekly detailed circulation of viruses (Figure 1 and Table 2), showed two successive winter epidemics. A RSV epidemic (24 RSV A, 1 RSV B) occurred between mid-September and end of October, with six co-infections including five rhinoviruses/enteroviruses. Nineteen of the 25 children infected with RSV were hospitalized which correspond to 14% of all the inpatients and 8% of the outpatients without significant difference (p = 0.2517). Children with RSV had significantly more bronchiolitis than the others (p = 0.0006) (table 1). RSV was found in the samples of 16 of the 70 children (22.9%) under the age of 6 months and in 9 of the 139 children above 6 months (6.5%) with significant difference (p = 0.0012).

This epidemic of RSV infection was followed by an epidemic of influenza A infection (H1N1pdm09, n = 8 and H3N2, n = 4) from mid-December to mid-February. These viruses were frequently associated with a rhinovirus or enterovirus (38.4%). Six children were hospitalized.

One hundred and nineteen children (56.9%) had a rhinovirus or an enterovirus which was detected during the year, with higher rates of rhinoviruses in April, May and June 2011. Rhinovirus and enterovirus were detected in 56.6% of the inpatients and 57.5% of the outpatients without significant difference (p = 0,8353). Of the 97 samples that underwent both bacteriological and virological investigation, 44 were positive for only enterovirus or human rhinovirus. A total of 56.5% of these children were under the age of 1 year and 39% were hospitalized.

Three adenovirus infections were detected at the end of February and five infections with parainfluenza virus 3 from March to June 2011. Only one of the three children infected with adenovirus was co-infected with a rhinovirus. The five children infected with parainfluenza virus 3 were co-infected with a rhinovirus or enterovirus and four of the five children were hospitalized.

An effect of climate has often been put forward as an explanation for the circulation patterns of respiratory viruses. A comparison of our findings for influenza and RSV with the available climatic data (Figure 2) showed that the influenza epidemic coincided with the period in which nighttime temperature (p = 0.0007) and relative humidity (p = 0.0343) were lowest. No significant climatic data were related to RSV epidemic.

Discussion

The epidemiology of respiratory virus infections is unknown in Burkina Faso, although suspected considering previous studies conducted in neighboring countries [13,14]. Firstly, this study provides evidence of the role of viruses in upper and lower airway diseases in this country. Our findings highlight the fact that three quarters of infants or young children with any respiratory symptoms carry at least one virus. This rate of detection concords with previous studies in developed and African countries [15,16,17,18]. Most of the viruses were identified by molecular diagnosis, and direct immunofluorescence yield was low but concordant with previous work [19], achieving only 10% of positive results. One discrepancy has been observed with a sample positive by DFA and negative by PCR without possible control. It has been verified that the exclusion of this sample would not have changed the statistical conclusions of the study. RSV must be considered as a main etiologic agent even if rhinoviruses or enteroviruses were most frequently detected. RSV is well known for being one of the main agents associated with upper or lower airway infections in infants, and it has been demonstrated that RSV causes more severe diseases than other respiratory viruses [6]. Although it is a universal virus, data on RSV circulation are still limited in Africa. In a previous review, *Stensballe et al.* suggested that RSV outbreaks begin on the southern coast and move northward from January to July [20]. In our study, the RSV outbreak in Burkina Faso was observed during the fall. This was consistent with data on RSV epidemics occurring in the fall or winter in neighboring countries like Senegal [13], Nigeria [21] and Cameroon [17]. In Ghana [14], another neighboring country to the south, RSV circulation was however observed throughout the year with a peak rate in summer. The influence of the climate remains difficult to demonstrate, and the various climates associated with RSV epidemics tend to prove the lack of impact of climate on their onset. In Burkina Faso, the peak for RSV infections coincided with the dry season, as reported in Nigeria and South Africa [21]. In contrast, RSV epidemics occur during

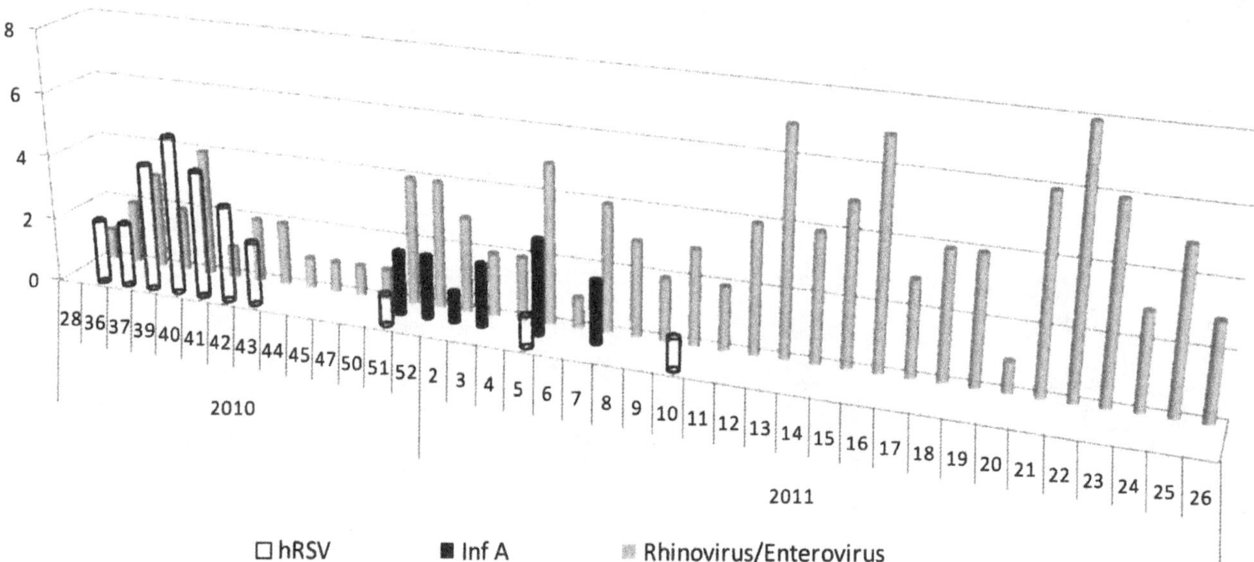

Figure 1. Weekly distribution of the three main detected viruses.

Table 2. Monthly distribution of viruses.

Year/Month	AdV	Inf A	Inf C	hRSV	hMPV	PIV 1	PIV 2	PIV 3	RhV	EnV	Total	
2010/07									1		1	0.6%
2010/09				6					5		11	6.3%
2010/10				16	1				5	6	28	15.9%
2010/11									3		3	1.7%
2010/12		4		1		1			7	2	15	8.5%
2011/01		3							6	3	12	6.8%
2011/02	2	5		1					6	6	20	11.4%
2011/03				1		1		2	10	4	18	10.2%
2011/04	1							1	14	8	24	13.6%
2011/05								1	14	4	19	10.8%
2011/06			1				1	1	17	5	25	14.2%
	3	12	1	25	1	2	1	5	88	38	176	
	1.7%	6.8%	0.6%	14.2%	0.6%	1.1%	0.6%	2.8%	50.0%	21.6%		

the rainy season in Mozambique [21] and Ghana [14]. Lastly in Kenya the duration of RSV seasons was long, but there were no clear climate patterns that appeared to coincide with changes in RSV circulation [19,22].

The second main finding of our study was the high rate of picornaviruses, and more than half of this population carried rhinoviruses or enteroviruses. The technique that we used for virus detection was not based on sequencing, and discrimination between the two species cannot be guaranteed. Nevertheless, it is clear that these viruses circulated throughout the year and were mainly isolated alone, although they are implicated in all but one viral co-infections. This high rate underlines the major involvement of these viruses in respiratory tract infections, as previously reported elsewhere in the world [23]. Picornaviruses are not the focus of the rare epidemiological studies conducted in Africa. They also appear to be the most frequent viruses identified in Cameroon, and Kenya [24], and a recent molecular study [25] detected all three (A, B and C) strains of rhinovirus in up to 35% of samples collected, as previously described in developing countries.

The bacteriological examinations were carried out during only 3 months, which is an important limitation for data analysis. During this period more than one quarter of this young population had a bacteria/virus co-infection. These co-infections associated an enterovirus or a rhinovirus with common potentially pathogenic bacteria encountered in childhood. When co-infections are identified, the respective contribution of each microbiological agent in the pathogenesis of respiratory tract infections remains unclear. Among the virus/virus co-infections, RSV was clearly identified as the most virulent agent, and its pathogenic effect predominated rhinovirus [6]. It is more difficult however to assess the respective pathogenic effect of bacteria or viruses detected simultaneously. Positive nasopharyngeal bacterial culture is a weak predictor of upper airway infections since healthy individuals often carry pathogenic bacteria. The presence of bacteria does not allow to conclude or to exclude to an isolated bacterial infection in upper airway infections. Conversely, Rhinovirus was detected as the sole causal agent in severe acute respiratory distress [24] and pneumonia [26] in Kenya and South Africa, respectively. This latter is in contrast with the better outcome attributed to Rhinovirus in developed countries [23], which is not necessarily associated with more severe disease.

Clinical diagnoses involving life-threatening infections such as malaria and meningitis were mentioned in the data collected. However, laboratory confirmation of these diagnoses was not part of our study and it was not possible to further analyze these cases.

Lastly, influenza A appeared as the fourth most prevalent virus in Ouagadougou, and was detected from mid December to the end of February. This result has not been compared with the Global Influenza Surveillance and Response System database, as no data on influenza epidemics was available from Burkina Faso for this season. This winter epidemic period of influenza A infection does not match that reported for neighboring countries. Nevertheless, this influenza epidemic occurred during the coldest period of the year, when relative humidity was low. This agreed with recent reports, showing that survival of the influenza virus in the external environment is related to low relative humidity and temperature [27,28,29]. No influenza B virus was identified in this study, contrasting with the high rates observed in neighboring countries over the same period. As our study mainly included very young children, for whom influenza virus was not reported as a major pathogenic agent [6], the likelihood of detecting either influenza A or B was reduced. Moreover, we are not able to rule out a concomitant circulation of influenza B in older populations.

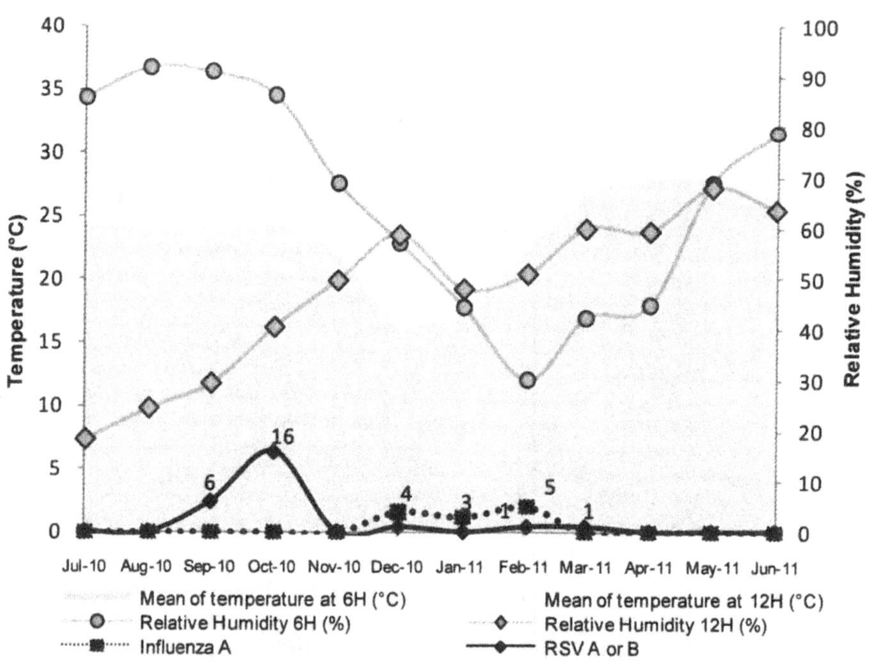

Figure 2. Progression of the epidemics of RSV and influenza virus infections related to temperature and relative humidity values recorded at 6 AM and 12 noon.

Our study is the first of its type in Burkina Faso and warrants follow-up to confirm the seasonality of RSV infection and the period during which this virus circulates. The results presented here assess the involvement of the most frequent pathogenic viruses in upper and lower respiratory tract infections in young children from Burkina Faso. Our findings raise the question of sparing antibiotics by introducing routine detection of viruses. Such a strategy would be supported by the weak mortality attributed to RSV, which is the most aggressive viral agent in Africa [21]. However, the expensive cost of multiplex PCR testing prevents feasibility in routine practice. The less costly direct immunofluorescence assay has shown very low yield in this study, and consequently can not be recommended as an alternative routine test. Further studies are warranted to achieve the best strategy for management of childhood respiratory tract infections in Burkina Faso. More extensive research on the etiological agents of ARIs can only be beneficial, facilitating early adoption of appropriate treatment strategies.

Acknowledgments

The authors are grateful to Nikki-Sabourin-Gibbs, Rouen University Hospital, for editing the manuscript. We also thank Mrs Krystyna Astier for her constant support of the cooperation between the university hospitals of Rouen and Ouagadougou.

Author Contributions

Conceived and designed the experiments: MG SO CM RO DY. Performed the experiments: RO AV BT ZABNB FTY. Analyzed the data: MG SO. Contributed reagents/materials/analysis tools: DK PB LC. Wrote the paper: SO MG CM JCP.

References

1. Williams BG, Gouws E, Boschi-Pinto C, Bryce J, Dye C (2002) Estimates of world-wide distribution of child deaths from acute respiratory infections. Lancet Infect Dis 2: 25–32.
2. Tall FR, Valian A, Curtis V, Traore A, Nacro B, et al. (1994) [Acute respiratory infections in pediatric hospital at Bobo-Dioulasso (Burkina Faso)]. Arch Pediatr 1: 249–254.
3. Liu L, Johnson HL, Cousens S, Perin J, Scott S, et al. (2012) Global, regional, and national causes of child mortality: an updated systematic analysis for 2010 with time trends since 2000. Lancet 379: 2151–2161.
4. Tregoning JS, Schwarze J (2010) Respiratory viral infections in infants: causes, clinical symptoms, virology, and immunology. Clin Microbiol Rev 23: 74–98.
5. Ruuskanen O, Lahti E, Jennings LC, Murdoch DR (2011) Viral pneumonia. Lancet 377: 1264–1275.
6. Marguet C, Lubrano M, Gueudin M, Le Roux P, Deschildre A, et al. (2009) In very young infants severity of acute bronchiolitis depends on carried viruses. PLoS One 4: e4596.
7. Kouni S, Karakitsos P, Chranioti A, Theodoridou M, Chrousos G, et al. (2012) Evaluation of viral co-infections in hospitalized and non-hospitalized children with respiratory infections using microarrays. Clin Microbiol Infect.
8. Simoes EAF, Cherian T, Chow J, Shahid-Salles SA, Laxminarayan R, et al. (2006) Acute Respiratory Infections in Children.
9. Ho A, Fox R, Seaton RA, MacConnachie A, Peters E, et al. (2010) Hospitalised adult patients with Suspected 2009 H1N1 Infection at Regional Infectious Diseases Units in Scotland–most had alternative final diagnoses. J Infect 60: 83–85.
10. Lillie PJ, Duncan CJ, Sheehy SH, Meyer J, O'Hara GA, et al. (2012) Distinguishing malaria and influenza: early clinical features in controlled human experimental infection studies. Travel Med Infect Dis 10: 192–196.
11. Gessner BD, Shindo N, Briand S (2011) Seasonal influenza epidemiology in sub-Saharan Africa: a systematic review. Lancet Infect Dis 11: 223–235.
12. Bellau-Pujol S, Vabret A, Legrand L, Dina J, Gouarin S, et al. (2005) Development of three multiplex RT-PCR assays for the detection of 12 respiratory RNA viruses. J Virol Methods 126: 53–63.
13. Niang MN, Diop OM, Sarr FD, Goudiaby D, Malou-Sompy H, et al. (2010) Viral etiology of respiratory infections in children under 5 years old living in tropical rural areas of Senegal: The EVIRA project. J Med Virol 82: 866–872.
14. Kwofie TB, Anane YA, Nkrumah B, Annan A, Nguah SB, et al. (2012) Respiratory viruses in children hospitalized for acute lower respiratory tract infection in Ghana. Virol J 9: 78.
15. Laurent C, Dugue AE, Brouard J, Nimal D, Dina J, et al. (2012) Viral epidemiology and severity of respiratory infections in infants in 2009: a prospective study. Pediatr Infect Dis J 31: 827–831.

16. Marcone DN, Ellis A, Videla C, Ekstrom J, Ricarte C, et al. (2013) Viral etiology of acute respiratory infections in hospitalized and outpatient children in Buenos Aires, Argentina. Pediatr Infect Dis J 32: e105–110.
17. Njouom R, Yekwa EL, Cappy P, Vabret A, Boisier P, et al. (2012) Viral etiology of influenza-like illnesses in Cameroon, January-December 2009. J Infect Dis 206 Suppl 1: S29–35.
18. D'Acremont V, Kilowoko M, Kyungu E, Philipina S, Sangu W, et al. (2014) Beyond malaria–causes of fever in outpatient Tanzanian children. N Engl J Med 370: 809–817.
19. Okiro EA, Ngama M, Bett A, Nokes DJ (2012) The incidence and clinical burden of respiratory syncytial virus disease identified through hospital outpatient presentations in Kenyan children. PLoS One 7: e52520.
20. Stensballe LG, Devasundaram JK, Simoes EA (2003) Respiratory syncytial virus epidemics: the ups and downs of a seasonal virus. Pediatr Infect Dis J 22: S21–32.
21. Robertson SE, Roca A, Alonso P, Simoes EA, Kartasasmita CB, et al. (2004) Respiratory syncytial virus infection: denominator-based studies in Indonesia, Mozambique, Nigeria and South Africa. Bull World Health Organ 82: 914–922.
22. Haynes AK, Manangan AP, Iwane MK, Sturm-Ramirez K, Homaira N, et al. (2013) Respiratory syncytial virus circulation in seven countries with Global Disease Detection Regional Centers. J Infect Dis 208 Suppl 3: S246–254.
23. Debiaggi M, Canducci F, Ceresola ER, Clementi M (2012) The role of infections and coinfections with newly identified and emerging respiratory viruses in children. Virol J 9: 247.
24. Feikin DR, Njenga MK, Bigogo G, Aura B, Aol G, et al. (2013) Viral and bacterial causes of severe acute respiratory illness among children aged less than 5 years in a high malaria prevalence area of western Kenya, 2007–2010. Pediatr Infect Dis J 32: e14–19.
25. Onyango CO, Welch SR, Munywoki PK, Agoti CN, Bett A, et al. (2012) Molecular epidemiology of human rhinovirus infections in Kilifi, coastal Kenya. J Med Virol 84: 823–831.
26. Pretorius MA, Madhi SA, Cohen C, Naidoo D, Groome M, et al. (2012) Respiratory viral coinfections identified by a 10-plex real-time reverse-transcription polymerase chain reaction assay in patients hospitalized with severe acute respiratory illness–South Africa, 2009–2010. J Infect Dis 206 Suppl 1: S159–165.
27. Azziz Baumgartner E, Dao CN, Nasreen S, Bhuiyan MU, Mah EMS, et al. (2012) Seasonality, timing, and climate drivers of influenza activity worldwide. J Infect Dis 206: 838–846.
28. Lowen AC, Mubareka S, Steel J, Palese P (2007) Influenza virus transmission is dependent on relative humidity and temperature. PLoS Pathog 3: 1470–1476.
29. Tamerius J, Nelson MI, Zhou SZ, Viboud C, Miller MA, et al. (2011) Global influenza seasonality: reconciling patterns across temperate and tropical regions. Environ Health Perspect 119: 439–445.

11

Personalized Tacrolimus Dose Requirement by CYP3A5 but Not ABCB1 or ACE Genotyping in Both Recipient and Donor after Pediatric Liver Transplantation

Yi-kuan Chen[¶], **Long-zhi Han**[¶], **Feng Xue***, **Cong-huan Shen**, **Jun Lu**, **Tai-hua Yang**, **Jian-jun Zhang**, **Qiang Xia***

Department of Liver Surgery and Liver Transplantation, Ren Ji Hospital, School of Medicine, Shanghai Jiao Tong University, Shanghai, P.R. China

Abstract

Tacrolimus (TAC) is the backbone of an immunosuppressive drug used in most solid organ transplant recipients. A single nucleotide polymorphism (SNP) at position 6986G>A in *CYP3A5* has been notably involved in the pharmacokinetic variability of TAC. It is hypothesized that *CYP3A5* genotyping in patients may provide a guideline for TAC therapeutic regimen. To further evaluate the impact of *CYP3A5* variants in donors and recipients, *ABCB1* and *ACE* SNPs in recipients on TAC disposition, clinical and laboratory data were retrospectively reviewed from 90 pediatric patients with liver transplantation and their corresponding donors after 1 year of transplantation. The recipients with *CYP3A5* *1/*1 or *1/*3 required more time to achieve TAC therapeutic range during the induction phase, and needed more upward dose during the late induction and the maintained phases, with lower C/D ratio, compared with those with *CYP3A5* *3/*3. And donor *CYP3A5* genotypes were found to impact on TAC trough concentrations after liver transplantation. No association between *ABCB1* or *ACE* genotypes and TAC disposition post-transplantation was found. These results strongly suggest that *CYP3A5* genotyping both in recipient and donor, not *ABCB1* or *ACE* is necessary for establishing a personalized TAC dosage regimen in pediatric liver transplant patients.

Editor: Lorna Marson, Centre for Inflammation Research, United Kingdom

Funding: This project was supported by National Ministry of Public Health grant (IHECCO8-201213) (http://www.nhfpc.gov.cn/gjhzs/index.shtml) and Shanghai Science and Technology Committee grant (12ZR1418300) (http://www.stcsm.gov.cn/). The funders had roles in study design, data collection and analysis.

Competing Interests: The authors have declared that no competing interests exist.

* Email: fengxue6879@163.com (FX); xiaqiang@medmail.com.cn (QX)

¶ These authors contributed equally to this work.

Introduction

Tacrolimus (TAC) is the backbone of immunosuppressive drug used worldwide in organ transplantation and characterized by a narrow therapeutic range and high inter-individual variability in its pharmacokinetics [1,2]. To achieve the desired target blood concentrations is of critical importance to avoid rejection and dose-related adverse effects after transplantation [3]. The variability makes it difficult to establish an empirical dose regimen for this drug, especially in pediatric patients, in whom 100-fold variability in pharmacokinetic parameters and blood concentration after a fixed dose is routinely observed [4,5]. Underexposure to TAC may result in immunosuppression failure and acute rejection in recipients. On the other hand, overexposure to it may put patients at risk for its considerable toxicity. Therefore, maintaining the drug exposure within this narrow safe therapeutic window becomes a critical aspect in patient management. Concerning the concept that young children need a higher TAC dose than adult patients [4,6], the blood TAC concentration should be monitored regularly to maintain a therapeutic range, especially during the induction phase post-transplantation therapy, when the risk of rejection is the highest. Although various factors, such as age, sex, body weight, drug interactions and other factors lead to the wide range of interpatient variability ineffective dosage of TAC [7], among them genetic factors play a critical role in the pharmacokinetic properties and therapeutic levels of TAC.

Cytochrome P450 (CYP) 3A5 is the major enzyme responsible for the metabolism of TAC and is found in small intestine as well as in the liver [8]. A single nucleotide polymorphism (SNP) in the *CYP3A5* gene involving an A to G transition at position 6986 within intron 3 was found strongly associated with CYP3A5 protein expression. At least one *CYP3A5**1 allele were found to express large amounts of CYP3A5 protein, whereas homozygous for the *CYP3A5**3 allele did not express significant quantities of CYP3A5 protein, which causes alternative splicing and results in a truncated protein and a severe decrease of functional *CYP3A5* [9]. It has become clear that *CYP3A5**1/*1 or *1/*3 (hereinafter defined 'expressor') are significantly associated with lower dose-adjusted TAC exposure and increased TAC dose requirements in order to achieve target blood concentrations compared with variant *CYP3A5**3/*3 (hereinafter defined 'nonexpressor') [7,9–12]. However, it is controversial that, for liver transplantation, the impact of the *CYP3A5* genotype of both the recipients (intestine) and the donors (graft liver) should be taken into account when evaluating TAC pharmacokinetics.

TAC is also substrate of P-glycoprotein, a member drug efflux transporter encoded by the multidrug resistance *ABCB1* gene [13,14]. It has been suggested that some SNPs of the *ABCB1* gene in exons 12 (1236C>T), 21 (2677G>A/T) and 26 (3435C>T) maybe affect synthesis and function of P-glycoprotein. In addition, angiotensin converting enzyme (ACE), which is a key enzyme in the renin-angiotensin system, catalyzes the conversion of angiotensin I to II in the liver and kidney. A line of evidence suggests that variation in intron 16 of the ACE gene (14091–14378) may impact on pharmacokinetics and pharmacodynamics of TAC [15]. However, the impact of SNPs of *ABCB1* and *ACE* on pediatric liver transplants remains unclear.

Although much effort has been devoted to the better understanding of inter-individual differences in response to TAC, little data are available about these relationships in Chinese liver transplanted recipients [16,17], particularly in the pediatric population. Moreover, the effects of *CYP3A5, ABCB1* and *ACE* variants on clinical outcomes are not well established in China. The aim of this study was, therefore to retrospectively determine the impact of *CYP3A5* genotype of recipients (intestine) and donors (graft liver), age, sex, body weight, primary diseases and other factors on TAC dosing requirements and disposition in a cohort of pediatric liver recipients during the 12 months following transplantation. We evaluated the effect of *CYP3A5, ABCB1* and *ACE* variants on the clinical outcomes in our pediatric liver recipients, and attempted understanding the relationship between *CYP3A5*, *ABCB1* or *ACE* genotype and TAC pharmacokinetics may improve our knowledge of how to most effectively administer this drug, leading to considerable benefit to pediatric liver transplant patients.

Materials and Methods

1. Patients

The patients in this retrospective study were 90 consecutive de novo liver graft recipients who underwent living-donor liver transplantation at Shanghai Ren Ji Hospital between October 2008 and December 2012. Median age of the pediatric patients at liver transplantation was 10 months (range, 5–72 months). This study was reviewed and approved by Shanghai Jiao Tong University School of Medicine Ren Ji Hospital Ethical Board (Approval No.: 2013010), and written informed consent was obtained from all their parents during enrollment.

All pediatric patients were administered the immunosuppressive therapy on day 2 to 3 after liver transplantation. TAC (Astella Pharma Co., Limited) was administered orally (dissolved in water for young children) twice daily with an initial dose of 0.15 mg/kg/day, and subsequently adjusted to archiving target blood trough concentration (termed C_0) through routine monitoring. The target C_0 was between 10 and 15 ng/ml during the first month, between 8 and 12 ng/ml during 2–6 months, and between 5 and 8 ng/ml thereafter. In general, repeat or multiple post-operative infections were considered as over-immunosupressive, which needs to reduce the dose of TAC, whereas when an acute cellular rejection happens, it was considered as under-immunosupressive, which needs to increase the dose of TAC. For acute cellular rejection cases, additional immunosuppressive therapy consisted of a maintenance dose of mycophenolate mofitil and steroid.

2. Tacrolimus C_0 monitoring and C/D ratio assessment

Analysis of all patients' clinical and laboratory assessments on day 3, 7, 14, and in month 1, 3, 6, and 12 post-transplantation were performed. EDTA-treated blood (1 ml) was collected every 12 h after the previous dose and then blood TAC C_0 was measured by a microparticulate enzyme immunoassay (Abbott Co., Ltd, Tokyo, Japan). The daily dose of TAC was recorded and weight-adjusted dosage (mg/kg/day) was calculated. The blood concentration was measured and normalized using the corresponding dose. A dose ratio was obtained by the concentration/dose (C/D) ratio, which was used for estimating TAC concentration. When the blood TAC C_0 was not measured at a given time point, the data were excluded.

3. Genotyping of *CYP3A5, ABCB1* and *ACE*

The 90 pediatric recipients and 90 adult donors were genotyped for the single nucleotide polymorphism of *CYP3A5* at position 6986A>G (the *3 or *1 allele, rs776746), *ABCB1* at exons 12 (1236C>T, rs1128503), 21 (2677G>A/T, rs2032582) and 26 (3435C>T, rs1045642) and *ACE* at intron 16 (14091–14378). The genotyping was detected using the PCR-based sequencing. In brief, whole blood samples (1.0 ml) were collected in EDTA-treated tubes. The genomic DNAs were extracted from leukocytes with a QIAamp Blood kit (Qiagen, Hilden, Germany). A fragment containing the 6986A>G polymorphism was amplified in ABI 7900 system (Applied biosystems, Foster City, CA, USA), using Taq polymerase qPCR kit (TaKaRa Bio. Inc., Dalian, China). The primers 5′-ACTGCCCTTGCAGCATTTA-3′ (forward) and 5′-CCAGGAAGCCAGACTTTGA-3′ (reverse) for *CYP3A5*, primers 5′-ACTTCAGTTACCCATCTCG-3′ (forward) and 5′-TTTCCCGTAGAAACCTTAC-3′ (reverse) (1236C>T), primers 5′-ATAGCAAATCTTGGGACAG-3′ (forward) and 5′-GCA-TAGTAAGCAGTAGGGA-3′ (reverse) (2677G>A/T), primers 5′-TGGCAGTTTCAGTGTAAGA-3′ (forward) and 5′-CTCCCAGGCTGTTTATTTG-3′ (reverse) (3435C>T) for *ACBC1* and primers 5′-GCCCTGCAGGTGTCTGCAG-CATGT-3′ (forward) and 5′-GGATGGCTCTCCCCGCCTTGTCTC-3′ (reverse) (1st), primers 5′-TGGGACCACAGCGCCCGCCACTAC-3′ (forward) and 5′-TCGCCAGCCCTCCCATGCCCATAA-3′ (reverse) (2nd) for *ACE* were employed. The qPCR process was carried out as following: 95°C for 10 min, then 94°C for 30 s, 55°C for 30 s, 72°C for 60 s for total 40 cycles and finally 72°C for 7 min. The products were then purified with a QIAquick PCRPurification kit (Qiagen, Hilden, Germany) and run on an ABI 3730XL Genetic Analyzer (Applied biosystems, Foster City, CA, USA) according to the manufacturer's recommendations.

4. Outcome measures

The primary outcomes were TAC dosing requirement (normalized for body weight) and C/D ratio (the latter as surrogate marker) at indicated time points of day (d) 3, d 7, d 14, month (m) 1, m 3, m 6 and m12 for TAC clearance. Secondary outcome measures were acute rejection, acute and chronic infection, as well as liver function.

A one-year follow up after liver transplantation was performed to investigate the possible correlation of various infections with the *CYP3A5**1 status of donors and recipients, and with the SNPs of *ABCB1* and *ACE* of recipients. Incidence of post-operative infections and acute cellular rejection were determined by double-blind physicians. Viral infections were classified by viral pathogens, including CMV, EBV, rotavirus, herpes virus, and HBV. The overlap and relative severity of these infections were also recorded. Viral infections differed according to the intensity of immunosuppression and the serologic status of the recipient. Diagnosis of acute cellular rejection or immunosuppressant-induced hepatic toxicity was based on pathological criteria.

Table 1. Demographic characteristics of recipients and donors.

	Recipient	Donor
Age (Median, Range)	**10 (4–120 month)**	**30 (21–56 year)**
Sex		
Male (%)	52 (57.8)	37 (41.1)
Female (%)	38 (42.2)	53 (58.9)
Body weight (Mean ± Sd; kg)	8.88±3.28	59.35±9.47
Height (Mean ± Sd; cm)	72.97±13.69	162±8.48
Surface area (m^2)	0.41±0.12	
CYP3A5 genotype		
AA, *1/*1 (%)	3 (3.3)	11 (12.2)
AG, *1/*3 (%)	37 (41.1)	34 (37.8)
GG, *3/*3 (%)	50 (55.6)	45 (50.0)
ABCB1 genotype		
1236C>T CT (%)	38 (42.2)	
TT (%)	42 (46.7)	
CC (%)	10 (11.1)	
2677G>AT AT (%)	13 (14.4)	
GA (%)	11 (12.2)	
GG (%)	21 (23.4)	
GT (%)	33 (36.7)	
TT (%)	12 (13.3)	
3435C>T CC (%)	36 (40.0)	
CT (%)	40 (44.4)	
TT (%)	14 (15.6)	
ACE genotype		
I/I (%)	40 (44.4)	
D/I (%)	37 (41.1)	
D/D (%)	13 (14.5)	
Primary diseases		
Congenital biliary atresia (%)	89 (98.9)	
Postoperative cholagenic infection (%)	1 (1.1)	

5. Statistical analyses

All data were collected and expressed as the mean ± standard deviation or the median with deviation range. Data among several groups or continuous variables between two groups were compared using one-way ANOVA, while continuous variables among several groups were compared using two-way ANOVA analysis and followed by Bonferroni adjustment. Categorical variables were compared using Chi-square test or Fisher's exact test. Other data between two groups was analyzed with T-test. A value $p<0.05$ was considered statistically significant in all analyses, which were performed using SPSS 19.0 soft (SPSS inc., Chicago, IL).

Results

1. Pediatric patient clinical characteristics

We summarized the demographic characteristics of the patients and showed them in Table 1. The total of 90 eligible Chinese pediatric liver transplant recipients (52 boys and 38 girls) and 90 Chinese healthy donors (37 men and 53 women) were enrolled. The median age of patient age was 10 months (between 4 months and 10 years), whereas that of donor age median was 30 years (between 21 and 56 years). The primary diseases of the pediatric recipients included 89 congenital biliary atresias (98.9%) and 1 postoperative cholagenic infection (1.1%). *CYP3A5**1/*1 (AA allele), *CYP3A5**1/*3 (AG allele) and *CYP3A5**3/*3 (GG allele) were 3 (3.3%), 37 (41.1%) and 50 (55.6%) cases respectively in recipients, whereas three variants were 11 (12.2%), 34 (37.8%) and 45 (50%) cases in donors. The allele frequencies of *ABCB1* 1236CT, TT, CC, 2677AT, GA, GG, GT, TT, 3435CC, CT and TT were 42.2%, 46.7%, 11.1%, 14.4%, 12.2%, 23.4%, 36.7%, 13.3%, 40.0%, 44.4% and 15.6% in recipients respectively. While the allele frequencies of *ACE I/I*, *D/I*, and *D/D* were 44.4%, 41.1% and 14.5% in recipients respectively. The allele frequencies of *CYP3A5*, *ABCB1* at 1236C>T, 2677G>AT and 2677G>AT, and *ACE* were detailedly shown in Table 2.

2. Effect of *CYP3A5* genotype in recipient (intestine) on TAC dosing requirements and disposition

According to *CYP3A5* genotypic results, pediatric recipients were divided into tow groups: expressor (*1/*1 and *1/*3 allele),

Table 2. Frequency of Genotyping from recipients and donors.

Genotype	Recipient	Donor	Tolerance/Total
CYP3A5	AA	AA	1/2
	AA	AG	0/1
	AA	GG	0/0
	AG	AA	2/8
	AG	AG	7/18
	AG	GG	5/11
	GG	AA	0/1
	GG	AG	7/15
	GG	GG	9/34
ABCB1 (1236C>T)	CC	CC	1/2
	CC	CT	3/8
	CC	TT	0/0
	CT	CC	2/7
	CT	CT	7/20
	CT	TT	3/11
	TT	CC	0/1
	TT	CT	8/19
	TT	TT	7/22
ABCB1 (2677G>AT)	AA	AA	0/0
	AA	AT	0/0
	AA	GA	0/0
	AA	GG	0/0
	AA	GT	0/0
	AA	TT	0/0
	AT	AA	1/2
	AT	AT	1/3
	AT	GA	2/4
	AT	GG	0/0
	AT	GT	1/2
	AT	TT	1/2
	GA	AA	0/0
	GA	AT	1/2
	GA	GA	1/1
	GA	GG	0/5
	GA	GT	0/3
	GA	TT	0/0
	GG	AA	0/0
	GG	AT	1/1
	GG	GA	2/5
	GG	GG	1/4
	GG	GT	3/9
	GG	TT	0/2
	GT	AA	0/0
	GT	AT	2/2
	GT	GA	0/2
	GT	GG	3/6
	GT	GT	5/15
	GT	TT	2/8
	TT	AA	0/0
	TT	AT	1/1

Table 2. Cont.

Genotype	Recipient	Donor	Tolerance/Total
	TT	GA	0/0
	TT	GG	0/0
	TT	GT	2/5
	TT	TT	1/6
ABCB1 (3435C>T)	CC	CC	6/19
	CC	CT	3/17
	CC	TT	0/0
	CT	CC	3/11
	CT	CT	9/21
	CT	TT	3/8
	TT	CC	0/1
	TT	CT	5/7
	TT	TT	2/6
ACE	D/D	D/D	1/4
	D/D	D/I	1/9
	D/D	I/I	0/0
	D/I	D/D	2/9
	D/I	D/I	7/17
	D/I	I/I	4/11
	I/I	D/D	0/0
	I/I	D/I	3/8
	I/I	I/I	12/32

and nonexpressor (*3/*3 allele). We compared clinical characteristics between two groups and showed them in Table 3. There was no significant difference in age, sex, body weight, height, primary diseases and postoperative complications between the recipients with expressor and those with nonexpressor. And there was no significant difference in donors' age, sex, body weight and height between the recipients with expressor and those with nonexpressor.

However, the peak time of TAC in the recipients with expressor was significantly longer than that in the recipients with nonexpressor (9.95±8.25 *vs.* 5.90±4.23, $p<0.01$; **Table 3**). We further investigated the difference of dose and C/D ratio between the recipients with expressor and those with nonexpressor. As shown in Figure 1, although the two groups had the same TAC initial dose (ng/kg/day) and early induction dose (from day 3 to day 14, **Fig. 1A and 1B**), the C/D ratio in the recipients with nonexpressor was significantly higher than those with expressor (**Fig. 1C and 1D**). And then a higher TAC dose was adjusted on day 14 after transplantation according to their C/D ratio in both expressor and nonexpressor groups. Importantly, the highest dose used on day 30 was almost two-fold of the initial dose in the recipients with expressor, which was significantly higher than that in the recipients with nonexpressor at the same time point (0.27±0.12 *vs.* 0.22±0.09, $p=0.013$; **Fig. 1A**). Then the TAC maintenance dose was progressively reduced in both groups. At the month12 time point, the TAC dose was almost reached the initial dose in the recipients with expressor (0.14±0.06), whereas the dose was lower than the initial dose in those with nonexpressor (0.10±0.06; **Fig. 1A**). While the normalized trough concentrations, the C/D ratios in the recipients with nonexpressor were significantly higher than those in the recipients with expressor at every time points during a year following transplantation (**Fig. 1C**). Therefore, the correlation between *CYP3A5* genotype and TAC late induction and maintenance doses was observed: expressor group had higher doses and lower C/D ratios, whereas nonexpressor group had lower doses and higher C/D ratios (**Fig. 1B and 1D**). Those results indicate that the recipients with expressor require more time to achieve TAC therapeutic range during the induction phase, need more upward dose during the late induction and the maintained phases, and have lower C/D ratio. In contrast, the recipients with nonexpressor require less time to achieve TAC therapeutic range during the induction phase, need lower dose during the late induction and the maintained phases, and have higher C/D ratio.

3. Impact of *CYP3A5* genotype in donors (graft liver) on TAC dosing requirements and disposition

There was significant difference in donors' *CYP3A5* genotypes between the recipients with expressor and those with nonexpressor, when Chi-square test was used (**Table 3**). We therefore further investigated whether *CYP3A5* expressor and nonexpressor from donors affect TAC dosing requirements and C/D ratio of recipients. According to recipients' and donors' *CYP3A5* genotyping, pediatric recipients were divided into four groups: the recipients with expressor/the donor with expressor (ReDe), the recipients with expressor/the donor with nonexpressor (ReDn), the recipients with nonexpressor/the donor with expressor (RnDe) and the recipients with nonexpressor/the donor with nonexpressor (RnDn). We found that the initial, induction and maintenance doses are very close to those in ReDe, ReDn and RnDe groups,

Table 3. Comparison of characteristics of recipients by *CYP3A5* genotyping.

	Expressor	Nonexpressor	P value
Age (Mean ± Sd; month)	19.0±23.0	16.0±14.4	0.448
Sex			0.702
Male (%)	24 (60.0)	28 (56.0)	
Female (%)	16 (40.0)	22 (44.0)	
Body weight (Mean ± Sd; kg)	9.2±3.7	8.6±2.9	0.426
Height (Mean ± Sd; cm)	73.4±14.6	72.7±13.1	0.809
Surface area (m^2)	0.41±0.13	0.40±0.12	0.663
CYP3A5 genotype			
AA, *1/*1 (%)	3 (3.3)	0 (0)	
AG, *1/*3 (%)	37 (41.1)	0 (0)	
GG, *3/*3 (%)	0 (0)	50 (55.6)	
Primary diseases			0.368
Congenital biliary atresia (%)	40 (100.0)	49 (98.0)	
Postoperative chologenic infection (%)	0 (0)	1 (2.0)	
TAC peak time (day)	9.95±8.25	5.90±4.23	0.004
Donor			
Age (Mean ± Sd; year)	32.4±8.9	30.5+5.3	0.260
Male (%)	21 (52.5)	16 (32)	0.050
Female (%)	19 (47.5)	34 (68)	
Body weight (Mean ± Sd; kg)	59.2±9.9	59.5±9.2	0.891
Height (Mean ± Sd; cm)	164.4±8.0	164.2±8.9	0.929
AA, *1/*1 (%)	10 (25.0)	1 (2.0)	
AG, *1/*3 (%)	19 (47.5)	15 (30.0)	
GG, *3/*3 (%)	11 (27.5)	34 (68.0)	0.000

Note: Expressor, *CYP3A5* *1/*1 and *1/*3; Nonexpressor, *CYP3A5* *3/*3.

respectively, while the late induction and the maintenance doses in RnDn group were significantly less than those in other three groups (**Fig. 2A and 2B**). However, TAC C/D ratios were observed with a different phenotype compared with TAC dosing phenotypes. With time, C/D ratio in RnDn group significantly increasingly higher than those in other three groups, especially in the maintenance phase (**Fig. 2C**). Moreover, ReDn group had higher C/D ratio than ReDe at month1, month3 and month12 time points (**Fig. 2C**). The overall dosing in very group was analyzed and showed in Figure 2D. The RnDn group had significantly higher TAC C/D ratio than other three groups. Although ReDn and RnDe groups had higher C/D ratio than ReDe group, no statistically significant relationship was observed among them (**Fig. 2D**). More importantly, the RnDe group had significantly lower C/D ratio than RnDn group (**Fig. 2D**), suggesting that although two groups share the same intestine *CYP3A5* expressor, graft livers with *CYP3A5* expressor or with *CYP3A5* nonexpressor play important impact on TAC trough concentrations after liver transplantation.

4. Effects of *ABCB1* and *ACE* genotypes in recipient (intestine) on TAC dosing requirements and disposition

Considering the possible influence of *ABCB1* and *ACE* SNPs in recipients on TAC pharmacokinetics, we finally assessed the effects of SNPs of *ABCB1* and *ACE* in intestine on TAC. As shown in Figure 3, we didn't find any significant difference of the C/D ratios among the recipients with *ABCB1* at position 1236CT, TT and CC (**Fig. 3A**), among those with *ABCB1* at position 2677AT, GT, GG, GT and TT (**Fig. 3B**), among those with ABCB1 at position 3435CC, CT and TT (**Fig. 3C**), and among those with *ACE* at intron 16 (14901–14378) (**Fig. 3D**). These results indicate that the variants of *ABCB1* and *ACE* have minimal impact on TAC disposition in pediatric liver transplant patients.

5. Analysis of relationship between donors and recipients

We investigated the family relationship between donors and recipients. As shown in Table 4, parental relationship between donors and recipients with *CYP3A5**1/*1, *CYP3A5**1/*3 and *CYP3A5**3/*3 were 2 (2.2%), 35 (38.9%) and 48 (53.3%) cases respectively, whereas grandparental relationship between those were 1 (1.1%), 2 (2.2%) and 2 (2.2%) cases respectively. Parental relationship between those with *ABCB1* 1236CT, TT, CC, 2677AT, GA, GG, GT, TT, 3435CC, CT and TT were 37 (41.1%), 39 (43.3%), 9 (10.0%), 12 (13.3%), 11 (12.2%), 20 (22.2%), 31 (34.4%), 11 (12.2%), 34 (37.8%), 38 (42.2%) and 13 (14.4%) respectively, whereas grandparental relationship between those were 1 (1.1%), 3 (3.3%), 1 (1.1%), 1 (1.1%), 0 (0%), 1 (1.1%), 2 (2.2%), 1 (1.1%), 2 (2.2%), 2 (2.2%) and 1 (1.1%) cases respectively. Parental relationship between those with *ACE I/I*, *D/I*, and *D/D* were 38 (42.2%), 36 (40.0%) and 11 (12.2%) cases respectively, whereas grandparental relationship between those were 2 (2.2%), 1 (1.1%) and 2 (2.2%) cases respectively.

We further analyzed frequency and rejection of pairing genotype of donors and recipients. As shown in Table 5, recipients

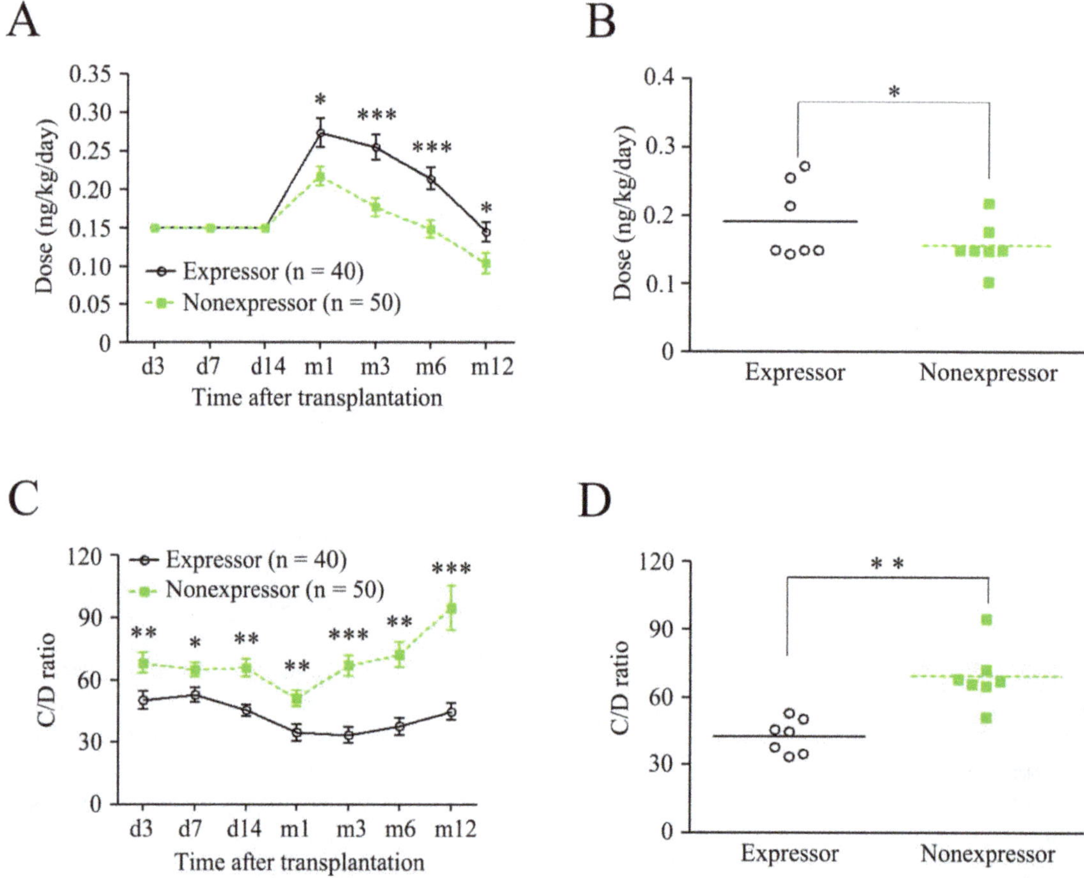

Figure 1. Doses and C/D ratios of TAC compared between recipients with *CYP3A5* expressor and those with nonexpressor. (A) Dose-time curves; (B) Doses in dots, every dot represents a dose at a time point; (C) C/D ratio-time curves; (D) C/D ratios in dots, every dot represents a C/D ratio at a time point. TAC, tacrolimus; Expressor, *CYP3A5* *1/*1 and *1/*3; Nonexpressor, *CYP*3A5 *3/*3; *$p<0.05$; **$p<0.01$; ***$p<0.001$.

with concomitant rejection in the same and different genotyping of donors with recipients in *CYP3A5* were 15 (34.1%) and 11 (30.6%) cases respectively. Recipients with concomitant rejection in the same and different genotyping of donors and recipients in *ABCB1* at 1236, 2677 and 3435 sites were 15 (34.1%), 11 (23.9%), 6 (20.7%), 21 (34.4%), 14 (30.4%) and 12 (27.3%) respectively. While recipients with concomitant tolerance in the same and different genotyping of donors and recipients in *ACE* were 12 (22.6%) and 14 (37.8%) respectively. Interestingly, no statistical difference between those with and without concomitant rejection in the same and different genotyping, including *CYP3A5*, *ABCB1* and *ACE*, was observed.

Discussion

Therapeutic drug monitoring of TAC in blood is necessary to provide an effective immunosuppression and avoid adverse effects after organ transplantation. With regard to TAC pharmacokinetic variability, *CYP3A5* genotype has been reported to consistently associate with TAC dosing requirement [9]. In pediatric recipients, however, it is difficult to perform frequently blood samplings for measurement. Therefore, it is very important to investigate the relationship of *CYP3A5* genotyping with TAC pharmacokinetics for establishing a personalized dosage regimen including the initial, the induction and the maintenance doses. In this study, the general consistency in the concept that *CYP3A5* expressor requires higher TAC doses than nonexpressor to reach target trough concentrations strongly suggests that *CYP3A5* genotyping not only in recipient (intestine) but also in donor (graft liver) is necessary for establishing a personalized dosage regimen in pediatric liver transplant patients. In addition, we didn't find any significant impact of *ABCB1* and *ACE* SNPs on TAC disposition. Although a recent study suggested a safer dosing and monitoring of TAC coadministered with rabeprazole early on after liver transplantation regardless of *CYP3A5* genotypes of recipients and their donors [18], our finding in this study is important as it emphasizes the combined effects of recipient's and donor's genetic variation in relation to TAC disposition. Moreover, although primary outcome time focused on the early postoperative period in most studies, we set one year of primary outcome time. It is necessary, we think, because impact on recipients, especially for pediatric liver transplant patients, will be long time period because of immunosuppressive regimen for his whole life.

TAC is characterized by narrow therapeutic index and interindividual variability in its exposure, and achieving target therapeutic level is difficult, especially during the early period of transplantation. Therefore, the TAC dosing regimens require a regular drug monitoring system based on its trough blood concentration [9]. On the other hand, TAC blood concentration is monitored to allow therapeutic levels to be maintained, to avoid toxicity and to improve efficacy. In general, post-operative infections were considered as over-immunosupressive, which needs to reduce the dose of TAC, whereas acute cellular rejection was

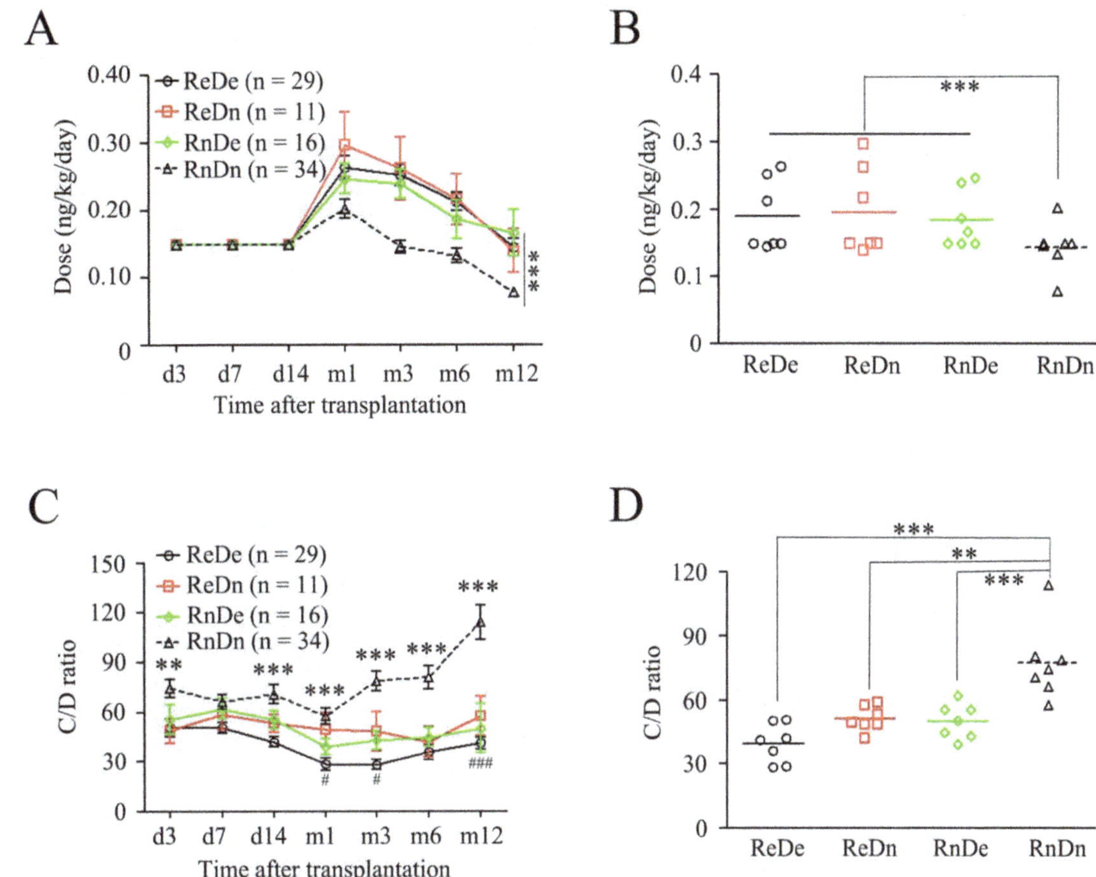

Figure 2. Doses and C/D ratios of TAC compared among four groups: ReDe, ReDn, RnDe and RnDn. (A) Dose-time curves; (B) Doses in dots, every dot represents a dose at a time point; (C) C/D ratio-time curves; * compared with ReDe; # compared with ReDn; (D) C/D ratios in dots, every dot represents a C/D ratio at a time point. TAC, tacrolimus; Expressor, *CYP3A5* *1/*1 and *1/*3; Nonexpressor, *CYP3A5* *3/*3; ReDe, recipient with expressor/donor with expressor; ReDn, recipient with expressor/donor with nonexpressor; RnDe, recipient with nonexpressor/donor with expressor; RnDn, recipient with nonexpressor/donor with nonexpressor; *p<0.05; **p<0.01; ***p<0.001; #p<0.05, ###p<0.001.

considered as under-immunosupressive, which needs to increase the dose of TAC. But the former needs to exclude the ordinary post-operative infections. Although the same initial TAC dose and the same early induction dose (~two weeks) were used, we were surprised to find a *CYP3A5* genotype effect so early after transplant, in which the C/D ratio was significantly higher in nonexpressor than expressor on day 3 (**Fig. 1**). For pediatric liver recipients, in contrast, another study claimed that they did not identify any relationship between recipient *CYP3A5* genotype and TAC dosing [19]. They supposed that the main reason for this lack of association was probably that variations in TAC deposit are largely dependent on hepatic metabolism and to a lesser extent on intestinal metabolism in the first 14 days after transplantation [19]. In addition, a similar data in pediatric renal transplant recipients have also shown that the independent impact of *CYP3A5* genotype on TAC pharmacogenetic was not evident [20]. We postulate that the main reason for this inconsistence with our results is probably that we had enrolled more cases, demonstrating a further large-scale study is necessary. Although CYP3A5 genotype has been convincingly impacted on TAC clearance in many ethic groups [1–3,5–7,9–12,16,17,19,21,22], there is limited evidence to prove that *CYP3A5* genotype-guided TAC dosing will benefit clinical outcomes.

In this study, we found that the association between TAC dosing and *CYP3A5* genotyping not only in recipients but also in donors for liver transplantation (**Fig. 1** and **Fig. 2**). Recent a report has also shown that a more significant effect of donor genotype as early as 2 weeks after transplantation in liver transplant recipients [23]. In any case, the relative importance of recipient and donor genotyping during the early post-transplantation period is of particular significance, especially in liver transplantation, concerning the risk of graft rejection is the highest in this period. To maximize the immunosuppressive effect and minimize adverse effects, TAC dosing regimen of in the induction phase (~3 months after transplantation) and the maintenance phase (3–12 months after transplantation) should be changed [7]. Generally, TAC dosing requirement for the induction phase is higher than that requirement for the maintenance phase. In the present study, a higher TAC dose was adjusted on day 14 after transplantation basing on C/D ratio monitor. The highest dose used on day 30 was almost two-fold of the initial dose in the recipients (**Fig. 1A**), then the TAC maintenance dose was progressively reduced, and on day 365 after transplantation, the TAC dose was almost reduced to the initial dose in the recipients (**Fig. 1A**). It is very clear that pharmacogenetics-based approach to TAC dosing may prove to be more clinically relevant in terms of preventing early overexposure and toxicity. Possibly, starting with a lower TAC dose in such patients may prevent early nephrotoxicity or the development of new-onset diabetes after transplantation.

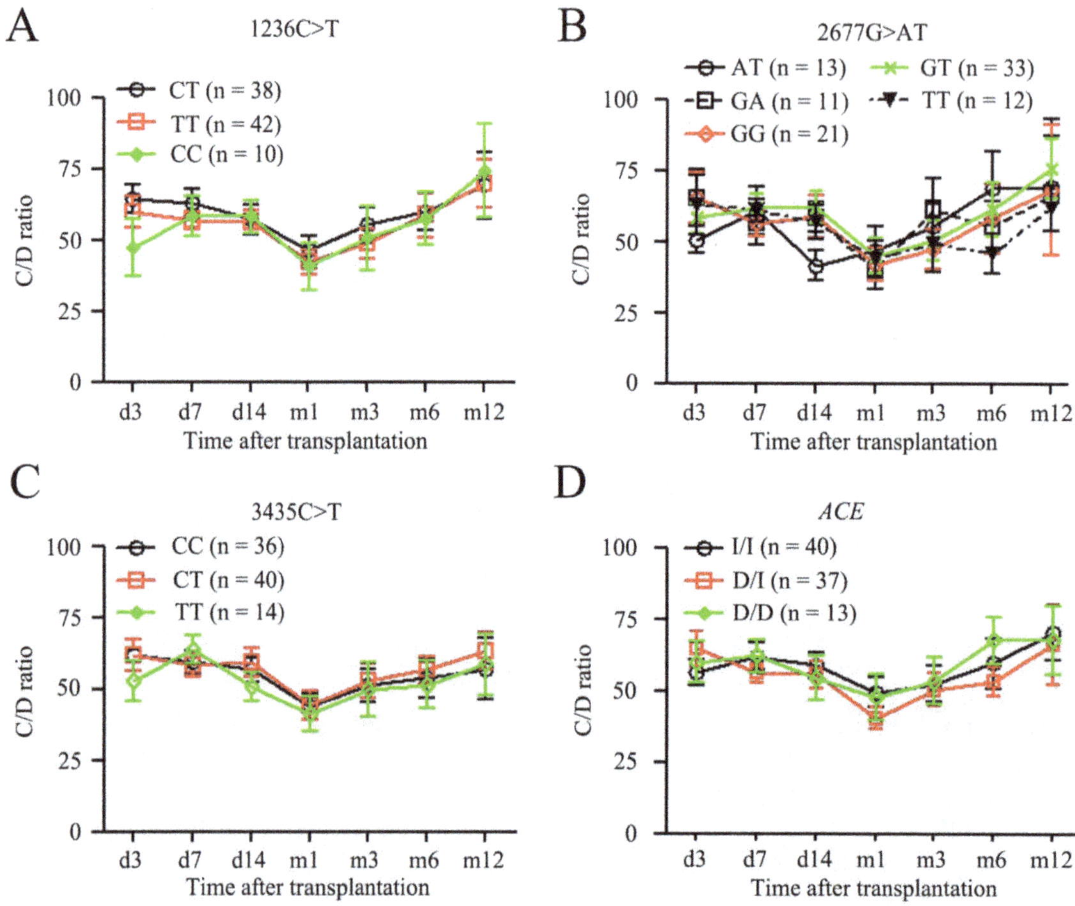

Figure 3. C/D ratios of TAC compared among *ABCB1* genotypes and among *ACE* genotypes. (A) C/D ratio-time curves of *ABCB1* variants at 1236C>T; (B) C/D ratio-time curves of *ABCB1* variants at 2677G>AT; (C) C/D ratio-time curves of *ABCB1* variants at 3435C>T; (D) C/D ratio-time curves of *ACE* variants. TAC, tacrolimus.

Patients with *CYP3A5* expressor require a higher TAC dose than *CYP3A5* nonexpressers to reach the same whole-blood exposure. Therefore, these expressor patients are prone to have subtherapeutic drug concentrations in the early phase after surgery and theoretically maybe increase acute rejection risk [9]. It is not surprising that, from a clinical point of view, TAC is prescribed to prevent acute rejection. However, an exception to this general pattern is a study of Korean kidney graft patients, which found a greater incidence of acute rejection with *CYP3A5* expressor [11]. A previous study reported that children younger than five years of age needed higher TAC doses than older children after both kidney and liver transplant and suggested that TAC starting dosing guidelines in children should reflect both age and *CYP3A5* genotype to quickly reach therapeutic concentrations after transplantation [19]. However, we didn't find an association between age and *CYP3A5* genotype (Table 3). We supposed that pediatric recipients in our study caused this inconsistence, which are almost younger children with only few cases above 5 years of age. Regarding that our results revealed the influence of CYP3A5 variant recipient or donor genotypes on TAC metabolic variables, we did not agree the idea that the impact of age and genetic variation appears to be weakened in the immediate post-transplantation period, while intraindividual variation appears larger [21].

The wide range of interpatient variability in effective dosage of TAC is caused by various factors, such as age, weight, and drug interactions. Similarly, inflammation and/or organ failure maybe reduce drug metabolism in patients [19]. In particular, genetic factors play an important role in the pharmacokinetic properties and therapeutic levels of TAC. The *CYP3A5* genotype is currently the strongest predictor of an individual's TAC dose requirement. However, it does not explain all variability. Other genetic variants may explain additional variation in TAC dose requirement. As has been illustrated in adults, the drug transporter ABCB1, the CYP3A4, the human pregnane X receptor (NR1I2), interleukin 6 and COMT SNP may be associated with early TAC exposure [9,24–26]. Although the association of *ABCB1*, *ACE* with the C/D ratios of TAC was investigated, we didn't observe any significant impact on TAC disposition in pediatric liver transplants (**Fig. 3**). Although a few reports found that high intestinal levels of P-glycoprotein were associated with TAC disposition after liver transplantation [16,27], most studies didn't find any influence of ABCB1 genotypes on TAC pharmacokinetics [28–30], especially in pediatric recipients [6,31,32]. Consistent with the majority, we couldn't find any significant association between ABCB1 genotypes and the disposition of TAC (**Fig. 3**). With regard to *ACE* SNPs, although the *ACE* study suggested an association between *ACE* and renal dysfunction in adult liver recipients who receive TAC [32], we couldn't find any significant association between its genotypes and the disposition of TAC too (**Fig. 3**). Taken together, their influence appears to be smaller than that of *CYP3A5* SNPs. If these additional genetic variants do indeed

Table 4. Relationship between recipients and donors.

Genotype of recipients	Recipients' relationship to donors	
	Parents (%)	**Grandparents (%)**
CYP3A5 genotype		
AA, *1/*1	2 (2.2)	1 (1.1)
AG, *1/*3	35 (38.9)	2 (2.2)
GG, *3/*3	48 (53.3)	2 (2.2)
ABCB1 genotype		
1236C>T CT	37 (41.1)	1 (1.1)
TT	39 (43.3)	3 (3.3)
CC	9 (10.0)	1 (1.1)
2677G>AT AT	12 (13.3)	1 (1.1)
GA	11 (12.2)	0 (0)
GG	20 (22.2)	1 (1.1)
GT	31 (34.4)	2 (2.2)
TT	11 (12.2)	1 (1.1)
3435C>T CC	34 (37.8)	2 (2.2)
CT	38 (42.2)	2 (2.2)
TT	13 (14.4)	1 (1.1)
ACE genotype		
I/I	38 (42.2)	2 (2.2)
D/I	36 (40.0)	1 (1.1)
D/D	11 (12.2)	2 (2.2)

explain residual variability in TAC dose requirement, it may become possible to develop personalized therapeutic strategy that helps clinicians to decide on an individual's initial dose. It is to be expected that with such an approach early TAC overexposure and toxicity may be expectantly prevented [9]. Further prospective studies of liver transplant recipients are needed to evaluate the impact of these genetic polymorphisms on TAC dosing requirement and determine whether routine genotyping would be improve in personalized TAC therapy. Since the actions of these genes appear to be cooperative. Moreover, the combination of some drugs with lower TAC dose may be safely coadministered [33]. However, our results provided evidence that *CYP3A5* plays a more dominant role than other genetic variants in the metabolism of TAC in pediatric liver transplant recipients and their donors.

In this study, we analyzed the relationship of pairing of donors and recipients. Among pairing of donors and recipients, parental relationship cases were more than grandparental those (Table 4). In addition, there were not significantly different in occurrence of rejection between the same or different genotypes in pairing of donors and recipients (Table 5). In additional, not only donors but also recipients were genotyped with their peripheral blood samples. It seems no difference for genotyping regardless of basing

Table 5. Profiles of pairing genotypes of donors and recipients on Rejection of TAC.

Genes		Donor and recipient	Rejection (total)	Non-rejection (total)	P value
CYP3A5		Same genotype	15 (54)	39 (54)	
		Different genotypes	11 (36)	25 (36)	0.776
ABCB1					
	1236C>T	Same genotype	15 (44)	29 (44)	
		Different genotypes	11 (46)	35 (46)	0.175
	2677G>AT	Same genotype	6 (29)	23 (29)	
		Different genotypes	21 (61)	40 (61)	0.170
	3435G>AT	Same genotype	14 (46)	32 (46)	
		Different genotypes	12 (44)	32 (44)	0.110
ACE		Same genotype	12 (53)	41 (53)	
		Different genotypes	14 (37)	23 (37)	0.105

on intestinal biopsies or blood samples, but using intestinal biopsies will have high novelty, especially for recipients. More importantly, intestinal biopsies from recipients will provide us more valued information about mRNA transcription and protein expression of interesting genes and second pass of metabolism of TAC.

The main limitations of this study are the retrospective design from a single center and a limited number of patients. Also, the confounding effects of *CYP3A4* with *ABCB1* or *ACE* variants that may affect TAC pharmacokinetics were not examined. A prospective study with a large number of pediatric recipients and standard timing of ImmuKnow assay is required to establish an effective monitoring tool of immune response in children following liver transplantation. Furthermore, for recipient genotyping, periphery blood has limited novelty.

In conclusion, this study further confirmed that the *CYP3A5* polymorphism at position 6986G>A of pediatric liver transplants and their donors, but not *ABCB1* or *ACE* SNPs in recipients, impacts on TAC dosing requirement, suggesting that early determination of the *CYP3A5* genotype in both recipients and donors would be helpful in the design of adequate immunosuppressive treatment and in lower adverse effects by predicting TAC dosing requirement for the induction and maintenance phases in individual liver transplant recipients.

Author Contributions

Conceived and designed the experiments: FX JJZ QX. Performed the experiments: YKC LZH. Analyzed the data: FX YKC. Contributed reagents/materials/analysis tools: LZH CHS JL THY. Contributed to the writing of the manuscript: YKC FX.

References

1. Penninga L, Moller CH, Gustafsson F, Steinbruchel DA, Gluud C (2010) Tacrolimus versus cyclosporine as primary immunosuppression after heart transplantation: systematic review with meta-analyses and trial sequential analyses of randomised trials. Eur J Clin Pharmacol 66: 1177–1187.
2. Kim JS, Aviles DH, Silverstein DM, Leblanc PL, Matti Vehaskari V (2005) Effect of age, ethnicity, and glucocorticoid use on tacrolimus pharmacokinetics in pediatric renal transplant patients. Pediatr Transplant 9: 162–169.
3. Provenzani A, Notarbartolo M, Labbozzetta M, Poma P, Biondi F, et al. (2009) The effect of CYP3A5 and ABCB1 single nucleotide polymorphisms on tacrolimus dose requirements in Caucasian liver transplant patients. Ann Transplant 14: 23–31.
4. Kausman JY, Patel B, Marks SD (2008) Standard dosing of tacrolimus leads to overexposure in pediatric renal transplantation recipients. Pediatr Transplant 12: 329–335.
5. Ferraris JR, Argibay PF, Costa L, Jimenez G, Coccia PA, et al. (2011) Influence of CYP3A5 polymorphism on tacrolimus maintenance doses and serum levels after renal transplantation: age dependency and pharmacological interaction with steroids. Pediatr Transplant 15: 525–532.
6. Gijsen V, Mital S, van Schaik RH, Soldin OP, Soldin SJ, et al. (2011) Age and CYP3A5 genotype affect tacrolimus dosing requirements after transplant in pediatric heart recipients. J Heart Lung Transplant 30: 1352–1359.
7. Vannaprasaht S, Reungjui S, Supanya D, Sirivongs D, Pongskul C, et al. (2013) Personalized tacrolimus doses determined by CYP3A5 genotype for induction and maintenance phases of kidney transplantation. Clin Ther 35: 1762–1769.
8. Iwasaki K (2007) Metabolism of tacrolimus (FK506) and recent topics in clinical pharmacokinetics. Drug Metab Pharmacokinet 22: 328–335.
9. Hesselink DA, Bouamar R, Elens L, van Schaik RH, van Gelder T (2014) The role of pharmacogenetics in the disposition of and response to tacrolimus in solid organ transplantation. Clin Pharmacokinet 53: 123–139.
10. Macphee IA, Fredericks S, Mohamed M, Moreton M, Carter ND, et al. (2005) Tacrolimus pharmacogenetics: the CYP3A5*1 allele predicts low dose-normalized tacrolimus blood concentrations in whites and South Asians. Transplantation 79: 499–502.
11. Min SI, Kim SY, Ahn SH, Min SK, Kim SH, et al. (2010) CYP3A5 *1 allele: impacts on early acute rejection and graft function in tacrolimus-based renal transplant recipients. Transplantation 90: 1394–1400.
12. Cho JH, Yoon YD, Park JY, Song EJ, Choi JY, et al. (2012) Impact of cytochrome P450 3A and ATP-binding cassette subfamily B member 1 polymorphisms on tacrolimus dose-adjusted trough concentrations among Korean renal transplant recipients. Transplant Proc 44: 109–114.
13. Saeki T, Ueda K, Tanigawara Y, Hori R, Komano T (1993) Human P-glycoprotein transports cyclosporin A and FK506. J Biol Chem 268: 6077–6080.
14. Glowacki F, Lionet A, Buob D, Labalette M, Allorge D, et al. (2011) CYP3A5 and ABCB1 polymorphisms in donor and recipient: impact on Tacrolimus dose requirements and clinical outcome after renal transplantation. Nephrol Dial Transplant 26: 3046–3050.
15. Gijsen VM, Madadi P, Dube MP, Hesselink DA, Koren G, et al. (2012) Tacrolimus-induced nephrotoxicity and genetic variability: a review. Ann Transplant 17: 111–121.
16. Wei-lin W, Jing J, Shu-sen Z, Li-hua W, Ting-bo L, et al. (2006) Tacrolimus dose requirement in relation to donor and recipient ABCB1 and CYP3A5 gene polymorphisms in Chinese liver transplant patients. Liver Transpl 12: 775–780.
17. Li L, Li CJ, Zheng L, Zhang YJ, Jiang HX, et al. (2011) Tacrolimus dosing in Chinese renal transplant recipients: a population-based pharmacogenetics study. Eur J Clin Pharmacol 67: 787–795.
18. Hosohata K, Masuda S, Yonezawa A, Sugimoto M, Takada Y, et al. (2009) Absence of influence of concomitant administration of rabeprazole on the pharmacokinetics of tacrolimus in adult living-donor liver transplant patients: a case-control study. Drug Metab Pharmacokinet 24: 458–463.
19. de Wildt SN, van Schaik RH, Soldin OP, Soldin SJ, Brojeni PY, et al. (2011) The interactions of age, genetics, and disease severity on tacrolimus dosing requirements after pediatric kidney and liver transplantation. Eur J Clin Pharmacol 67: 1231–1241.
20. Shilbayeh S, Zmeili R, Almardini RI (2013) The impact of CYP3A5 and MDR1 polymorphisms on tacrolimus dosage requirements and trough concentrations in pediatric renal transplant recipients. Saudi J Kidney Dis Transpl 24: 1125–1136.
21. Satoh S, Kagaya H, Saito M, Inoue T, Miura M, et al. (2008) Lack of tacrolimus circadian pharmacokinetics and CYP3A5 pharmacogenetics in the early and maintenance stages in Japanese renal transplant recipients. Br J Clin Pharmacol 66: 207–214.
22. Xue F, Zhang J, Han L, Li Q, Xu N, et al. (2010) Immune cell functional assay in monitoring of adult liver transplantation recipients with infection. Transplantation 89: 620–626.
23. Yu S, Wu L, Jin J, Yan S, Jiang G, et al. (2006) Influence of CYP3A5 gene polymorphisms of donor rather than recipient to tacrolimus individual dose requirement in liver transplantation. Transplantation 81: 46–51.
24. Jacobson PA, Oetting WS, Brearley AM, Leduc R, Guan W, et al. (2011) Novel polymorphisms associated with tacrolimus trough concentrations: results from a multicenter kidney transplant consortium. Transplantation 91: 300–308.
25. Chen D, Fan J, Guo F, Qin S, Wang Z, et al. (2013) Novel single nucleotide polymorphisms in interleukin 6 affect tacrolimus metabolism in liver transplant patients. PLoS One 8: e73405.
26. Uesugi M, Hosokawa M, Shinke H, Hashimoto E, Takahashi T, et al. (2013) Influence of cytochrome P450 (CYP) 3A4*1G polymorphism on the pharmacokinetics of tacrolimus, probability of acute cellular rejection, and mRNA expression level of CYP3A5 rather than CYP3A4 in living-donor liver transplant patients. Biol Pharm Bull 36: 1814–1821.
27. Fukudo M, Yano I, Masuda S, Goto M, Uesugi M, et al. (2006) Population pharmacokinetic and pharmacogenomic analysis of tacrolimus in pediatric living-donor liver transplant recipients. Clin Pharmacol Ther 80: 331–345.
28. Hawwa AF, McElnay JC (2011) Impact of ATP-binding cassette, subfamily B, member 1 pharmacogenetics on tacrolimus-associated nephrotoxicity and dosage requirements in paediatric patients with liver transplant. Expert Opin Drug Saf 10: 9–22.
29. Staatz CE, Goodman LK, Tett SE (2010) Effect of CYP3A and ABCB1 single nucleotide polymorphisms on the pharmacokinetics and pharmacodynamics of calcineurin inhibitors: Part II. Clin Pharmacokinet 49: 207–221.
30. Gomez-Bravo MA, Salcedo M, Fondevila C, Suarez F, Castellote J, et al. (2013) Impact of donor and recipient CYP3A5 and ABCB1 genetic polymorphisms on tacrolimus dosage requirements and rejection in Caucasian Spanish liver transplant patients. J Clin Pharmacol 53: 1146–1154.
31. Grenda R, Prokurat S, Ciechanowicz A, Piatosa B, Kalicinski P (2009) Evaluation of the genetic background of standard-immunosuppressant-related toxicity in a cohort of 200 paediatric renal allograft recipients–a retrospective study. Ann Transplant 14: 18–24.
32. Hawwa AF, McKiernan PJ, Shields M, Millership JS, Collier PS, et al. (2009) Influence of ABCB1 polymorphisms and haplotypes on tacrolimus nephrotoxicity and dosage requirements in children with liver transplant. Br J Clin Pharmacol 68: 413–421.
33. Hosohata K, Masuda S, Katsura T, Takada Y, Kaido T, et al. (2009) Impact of intestinal CYP2C19 genotypes on the interaction between tacrolimus and omeprazole, but not lansoprazole, in adult living-donor liver transplant patients. Drug Metab Dispos 37: 821–826.

12

Local Modelling Techniques for Assessing Micro-Level Impacts of Risk Factors in Complex Data: Understanding Health and Socioeconomic Inequalities in Childhood Educational Attainments

Shang-Ming Zhou[1*¶], Ronan A. Lyons[1], Owen G. Bodger[1], Ann John[1], Huw Brunt[2], Kerina Jones[1], Mike B. Gravenor[1¶], Sinead Brophy[1¶]

1 Institute of Life Science, College of Medicine, Swansea University, Swansea, United Kingdom, **2** Public Health Wales, Temple of Peace and Health, Cathays Park, Cardiff, United Kingdom

Abstract

Although inequalities in health and socioeconomic status have an important influence on childhood educational performance, the interactions between these multiple factors relating to variation in educational outcomes at *micro-level* is unknown, and how to evaluate the many possible interactions of these factors is not well established. This paper aims to examine multi-dimensional deprivation factors and their impact on childhood educational outcomes at micro-level, focusing on geographic areas having widely different disparity patterns, in which each area is characterised by six deprivation domains (*Income*, *Health*, *Geographical Access to Services*, *Housing*, *Physical Environment*, and *Community Safety*). Traditional health statistical studies tend to use one global model to describe the whole population for *macro-analysis*. In this paper, we combine linked educational and deprivation data across small areas (median population of 1500), then use a *local modelling* technique, the Takagi-Sugeno fuzzy system, to predict area educational outcomes at ages 7 and 11. We define two new metrics, "*Micro-impact of Domain*" and "*Contribution of Domain*", to quantify the variations of local impacts of multidimensional factors on educational outcomes across small areas. The two metrics highlight differing priorities. Our study reveals complex multi-way interactions between the deprivation domains, which could not be provided by traditional health statistical methods based on single global model. We demonstrate that although *Income* has an expected central role, all domains contribute, and in some areas *Health*, *Environment*, *Access to Services*, *Housing* and *Community Safety* each could be the dominant factor. Thus the relative importance of health and socioeconomic factors varies considerably for different areas, depending on the levels of each of the other factors, and therefore each component of deprivation must be considered as part of a wider system. Childhood educational achievement could benefit from policies and intervention strategies that are tailored to the local geographic areas' profiles.

Editor: David O. Carpenter, Institute for Health & the Environment, United States of America

Funding: The work was undertaken with the support of The Centre for the Development and Evaluation of Complex Interventions for Public Health Improvement (DECIPHer), a UKCRC Public Health Research Centre of Excellence. Joint funding (MR/KO232331/1) from the British Heart Foundation, Cancer Research UK, Economic and Social Research Council, Medical Research Council, the Welsh Government and the Wellcome Trust, under the auspices of the UK Clinical Research Collaboration, is gratefully acknowledged. This research was also supported by the Farr Institute of Health Informatics Research. The Farr Institute is funded by a consortium of ten UK research organizations (MR/K006525/1): Arthritis Research UK, the British Heart Foundation, Cancer Research UK, the Economic and Social Research Council, the Engineering and Physical Sciences Research Council, the Medical Research Council, the National Institute of Health Research, the National Institute for Social Care and Health Research (Welsh Government), and the Chief Scientist Office (Scottish Government Health Directorates). The funders had no role in study design, data collection and analysis, decision to publish, or preparation of the manuscript.

Competing Interests: The authors have declared that no competing interests exist.

* Email: s.zhou@swansea.ac.uk

¶ SMZ, MBG, and SB are joint lead authors on this work.

Introduction

Increasing evidence shows that childhood health and socioeconomic inequalities have strong impact on educational attainments [1]–[7]. It is often the case, however, that existing studies focus on the impact of *either* health *or* socioeconomic status, and research results are often obtained at a *macro-level*, whereas the subtle analysis of risk factor interactions at a *micro-level* across different subgroups is much less understood in epidemiological and public health studies. Such considerations might reveal more complex relationships and provide important insights for targeted policy development and intervention. However, currently few statistical analytics methods and modelling techniques can fulfil the tasks of conducting subtle analysis of risk factor interactions at the *micro-level* while maintaining the *macro-level* system performance.

This paper offers a local modelling technique, the Takagi-Sugeno (TS) fuzzy system [8] for characterising subtle relationships between independent variables (inputs) and the dependent variable (output) across different local data regions while constructing a global system model. As a popular modelling technique, TS fuzzy models have gained successful applications in many areas [9]–[11], but few studies have examined the roles of TS fuzzy models in characterising subtle relationships between inputs and output across local data regions. There are a number of challenges in applying TS fuzzy models to local characterisation of data space. First, the number of TS fuzzy rules (corresponding to local linear models) increases exponentially along with the growth of the number of independent variables (the *curse of dimensionality*). In order to tackle this challenge, Zhou et al proposed a method of constructing compact TS model [12], in which the redundant local linear models (LLMs) are removed, and only important ones are used in the final model. Second, currently there are no effective analytic tools for TS fuzzy models to quantitatively assess the impacts of input variables on output across different local data regions. To this end, this paper proposes two new metrics: One is called "*Micro-impact of Domain*" (*MiD*) to assess the expected impact of changes in an input variable on outcome at a micro-level by fusing the coefficients of dominated LLM and all other LLMs in a given data sub-region. We further propose a second metric: "*Contribution of Domain*" (CoD) to assess the gross contribution of each domain at the corresponding sub-region.

Using the two new metrics we aim to provide new insights into the complex relationships between health and socioeconomic status, and educational attainments at the small area level based on data linked across routine databases. The significance of research on area-based effects lies in the need to focus public health and socioeconomic promotion initiatives on the broader characteristics of places where disadvantaged people live [13]–[20]. Understanding how drivers such as poor health, poor housing, poor local environment, unstable communities and poor public service support, interact to create a cycle of decline and underachievement is vital to identify the most appropriate policy responses.

Materials and Methods

Indices of childhood deprivation

We performed a cross-sectional study linking routine data from the Welsh Child Index for Multiple Deprivation (WCIMD) [21] with data from the UK National Pupil Database (NPD) [22]. In the UK, a considerable amount of data is produced at the so-called Lower Super Output Area (LSOA) level. LSOAs have a median population of approximately 1500 people, and were created by the UK Office for National Statistics as permanent census geographies, taking into account population size, proximity, and social homogeneity [23].

A variety of indices of area level deprivation have been created for LSOAs, by governments in different parts of the UK. The WCIMD was designed specifically for childhood policy development as part of the Neighbourhood Statistics programme in England and Wales, UK [21]. The WCIMD is based on seven separate domains of deprivation: *Income*, *Health*, *Access (Geographic) to Services*, *Housing*, *Physical Environment*, *Community Safety* and *Education (including skills and training)* at the LSOA level [21]. The indicators for each domain are based on comprehensive and robust criteria, and are regularly updated. The 2008 recently revised version of WCIMD [24][25] is calculated for each of the 1896 LSOAs across Wales. Each domain of the index is scored on a scale of 0 to 100 (highest level of deprivation) and is itself a composite variable. For example: *Income* captures the proportion of children living in households with income below a defined threshold or claiming benefits relating to low incomes. *Health* measures the degree to which children are deprived of good health, as determined by the area prevalence of limiting long-term illness and low birth weight. *Housing* captures deprivation though lack of central heating and indicators of overcrowding. *Environment* represents physical environmental risk factors that may impact quality of life, including air quality, air emissions, flood risk and proximity to waste disposal and industrial sites. *Access* represents deprivation resulting from difficulties in accessing a range of necessary services (average travel time to primary care centres, schools, libraries, leisure facilities). *Community* represents safety, based on police recorded crime, numbers of youth and adult offenders and incidents of fire. Since our target outcome variable is educational achievement, which is itself a component of the seventh WCIMD domain, we excluded the *Education* component of WCIMD from our analysis.

Simple investigation of the data may reveal that some of the domains (e.g. *Access* and *Environment*) are not strongly associated with educational attainment. However, in practice, the indicators used to define the two deprivation indices can potentially have direct or indirect impact on educational performances. For example, long distances to schools and transport nodes could worsen educational performances for children from poor family backgrounds. The *Environment* indicators, such as air quality, can significantly affect child's health, then impact educational performance indirectly. This is particularly true for children with existing poor health conditions. Substantial evidence has shown the adverse effects of exposure to ambient air pollutants on the development of lung function, and aggravation of asthma [26]. These effects may only be apparent at certain local regions, and also in combination (interaction) with other deprivation domains. Such subtle local effects, that are missed at the global level and that may exist across and between all deprivation domains, are the motivation and target of our study.

Educational under-attainment rates

The UK NPD [22] matches information from the Pupil Level Annual School Census (PLASC) with records on key stage (KS) educational attainment. We focused on educational attainment at KS1 (age 6–7) and KS2 (age 10–11). Categorisation is based on whether a pupil attains an expected level of attainment for all three core subjects: *Mathematics*, *Science*, and *English* or *Welsh* (depending on first language). Here, we defined the overall *education under-attainment rate* (EUR) at the LSOA level as a proportion, being the total number of children achieving lower than expected levels (KS1 and KS2) divided by the total number of child assessments made during the same period represented by the WCIMD indices. Education data at the LSOA level was collected from anonymised individual records, and linked to deprivation indices, using the *SAIL (Secure Anonymised Information Linkage)* databank [27][28] (Figure 1).

TS fuzzy modelling framework

This study is based on a local modelling technique, the TS fuzzy rule system [8] and a recently developed tool suited for detection of complex interactions in epidemiological data [12].

Different from the traditional health statistics for macro analyses, the TS fuzzy system decomposes the whole data space into individual regions, a local linear model (LLM) is fitted in every region, with the overall system output given as a global model which is obtained by fusing the submodels. Specifically, a TS fuzzy model is expressed as follows:

$$\begin{aligned} Rule_i: &\text{ If } x_1 \textit{ is } A_{i,1} \textit{ and } \cdots x_p \textit{ is } A_{i,p} \\ &\text{then } y_i = a_{0i} + a_{1i}x_1 + \cdots + a_{ni}x_p \end{aligned} \qquad (1)$$

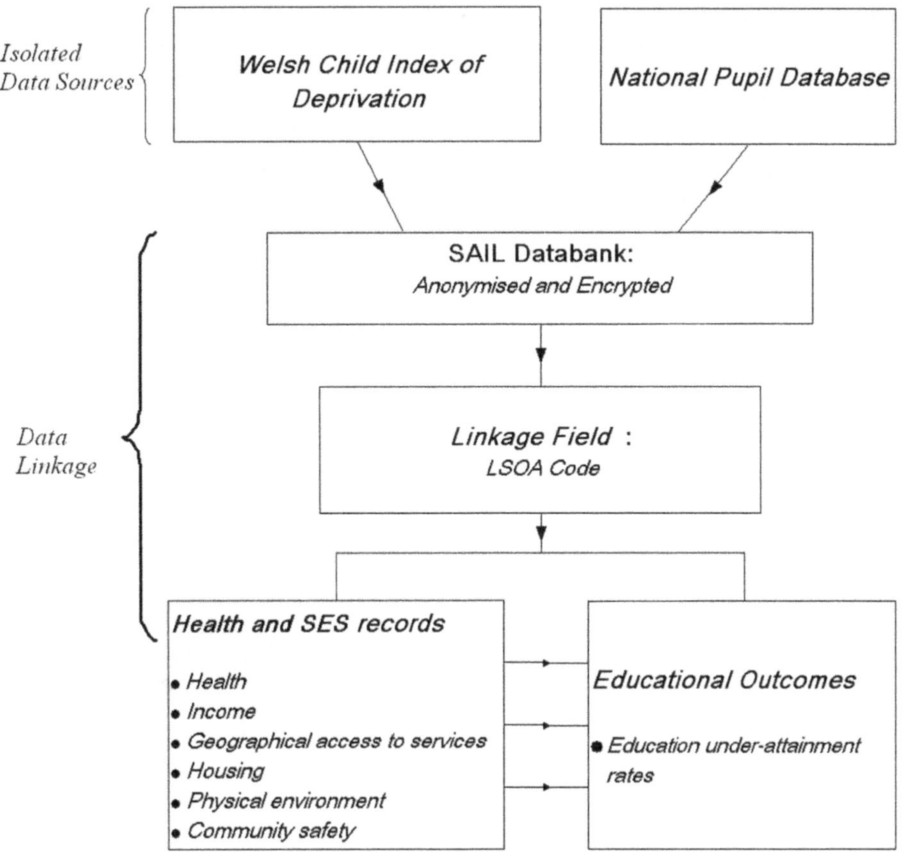

Figure 1. Linkage of data from Welsh Child Index of Multiple Deprivation with educational outcomes (under-attainment rate) at Lower Super Output Area level via Secure Anonymised Information Linkage (SAIL) databank.

where, $i=1, \cdots, L$, y_i is the output variable of the ith rule, $A_{i,j}$ is a fuzzy set of the jth domain in the ith rule, and $a_{0i}, \cdots, a_{pi}$ are consequent coefficients of the ith rule. An overall output y is produced by fusing together these *LLMs* y_i as

$$\begin{aligned} y &= \sum_{i=1}^{L} \tau_i(x) y_i \\ &= \sum_{i=1}^{L} \tau_i(x)(a_{0i} + a_{1i}x_1 + \cdots + a_{pi}x_p) \end{aligned} \tag{2}$$

where

$$\tau_i(x) = r_i(x) \Big/ \sum_{i=1}^{L} r_i(x) \tag{3}$$

is the normalized firing strength of the ith rule, and r_i is usually defined by

$$r_i(x) = \prod_j A_{i,j}(x_j) \tag{4}$$

in which the $A_{i,j}(x_j)$is the membership function of the fuzzy set $A_{i,j}$. The overall fused system model (2) is also called the *global* model. The coefficients determine the size and direction of the effects in the local fuzzy region. For example, for the 6 deprivation domains, if each is categorized into regions "high" and "low", there would be 64 ($=2^6$) sub-regions representing all combinations of each domain. The overall system output is obtained by fusing the outputs of all these submodels. The output is a predicted (fitted) education under-attainment rate for each LSOA (geographic area).

In essence, we might say "*if all deprivation levels are 'low', then use Rule (LLM) 1*". But in practice we wish to utilise our continuous data for deprivation, and might not be able to confidently classify each deprivation level as 'low'. Therefore the specific LSOA prediction is obtained as a weighted average of *all* LLMs with the weights determined by how closely the specific LSOA fits into each sub-region characterised by fuzzy sets. The complexity of the model is reduced, by fitting local simple models to partitions of the data space, a *micro characterizations of input space* [29][30]. In practice, one may tend to find a dominant rule for each sub-region. In this manner, TS rule modelling technique offers a novel way of revealing the subtle relationships between independent variables (inputs, the domains of deprivation) and dependent variable (output, the education under attainment rate) across very many small geographic regions.

Although the method is appealing, a cost is the "curse of dimensionality" whereby for many variables or sub-regions, there may be a large number of LLMs, which can lead to over-fitting and poor out-of-sample performance. Zhou et al have developed a method to identify a parsimonious set of rules that capture the key interactions between the variables whilst avoiding such over-fitting [12].

Table 1. Core cut-off points for fuzzy sets to characterise "non-deprived" and "highly deprived" scores.

Input variables	*Non-deprived core scores*	*Highly deprived core scores*
Income	[0, 11.71]	[36.56, 100]
Health	[0, 13.14]	[35.2, 100]
Access	[0, 14.66]	[26.05, 100]
Housing	[0, 14.77]	[31.77, 100]
Environment	[0, 18.80]	[25.91, 100]
Community	[0, 12.24]	[36.63, 100]

Output metrics for the TS model

In this paper we propose two new metrics to quantitatively assess how the impacts of domain factors on outcome vary across these local regions at micro-level.

1. MiD: micro-impact of domain. First note that in a TS fuzzy system, each LLM describes the relationship between domain factors and outcome in a certain data sub-region. The coefficients of these LLMs represent, for each deprivation domain,

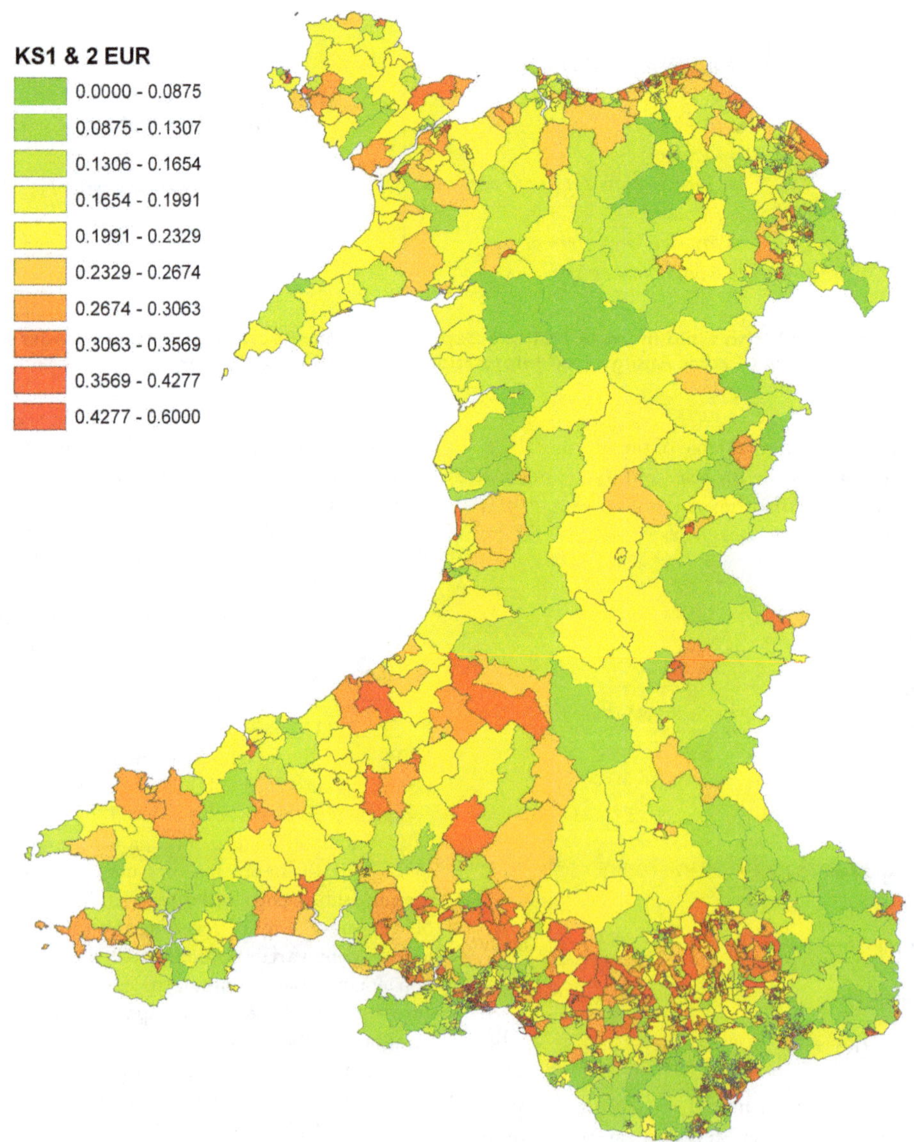

Figure 2. Educational under-attainment rates (EUR) in each LSOA across Wales.

the rates and directions of expected change of the conditional mean of the outcome (e.g. education under-attainment rate) with respect to each deprivation domain. To make a prediction for a specific LSOA, the coefficients across all LLM are fused with the weights determined by how well the LSOA fits to each LLM data space region. These averaged coefficients are unique to each LSOA and give an indication of how the educational achievement would be expected to change given changes in deprivation scores. We denote this metric by the term "*Micro-impact of Domain*" (*MiD*) at the given sample point.

Specifically, given an LLM $y_i = a_{0i} + a_{1i}x_1 + \cdots + a_{pi}x_p$, the slope coefficient vector $E = (a_{1i}, \cdots, a_{pi})^T$ is be normalized into a unitary vector:

$$e_{ji} = \frac{a_{ji}}{\|E\|} \tag{5}$$

Then given an input (e.g. vector of WCIMD deprivation scores) $\widehat{x} = \left(\widehat{x}_1, \cdots, \widehat{x}_p\right)^T$, the overall influence of the jth domain on output at the point $\widehat{x}$ is defined as

$$MiD_j(\widehat{x}) = \sum_{i=1}^{L} \tau_i(\widehat{x}) e_{ji} \tag{6}$$

Hence the *MiD* defines *the overall expected change in the output (e.g. education under-attainment rate), on average, for a one-unit change in the jth domain at the point $\widehat{x}$, while holding all the other domains fixed*. It gives the size and direction of the effect that the jth domain is having on the output at the point $\widehat{x}$. Note that x represents a general variable, while $\widehat{x}$ denotes the values of x at a specific point.

2. CoD: contribution of domain. The MiD coefficient represents the slope of the relationship between deprivation and education, hence a standardised effect size for a given change in deprivation. In practice, domain scores for certain LSOAs may differ widely in magnitude, and potential changes in deprivation score via policy intervention may also differ widely, hence the absolute change in educational score needs to take this into account. The "*Contribution of Domain*" (CoD) is defined as the product of the MiD and the actual domain value.

Specifically, given an input sample, $\widehat{x} = \left(\widehat{x}_1, \cdots, \widehat{x}_p\right)^T$, the overall influence of the jth domain on $\widehat{x}$ is defined as

$$CoD_j(\widehat{x}) = \widehat{x}_j \sum_{i=1}^{L} \tau_i(\widehat{x}) e_{ji} \tag{7}$$

Fitting the TS model

First, given the 1896 LSOA samples across Wales, a 9-fold cross validation scheme was used to evaluate the performance of the TS model. In each data partition, 1400 samples were used for training, 200 samples for validation, and 296 samples for testing. The 1400 training samples were used to fit the initial TS model with inputs representing the various indices of deprivation: *income* (x_1), *health* (x_2), *access to services* (x_3), *housing* (x_4), *physical environment* (x_5), *community safety* (x_6) and one output: *education educational under-attainment rate* (y). In this study, each of the deprivation domains was characterised into 'low' *non-deprived* scores and 'high' *highly deprived* categories. Since such classification has uncertainty associated with it, fuzzy sets were used to characterise these linguistic terms. First, the fuzzy c-means unsupervised clustering algorithm [31] was used to partition input space. By projecting the multi-dimensional prototypes on the input variable space [32], the membership functions of fuzzy sets were generated with the core cut-off points shown in the Table 1. In this way, this initial TS model consists of 64 rules representing all combinations of each domain in partitioning the input space. Then the validation data set was used to select the important rules and remove the redundant ones in the interest of constructing compact model using the ω-index of TS fuzzy rules proposed in [12]. The generalisation performance of the constructed compact TS model was evaluated by applying to the testing data set. Then the most compact TS model with good global prediction performance was used to analyse the micro-impacts of deprivation domains on educational under-attainment rate across different data sub-regions. All models were implemented in Matlab, and code is available upon request from the corresponding author.

Ethics

The data used in this study was collected via national databases held in the *SAIL (Secure Anonymised Information Linkage)* databank [27][28]. No ethical review was required because the SAIL databank holds the data which has been anonymised and granted with the permission of relevant Caldicott Guardian/Data Protection Officer [33], however, approval to proceed with the

Table 2. The eight most important *"if-then"* input components of the rules ($W_1 \sim W_8$) for the final TS fuzzy model.

Rule ID	Access	Community	Environment	Health	Housing	Income
W_1	-	-	-	-	-	-
W_2	D	-	-	-	-	-
W_3	-	-	D	-	-	-
W_4	D	-	-	-	D	-
W_5	D	-	D	-	-	-
W_6	-	D	-	D	D	D
W_7	-	D	D	D	D	D
W_8	-	D	-	D	-	D

(These rules are selected from the 64 possible Local Linear Models according to our algorithm [12]. D = high deprivation, - = non-deprived).

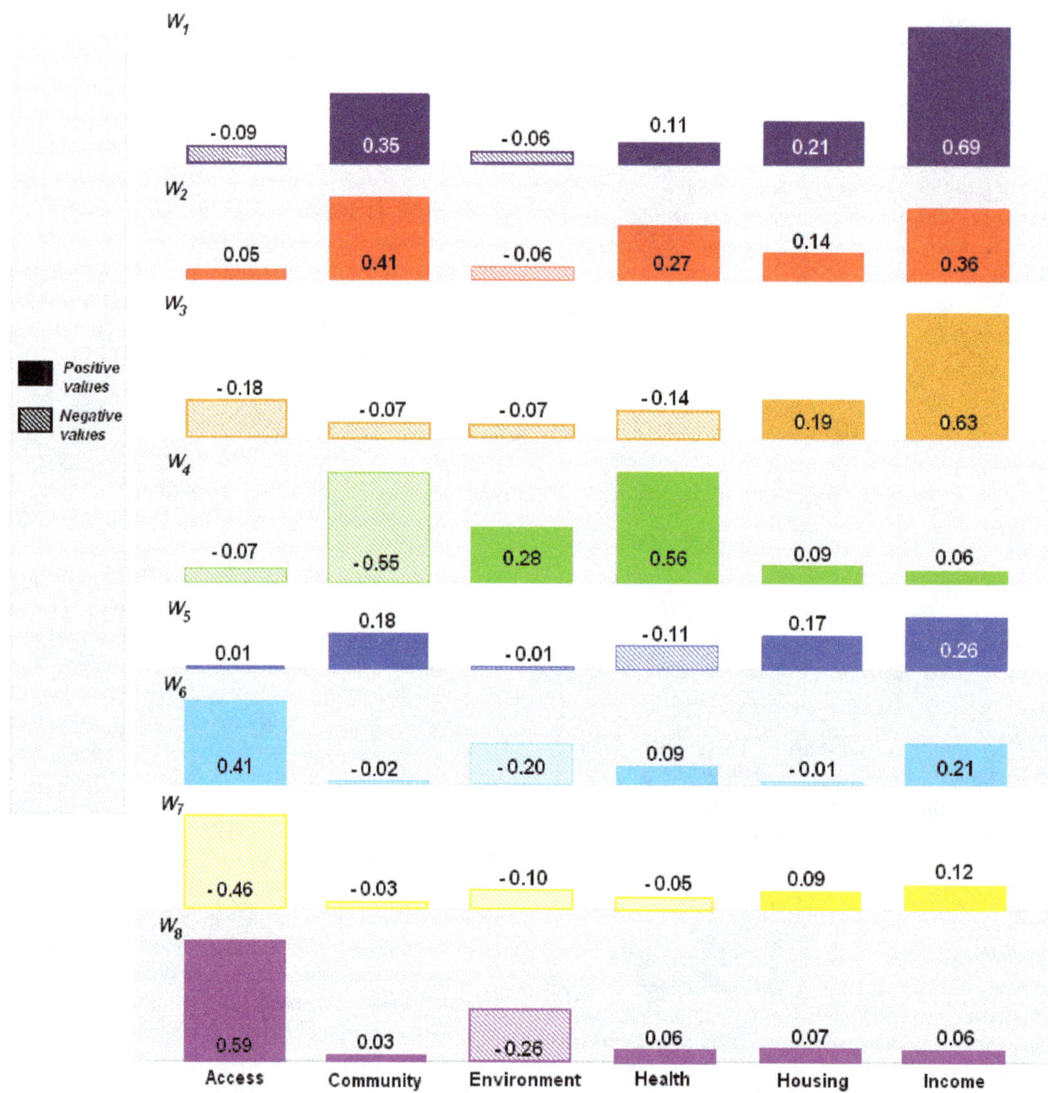

Figure 3. The coefficients of the eight local linear models in the parsimonious constructed compact TS system model. The rules are coded as W_1 to W_8 (see Table 2). Note that individual LSOAs have predicted values that are weighted averages of these 8 models, with the weights determined by the uncertainty of membership of the sub-regions.

study was given by the Information Governance Review Panel [28].

Results

There were 196,770 KS1 and KS2 childhood records for Wales during the relevant WCIMD period. The number of children with KS 1 or KS2 records in this study between 2005 and 2007 can be found in Table S1 of Data Supplement. Figure 2 depicts the educational under-attainment rate (EUR) across each of the 1896 LSOAs in Wales. The overall percentage failing to achieve the education target was 22.7%, with considerable geographical heterogeneity. The pair-wise linear correlation coefficients for all domains: *Income*, *Health*, *Access*, *Housing*, *Environment* and *Community*, can be found in Table S2 of Data Supplement. Fuzzy sets with the core cut-off points shown in the Table 1 were used to characterise the 'low' *non-deprived* scores and 'high' *highly deprived* categories. Uncertainty emerges for the areas whose deprivation scores lie between the cut-offs. For example, an LSOA with income deprivation score below 11.71 should belong, with high certainty, to the *non-deprived* category on *Income*, and one with deprivation score above 36.56 to the *highly deprived* category. In contrast an LSOA with income deprivation scores of 30 would have the membership of the *non-deprived* category with a "degree" (representing uncertainty) of 0.29 and at the same time, a degree of 0.84 belonging to the *highly-deprived* category. So in decision making about such areas, both high and low deprivation on *Income* (with their associated "*if-then*" rules) will contribute significantly, with the *weights* of each calculated from the degree of membership.

Using sub-regions of the data space based on the two sets of each of the 6 deprivation domains results in 64 rules (LLMs), and a risk of redundancy and over fitting of the data. Application of our recently developed algorithm [12] resulted in a compact, and parsimonious TS model. The 9 fold cross validation scheme showed an overall root-mean-squared-error (RMSE) of 0.0888 (95% confidence interval: [0.0845, 0.0931]). The best compact TS model had only 8 important rules (note that this is fewer than

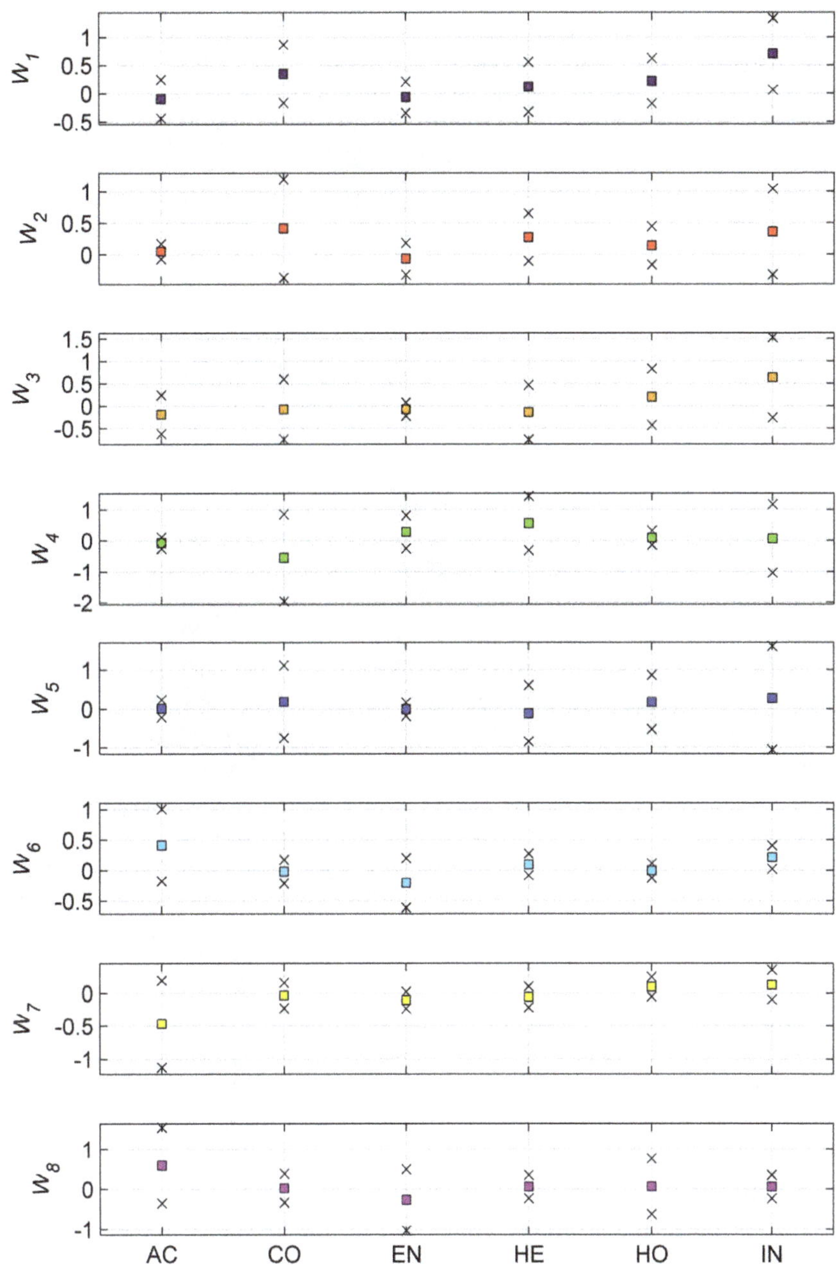

Figure 4. Properties of the coefficients of the eight selected "parsimonious" local linear models (LLMs). Green square represents point estimate, and "x" marks upper and lower 95% confidence intervals. (*IN- Income; HE- Health; AC- Access to Services; HO – Housing; EN – Physical Environment; CO- Community Safety*).

found in [12] as we are now using an updated version of the WIMCS data set). Taken together, these were sufficient to provide an accurate prediction of the education under-attainment rate in all LSOAs (generalization performance on testing data set with RMSE of 0.0842, see Figure S1 of Data Supplement). This means that the whole population of children attending the KS1 and KS2 across Wales can be grouped into 8 different clusters with similar characteristics in each cluster according to their combinations of deprivation domains of the WCIMD, and each cluster is dominated by an LLM.

The input conditions for each rule are outlined in Table 2, and the coefficients of each of the 8 local linear models are given in Figure 3, while Figure 4 depicts the 95% confidence intervals (CIs) of these coefficients. The colours in Figure 3 are used to differentiate these LLMs and the corresponding clusters of LSOAs revealed in Figure 5. It can be seen that based on the given WCIMD training dataset, some coefficients of the LLMs have the negative values. These negative values represent the "unexpected" conclusion that education scores tend to *improve* with increased deprivation of corresponding domain, and tend to have wide confidence intervals associated with them. Hence although these trends are present in certain sub-regions of the data, evidence for such an effect is not very strong. The 95% CIs in Figure 4 show the range of plausible values that can act as estimates for the coefficients of each deprivation score in each LLM. *Income* domain in the LLMs W_1 and W_6 is clearly statistically significantly

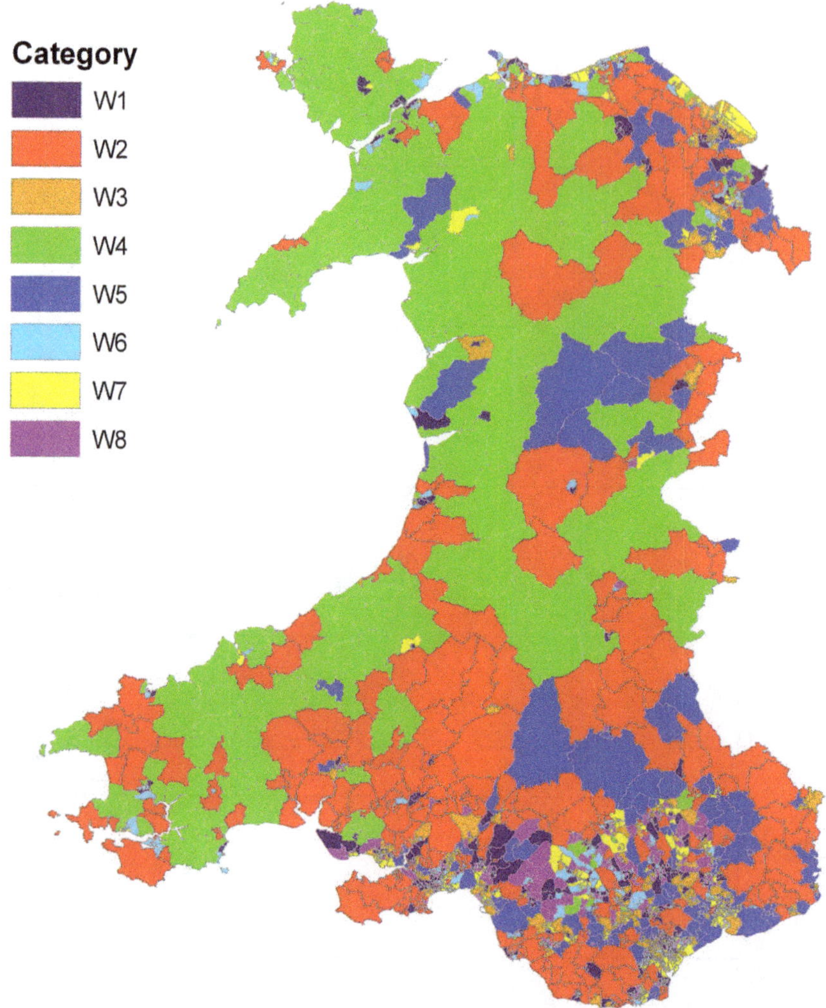

Figure 5. Map of Wales showing Lower Super Output Areas (LSOAs) coded according to the dominant rule at each LSOA that represents the relationship between deprivation domains and education under-attainment rate.

different from zero. The CIs for the domains of *Access* in W_2, *Environment* in W_3, *Health* in W_6, and *Housing* in W_7 all also indicate statistical significance. We note that even small coefficients can make considerable contributions to the predicted education failure rate in local areas of high deprivation. This is because the expected education failure rate is obtained from the product of the coefficient and the deprivation score. This is part of the rationale for the choice of the CoD metric as a key output.

As indicated above, each data sub-region has one dominating LLM while the rest of other LLMs play minor roles in prediction for the samples in this sub-region. Summarising the LLMs in the whole data space, Table 3 shows the values of mean, minimum and maximum of the LLMs' coefficients and corresponding 95% CIs. The Table 3 indicated that in overall, the *Income* and *Housing* domains are statistically significant, as might be expected, *Income* was the most influential domain.

To further interpret these LLMs, the input conditions from Table 2 (the "*if*" component of the rules) can be combined with the coefficients from Figure 3 (the "*then*" component of the rules) to illustrate the extremely complicated interactions that emerge from the data mining. The effects of all individual deprivation domains were strongly dependent on the categories of all other domains in determining educational outcomes. This means that generalisations about the effect of any deprivation index to a local level could have poor performance if the other factors are not properly taken into account.

There are several outputs from the model that are of interest. First, a simple indicator that can be used to classify each LSOA is the "dominant rule". Figure 5 shows the distribution of these 8 types of relationship across Wales revealed by the 8 LLMs in Figure 3 (colours used in these two Figures to represent the LLMs and corresponding LSOAs are consistent). Several interesting patterns emerge. The urban and rural areas of Wales are naturally marked by the size of the LSOA, with very small LSOAs found in the north and south coastal cities, as well as the South Wales industrial valleys. If we concentrate instead on the remaining rural areas, there remains a general north-west (NW) to south-east (SE) divide, with the NW characterised by rule 4 (green) in which the relationship between education under attainment and deprivation is strongly influenced by *Health*, with a contribution from *Environment* but a surprisingly small role for *Income*. While in the SE rule 2 dominates (red) in which *Income* plays a much more central role, along with *Community* and, to a lesser extent, *Health*.

Table 3. Summary of coefficients of the local linear models in the constructed TS system model.

Variable	*Baseline*	*Access score*	*Community score*	*Environment score*	*Health score*	*Housing score*	*Income score*
Minimum	7.09	−0.47	−0.55	−0.26	−0.14	−0.00	0.06
Maximum	30.88	0.60	0.42	0.28	0.56	0.22	0.7
Mean	16.31	0.03	0.04	−0.06	0.10	0.12	0.30
95%CI	[9.96, 22.66]	[−0.25, 0.31]	[−0.21, 0.29]	[−0.20, 0.07]	[−0.10, 0.29]	[0.06, 0.19]	[0.10, 0.51]

Recall however, that the fitted value for each LSOA is a weighted average of all 8 rules (LLMs). Hence the need for the proposed metrics to reveal the unique local picture. The MiD values across all LSOAs are illustrated in Figure 6, in which a positive MiD indicates higher levels of deprivation are associated with higher education failure rates. Figure 7 shows the domain factor for each LSOA that has the strongest MiD across Wales. Moreover, Figure 8 illustrates the geographical trends of the CoD for each LSOA. The number of observations here are large. Based on our knowledge concerning specific LSOAs, we provide some case studies highlighting the insights from the new model and metrics.

Case Study 1: Affluent area, with only poor access to services. For this region, the dominant rule is W_2, which suggests that in terms of the MiD metric the domain factors - *Community*, *Income* and *Health* have strong associations with educational outcomes (highest coefficients in Figure 3). However, for this area, all these domains are already at extremely low deprivation levels, making them unlikely targets for improvement. In contrast, the CoD metric shows that *Access* is overall the most important determinant of under-attainment performance (>33% contribution to the predicted educational under-attainment score), and should be the key target. This case study represents a "straightforward" situation, in which the most important target domain is simply the standout value from the WCIMD data. Here, all deprivation scores are very low, apart from *Access*. Despite the obvious main conclusion, the MiD values highlight higher than expected roles for certain domains (*Income*, *Community* and *Health*, reflected in high MiD coefficients, and moderate CoD scores).

Case Study 2: Area with poor access to services, and moderate levels of deprivation for other domains. This is another area for which the dominant rule is W_2, and might be expected to have similar problems to the Case Study 1. It is in fact the next most deprived area in their region for *Access* (98th percentile). However, despite *Access* being the standout value in the raw WCIMD data, this time a simple interpretation does not hold. Since there are moderate deprivation levels for *Health* (37th percentile), and MiD coefficients show that the effect of *Health* in this region to be highest, then *Health* is classified as by far the most important target in the area.

Case Study 3: Deprived area, with especially poor income, health and community safety domains (but good access to services). The dominant rule is W_6 (also with significant weighting from W_7), which implies an expected impact (according to MiD) from *Access*, *Income* and *Health*. However, due to the great disparity between high deprivation on the *Income* (94th percentile) and good *Access* (39th percentile), then in the CoD metric the *Income* domain (and to a lesser extent *Health*) dominates and is highlighted as the key priority.

Case Study 4: Area of moderate deprivation across all domains. Here, the dominant local model is W_1 (although with significant contribution from several other models). According to the MiD metric, *Income*, *Community* and *Housing* are expected to have the strongest relationship with educational outcome. Both metrics suggests that *Income* is the target domain, having the strongest coefficient (MiD) value and with a CoD value contributing 67% to the expected under-attainment rate.

The last two Case Studies focus on *Housing* and *Environment*. Although these factors tend to have a smaller role than the other domains, it is not difficult to identify cases in which they play important roles. *Case Study 5* represents an LSOA with generally very low deprivation (*Income*, *Health*, *Community*), but with roughly average levels of *Housing*, *Environment* and *Access*. This area is dominated by rule W_3 (though with significant contribu-

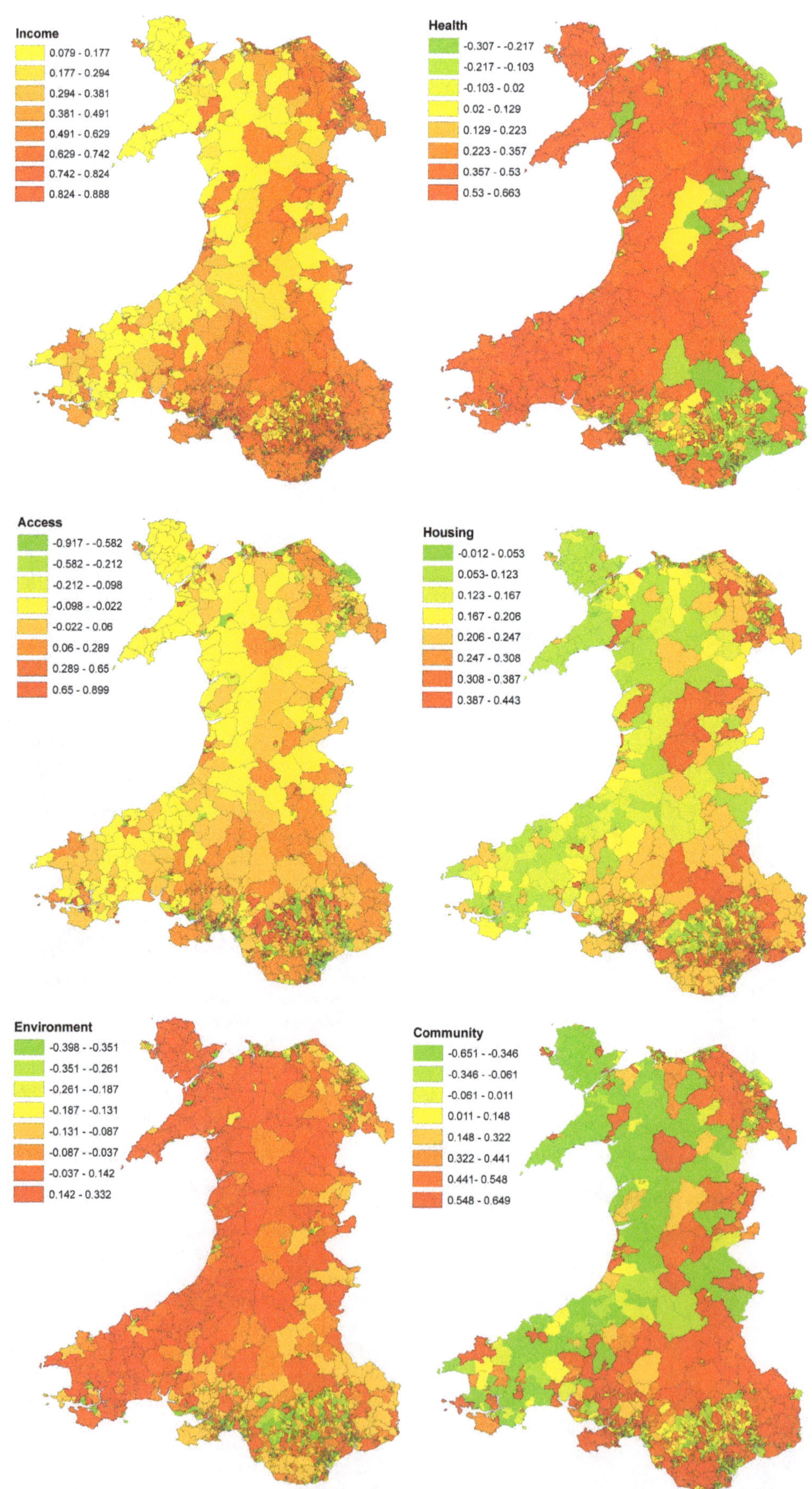
Income
0.079 - 0.177
0.177 - 0.294
0.294 - 0.381
0.381 - 0.491
0.491 - 0.629
0.629 - 0.742
0.742 - 0.824
0.824 - 0.888
Health
-0.307 - -0.217
-0.217 - -0.103
-0.103 - 0.02
0.02 - 0.129
0.129 - 0.223
0.223 - 0.357
0.357 - 0.53
0.53 - 0.663
Access
-0.917 - -0.582
-0.582 - -0.212
-0.212 - -0.098
-0.098 - -0.022
-0.022 - 0.06
0.06 - 0.289
0.289 - 0.65
0.65 - 0.899
Housing
-0.012 - 0.053
0.053- 0.123
0.123 - 0.167
0.167 - 0.206
0.206 - 0.247
0.247 - 0.308
0.308 - 0.387
0.387 - 0.443
Environment
-0.398 - -0.351
-0.351 - -0.261
-0.261 - -0.187
-0.187 - -0.131
-0.131 - -0.087
-0.087 - -0.037
-0.037 - 0.142
0.142 - 0.332
Community
-0.651 - -0.346
-0.346 - -0.061
-0.061 - 0.011
0.011 - 0.148
0.148 - 0.322
0.322 - 0.441
0.441- 0.548
0.548 - 0.649

Figure 6. Variations in Micro-impact of Domain (MiD). Overall rates and directions of expected changes in education under attainment rate, for unit change in domain deprivation score.

tions from the other rules). In terms of MiD coefficient, *Income* appears to have the strongest correlation with educational performance. However, due to the very low WCIMD values for *Income*, the largest component of under-attainment, CoD value, is *Housing*.

Case Study 6 represents a set of rural areas, which are very affluent, yet have high deprivation scores at the *Environment* and *Access* domains. They are described predominately by rule W_4, which suggests a strongest coefficient (MiD) for *Health*. However, the CoD value shows that the greatest deprivation contribution to under-attainment comes from the *Environment* domain.

We note that these examples are not easily generalized. There is a role for all aspects of deprivation, including *Environment*, *Housing*, *Access* and *Community*, in addition to the factors of *Income* and *Health* that are usually focused on. The importance in a given region is not simply revealed by the deprivation scores alone, and consequently there are very many different spatial patterns that can be found in the data, and contrasting effects found across areas that initially appear quite similar. A need for area-based interpretation is clear.

Our investigations so far suggest that, although in our modelling each LSOA is considered as independent one from another, regional characteristics (urban, rural, industrial areas, etc.) can play important roles in explaining the variations of spatial patterns. For rural areas with scattered population, such as those dominated by rule W_2, *Access to Services* emerges as a key domain for improving educational performance. Areas, such as the ex-coalfields in South Wales Valleys, have the key priority in the domains of *Income* and *Health*. An extension of the approach to formally include spatial statistics would be a potential area of future research.

Discussion

On first encounter, the algorithm for fitting the TS model can appear complicated. However it is little more than a trick for finding sub-regions of the multidimensional data space that are

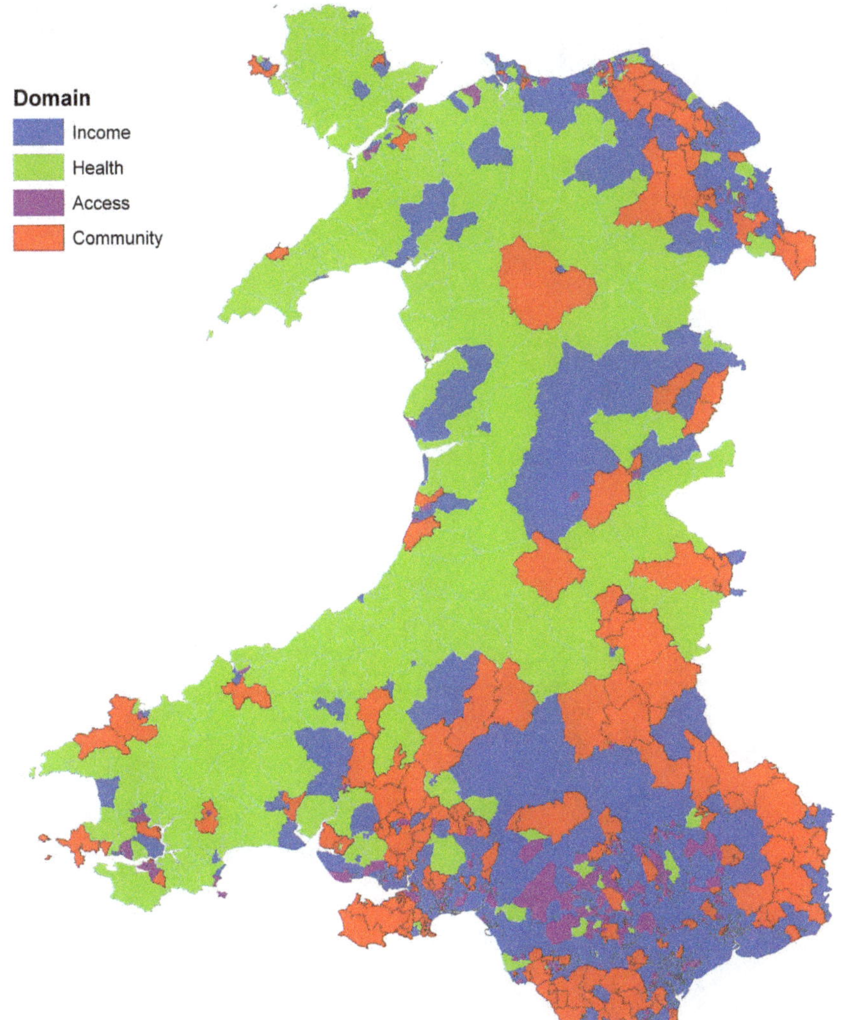

Figure 7. Highlighting key domains having strong association with educational performance (defined by largest MiD) across Wales.

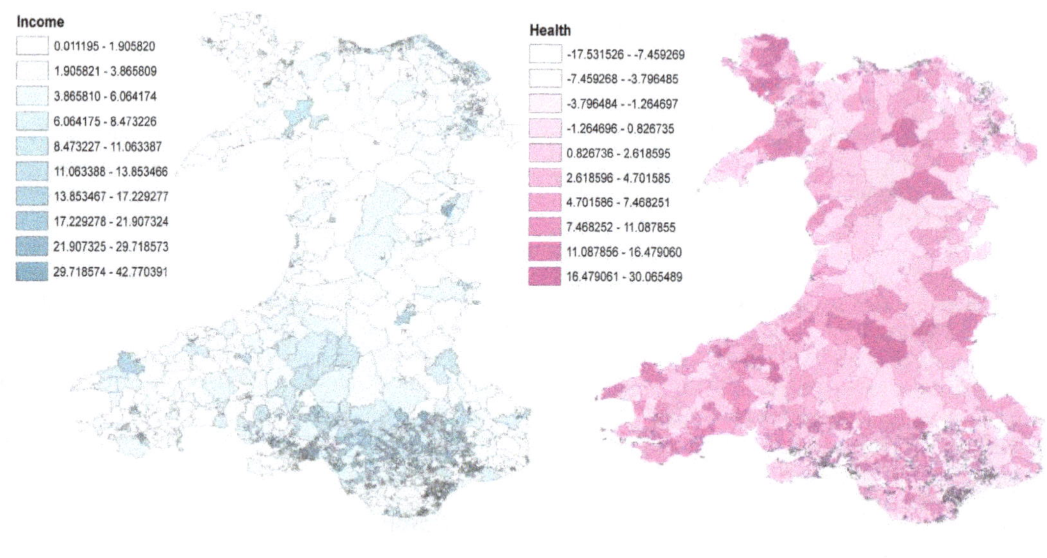
Income
0.011195 - 1.905820
1.905821 - 3.865809
3.865810 - 6.064174
6.064175 - 8.473226
8.473227 - 11.063387
11.063388 - 13.853466
13.853467 - 17.229277
17.229278 - 21.907324
21.907325 - 29.718573
29.718574 - 42.770391
Health
-17.531526 - -7.459269
-7.459268 - -3.796485
-3.796484 - -1.264697
-1.264696 - 0.826735
0.826736 - 2.618595
2.618596 - 4.701585
4.701586 - 7.468251
7.468252 - 11.087855
11.087856 - 16.479060
16.479061 - 30.065489

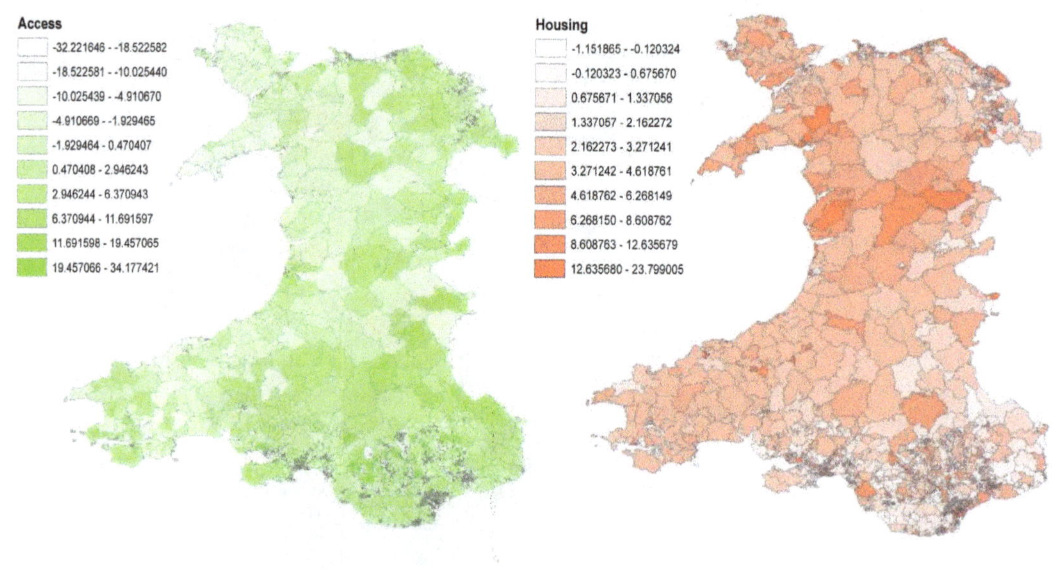
Access
-32.221646 - -18.522582
-18.522581 - -10.025440
-10.025439 - -4.910670
-4.910669 - -1.929465
-1.929464 - 0.470407
0.470408 - 2.946243
2.946244 - 6.370943
6.370944 - 11.691597
11.691598 - 19.457065
19.457066 - 34.177421
Housing
-1.151865 - -0.120324
-0.120323 - 0.675670
0.675671 - 1.337056
1.337057 - 2.162272
2.162273 - 3.271241
3.271242 - 4.618761
4.618762 - 6.268149
6.268150 - 8.608762
8.608763 - 12.635679
12.635680 - 23.799005

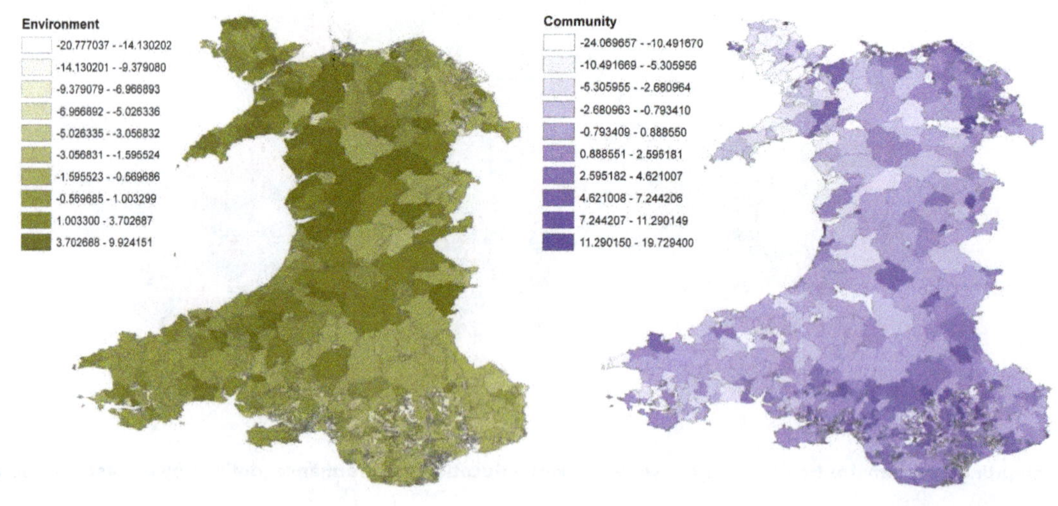
Environment
-20.777037 - -14.130202
-14.130201 - -9.379080
-9.379079 - -6.966893
-6.966892 - -5.026336
-5.026335 - -3.056832
-3.056831 - -1.595524
-1.595523 - -0.569686
-0.569685 - 1.003299
1.003300 - 3.702687
3.702688 - 9.924151
Community
-24.069657 - -10.491670
-10.491669 - -5.305956
-5.305955 - -2.680964
-2.680963 - -0.793410
-0.793409 - 0.888550
0.888551 - 2.595181
2.595182 - 4.621007
4.621008 - 7.244206
7.244207 - 11.290149
11.290150 - 19.729400

Figure 8. Variations in Contribution of Domain (CoD). These values represent a product of the observed WCIMD deprivation scores, and the domain coefficient scores (MiD values) in each LSOA, and represents the contribution of each type of deprivation domain to the expected education under-attainment rate in each LSOA.

distinct, and can then be well described by a small set of simple models (LLMs). Then for a specific area, one uses an average of these models that reflects how well the area 'belongs' to the sub region of the data. Using if-then rules and local modelling technique, we suggest that the TS model offers greater transparency than fitting interactions and complex non-linear terms in, for example, regression models, because we are always dealing with a simple model in a relevant data space, rather than a complex model that tries to capture all the subtleties at once.

A statistical interaction can be defined as a relationship in which the influence of a variable on an outcome measure is dependent on the value of other (interacting) variables. In the fitting of a TS system, if there is a requirement for several LLMs this, by definition, represents interaction (or non-linearity) in the data. It means that the coefficients for a certain variable will be different (specified by a different LLM) across different regions of the data space. Hence, this approach is natural for revealing complex interactions between variables, while remaining fairly easy to interpret at the local level, where the effects are approximately linear.

As a comparison to our data mining approach, a standard linear regression analysis finds that *Access* and *Community* are not statistically significantly associated (at the 5% level) with educational attainment (in univariate analysis) and the majority of two-way interactions were not significant (see Table S3 and Table S4 of Data Supplement). Some of the complexity of the data can indeed be recovered from the presence of several significant multi-way interactions, however we argue that these models are much more difficult to interpret than the straightforward "*if-then*" linear models presented here. Nevertheless, this study has some potential limitations. First our data mining approach adopted in this study involves higher computing overhead for the purpose of constructing a parsimonious model. Moreover designing the fuzzy sets for linguistic terms needs skills and additional efforts for appropriate generation of hyper-parameter values via a trial-and-error approach.

To put some of these findings in context, the World Health Organization (WHO) has promoted the importance of early area-based interventions in health and educational attainment worldwide [34], leading to community-based initiatives to improve developmental outcomes among socio-economically disadvantaged children [35]–[37]. These initiatives reflect the WHO's principles of the Health for All (HFA) [34]. For example, the Best Start project in Australia aims to improve the overall health, development, learning and wellbeing of Victoria's young children and their families in some of the most socially disadvantaged communities through local partnerships and improved service co-ordination [38]. After several years, the findings suggest that improvements in access to services in disadvantaged areas can be achieved by area-based interventions, such as optimising the use of existing resources, and that the potential health benefits of area-based interventions might be better assessed by examining steps along the pathway between intervention and outcome [35][39]. In the UK, improving education and skills is one of the five priority goals of the National Strategy for Neighbourhood Renewal and the New Deals for Communities Programme. This area-based approach has led to initiatives such as Sure Start, Excellence in Cities, Education Action Zones and Aim Higher which target education. The New Deals for Communities is unique in relation to previous initiatives by addressing not only education but the *other factors* that might impede progress in educational performance [37]. More specifically, it picks highly deprived neighbourhoods to tackle place based issues (crime, community, housing, physical environment) in order to address people based outcomes (education, health and worklessness) using school and community interventions. The findings of our study offer data mining evidence suggesting that a combined approach of tackling place based issues and educational attainment may be more effective than simply focusing on education alone.

In intervention evaluation, a general theme is that rigorous program evaluation is needed to determine which interventions will work most effectively and to spend scarce resources wisely [40]. However, evaluation of complex intervention is often difficult. For example, a review looking at housing improvements and health effects [41] found a large number of methodological difficulties in the before and after comparisons, especially in the response and follow-up rates among deprived communities and there is a lack of evidence on health gains that result in investment in housing. Thus, while this study suggests that tackling place and income barriers will improve children's education, there is currently a lack of evidence from intervention studies to confirm this. The scope of future evaluations must be carefully tailored and techniques must be properly selected to generate accurate information for policy makers.

Conclusions

Complex interactions are notoriously difficult to detect and interpret within a standard statistical regression framework. This paper provided a local modelling method that relies on sets of simple linear models, and proposed two new metrics, *MiD* and *CoD*, to quantify the variations of local level impacts of multidimensional factors on educational outcomes. This study revealed some intriguing findings to bolster the scanty evidence base around the complex inter-relationship between different domains of health and socio-economic status and educational achievement. The results are consistent with a growing literature on the importance of place characteristics on individual outcomes. The findings imply that a broad range of policies may have influence in reducing inequalities in educational achievement and that interventions tailored to fit in with local characteristic would help to increase their effectiveness. It is now important to exploit the opportunities posed by natural experiments where substantial changes are made to the distribution of deprivation domains as a result of planned or serendipitous circumstances. Such longitudinal effects would serve to validate predictions of the data mining models, and aid in the assessment of causality.

Supporting Information

Figure S1 The prediction by the constructed TS model (circles) vs observed child educational under-attainment rates (points) at testing LSOAs. A random sample of 50 LSOAs from the testing sample are shown here, to aid in clarity.

Table S1 Number of children with Key Stage 1 or 2 records in study, between 2005 and 2007.

Table S2 Pair-wise linear correlation coefficients for all domains. Note that negative association is common, and few of the domain scores are highly correlated.

Table S3 Results of linear regression applied to the same dataset.

Table S4 Linear regression with all pairwise interactions.

Author Contributions

Conceived and designed the experiments: SMZ SB MBG. Performed the experiments: SMZ MBG. Analyzed the data: SMZ MBG OGB RAL SB AJ HB KJ. Contributed reagents/materials/analysis tools: RAL SMZ MBG SB. Wrote the paper: SMZ MBG SB.

References

1. Webber R, Butler T (2005) Classifying pupils by where they live: how well do these predict variations in their GCSE results? CASA Working Paper No. 99. London: UCL.
2. Brownell M, Roos N, Fransoo R, Roos LL, Guevremont A, et al. (2006) Is the class half empty? A population-based perspective on socioeconomic status and educational outcomes. IRPP Choices 12:1–30.
3. Currie J (2007) Healthy, wealthy, and wise: is there a causal relationship between child health and human capital development. Workshop on The Long-run Impact of Early Life Events, December 13–14, Ford School of Public Policy, Weill Hall, Ann Arbor, MI, USA.
4. Black SE, Devereux PJ, Salvanes KG (2007) From the cradle to the labor market? The effect of birth weight on adult outcomes. Quarterly Journal of Economics 122: 409–439.
5. Malacova E, Li J, Blair E, Leonard H, de Klerk N, et al. (2008) Association of birth outcomes and maternal, school, and neighborhood characteristics with subsequent numeracy achievement. American Journal of Epidemiology 168: 21–29.
6. Schools Analysis and Research Division (2009) Deprivation and Education: The evidence on pupils in England, foundation stage to Key Stage 4. March 2009, Department for Children, Schools and Families, http://www.education.gov.uk/publications/eOrderingDownload/DCSF-RTP-09-01.pdf (accessed 29 Feb 2012).
7. Acheson D (Chairman) Independent Inquiry into Inequalities in Health Report. The Stationery Office, UK. http://www.archive.official-documents.co.uk/document/doh/ih/ih.htm (Accessed date: 9 April 2011)
8. Takagi T, Sugeno M (1985) Fuzzy identification of systems and its applications to modeling and control. IEEE Transactions on System, Man and Cybernetics 15: 116–132.
9. Chadli M, Borne P (2012) Multiple models approach in automation: Takagi-Sugeno fuzzy systems, Wiley.
10. Juang CF, Chen GC (2012) A TS fuzzy system learned through a support vector machine in principal component space for real- time object detection. IEEE Transactions on Industrial Electronics 59: 3309–3320.
11. Precup RE, Hellendoorn H (2011) A survey on industrial applications of fuzzy control. Computers in Industry 62: 213–226
12. Zhou SM, Lyons RA, Brophy S, Gravenor MB (2012) Constructing compact Takagi-Sugeno rule systems: identification of complex interactions in epidemiological data. PLoS ONE 7: e51468.
13. Popham F, Dibben C, Bambra C (2013) Are health inequalities really not the smallest in the Nordic welfare states? A comparison of mortality inequality in 37 countries. Journal of Epidemiology & Community Health 67:412–418
14. Dibben C, Popham F (2013) Are health inequalities evident at all ages? An ecological study of English mortality records. European Journal of Public Health 23:39–45
15. Ngo N, Paquet C, Howard NJ, Coffee NT, Adams RA, et al. (2014). Area-Level Socioeconomic Characteristics, Prevalence and Trajectories of Cardiometabolic Risk. International Journal of Environmental Research and Public Health 11: 830–848.
16. Ngo AD, Paquet C, Howard NJ, Coffee NT, Adams R, et al. (2013). Area-level Socioeconomic Characteristics and Incidence of Metabolic Syndrome: A Prospective Cohort Study. BMC Public Health. 13:681, Accessed at: biomedcentral.com/1471-2458/13/681.
17. Davey SG, Hart CL, Watt G, Hole DJ, Hawthorne VM (1998) Individual social class, area-based deprivation, cardiovascular disease risk factors, and mortality: the Renfrew and Paisley Study. Journal of Epidemiology and Community Health 52:399–405
18. Picciotto S, Forastiere F, Stafoggia M, D'Ippoliti D, Ancona C, et al. (2006) Associations of area based deprivation status and individual educational attainment with incidence, treatment, and prognosis of first coronary event in Rome, Italy, J Epidemiol Community Health 60:37–43.
19. Steenland K, Henley J, Calle E, Thun M (2004) Individual- and area-level socioeconomic status variables as predictors of mortality in a cohort of 179,383 persons. American Journal of Epidemiology 159:1047–1056.
20. Blanc PD, Yen IH, Chen H, Katz PP, Earnest G, et al. (2006) Area-level socioeconomic status and health status among adults with asthma and rhinitis, Eur Respir J 27: 85–94.
21. Welsh Statistical Directorate. Welsh Index of Multiple Deprivation 2008, Technical Report, Welsh Assembly Government.
22. Administrative Data Liaison Service. National Pupil Database (NPD), http://www.adls.ac.uk/department-for-education/dcsf-npd/?detail (accessed 10 Sept 2010).
23. UK Office for National Statistics. Super Output Areas, http://www.ons.gov.uk/ons/guide-method/geography/beginner-s-guide/census/super-output-areas-soas-/index.html (accessed 10 Sept 2010).
24. Welsh Assembly Government. Welsh Index of Multiple Deprivation 2008, Summary Report (http://wales.gov.uk/docs/statistics/2011/111220wimdsummaryreviseden.pdf) (accessed 29 Feb 2012).
25. Welsh Assembly Government. Analysis of the correction to the Welsh Index of Multiple Deprivation 2008 (http://wales.gov.uk/docs/statistics/2012/120628wimdincomeanalysisen.pdf) (accessed 16 November 2012).
26. Schwartz J (2004) Air Pollution and Children's Health. Pediatrics 13: 1037–1043
27. Lyons RA, Jones KH, John G, Brooks CJ, Verplancke JP, et al. (2009) The SAIL databank: linking multiple health and social care datasets. BMC Medical Informatics and Decision Making 9 (doi:10.1186/1472-6947-9-3)
28. Ford DV, Jones KH, Verplancke JP, John G, Brown G, et al. (2009) The SAIL databank: building a national architecture for e-health research and evaluation. BMC Health Services Research 9 (doi: 10.1186/1472-6963-9-157).
29. Zhou SM, Gan JQ (2008) Low-level interpretability and high-level interpretability: a unified view of interpretable fuzzy system modelling from data. Fuzzy Sets and Systems 159:3091–3131.
30. Zhou SM, Gan JQ (2009) Extracting Takagi-Sugeno fuzzy rules with interpretable submodels via regularization of linguistic modifiers. IEEE Transactions on Knowledge and Data Engineering 21: 1191–1204.
31. Bezdek JC (1981) Pattern Recognition with Fuzzy Objective Function Algorithms. Plenum Press.
32. Zhou SM, Gan JQ (2006) Constructing accurate and parsimonious fuzzy models with distinguishable fuzzy sets based on an entropy measure. Fuzzy Sets and Systems 157: 1057–1074.
33. Ford DV, Jones KH, Verplancke JP, et al., Data Anonymisation Policy and Process (DAPP). HIRU project document, Swansea University.
34. World Health Organisation (1998) Health21- Health for All in the 21st Century. Geneva: World Health Organisation; 1998.
35. Kelaher M, Dunt D, Feldman P, Nolan A, Raban B (2009) The effects of an area-based intervention on the uptake of maternal and child health assessments in Australia: A community trial. BMC Health Serv Res. 9: 53.
36. Abbema EA, van Assema P, Kok GJ, De Leeuw E, De Vries NK (2004) Effect evaluation of a comprehensive community intervention aimed at reducing socioeconomic health inequalities in the Netherlands. Health Promot Int 19: 141–156.
37. Whitworth A, Wilkinson K, McLennan D, Noble M, Anttila C. Raising educational attainment in deprived areas: the challenges of geography and residential mobility for area-based initiatives. Evidence from the New Deal for Communities Programme. Department for Communities and Local Government 2009.
38. Best Start atlas-children 0–8 year in Victoria: http://www.education.vic.gov.au/ecsmanagement/beststart/#eval (accessed 29 Feb 2012).
39. Victorian Auditor-general (2007) Giving Victorian children the best start in life. Melbourne: Victorian Government Printer 2007.
40. Wynn BO, Dutta A, Nelson MI (2005) Challenges in program evaluation of health interventions in developing countries, Report, RAND Center for Domestic and International Health Security.
41. Thomson H, Petticrew M, Morrison D (2001) Health effects of housing improvement: systematic review of intervention studies. BMJ 323:187–90.

13

Methodological Quality and Reporting of Generalized Linear Mixed Models in Clinical Medicine (2000–2012)

Martí Casals[1,2,3,4]*, Montserrat Girabent-Farrés[5], Josep L. Carrasco[2]

1 CIBER de Epidemiología y Salud Pública (CIBERESP), Barcelona, Spain, **2** Bioestadística, Departament de Salut Pública, Universitat de Barcelona, Barcelona, Spain, **3** Departament de Ciencies Basiques, Universitat Internacional de Catalunya, Barcelona, Spain, **4** Servei d'Epidemiologia, Agència de Salut Pública de Barcelona, Barcelona, Spain, **5** Departament de Fisioteràpia (unitat de Bioestadística), Universitat Internacional de Catalunya, Barcelona, Spain

Abstract

Background: Modeling count and binary data collected in hierarchical designs have increased the use of *Generalized Linear Mixed Models (GLMMs)* in medicine. This article presents a systematic review of the application and quality of results and information reported from GLMMs in the field of clinical medicine.

Methods: A search using the Web of Science database was performed for published original articles in medical journals from 2000 to 2012. The search strategy included the topic *"generalized linear mixed models","hierarchical generalized linear models", "multilevel generalized linear model"* and as a research domain we refined by science technology. Papers reporting methodological considerations without application, and those that were not involved in clinical medicine or written in English were excluded.

Results: A total of 443 articles were detected, with an increase over time in the number of articles. In total, 108 articles fit the inclusion criteria. Of these, 54.6% were declared to be longitudinal studies, whereas 58.3% and 26.9% were defined as repeated measurements and multilevel design, respectively. Twenty-two articles belonged to environmental and occupational public health, 10 articles to clinical neurology, 8 to oncology, and 7 to infectious diseases and pediatrics. The distribution of the response variable was reported in 88% of the articles, predominantly Binomial (n = 64) or Poisson (n = 22). Most of the useful information about GLMMs was not reported in most cases. Variance estimates of random effects were described in only 8 articles (9.2%). The model validation, the method of covariate selection and the method of goodness of fit were only reported in 8.0%, 36.8% and 14.9% of the articles, respectively.

Conclusions: During recent years, the use of GLMMs in medical literature has increased to take into account the correlation of data when modeling qualitative data or counts. According to the current recommendations, the quality of reporting has room for improvement regarding the characteristics of the analysis, estimation method, validation, and selection of the model.

Editor: Antonio Guilherme Pacheco, FIOCRUZ, Brazil

Funding: The authors received no specific funding for this work.

Competing Interests: The authors have declared that no competing interests exist.

* Email: marticasals@gmail.com

Introduction

Statistical modeling is a highly important tool that receives a lot of attention in any scientific field. In health sciences, statistical models arise as an important methodology to predict outcomes and assess association between outcomes and risk factors as well. Thus, one important aspect is to efficiently test the investigational hypothesis by avoiding biases and accounting for all the sources of variability present in data. This usually leads to complex designs where data is hierarchically structured. Multilevel, longitudinal or cluster designs are examples of such structure. In health sciences, longitudinal studies probably are more common, where measurements are grouped in subjects who are followed over time. Furthermore, other possibilities are studies where measurements are hierarchically grouped in subgroups such as schools, hospitals, neighborhoods, families, geographical areas or place of employment.

In the classic linear model (linear regression analysis, ANOVA, ANCOVA), the variable response is continuous and it is assumed that the response conditioned to covariates follows a normal distribution with maximum likelihood based approaches as the principal estimation methods [1–3]. However, the general linear model is not appropriate for non-continuous responses (e.g. binary, counts) because the underlying assumptions of the model do not hold.

Generalized linear models (GLMs) arose as an extension of the classic linear model that allowed for the accommodation of non-normal responses as well as a non-linear relationship between the expectation of the response and the covariates [2,4,5]. GLMs are most often applied to count or binary responses in health sciences [6], assuming Poisson, Binomial or Bernoulli as probability distributions for the response.

Similar to the classic linear model (which is indeed a particular type of GLM), GLMs also assume that the observations (conditioned to covariates) are independent and identically distributed. Regarding study designs with hierarchical structure, the assumption of independence is usually violated because measurements within the same cluster are correlated. The main disadvantage of ignoring within-cluster correlation is the bias in point estimates and standard errors. These biases might cause a loss of statistical power and efficiency of hypothesis testing on fixed effects [7,8]. Thus, the statistical significance could be wrongly assessed [9] and the type I error rate could be different than that *a priori* determined in hypothesis testing.

Generalized linear mixed models (GLMMs) are a methodology based on GLMs that permit data analysis with hierarchical GLMs structure through the inclusion of random effects in the model. The GLMMs are also known in the literature as hierarchical generalized linear models (HGLMs) and multilevel generalized linear models (MGLMs) depending on the field [10–12]. For the sake of simplicity we will use the term GLMMs throughout the text. The first estimation method of GLMMs was introduced in the early 1990 s [13]. Nowadays various estimation methods can be found for GLMMs, such as the penalized quasi-likelihood method (PQL) [14], the Laplace method [14], Gauss-Hermite quadrature [15], hierarchical-likelihood methods [11], and Bayesian methods based on the Markov chain Monte Carlo technique [16,17], and, recently also based on the integrated nested Laplace approximation [18].

Furthermore, GLMM methodology is now available in the main statistical packages, though estimation methods as well as statistical packages are still under development [19,20].

The increasing interest in GLMMs is reflected by the publication of tutorials in various fields, such as ecology [19], psychology [21], biology [22], and medicine [23–26]. Nowadays, original articles, academic work and reports which utilize GLMMs exist, and methodological guidelines and revisions are also available for the analysis of GLMMs in each field [19,27–29].

However, it is not possible to find guidelines that specifically address the appropriate reporting of population modeling studies [30]. In addition, no reviews of the use and quality of reported information by GLMMs exist despite an important increase in quantitative analyses in the academic and professional science settings.

Reporting guidelines are evidence-based tools that employ expert consensus to help authors to report their research such that readers can both critically appraise and interpret study findings [30–34]. Recently, minimal rules that can serve as standardized guidelines should be established to improve the quality of information and presentation of data in medical scientific articles [35]. Only Thiele [22] has made reference to GLMMs in the field of biology and still no standardized guidelines indicate what information is relevant to present in medical articles.

For this reason, the objective of the present study is to review the application of GLMMs and to evaluate the quality of reported information in original articles in the field of clinical medicine during a 13-year period (2000–2012), while analyzing the evolution over time, journals, and areas of publication.

Methods

This review was conducted according to the Preferred Reporting Items for Systematic Reviews and Metanalyses (PRISMA) Statement [36,37]. We also report the review in accordance with PRISMA guidelines (Checklist S1).

With the objective to obtain and analyze the existing scientific literature related to the use of GLMMs in clinical medicine, a strategic search of original published articles in this field from 2000 to 2012 was performed using the Web of Science database.

The search strategy included the topic "*generalized linear mixed models*", "*hierarchical generalized linear models*", "*multilevel generalized linear model*" and as a research domain we refined by science technology (Appendix S1).

The following fields of clinical medicine were included in the search:

Endocrinology Metabolism, Urology Nephrology, Public environmental occupational health, Orthopedics, Respiratory system, Entomology, Health care sciences services, Medical laboratory technology, Pediatrics, Pathology, Life sciences biomedicine other topics, Hematology, Geriatrics gerontology, Gastroenterology hepatology, Rheumatology, Critical care medicine, Medical informatics, Emergency medicine, Integrative complementary medicine, Obstetrics gynecology, Neurosciences neurology, Cardiovascular system cardiology, Infectious diseases, Radiology nuclear medicine medical imaging, Transplantation, Tropical medicine, Allergy, Anesthesiology, Anatomy morphology, General internal medicine, Immunology, Research experimental medicine, Dermatology, Oncology, Surgery.

Selection of the studies included in the review

Articles were eligible for inclusion if they were original research articles written in English in peer-reviewed journals reporting an application of GLMM. We excluded articles of statistical methodology development and those that were not entirely involved in clinical medicine (biology, psychology, genetics, sports, dentistry, air pollution, education, economy, family and health politics, computer science, ecology, nutrition, veterinary and nursing).

Identification of studies

The information from Appendix S1 (Table) was extracted from the selected articles. Data were collected and stored in a database. Then, data were checked to find discrepancies between the two reviewers. Discrepancies were solved by consensus after reviewing again the conflictive articles.

Figure 1 uses the PRISMA flowchart to summarize all stages of the paper selection process [37]. In the first review phase, 462 articles were identified, nineteen of which were duplicates.

After inspection of the abstracts, we excluded the articles that were non-original articles (reviews, short articles or conferences) and those articles that did not have a GLMM as a key word in the abstract or in the title of the article.

In the second review phase, of the 428 articles, only 129 pertained to the aforementioned medical fields. Thus, 299 articles were excluded because they belonged to other fields, such as ecology, computer science, air pollution or statistical methodology. In the third review phase, we obtained full text versions of potentially eligible articles. Two articles were excluded due to inconsistency in the specification of the model applied because in the full text version they were not a GLMM as it was stated in the abstract. We then conducted a detailed review of the 127 articles and we excluded 19 articles because they were not published in an indexed journal included in Journal Citation Reports (JCR).

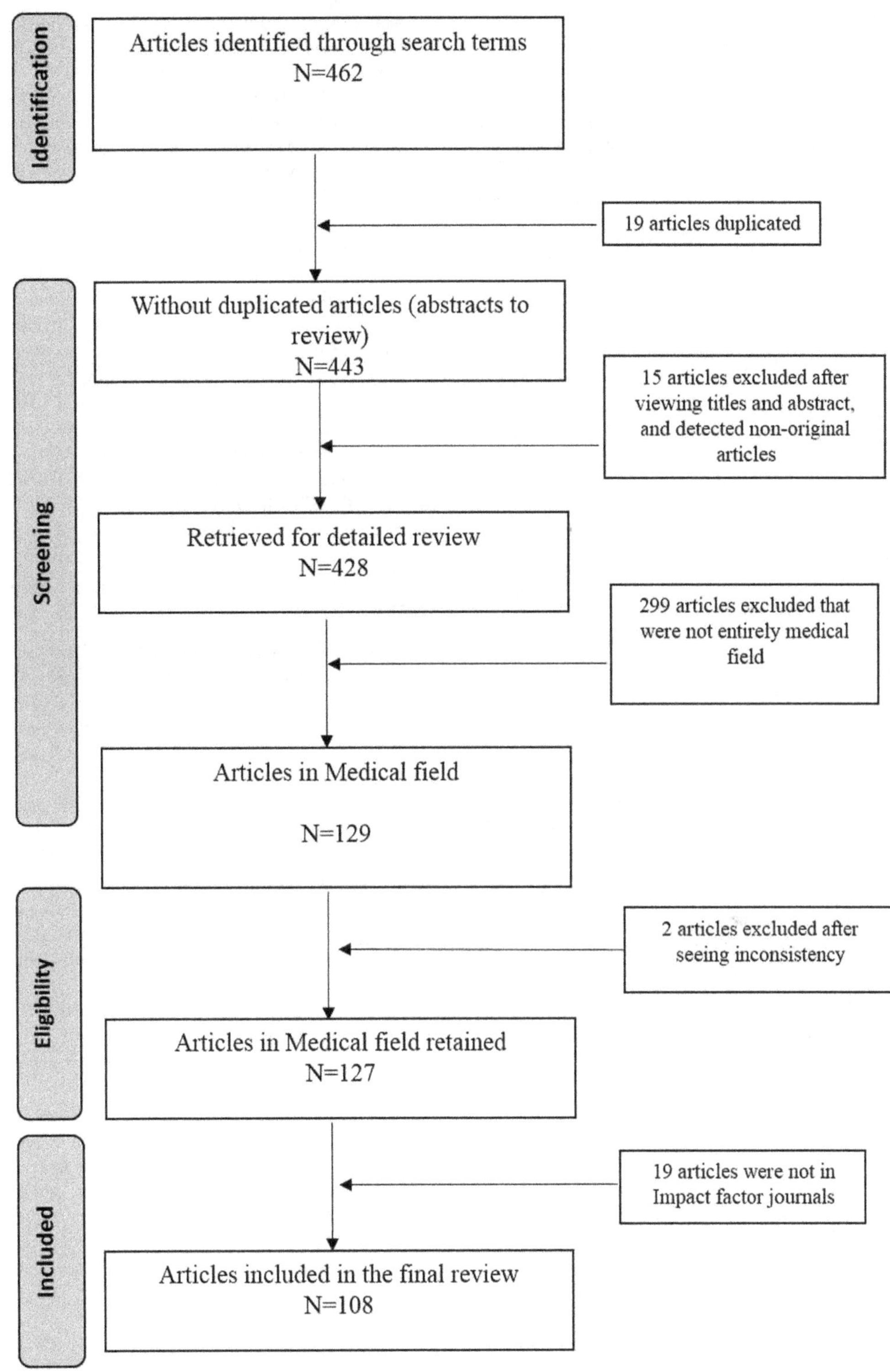

Figure 1. Flow chart of the selection of reviewed articles.

Finally, 108 articles were included in the final review (Appendix S2). Figure 1 summarizes the numbers of articles identified and the reasons for exclusion at each stage.

Information collected from the selected articles

Based on Thiele's and Bolker's works [22,38], a list of relevant information and basic characteristics of the study that should be reported in an article with GLMM analysis was suggested (Appendix S1).

Study characteristics

Regarding the study design, we refer to different aspects of each study, such as hierarchical structure of data and sample size. The hierarchical structure was used to differentiate between the different study designs that are not mutually exclusive, such as longitudinal, repeated measurements, and multilevel studies. Longitudinal data consist of outcome measurements repeatedly taken on each experimental unit over time. Longitudinal analysis is distinct from cross-sectional analysis as it addresses dependency among measurements taken on the same experimental unit [39]. The studies with repeated measurements usually involve only one level of clustering, where the repeated measurements are interchangeable (replicates).

Finally, multilevel studies present various levels of clusters, potentially providing hierarchical structure in each cluster, as seen in longitudinal or repeated measurement studies. We also took note of whether the probability distribution of the variable response was mentioned or easily deducible. Regarding sample size, the number of clusters, individuals or experimental units were collected.

Inferential issues

This section includes information regarding the GLMM model, as seen in Appendix S1 (Table).

The mixed models are characterized by including fixed and random effects in the linear predictor. Random effects are usually related to the cluster variable. Therefore, it is important to provide information about the cluster variable in the model.

It is also important to report the estimation method of the study and the software applied because they can influence the validity of the GLMM estimates [6,20,38]. Furthermore, the software implementations differ considerably in flexibility, computation time and usability [20].

Concerning the computational issues, the macro GLIMMIX from SAS (1992) was the first available software to fit GLMMs using penalized quasilikelihood (PQL) estimation method. The first production version of PROC GLIMMIX for SAS was first released in 2005 and became the standard procedure in version 9.2 in 2008 [40]. Nowadays, there are other available softwares to fit GLMMs. Among them the lme4 package was first implemented for R in 2003 [41]. Moreover, in R software, we can find other packages to fit GLMMs such as glmmML [42], MASS (with the glmmPQL function) [43] or gar (with the repeated function) [44,45]. Concerning SAS software besides the aforementioned PROC GLIMMIX, the PROC NLMIXED is also able to fit GLMMs [46]. Additionally, it is also possible to use ASReml [47], MLwiN [48] and STATA software (which uses the functions xtmixed and gllamm [22,28,49,50]) [22,28,49,50]. The SPSS (starting with SPSS 19) software now also includes a GLMM obtained in the GENLINMIXED procedure [51,52].

With respect to statistical inference, the hypotheses concerning fixed and random effects (or their variances) are tested in separated form. Thus, testing the hypotheses for fixed effects is commonly assessed by the Wald score tests. On the other hand, hypotheses concerning random effects variances can be tested using the likelihood ratio test [19] or by comparing the goodness of fit of the models using the Akaike's Information Criterion (AIC) or the Bayesian Information Criterion (BIC) [19].

Validation model

Similar to GLMs, validation of GLMMs is commonly based on the inspection of residuals to determine if the model assumptions are fulfilled.

An important point is related to the so-called scale parameter when it is fixed to a specific value because of the probability model assumed. For example, the scale parameter for Poisson and Binomial distribution should be equal to 1. A parameter different from 1 implies that the probability distribution of the responses conditioned to covariates is not correctly specified and the model is not valid. This phenomenon is known as over or underdispersion and causes incorrect standard errors that can produce different clinical conclusions [53]. Thus, it is relevant to evaluate the presence of over- or underdispersion and report the results of this analysis.

Finally, information on the use of a concrete strategy to select the variables in the model and its criterion was obtained. Variable selection strategy usually consist of stepwise selection of variables (forward or backward) [19]. Concerning the criterion, it can be based on entropy as the aforementioned AIC and BIC, or hypotheses testing (likelihood ratio test or Wald test). However, it is possible to find studies with no need of variable selection, for example confirmatory analysis where a particular hypothesized model is fit. This hypothesized model may be based on theory and/or previous analytic research [54,55]. In this latter case, the selection variable strategy was considered appropriately reported.

Results

The evolution of the use of GLMMs in medical journals of the 443 articles selected in the first phase is described in Figure 2. The remaining results (Tables 1, 2, 3 and Appendix S3 and S4) make reference to the 108 articles included in the final in-depth review. Of these, 92 (85.2%) were defined as GLMMs, 14 (13.0%) as HGLMs, and 2 (1.9%) as MGLMs.

Most of these articles were found in the following journals: *American Journal of Public Health*, which had 7 publications; *PLoS ONE, Cancer Causes & Control, BMC Public Health, Annals of Surgery,* and *Headache,* which had 3 publications each. Twenty-two articles pertained to environmental and occupational public health area, 10 articles pertained to clinical neurology, 8 to oncology, and 7 to infectious diseases and pediatrics (Appendix S3).

Forty-five articles (41.7%) were written by an author who was part of a biometric or statistical department and some co-authors (53.3%) were affiliated with a public health department.

Of the 108 selected articles, 59 (54.6%) declared to be longitudinal studies, whereas 56 (58.3%) and 29 (26.9%) were defined as repeated measurements and multilevel design, respectively (Table 1). It is important to note that over 8% of the articles were unclear when reporting the cluster design. Twenty-seven articles (25%) involved confirmatory analysis whereas 81 (75%) were declared as exploratory analysis. Ninety-five of the articles stated their sample size, which ranged from 20–785,385 with a median of 2,201 (Q1 = 408; Q3 = 25000). One random effect in the *intercept* was used in 61 articles, and two or more random effects were used in 36 articles. Of these, 61.1% of the articles had a random effect that pertained to a multilevel model. The size of the random effect or *cluster*, as the number of levels of random effects or the number of clusters, was clearly described in only 33 articles, which ranged from 9–16,230 clusters with a median of 167 (Q1 = 55; Q3 = 1187). The cluster was principally the individual (subject, patient, participant, etc) (n = 46), hospital (n = 15), center (n = 10), geographical area (n = 9) and family (n = 3).

The type of study design was described as cross-sectional (n = 31), cohort (n = 26), clinical trial (n = 18), case-control (n = 2) and *cross-over* (n = 1). Eight articles did not mention study design

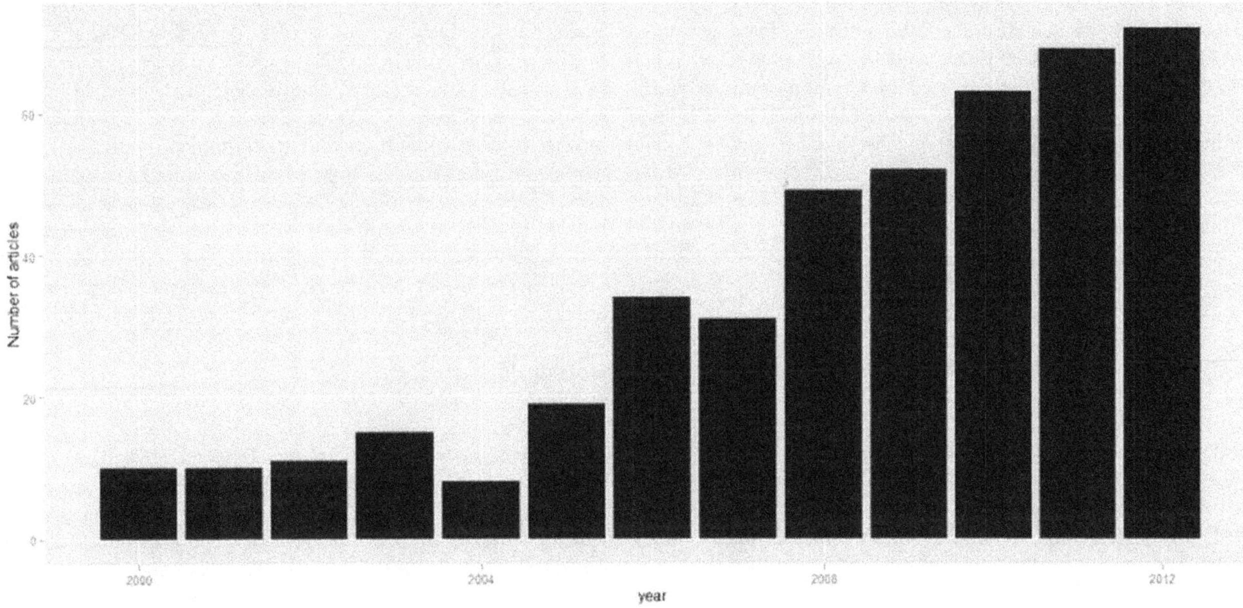

Figure 2. Number of reviewed articles by year of publication.

and 18 articles only described the characteristics of the study design (i.e. experimental, prospective, multicenter, etc) without specifying which study design was used (Table 1).

The response variable ('clinical') of the study differed in each of the reviewed articles, and thus there was no common illness or pathology. Available software can fit different response variables

Table 1. Characteristics of the study design in the reviewed articles.

	N = 108
Longitudinal study:	
NO	40 (37.0%)
Unclear	9 (8.30%)
YES	59 (54.6%)
Repeated measures:	
NO	34 (31.5%)
Unclear	11 (10.2%)
YES	56 (58.3%)
Multilevel (nested design):	
NO	79 (73.1%)
YES	29 (26.9%)
Type of analysis	
Exploratory	81 (75.0%)
Confirmatory	27 (25.0%)
Design	
Case-control	2 (2.30%)
Case-crossover	1 (1.10%)
Cluster Random Trial	18 (16.7%)
Cohorts	26 (24.1%)
Cross-sectional	31 (28.7%)
NR	8 (7.40%)
Unclear	22 (20.4%)

NR: Not reported.

for exponential family, such as Poisson, binomial, Gamma, and Inverse Gaussian, though Poisson and Binomial (or binary) are the most used in medicine. The distribution of the response variable was reported in 88% of the articles, and the most common was binomial (n = 64), Poisson (n = 22), negative binomial (n = 1) and multinomial (n = 2).

Furthermore, the estimation method for each model was reported in only 21 articles (19.4%), and the following estimation methods were used: *maximum likelihood* (n = 3), *penalized quasi-likelihood* (n = 8), pseudo-likelihood (n = 2), restricted maximum likelihood (n = 2), *adaptative quadrature likelihood approximation* (n = 1), and Markov chain Monte Carlo (MCMC; n = 5). It is important to mention that over 90% of the articles did not report the test used for the fixed nor random effects, which implies that the section on statistical methods was insufficiently described (Table 2).

The most used statistical software packages were SAS (n = 57), R (n = 13), Stata (n = 12), and HLM (n = 6). For SAS, the use of macro GLIMMIX was reported in 24 articles and the macro NLMIXED with PROC MIXED to fit the GLMM was used in five articles. For R, different packages were used to fit the GLMM, such as lme4 (n = 2), glmmPQL (n = 4), glmmML(n = 1), BayesX (n = 2) or repeated (n = 1). For Stata, the gllamm (n = 2) and xtmixed functions were also used (n = 1).

Overdispersion for models with counts or binary response which assume a Poisson or Binomial distribution was evaluated in 10 articles. Of these, different approaches were proposed to fit as alternatives (GEE, Negative Binomial, Quasi-Poisson, Zero-Inflated). For the articles that used Poisson or Binomial distribution of probability, 90.7% did not state if under-over-dispersion was evaluated, 99.1% did not report the magnitude of the scale parameter, and 92.6% did not suggest alternatives for possible under-overdispersion. Variance estimates of random effects were described in only 10 articles (9.3%). With respect to the fixed effects, the standard error and confidence interval were reported in 20% and 71.3%, respectively, whereas in the variance components, they were reported in 3.7% and 2.8%, respectively. The model validation, the method of covariate selection and the method of goodness of fit were reported in 6.5%, 35.2% and 15.7% of the articles, respectively (Table 3).

Discussion

The articles selected in this review showed that the number of bibliographical references that use GLMMs in medical journals increased from the year 2000 to 2012.

Our review also indicated that there is room for improvement in quality when basic characteristics about the GLMMs are reported in medical journals.

A predominance of the articles reviewed were in the fields of environmental and occupational public health. Furthermore, for 45 of the articles (41.7%) at least one of the co-authors was associated with a biometrics or statistical department. This result is consistent with the systematic review of Diaz-Ordaz that showed that trials having a statistician as co-author was associated with a increase in the methodological quality of the analyses [56].

In any scientific paper, the validity of the conclusions is linked to the adequacy of the methods used to generate the results. Thus, it is important to adequately describe the statistical methods used in the analysis. Hence, the reader is able to judge whether the methods used are appropriate, and by extension whether the conclusions are correct.

In the case of GLMM's, as we observed in the results section, the majority of the useful and relevant information about GLMMs that is proposed by Bolker [19] and Thiele [22] was not reported. Therefore, the main consequence is the difficulty to assess the reliability of the results and the validity of the conclusions. For example, the majority of the articles did not mention the estimation method or software that was used. The inferential issues (hypothesis testing, confidence interval estimation) and model validation are closely linked to the estimation method (for instance, bayesian or frequentist). As a consequence, the lack of reporting of the estimation method (or software) used makes it complicated to evaluate the adequacy of the approaches used to inference purposes. Furthermore, the estimation method may have important flaws depending on the situation. For example, PQL yields biased parameter estimates if the standard deviations of the random effects are large, especially with binary data [19].

Additionally, an important deficit regarding the inference of fixed and random effects was observed. Such inference may consist of : 1) hypothesis testing of a set of parameters; 2) competing models using entropy measures; 3) confidence interval of parameters. Here again the validity of the conclusions drawn from the analysis depends on the appropriateness of the procedures used in the inference. For example, the likelihood ratio test is only applicable to nested models. Another example arises when testing the existence of a random effect. This question could be solved by a common hypothesis testing using a null hypothesis whose variance is zero. However, the null hypothesis is set to the boundary of the parameter domain (variance must be positive). Therefore, it is necessary to modify the probability distribution function under the null hypothesis otherwise the p-value obtained is incorrect [57]. Additionally, as we mentioned above, the inferential procedures must be coherent with the estimation technique used.

Furthermore, the validity and model selection as proposed by Bolker and Thiele [19,22] were also not reported in most cases. Once again, the results of the inference and the conclusions of the study will be valid when the assumptions made on the model and estimation method are fulfilled. This is the aim of the validation and, thus, it is essential that the researchers report the results of such a validation and how it was made.

Therefore, in our opinion the methodological information reported in articles using GLMMs could be improved.

We also think that standardized guidelines to report GLMM characteristics in medicine could be beneficial, even though they would not imply by themselves a direct improvement on quality of the articles. As stated by Cobo [35] and Moher [58], it is necessary that both authors and reviewers are aware of recommendations to improve the quality of the manuscripts.

Limitations of the study

One of the limitations of our study could be that the number of identified articles was not high, despite the 13-years review. Nonetheless, the only similar existing review by Thiele [22] in the field of "invasion biology" included only 50 articles. One possible explanation for this number of articles that use GLMMs in health sciences is that medical literature frequently uses models with fixed effects in a hierarchical structure, even though the use of GLMMs is well known in statistical literature [6,59].

Another possible limitation of our review is the potential bias to disregard articles that use a GLMM but do not specify the term as a topic. However, we could assume that articles that use GLMM as topic are more sensitive to this methodology. Thus, it is expected that if this bias existed, the reporting quality would be even better in those potential articles that applied GLMM and used it as a topic.

Table 2. Characteristics of inference and estimation methods reported in the review articles.

	N = 108
Test for fixed effects:	
NR	103 (95.4%)
t-value	1 (0.90%)
Wald F test	4 (3.7%)
Test for random effects:	
LRT	3 (2.80%)
NR	105 (97.2%)
Variance estimates of random effects:	
NR	98 (90.7%)
YES	10 (9.30%)
Statistical software:	
SAS	57 (52.8%)
R	13 (12.0%)
Stata	12 (11.1%)
WinBugs	2 (1.90%)
S-plus	3 (2.80%)
HLM	6 (5.60%)
Statistical Analysis System	1 (0.90%)
SPSS	2 (1.90%)
SEER*Stat	1 (0.90%)
MLwiN	1 (0.90%)
NR	10 (9.30%)
Estimation method:	
Adaptative Quadrature likelihood Approximation	1 (0.90%)
Maximum Likelihood	3 (2.80%)
NR	87 (80.6%)
Penalized Quasi- likelihood	8 (7.50%)
Posterior mean	5 (4.60%)
Restricted Maximum Likelihood	2 (1.90%)
Pseudo likelihood	2 (1.90%)
Statistical software function or macro:	
PROC GLIMMIX	24 (22.2%)
glmmPQL	4 (3.70%)
Gllamm	2 (1.90%)
BayesX	2 (1.90%)
Xtmixed	1 (0.90%)
PROC MIXED/NLMIXED	5 (4.70%)
lme4	2 (1.90%)
glmmML	1 (0.90%)
Repeated	1 (0.90%)
NR	66 (61.1%)

NR: No reported; MCMC: Markov chain Monte Carlo.

There could be also a trend on the estimation methods according to the names given to GLMMs in the articles. Bayesians usually prefer the term hierarchical models instead of mixed effects models whereas frequentists are more likely to use mixed models, which seems to be consistent with our results (Appendix S4).

Conclusions

During recent years, the use of GLMMs in medical literature has increased to take into account the correlation of data when modeling binary or count data. Our review included articles from indexed medical journals included in JCR that mainly consisted of longitudinal studies in a medical setting.

Table 3. Characteristics of the specification, validation and construction of the model for the reviewed articles.

	N = 108
Variable response distribution:	
2 distributions: Binomial, Poisson	1 (0.90%)
2 distributions: Binomial, Multinomial	1 (0.90%)
Binomial	64 (59.2%)
Binomial count	1 (0.90%)
Negative Binomial with offset	1 (0.90%)
NR	11 (10.2%)
Poisson	22 (20.4%)
Poisson with offset	2 (1.90%)
Multinomial	2 (1.90%)
Ordinal	1 (0.90%)
Unclear	2 (1.90%)
Overdispersion evaluation:	
NR	98 (90.7%)
YES	10 (9.20%)
Overdispersion measurement:	
NR	107 (99.1%)
Pearson residuals	1 (0.90%)
Proposed alternative for overdispersion:	
GEE	2 (1.90%)
Negative Binomial	2 (1.90%)
NR	100 (92.6%)
Quasi-Poisson	1 (0.90%)
Variogram	1 (0.90%)
Dscale-adjusted	1 (0.90%)
Zero-inflated	1 (0.90%)
Method of variable selection:	
Backward	3 (2.80%)
Forward	1 (0.90%)
Forward stepwise	1 (0.90%)
NR	70 (64.8%)
Unnecessary (Confirmatory analysis)	27 (25.0%)
Stepwise	6 (5.60%)
Method of goodness of fit comparison model:	
AIC	12 (11.1%)
BIC	3 (2.80%)
DIC	1 (0.90%)
NR	91 (84.3%)
Pseudo R-squared	1 (0.90%)
GLMM Validation:	
NR	101 (93.5%)
YES	7 (6.50%)

NR: No reported; MCMC: Markov chain Monte Carlo; GEE: Generalized estimating equation;
DIC: Deviance information criterion; AIC: Akaike information criterion; BIC: Bayesian information criterion; df: freedom degree.

According to the current recommendations, the quality of reporting has room for improvement regarding the characteristics of the analysis, estimation method, validation and selection of the model.

After analyzing and reviewing the quality of the publications, we believe it is important to consider the use of minimal rules as standardized guidelines when presenting GLMM results in medical journals.

Supporting Information

Appendix S1 Search strategy protocol.

Appendix S2 Articles included in our study.

Appendix S3 Journals according to field of knowledge.

Appendix S4 Estimation methods according to the name used (GLMM, HGLM, MGLM).

Acknowledgments

We thank LLuís Jover and Klaus Langohr for helpful comments.

Author Contributions

Conceived and designed the experiments: MC MGF JLC. Performed the experiments: MC MGF JLC. Analyzed the data: MC MGF. Contributed reagents/materials/analysis tools: MC MGF JLC. Contributed to the writing of the manuscript: MC MGF JLC.

References

1. Davidson R, MacKinnon JG (1993) Estimation and inference in econometrics. OUP Catalogue.
2. Nelder JA, Wedderburn RW (1972) Generalized linear models. Journal of the Royal Statistical Society. Series A (General) : 370–384.
3. Diggle P, Heagerty P, Liang K, Zeger S (2013) Analysis of longitudinal data. : Oxford University Press.
4. MacCullagh P, Nelder JA (1989) Generalized linear models. : CRC press.
5. Draper N, Smith H (1998)Applied regression analysis new york.
6. Austin PC (2010) Estimating multilevel logistic regression models when the number of clusters is low: A comparison of different statistical software procedures. The international journal of biostatistics 6.
7. Littell RC, Pendergast J, Natarajan R (2000) Tutorial in Biostatistics modelling covariance structure in the analysis of repeated measures data.
8. Wang LA, Goonewardene Z (2004) The use of MIXED models in the analysis of animal experiments with repeated measures data. Canadian Journal of Animal Science 84: 1–11.
9. Campbell MJ (2008) Statistics at square two: Understanding modern statistical applications in medicine. : Wiley. com.
10. Garson GGD (2012) Hierarchical linear modeling: Guide and applications. : Sage Publications.
11. Lee Y, Nelder JA, Pawitan Y (2006) Generalized linear models with random effects: Unified analysis via H-likelihood. : CRC Press.
12. Stryhn H, Christensen J (2014) The analysis-Hierarchical models: Past, present and future. Prev Vet Med 113: 304–312.
13. Schall R (1991) Estimation in generalized linear models with random effects. Biometrika 78: 719–727.
14. Breslow NE, Clayton DG (1993) Approximate inference in generalized linear mixed models. Journal of the American Statistical Association 88: 9–25.
15. Aitkin M (1996) A general maximum likelihood analysis of overdispersion in generalized linear models. Statistics and computing 6: 251–262.
16. Zeger SL, Karim MR (1991) Generalized linear models with random effects; a gibbs sampling approach. Journal of the American statistical association 86: 79–86.
17. Gelman A, Hill J (2006) Data analysis using regression and multilevel/hierarchical models. : Cambridge University Press.
18. Rue H, Martino S, Chopin N (2009) Approximate bayesian inference for latent gaussian models by using integrated nested laplace approximations. Journal of the royal statistical society: Series b (statistical methodology) 71: 319–392.
19. Bolker BM, Brooks ME, Clark CJ, Geange SW, Poulsen JR, et al. (2009) Generalized linear mixed models: A practical guide for ecology and evolution. Trends in ecology \& evolution 24: 127–135.
20. Li B, Lingsma HF, Steyerberg EW, Lesaffre E (2011) Logistic random effects regression models: A comparison of statistical packages for binary and ordinal outcomes. BMC medical research methodology 11: 77.
21. Moscatelli A, Mezzetti M, Lacquaniti F (2012) Modeling psychophysical data at the population-level: The generalized linear mixed model. Journal of vision 12.
22. Thiele J, Markussen B (2012) Potential of GLMM in modelling invasive spread. CAB Reviews: Perspectives in Agriculture, Veterinary Science, Nutrition and Natural Resources 7.
23. Brown H, Prescott R (2006) Applied mixed models in medicine. : Wiley Chichester.
24. Platt RW, Leroux BG, Breslow N (1999) Generalized linear mixed models for meta-analysis. Stat Med 18: 643–654.
25. Cnaan A, Laird N, Slasor P (1997) Tutorial in biostatistics: Using the general linear mixed model to analyse unbalanced repeated measures and longitudinal data. Stat Med 16: 2349–2380.
26. Skrondal A, Rabe-Hesketh S (2003) Some applications of generalized linear latent and mixed models in epidemiology: Repeated measures, measurement error and multilevel modeling. Norsk epidemiologi 13.
27. Dean C, Nielsen JD (2007) Generalized linear mixed models: A review and some extensions. Lifetime Data Anal 13: 497–512.
28. Baayen RH, Davidson DJ, Bates DM (2008) Mixed-effects modeling with crossed random effects for subjects and items. Journal of memory and language 59: 390–412.
29. Tuerlinckx F, Rijmen F, Verbeke G, Boeck P (2006) Statistical inference in generalized linear mixed models: A review. Br J Math Stat Psychol 59: 225–255.
30. Bennett C, Manuel DG (2012) Reporting guidelines for modelling studies. BMC medical research methodology 12: 168.
31. Weinstein MC, Toy EL, Sandberg EA, Neumann PJ, Evans JS, et al. (2001) Modeling for health care and other policy decisions: Uses, roles, and validity. Value in Health 4: 348–361.
32. Kopec JA, Finès P, Manuel DG, Buckeridge DL, Flanagan WM, et al. (2010) Validation of population-based disease simulation models: A review of concepts and methods. BMC Public Health 10: 710.
33. Bagley SC, White H, Golomb BA (2001) Logistic regression in the medical literature: Standards for use and reporting, with particular attention to one medical domain. J Clin Epidemiol 54: 979–985. 10.1016/S0895-4356(01)00372-9.
34. Lang TA, Altman DG (2013) Basic statistical reporting for articles published in biomedical journals: The "Statistical analyses and methods in the published literature" or the SAMPL guidelines". Science Editors' Handbook, European Association of Science Editors.
35. Cobo E, Cortés J, Ribera J, Cardellach F, Selva-O'Callaghan A, et al. (2011) Effect of using reporting guidelines during peer review on quality of final manuscripts submitted to a biomedical journal: Masked randomised trial. BMJ: British Medical Journal 343.
36. Hutton B, Salanti G, Chaimani A, Caldwell DM, Schmid C, et al. (2014) The quality of reporting methods and results in network meta-analyses: An overview of reviews and suggestions for improvement. PloS one 9: e92508. 10.1371/journal.pone.0092508.
37. Moher D, Liberati A, Tetzlaff J, Altman DG, PRISMA Group (2010) Preferred reporting items for systematic reviews and meta-analyses: The PRISMA statement. International journal of surgery (London, England) 8: 336–341. 10.1016/j.ijsu.2010.02.007.
38. Bolker BM (2008) Ecological models and data in R. : Princeton Univ Pr.
39. Liu C, Cripe TP, Kim M (2010) Statistical issues in longitudinal data analysis for treatment efficacy studies in the biomedical sciences. Molecular Therapy 18: 1724–1730.
40. Institute Inc S (2008) SAS/STAT 9.2. user's guide.
41. Bates D., Sarkar D (2004) 1. lme4: Linear mixed-effects models using S4 classes. R package version 0.6–9.
42. Bröstrom G, Holmberg H. Glmmml: Generalized linear models with clustering. 2011; r package version 0.82–1. Available: http://CRAN. R-project.org/package = glmmML.
43. Venables WN, Ripley BD (2002) Modern applied statistics with S. : Springer.
44. Lindsey JK (1999) Models for repeated measurements. : Oxford University Press, UK.
45. Lindsey JK (2001) Nonlinear models in medical statistics. : Oxford University Press, Oxford, UK.
46. Wolfinger RD (1999) Fitting nonlinear mixed models with the new NLMIXED procedure. : 278–284.
47. Gilmour A, Gogel B, Cullis B, Welham S, Thompson R (2002) ASReml user guide release 1.0 VSN international ltd, hempstead, HP1 1ES, UK. Online im Internet unter.
48. Rowe K (2007) Practical multilevel analysis with MLwiN & LISREL: An integrated course.
49. Rabe-Hesketh S, Skrondal A, Pickles A (2002) Reliable estimation of generalized linear mixed models using adaptive quadrature. The Stata Journal 2: 1–21.
50. Rabe-Hesketh S, Skrondal A (2008) Estimation using xtmixed. In: Anonymous Multilevel and longitudinal modeling using Stata. : STATA press. 433–436.
51. Garson GD (2013) Fundamentals of hierarchical linear and multilevel modeling. GD Garson, Hierarchical linear modeling guide and applications. Raleigh, NC: North Carolina State University. Sage.
52. Heck RH, Thomas SL, Tabata LN (2013) Multilevel and longitudinal modeling with IBM SPSS. : Routledge.
53. Milanzi E, Alonso A, Molenberghs G (2012) Ignoring overdispersion in hierarchical loglinear models: Possible problems and solutions. Stat Med 31: 1475–1482.

54. Preedy VR, Watson RR (2010) Handbook of disease burdens and quality of life measures. : Springer New York.
55. Bender R, Lange S (2001) Adjusting for multiple testing–when and how? J Clin Epidemiol 54: 343–349.
56. Diaz-Ordaz K, Froud R, Sheehan B, Eldridge S (2013) A systematic review of cluster randomised trials in residential facilities for older people suggests how to improve quality. BMC medical research methodology 13: 127.
57. Molenberghs G, Verbeke G, Demetrio CGB (2007) An extended random-effects approach to modeling repeated, overdispersed count data. Lifetime Data Anal 13: 513–531. 10.1007/s10985-007-9064-y.
58. Moher D, Schulz KF, Simera I, Altman DG (2010) Guidance for developers of health research reporting guidelines. PLoS medicine 7: e1000217.
59. Austi PC, Alte DA (2003) Comparing hierarchical modeling with traditional logistic regression analysis among patients hospitalized with acute myocardial infarction: Should we be analyzing cardiovascular outcomes data differently? Am Heart J 145: 27–35.

14

Effect of a One-Off Educational Session about Enterobiasis on Knowledge, Preventative Practices, and Infection Rates among Schoolchildren in South Korea

Dong-Hee Kim[1], **Hak Sun Yu**[2,3]*

1 Department of Nursing, College of Nursing, Pusan National University, Yangsan, Gyeongsangnamdo, South Korea, 2 Department of Parasitology, School of Medicine, Pusan National University, Yangsan, Gyeongsangnamdo, South Korea, 3 Immunoregulatory therapeutics group in Brain Busan 21 project, Busan, South Korea

Abstract

Although health education has proven to be cost-effective in slowing the spread of enterobiasis, assessments of the effectiveness of health education to reduce infectious diseases specifically in children are rare. To evaluate the effect of health education on knowledge, preventative practices, and the prevalence of enterobiasis, 319 children from 16 classes were divided into experimental and control groups. Data were collected from May 2012 to March 2013. A 40-minute in-class talk was given once in the experimental group. There were significant differences over the time in the mean scores for children's knowledge of *Enterobius vermicularis* infection in the intervention group compared to the control group ($p<$ 0.001). After the educational session, the score for knowledge about *E. vermicularis* infection increased from 60.2±2.32 to 92.7±1.19 in the experimental group; this gain was partially lost 3 months later, decreasing to 83.6±1.77 ($p<0.001$). Children's enterobiasis infection prevention practice scores also increased, from 3.23±0.27 to 3.73±0.25, 1 week after the educational session, a gain that was partially lost at 3 months, decreasing to 3.46±0.36 ($p<0.001$). The overall *E. vermicularis* egg detection rate was 4.4%; the rates for each school ranged from 0% to 12.9% at screening. The infection rate at 3 months after the treatment sharply decreased from 12.3% to 0.8% in the experimental group, compared to a decrease from 8.5% to 3.7% in the control group during the same period. We recommend that health education on enterobiasis be provided to children to increase their knowledge about enterobiasis and improve prevention practices.

Editor: David Joseph Diemert, The George Washington University Medical Center, United States of America

Funding: This research was supported by Basic Science Research Program through the National Research Foundation of Korea funded by the Ministry of Education, Science and Technology (NRF-2013R1A1A1A05012615). The funders had no role in study design, data collection and analysis, decision to publish, or preparation of the manuscript.

Competing Interests: The authors have declared that no competing interests exist.

* Email: hsyu@pusan.ac.kr

Introduction

Although most parasitic infectious diseases have disappeared in developed countries, enterobiasis (pinworm infection) has still often been reported in many developed countries [1–3]. In South Korea, the prevalence of total intestinal helminthic parasitic infection rates has sharply decreased from 84.3% in 1971 to 2.4% in 1997 [4,5]. However, a relatively high egg positive rate of *Enterobius vermicularis* ranging from 4% to 10% has been reported in Korean children during the last decade [6–9].

Enterobiasis is transmitted through direct contact with infected (or egg-contaminated) persons or objects. Transmission of *E. vermicularis* commonly occurs by ingesting infectious pinworm eggs. Eggs are transmitted from the anus to the finger, fingernails, or hands when an individual scratches the perianal area where the gravid female worms emerge and deposit eggs. Eggs are spread to underwear and night-clothing and further transmitted to other objects including food and books, desks, and chairs [10]. When dislodged from such objects, the eggs can enter another individual's mouth and nose, thereby being ingested [10,11]. As a result of this transmission process, children's personal and hygiene habits, such as thumb sucking, overcrowded conditions, and inadequate sanitation, contribute to the spread of enterobiasis in primary schools, where close contact between children occurs [2,7,9].

Medication against *E. vermicularis*, such as albendazole, is very effective in treating enterobiasis [12]. However, reinfection is also common in spite of treatment, as the medication only kills the adult worm but not the worm larvae [10]. An important aspect in the failure of single-dose chemotherapy is the continuing presence of infectious eggs in the environment, which facilitate rapid reinfection. Therefore, individuals with enterobiasis require repeated doses of medication to cover the time taken for the eggs to become adult worms. Importantly, most parents in South Korea believe that antihelminthic medications can easily cure every helminthic infection, including those by *E. vermicularis*, by just a one-time treatment [9]. In addition, most kindergarten directors and teachers have limited knowledge of *E. vermicularis* infection [2].

Knowledge of disease has successfully improved many different health outcomes [13]. However, there has been little emphasis on the impact of health education on the prevalence of enterobiasis, despite the incidence of enterobiasis being reduced by encouraging habits of cleanliness in children. Health education promoting knowledge of enterobiasis has proven to be cost-effective in decreasing reinfection rates in schoolchildren [14]. Previously, we evaluated the impact of a health education among pre-school children [2]. We provided brochures on prevention, transmission, and treatment of enterobiasis to parents, as they are in charge of their child's personal hygiene since children younger than 6 years of age are not old enough to be responsible for self-care [2].

In the present study, we conducted an experimental health education session on enterobiasis at primary schools in South Korea and assessed its effect on knowledge about *E. vermicularis* infection, enterobiasis infection prevention practices, and the incidence rate of enterobiasis among primary school children in Korea.

Subjects and Methods

Subject recruitment and screening evaluation

Participants were Grade 1 and Grade 2 primary school students (aged 7−9 years) from separate school districts in three distinct regions: an industrial city, an urban site, and a suburban area of South Korea. Recruitment was conducted through the Office of Education websites at each of these sites with a letter informing about the nature, significance, and objectives of the study. Schools were approached with the help of an assistant. Once the assistant had obtained verbal consent from the principal of a school, investigators met with the principal and class teachers of each school to describe the details of the study. The class teachers sent a consent form, a letter of information, and a questionnaire to the parents of each child. A total of 3,840 children from 183 classes in 27 schools underwent a screening for enterobiasis via the sellotape anal swab technique. The parents were each given two pieces of sellotape and written instructions showing how to swab the perianal area of their child with the sellotape and other aspects of the screening procedure. The investigators emphasized that the examinations should be done before the child washed or went to the toilet in the morning to prevent any pinworms eggs from being washed from the area. We cautioned that the chances of making an incorrect diagnosis of enterobiasis increased when the parents did not swab their child's anus first thing in the morning before the child washed. We asked the parents to do this twice, on separate days.

Sample size was determined on the basis of the primary outcome, the score in the knowledge test after education. To have an 80% chance of detecting as significant (at the two sided 5% level) a 10 point difference between the two groups in the knowledge test scores after education, with an assumed standard deviation of 15, the overall sample size required is 74 individuals (37 in each arm of the study). Since this study is cluster-randomized, the sample size had to be larger than if simple randomization had been performed, in order to take into account the design effect. Assuming that the inter-cluster correlation coefficient is 0.1, and a mean cluster size is 21 individuals, the design effect is 3. Therefore, the number of individuals required in each group is 111 ('Cochrane Consumers and Communication Review Group: cluster randomized controlled trials'. http://cccrg.cochrane.org, March 2014). Assuming the expected drop-out rate of 10%, the final sample size required is 246 (123 in each arm) with a minimum of 6 clusters per arm.

Study design

The study was designed as a pretest-posttest experiment, with an equivalent control group. We excluded schools that had classes with an incidence rate of 0% at the screening evaluation, and then selected classes in which all students were tested at the screening evaluation. Based on a combination of similar egg positive rates and geographical locations, 10 schools in different regions were involved this study; two schools were in an industrial city, four schools were in an urban site, and four schools were in a suburban area. One or two classes participated at each school. Each school was identified as either an intervention or control group in order to control for the contamination of the control group. The schools were assigned to either the intervention (8 classes from 5 schools) or control (8 classes from 5 schools) arms through a coin toss. A total of 346 children from 16 classes were included at baseline. At post-treatment examination, 319 children (130 for the experimental and 189 for the control group) participated (Fig. 1). Blinding of investigators was not possible as the intervention was educational; however, the investigators were blinded to the exposure status of participants during data collection. In the intervention group, an educational session was given once, for 40 minutes, in a group setting for each class. In the control group, children received an *E. vermicularis* infection brochure. Knowledge of *E. vermicularis* infection and enterobiasis infection prevention practice and the *E. vermicularis* infection rate among children were evaluated at baseline and at 3 months after the intervention. Children's knowledge of *E. vermicularis* infection was assessed on the day of the educational session in order to ensure that their knowledge of *E. vermicularis* infection increased.

Intervention

The educational program was developed based on the Dick & Carey's Systematic Design of Instruction model [15]. A comprehensive review of the literature, a pilot study, and a focus group interview were used to develop the educational session. The session was comprised of topics such as the lifecycle of *E. vermicularis*, diagnosis of enterobiasis, symptoms and signs, infection and transmission, and treatment and prevention of enterobiasis. A trained teacher provided a 30-minute lecture using visual aids to stimulate interest and support explanations of the educational contents. The lecture included an example situation, describing how one student became infected with a pinworm, and showing how enterobiasis spread to other students in the same classroom. Key messages were reinforced with an interactive quiz, and there was a 10-minute session to answer students' questions.

Measurement

The main outcome variable is the improvement of 15 or more points in children's knowledge of *E. vermicularis* infection. As there are no currently published scales for children's knowledge on *E. vermicularis* infection and children's preventative practice against enterobiasis infection, the investigators composed a scale, which was validated by experts (including parasitologists, pediatric doctors, internal medicine doctors, school nurses, and school-teachers). Four pilot studies were conducted to assess comprehension of the questionnaire items. The instrument to measure children's knowledge of *E. vermicularis* infection included 10 dichotomous items (answered as either "correct" [1 point] or "incorrect" [0 points]).

The secondary outcome variables recorded are children's prevention practices and the infection rate 3 months later. The instrument to assess children's prevention practices consisted of 8 Likert-scale items; each Likert item ranged from 1 (never) to 4 (every time).

Study procedure

Children in both the education and control groups who tested positive for *E. vermicularis* eggs received medical treatment with 400 mg albendazole twice, at a 15-day interval. The pre-treatment structured questionnaire on knowledge of *E. vermicularis* infection was provided to the children by a class teacher. This questionnaire

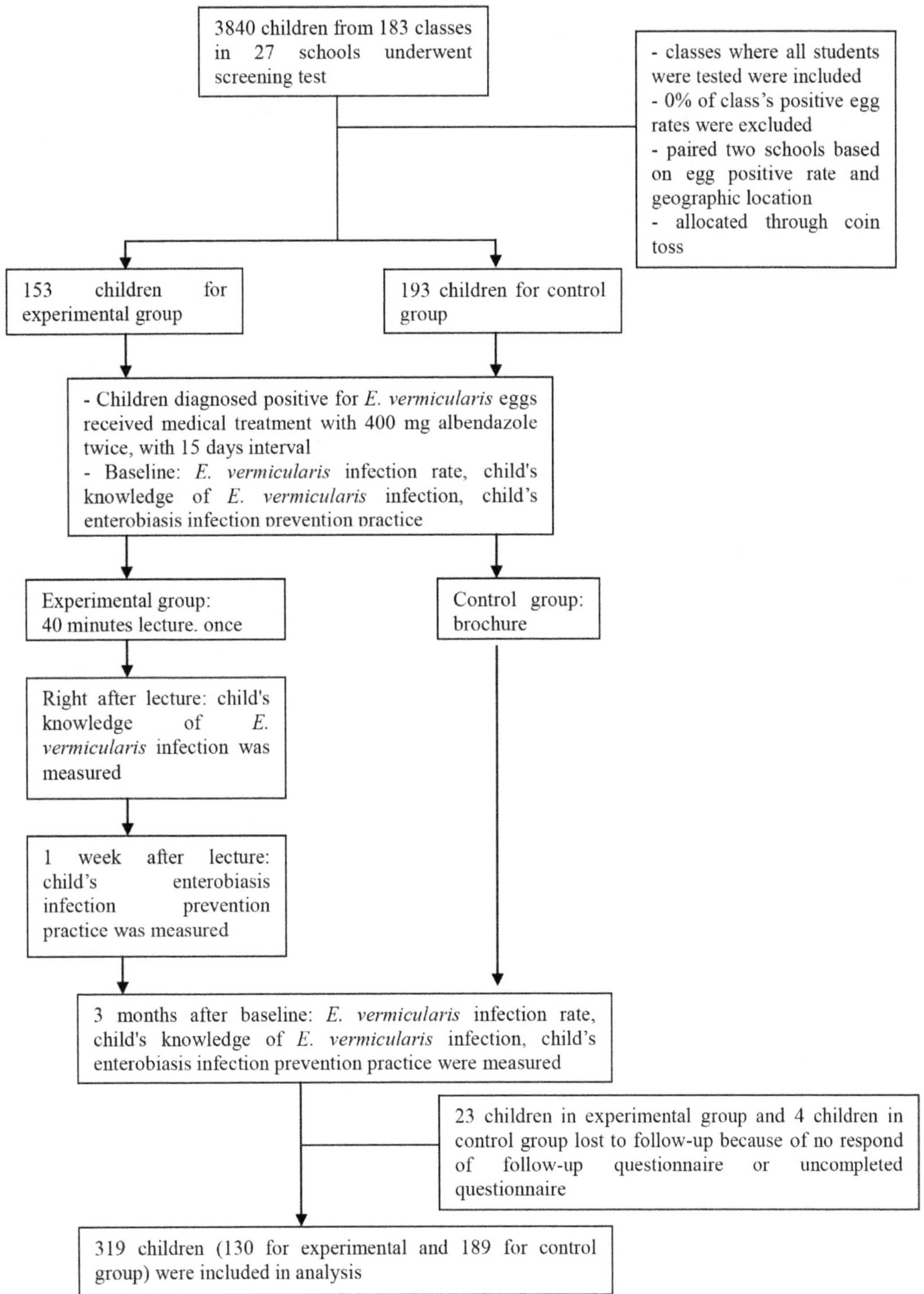

Figure 1. Study design including screening, group allocation, and follow-up. A total of 319 children from 16 classes were invited from among 3,840 children screened from 183 classes. The schools were assigned to either the intervention or the control arms by simple randomization using a coin toss.

was also provided to the parents of each child, enquiring about demographics and socioeconomic status, the child's enterobiasis infection prevention practices at home, and the parents' knowledge of enterobiasis. Children's knowledge of *E. vermicularis* infection was assessed the day they learned about enterobiasis and 3 months later. One week and three months after the intervention, parents were asked to complete another questionnaire on the children's enterobiasis infection prevention practices at home. *E. vermicularis* egg detection and the reinfection rates were evaluated using a sellotape anal swab 3 months after the intervention.

Ethics statement

The study was performed after receiving approval from the Ethical Review Committee of Yangsan Pusan National University Hospital, and after informed written consent was obtained from each participant before enrollment. Participation was entirely voluntary. Participants, including principals and teachers of schools, parents, and their children, were free to refuse to participate or withdraw from the study at any time, and were informed that only the aggregate data would be reported. Informed consent for the children in this study was provided by their parents or guardians and by the children. Once we obtained written consent from the parents or guardians to contact their children, the class teacher informed the children that permission to conduct the study had been granted. We briefed the individual children about the study and what they were being asked to do. Children who diagnosed positive for *E. vermicularis* eggs at screening received medical treatment with 400 mg albendazole twice, at a 15-day interval.

Statistical analysis

We report descriptive statistics for the characteristics of study sites and individual participants. To test the effectiveness of the education program in changing children's knowledge and prevention practices (continuous variables), we used multivariable mixed-effects analysis allowing random effects for clusters and controlling for gender and age. Each estimator was presented with its 95% confidence interval (95% CI). The prevalence of *E. vermicularis* eggs at baseline and after treatment in each group was compared using proportions and the McNemar test.

To examine the effectiveness of the education program in reducing infection (yes: 1; no: 0, binary response), we used multivariable logistic regression allowing random effects for clusters. All statistical analyses were performed using SAS 9.2 (SAS Institute, Inc., Cary, NC) statistical package and p values less than 0.05 were considered as statistically significant.

Results

Participant characteristics were compared between the experimental and control groups, most of which were similar. The small differences observed between groups were not statistically significant. Several characteristics of the participants are shown in Table S1. The overall *E. vermicularis* egg detection rate was 4.4%; the rate for each school ranged from 0% to 12.9% at screening (Table 1). Characteristics of study sites and individual participants are summarized in Table 2. Experimental and control groups enrolled 130 and 189 children, respectively. There were no statistically significant differences in children's baseline characteristics ($p>0.05$).

Between-group comparisons of knowledge of and prevention practices for *E. vermicularis* infection, as well as the prevalence of *E. vermicularis* egg positive rates, are show in Table 3. There were significant time effects in the mean scores for children's knowledge of *E. vermicularis* infection in the intervention group compared to the control group ($p<0.001$). Regarding *E. vermicularis* infection prevention practices, the experimental group increased from 3.22 to 3.45 (a difference of 0.23), whereas the control group increased from 3.19 to 3.23 (a difference of 0.04) between baseline and 3 months after treatment ($p<0.001$). The experimental group had a higher increase in knowledge test scores than the control group (adjusted difference = 1.95 [95% CI, 1.57–2.34]; $p<0.001$). The experimental group also had a higher increase in prevention practices than the control group (adjusted difference = 0.19 [95% CI, 0.13–0.25]; $p<0.001$). Clustering was considered in all logistic and multivariate regression models.

The incidence rate was lower in the experimental group, although this finding was not significant after adjustment for the clusters as random effects (adjusted odds ratio = 0.20, 95% CI = 0.02–2.41, $p=0.175$). The infection rate at 3 months after treatment sharply decreased from 12.3% to 0.8% in the experimental group ($p<0.001$), while that in the control group decreased from 8.5% to 3.7% ($p=0.049$) during the same period. Some children were diagnosed with new infections at 3 months after treatment; however, the number of new infections in the experimental group was lower than that in the control group. Moreover, although children who tested positive for *E. vermicularis* eggs were treated with antihelminthic drugs at baseline, *E. vermicularis* reinfection was observed in the control group.

We also jointly compared baseline, post-education, and 3-month changes in the experimental group. Correct answer rates on the *E. vermicularis* infection knowledge test in the experimental group are shown in Table 4. After the educational session, the score for knowledge about *E. vermicularis* infection increased from 60.2±2.32 to 92.7±1.19 in the experimental group; this gain was partially lost 3 months after the educational session, decreasing to 83.6±1.77 ($p<0.001$). The correct answer rate was 34.6% to 78.5% at baseline, 80.0% to 99.2% at post-education, and 75.4% to 93.1% 3 months after the intervention. At baseline, the item "Proper teeth brushing can prevent *E. vermicularis* infection" (34.6%) had the lowest rate of correct answers, followed by "Weekly change of underwear is important for preventing *E. vermicularis* infection" (36.9%), "*E. vermicularis* is not transmitted to other humans via hand contact" (47.7%), and "*E. vermicularis* infection can be treated by taking antihelminthic medication once" (50.0%); the rates for these items increased to over 80% correct responses at post-education, and over 75% correct 3 months later.

Results for children's practices for the prevention of *E. vermicularis* infection are shown in Table 5. Children's enterobiasis infection prevention practice scores also increased, from 3.23±0.27 to 3.73±0.25, 1 week after the educational session, and then partially decreased to 3.46±0.36 after 3 months ($p<0.001$). Items related to hand washing had lower scores than other items, such as keeping nails short and cleaning underwear. After 3 months, the item "My child does not bite his/her nails" had the lowest score of all items at both 1 week and 3 months after the health education session.

Discussion

Mass drug administration is the most effective means to control enterobiasis, but this method also has some limitations in that it does not prevent reinfections. In a previous study, we found new infection cases in the mass drug administration treatment group at both 3 and 6 months after treatment [2]. Moreover, reinfection increases the financial burden placed on preventative medicine programs. Consensus among government health employees and social workers might be necessary, because part of the cost of group treatment must be covered by the government. Furthermore, there is concern that mass drug administration might lead to the development of drug-resistant parasites [16]. The development of drug resistance in nematodes that infect humans is considered inevitable, given the number of species infecting livestock that are now resistant to antihelminthic agents due to continuous and extensive drug use [17,18]. Strategies to reduce the overall incidence of enterobiasis infection are likely to require an integrated approach, including pharmacological treatment to

Table 1. Egg positive rates of *E. vermicularis* infection among children in South Korea (n = 3840).

School	No. class	No. examined/total No. student (compliance %)	No. positive (%)
1	2	31/37 (83.8)	4(12.9)
2	11	260/287 (90.6)	21(8.1)
3	6	97/133 (72.9)	7(7.2)
4	2	15/19 (78.9)	1(6.7)
5	6	139/152 (91.4)	9(6.5)
6	6	122/136 (89.7)	7(5.7)
7	4	57/57 (100.0)	3(5.3)
8	13	317/361 (87.8)	16(5.0)
9	6	142/155 (91.6)	7(4.9)
10	10	238/256 (93.0)	11(4.6)
11	9	160/203 (78.8)	7(4.4)
12	6	115/149 (77.2)	5(4.3)
13	8	189/242 (78.1)	8(4.2)
14	10	288/309 (93.2)	12(4.2)
15	9	135/220 (61.4)	5(3.7)
16	10	202/259 (78.0)	7(3.5)
17	8	145/182 (79.7)	5(3.4)
18	8	134/189 (70.9)	4(3.0)
19	12	277/316 (87.7)	8(2.9)
20	9	272/272 (100.0)	8(2.9)
21	4	82/100 (82.0)	2(2.4)
22	6	127/158 (80.4)	3(2.4)
23	4	84/89 (94.4)	2(2.4)
24	7	134/169 (79.3)	1(0.7)
25	2	33/33 (100.0)	0(0.0)
26	2	17/17 (100.0)	0(0.0)
27	3	28/59 (47.5)	0(0.0)
Total	183	3840/4559 (84.2)	163
Mean positive rate			4.4%

reduce the infection rate and health education for prevention and sustainable control.

Our results showed that health-education increased students' knowledge about enterobiasis transmission and changed their behavior. Notably, students washed their hands more frequently and sucked their fingers or toys less after the health education session (Tables 4 and 5). Most instances of infection transmission could be effectively prevented by repeated hand washes; therefore, behavioral changes might contribute to a reduction in enterobiasis rates. Interestingly, most students remembered general facts about enterobiasis (life cycle, transmission route, prevention, etc.) 3 months after receiving an educational lecture (Table 4).

In Korea, over 80% of people were infected with intestinal helminthic parasites in the 1960s [19]. Most people at the time lived in poor environments in which parasitic infections were easily transmitted [20]. Additionally, farmers at the time used "Night-soil" (human feces and urine) as fertilizer on food crops. Furthermore, underground water was easily contaminated by parasite eggs found in human and animal feces; therefore, parasites were not easily eradicated in humans by mass drug administration. However, after the South Korean government launched a life environmental improvement project ("Saemaeul" [new village] Movement) and established the Korean Parasite Eradiation Association (KPEA), parasitic infection rates rapidly decreased. The Saemaeul Movement improved the drinking water supply system and sewage treatment system. The KPEA (now, Korea Association of Health Promotion) strived to eradicate parasite infections by conducting periodic examinations of the parasite infection rate, treating infected people, and providing preventative education for inhabitants in endemic areas. After the 1990s, most intestinal parasitic infection rates decreased to less than 3.0% in South Korea, with soil-transmitted helminthic infection rates decreasing to less than 1.0% [2,9].

However, in spite of the struggles of the government, enterobiasis has yet to be eliminated. One of the reasons for this is that there are misconceptions about enterobiasis in South Korea [2,9]. The first is the belief that parasitic infections, including enterobiasis, have already disappeared in South Korea; due to this belief, approximately half of children have not taken medication against helminthic parasites, including pinworms. The second misconception is that enterobiasis can easily be cured by a one-time anti-helminthic medication, as is the case for other intestinal nematodes. It was recently shown that the numbers of young children being cared for in group facilities, including private

Table 2. Characteristics of study sites and individual participants (n = 319).

Characteristic		Experimental (n = 130)	Control (n = 189)	P value
Site's characteristic				
Cluster size				
	mean ± SD	19.13±3.94	24.25±2.25	
No. of Conforming Requests/Total				
		11/14(78.6%)	25/26 (96.2%)	
		21/23 (91.3%)	21/21 (100.0%)	
		18/21 (85.7%)	27/27 (100.0%)	
		18/21 (85.7%)	21/21 (100.0%)	
		16/20 (80.0%)	23/24 (95.8%)	
		19/24 (79.2%)	23/24 (95.8%)	
		14/16 (87.5%)	26/26 (100.0%)	
		13/14 (92.9%)	23/25 (92.0%)	
Total		130/153 (85.0%)	189/194 (97.4%)	
Children's characteristics				
Sex				
	Male	69 (53.9%)	104 (57.1%)	0.581
	Female	59 (46.1%)	78 (42.9%)	
Age				
	Mean ± SD	8.22±0.70	8.24±0.67	0.827
House type				
	Apartment	109 (85.2%)	158 (86.8%)	0.823
	Non-apartment	19 (14.8%)	24 (13.2%)	
Job of parents				
	Single	71 (55.5%)	99 (54.4%)	0.261
	Both	57 (44.5%)	83 (45.6%)	
Family size				
	≤3 persons	96 (76.8%)	142 (78.5%)	0.583
	>4 persons	29 (23.2%)	39 (21.5%)	

educational institutes, have increased, and the employees and teachers of these facilities have such misconceptions [2]. Therefore, opportunities for infection and transmission from child to child have increased as a result. These misconceptions should be rectified through health education providing the correct information, which would be expected to result in a rapid decrease in infection rates [2,9].

Visual educational materials targeting schoolchildren have been shown to have a positive effect on knowledge and attitudes [18,21,22]. In this study, the educational information on enterobiasis included cartoon materials and real-life visual representations, such as microscopic images of pinworms, sellotape used for the diagnosis of enterobiasis, and the medications used to treat it. Most students who participated in this study were interested and immersed in the example situation as if he/she was the infected student. We believe that storytelling using cartoon materials was effective in helping children to focus on the educational contents. Moreover, descriptions of other aspects, such as the sellotape anal swab technique for diagnosis, elicited a response from the students, as they had themselves experienced this during the baseline data collection period. Finally, the interactive quiz emphasized the major educational content. This interactive health education session might lead to behavioral changes that result in decreasing the risk of *E. vermicularis* infection.

The health education session increased knowledge about enterobiasis. We were worried that at the 3-month follow-up assessment children would not remember the information acquired earlier. However, interestingly, the majority of children remembered most of the information they had learned on the subject. In addition, their prevention practices against *E. vermicularis* infection were maintained in their daily lives. Some children were administered the antihelminthic drug (albendazole) at the same time as their family members (personal communication), indicating that educating children may also have an indirect influence on their family members. These results could provide substantial gains in the elimination of enterobiasis in Korea, since Grade 1 and 2 primary school students are the most commonly infected population [6,23].

The prevalence of the *E. vermicularis* egg positive rate was not significant after adjusting for clusters as a random effect in this study, although the infection rates in the experimental group showed larger changes than in the control group. In a previous study, Gai et al. reported the negative relationship between the rate of parasitic infection and knowledge of prevention [24]. Enterobiasis was successfully treated with an anthelminthic agent.

Table 3. Comparison of the prevalence of *E. vermicularis* egg positive rates, knowledge, and prevention practices for *E. vermicularis* infection between groups (n = 319).

	Time	Experimental (n = 130)	Control (n = 189)	P value of Difference	Treatment Difference
		n (%)/mean ± SD	n (%)/mean ± SD		(95% CI)
Knowledge					
Baseline		6.02±2.32	6.12±2.09		
3 months after		8.36±1.77	6.45±2.04		
Difference		2.35±2.43	0.33±0.97	<0.001	1.96‡ (1.57–2.34)
Preventing Practice					
Baseline		3.22±0.28	3.19±0.43		
3 months after		3.45±0.36	3.23±0.40		
Difference		0.23±0.37	0.04±0.18	<0.001	0.19‡ (0.13–0.25)
Infection rate					
Baseline	Positive	16(12.3%)	16 (8.5%)	0.263	
3 months after	Positive	1(0.8%)*	7 (3.7%)*	0.175	0.20†(0.02–2.41)
Baseline - 3 months after	Positive - positive (re-infection case)	0(0.0%)	3(1.6%)		
	Negative - positive (New infected case)	1(0.8%)	4(2.1%)		

*Statistically significant between baseline and 3 months in experimental group (p<0.001) and control group (*p* = 0.049), based on the McNemar test.
†OR was adjusted for clusters as a random effect.
‡Mean difference was adjusted for clusters as a random effect, as well as gender and age.

Children in both the education and control groups who tested positive for *E. vermicularis* eggs received medical treatment with albendazole at baseline according to ethical considerations. Moreover, we evaluated the effect of the intervention for 3 months since participants changed classes as they advanced into the next grade. Future long-term evaluation studies need to assess whether health education increasing students' knowledge about enterobiasis transmission impacts infection rates.

Our study has a few limitations. First, there was potential confounding effect due to interaction between teachers in the experimental and control groups, despite our attempts to maintain a distance between groups by selecting them from different districts. Second, we asked the parents to assess their children's enterobiasis infection prevention practices, that is an indirect measure and might not be accurate. In addition, we asked the parents to do the Sellotape swab of their child's anus first thing in the morning, before the child had washed. There is a possibility that the children's parents decided to wash their child first, before preparing the swab, to show that their child had not become reinfected. This would influence the infection rates 3 months after the educational session. Third, as the study could not be double-blinded, other factors may have affected the results. Furthermore,

Table 4. Assessment of children's correct answer rates on *E. vermicularis* infection knowledge test (Experimental group: n = 130).

Items	Correct answer rate (%)		
	Baseline	After education	3 month after
E. vermicularis is parasitic worm that can live inside the human	74.6	99.2	88.5
E. vermicularis is not transmitted to other human via hands	47.7	86.9	88.5
Enterobius vermicularis infection can be diagnosed by using sellotape anal technique	68.5	98.5	83.1
Child with *E. vermicularis* may have anal itching	71.5	98.5	93.1
The habits of sucking fingers or biting nails is associated with *E. vermicularis* infection	65.4	93.1	89.2
Good hand hygiene can help prevent the spread of *E. vermicularis* infection	78.5	95.4	91.5
Proper brushing teeth can be preventive *E. vermicularis* infection	34.6	91.5	79.2
Anal cleansing can help prevent *E. vermicularis* infection	73.8	95.4	86.2
Weekly change of underwear is good for preventing *E. vermicularis* infection	36.9	80.0	75.4
E. vermicularis infection can be treated by taking antihelminthic medication once	50.0	88.5	80.0
Over all M± SD	60.2±2.32	92.7±1.19	83.6±1.77
Generalized linear mixed model test statistic (*p*)	157.230 (<0.001)		

Table 5. Children's prevention practices for *E. vermicularis* infection (Experimental group: n = 130).

Items	Baseline	1 week after	3 month after
My child practices hand washing after defecation	3.00±0.29	3.71±0.47	3.32±0.60
My child practices hand washing before eating	2.72±0.51	3.57±0.53	3.32±0.61
My child practices hand washing after coming in from outside	2.89±0.44	3.77±0.48	3.51±0.59
My child does not sucking fingers or toys	3.30±0.86	3.68±0.62	3.50±0.79
My child does not biting nails	3.12±0.97	3.45±0.82	3.28±0.96
My child keeps the nails short	3.58±0.75	3.78±0.54	3.40±0.55
My child practices proper anal cleansing	3.49±0.61	3.96±0.20	3.59±0.55
My child wears clean underwear	3.63±0.60	3.96±0.20	3.65±0.48
Over all M± SD	3.23±0.27	3.73±0.25	3.46±0.36
Generalized linear mixed model test statistic (*p*)		149.486 (<0.001)	

it was not clear whether the educational session would have an impact on infection rates due to lack of previous studies. That is why we tested children's knowledge as a primary outcome. To detect the infection rate difference of 2.9 derived in this study, the total number of clusters required is 117. Due to the lack of statistical power, the result regarding infection rates need to be interpreted with caution and future studies with large sample sizes are required.

In spite of these limitations, we believe that health education can be a cost-effective and safe strategy to decrease enterobiasis and other childhood diseases through to adulthood, as behaviors obtained early in life can result in long-term favorable sanitary habits later in life.

Acknowledgments

We would like to thank J. M. Choi at ACE statistical consulting for his valuable recommendations on statistical aspects of this paper.

Author Contributions

Conceived and designed the experiments: DHK HSY. Performed the experiments: DHK HSY. Analyzed the data: DHK HSY. Contributed reagents/materials/analysis tools: DHK HSY. Wrote the paper: DHK HSY.

References

1. Degerli S, Malatyali E, Ozcelik S, Celiksoz A (2009) Enterobiosis in Sivas, Turkey from past to present, effects on primary school children and potential risk factors. Turkiye Parazitol Derg 33: 95–100.
2. Kang IS, Kim DH, An HG, Son HM, Cho MK, et al. (2012) Impact of health education on the prevalence of enterobiasis in Korean preschool students. Acta Trop 122: 59–63.
3. Bager P, Vinkel Hansen A, Wohlfahrt J, Melbye M (2012) Helminth infection does not reduce risk for chronic inflammatory disease in a population-based cohort study. Gastroenterology 142: 55–62.
4. Report of Ministry of Health and Welfare of Republic of Korea and the Korea Association of Health (1971) Prevalence of intestinal parasitic infections in Korea—1st report. Ministry of Health and Welfare of Republic of Korea and the Korea Association of Health.
5. Report of Ministry of Health and Welfare of Republic of Korea and the Korea Association of Health (1997) Prevalence of intestinal parasitic infections in Korea -6th report. Ministry of Health and Welfare of Republic of Korea and the Korea Association of Health.
6. Kim BJ, Lee BY, Chung HK, Lee YS, Lee KH, et al. (2003) Egg positive rate of Enterobius vermicularis of primary school children in Geoje island. The Korean J Parasitol 41: 75–77.
7. Song HJ, Cho CH, Kim JS, Choi MH, Hong ST (2003) Prevalence and risk factors for enterobiasis among preschool children in a metropolitan city in Korea. Parasitol Res 91: 46–50.
8. Kang S, Jeon HK, Eom KS, Park JK (2006) Egg positive rate of Enterobius vermicularis among preschool children in Cheongju, Chungcheongbuk-do, Korea. Korean J Parasitol 44: 247–249.
9. Kim DH, Son HM, Kim JY, Cho MK, Park MK, et al. (2010) Parents' knowledge about enterobiasis might be one of the most important risk factors for enterobiasis in children. Korean J Parasitol 48: 121–126.
10. Roberts LS, Schmidt GD, Janovy J (2009) Foundations of parasitology. Boston: McGraw-Hill Higher Education. xvii, 701 p.
11. Cook GC (1994) Enterobius vermicularis infection. Gut 35: 1159–1162.
12. St Georgiev V (2001) Chemotherapy of enterobiasis (oxyuriasis). Expert Opin pharmacother 2: 267–275.
13. Owais A, Hanif B, Siddiqui AR, Agha A, Zaidi AK (2011) Does improving maternal knowledge of vaccines impact infant immunization rates? A community-based randomized-controlled trial in Karachi, Pakistan. BMC Public Health 11: 239.
14. Nithikathkul C, Akarachantachote N, Wannapinyosheep S, Pumdonming W, Brodsky M, et al. (2005) Impact of health educational programmes on the prevalence of enterobiasis in schoolchildren in Thailand. J Helminthol 79: 61–65.
15. Dick W, Carey L, Carey JO (2005) The systematic design of instruction. Boston; London: Pearson/Allyn & Bacon. xx, 376 p.
16. Keiser J, Utzinger J (2010) The drugs we have and the drugs we need against major helminth infections. Adv Parasitol 73: 197–230.
17. Albonico M (2003) Methods to sustain drug efficacy in helminth control programmes. Acta Trop 86: 233–242.
18. Bieri FA, Gray DJ, Williams GM, Raso G, Li YS, et al. (2013) Health-education package to prevent worm infections in Chinese schoolchildren. N Engl J Med 368: 1603–1612.
19. Seo BS, Rim HJ, Loh IK, Lee SH, Cho SY, et al. (1969) [Study On The Status Of Helminthic Infections In Koreans]. Kisaengchunghak chapchi 7: 53–70.
20. Kim CH, Park CH, Kim HJ, Chun HB, Min HK, et al. (1971) [Prevalence Of Intestinal Parasites In Korea]. Kisaengchunghak chapchi 9: 25–38.
21. Myint UA, Bull S, Greenwood GL, Patterson J, Rietmeijer CA, et al. (2010) Safe in the city: developing an effective video-based intervention for STD clinic waiting rooms. Health Promot Pract 11: 408–417.
22. Naldi L, Chatenoud L, Bertuccio P, Zinetti C, Di Landro A, et al. (2007) Improving sun-protection behavior among children: results of a cluster-randomized trial in Italian elementary schools. The "SoleSi SoleNo-GISED" Project. J Invest Dermatol 127: 1871–1877.
23. Lee KJ, Ahn YK, Ryang YS (2001) *Enterobius vermicularis* egg positive rates in primary school children in Gangwon-do (province), Korea. Korean J Parasitol 39: 327–328.
24. Gai L, Ma X, Fu Y, Huang D (1995) [Relationship between the rate of parasitic infection and the knowledge of prevention]. Zhongguo ji sheng chong xue yu ji sheng chong bing za zhi 13: 269–272.

15

Pediatric Health-Related Quality of Life: A Structural Equation Modeling Approach

Ester Villalonga-Olives[1,2]*, Ichiro Kawachi[2], Josué Almansa[3], Claudia Witte[1], Benjamin Lange[1], Christiane Kiese-Himmel[1], Nicole von Steinbüchel[1]

1 Institute of Medical Psychology and Medical Sociology, Georg-August-University Göttingen, Göttingen, Germany, **2** Department of Social and Behavioral Sciences, Harvard School of Public Health, Boston, Massachusetts, United States of America, **3** Department of Health Sciences, Community and Occupational Medicine, University of Groningen, University Medical Center Groningen, Groningen, The Netherlands

Abstract

Objectives: One of the most referenced theoretical frameworks to measure Health Related Quality of Life (HRQoL) is the Wilson and Cleary framework. With some adaptions this framework has been validated in the adult population, but has not been tested in pediatric populations. Our goal was to empirically investigate it in children.

Methods: The contributory factors to Health Related Quality of Life that we included were symptom status (presence of chronic disease or hospitalizations), functional status (developmental status), developmental aspects of the individual (social-emotional) behavior, and characteristics of the social environment (socioeconomic status and area of education). Structural equation modeling was used to assess the measurement structure of the model in 214 German children (3–5 years old) participating in a follow-up study that investigates pediatric health outcomes.

Results: Model fit was $\chi 2 = 5.5$; $df = 6$; $p = 0.48$; SRMR $= 0.01$. The variance explained of Health Related Quality of Life was 15%. Health Related Quality of Life was affected by the area education (i.e. where kindergartens were located) and development status. Developmental status was affected by the area of education, socioeconomic status and individual behavior. Symptoms did not affect the model.

Conclusions: The goodness of fit and the overall variance explained were good. However, the results between children' and adults' tests differed and denote a conceptual gap between adult and children measures. Indeed, there is a lot of variety in pediatric Health Related Quality of Life measures, which represents a lack of a common definition of pediatric Health Related Quality of Life. We recommend that researchers invest time in the development of pediatric Health Related Quality of Life theory and theory based evaluations.

Editor: Enrique Hernandez-Lemus, National Institute of Genomic Medicine, Mexico

Funding: This study is funded by the Niedersächsisches Institut für frühkindliche Bildung und Entwicklung (nifbe FP17-09); the Albert and Barbara von Metzler Stiftung, Gemeinnützige Hertie-Stiftung, Adolf Messer-Stiftung (all in Frankfurt/Main). The funders had no role in study design, data collection and analysis, decision to publish, or preparation of the manuscript.

Competing Interests: The authors have declared that no competing interests exist.

* Email: ester.villalonga@gmail.com

Introduction

To evaluate outcomes in terms of prevention, treatment and rehabilitation in children, it is important to test Health Related Quality of Life (HRQoL) [1]. Measures of HRQoL provide a broad view of child health, encompassing aspects of perceived health, health behavior, and well-being. Therefore, HRQoL has the potential to describe the health of children in the general and specific population more comprehensively than conventional health measures and provide better identification of specific groups with high rates of unrecognized conditions, social and emotional problems, and poor well-being and functioning [2]. Several variables have been identified as associated with HRQoL, including functional status, symptom status, biological status, and health perception [3].

The World Health Organization has proposed that the theoretical frameworks for conceptualizing the health of children and adults should be harmonized. One example is the International Classification of Functioning, Disability and Health (ICF) [4], in which the bio-psycho-social models for adults and children/youths do not vary. The WHO argues that what differs are the indicators for each component of the classifications. Differences between these populations have been summarized based on stage of human development, dependency, differential epidemiology, and demographics [5]. This means that, for example, the component body function of the ICF checklist for adults measures sexual functioning, while the ICF-CY (children/youths) measures genital functions. Another example would be in the activity limitations and performance component. There, language acquisition is an indicator in the checklist for children, whereas in the checklist version for adults, solving problem ability is emphasized.

One of the most referenced theoretical frameworks to measure HRQoL in the literature is the Wilson and Cleary model [3,6–8], which presents a conceptual model, a taxonomy of patient outcomes that categorizes patient outcomes according to the underlying health concepts they represent; it proposes specific causal relationships between the different health concepts [9] and focuses on relationships among different domains of health; its principal goal is to specify a series of critical concepts along a causal pathway. It proposes a linear sequence of causal relationships that proceeds from biological/physiological perturbance → symptoms → function → perceptions → overall Health Related Quality of Life. The theoretical framework's implication is that researchers need to measure these various outcomes and develop statistical models that explicitly estimate the size of the effects specified within the model. Sousa et al. [7] tested the model in an adult population with HIV-associated illness, to validate it as suggested by the original authors, using Structural Equation Modeling. However, it has never been tested in the pediatric population.

Our aim was to investigate the applicability of the framework of Wilson and Cleary in children by empirically testing the dominant causal associations they propose, using pediatric data available in our study.

Materials and Methods

Participants

The participants of the study comprised the baseline data of a longitudinal study whose main aim was to investigate developmental outcomes and well-being in children from 3 to 5 years old with predominantly migrant backgrounds (second generation migrants).The study was conducted in five kindergartens in Frankfurt/Main and Darmstadt, Germany, located in different neighborhoods. Participants were enrolled at the kindergartens. The parents of 96% of the children enrolled in these kindergartens consented to their children taking part of the study (N = 220 children).

The project was approved by the local ethics committee of the University Medical Center Göttingen. Written informed consent was obtained from the participating families (directly from the parents), together with the approval of the kindergarten councils. Families received detailed information regarding the background and implementation of the study and were offered the opportunity to withdraw their children from the study at any time. No incentives were given.

Investigation Tools and Questionnaires

Socioeconomic variables. We collected information about occupation and level of education of the main sustainer of the family to characterize the family's socioeconomic status. Here the international ISCO categorization was followed [10]. To perform the analysis of these data, we created a final categorical variable: out of work (0), unskilled workers (1), skilled workers (2), professionals (3) and professionals with advanced qualifications (4).

Kiddy-KINDL *(KK; Ravens-Sieberer et al., 1998).* The "Kiddy-KINDL (KK)" is an instrument designed to measure general HRQoL in children aged between 4 and 7 [1,11]. The recall period of the questionnaire is the past week. The short version of this questionnaire comprises 12 items belonging to 6 dimensions: physical well-being, psychological well-being, self-esteem, family, friends, and everyday functioning at the kindergarten. Response categories are arranged on a 3 point Likert scale (never, sometimes, very often). The final scores are T-scores that range from 20–80, with higher scores indicating better HRQoL. We used KK in interviews to collect self-reports from children who were 3–5 years old. We previously tested the psychometric properties of the instrument in the present sample and found their overall validity and overall reliability scores to be acceptable to very good. The work is under review elsewhere.

Symptom status. As an indicator of symptom status, we asked whether the child had recently been in a hospital or had a chronic disease (Table 1). Response categories were yes/no.

Wiener Entwicklungstest *(WET - Vienna Development Test; Kastner-Koller and Deimann, 2002).* The WET is a widely used instrument which measures the developmental status of children aged 3 to 6 years [12]. The WET consists of 13 subtests and a parent questionnaire, covering 6 functional areas of development: visual, motor, learning/memory, cognitive stage, language, and socio-emotional development, and a final score that measures overall development. The variables and the final score range from 0 to 9, with higher scores indicating better development. We used C scores in the analysis. The instrument has good face validity and construct validity [12].

Verhaltensbeurteilungsbogen für Vorschulkinder *(Behavioral Assessment Rating Scale for Preschool Children. VBV 3–6; M.Döpfner, W Berner, T. Fleischmann et al., 1993).* The VBV is an observation- and rating scale for behavioral problems that has 93 items organized in 4 scales: social-emotional competence, oppositional-aggressive behavior, attention deficit/hyperactivity versus playing time and emotional disorders. Responses are arranged on a 5 point rating-scale (never; once a week; several times a week; every day and several times a day). A sum score for every scale and an overall sum score can be calculated and these can be transferred into stanine norm scores (ranging from 1 to 9) with higher scores indicating more appropriate behavior. In this study, only information about the social-emotional behavior was collected. Kindergarten teachers rated the scales based on observed behavior in the last 4 weeks. The psychometrical properties are acceptable [13].

In this study we have included area-level education in the model. This variable is considered an environmental factor because every kindergarten is located in a different neighborhood. We selected this variable to account for the potential contextual effect of neighborhoods [14]. We used the WET developmental score and the social-emotional behavior score of the VBV 3–6 scale. More information is provided at Table 1.

Procedure

Data were collected at the kindergartens during day care. Children were interviewed and tested by psychologists and educational scientists. The same interviewers assessed the socio-economic status of the family in an interview with the parents at the kindergartens. Information was gathered following time sequence of variables, and the information of the Kiddy-KINDL was reported between 10 and 15 days after the collection of the other variables.

Adaptation of the Wilson and Cleary framework

Wilson and Cleary postulated that six categories of variables were directly or indirectly related to overall Quality of Life: health perception, symptom status, functional status, biological/physiologic status, characteristics of individual behavior, and environmental characteristics (Figure 1). We sought to test a reduced version of the model with the data available in our study: symptom status, functional status, individual and environmental characteristics (Figure 2). The variables 'health perceptions' and 'biological/

Table 1. Indicators used in the study to test the Wilson and Cleary theoretical framework in pediatric data: concepts, measured variables and details of the instruments used.

Concepts	Measured variables	Instrument	Recall period	Respondent	Content example
HRQoL	HRQoL	Kiddy-KINDL	Past week	Children	Had fun at the kindergarten
Environmental factors	Socioeconomic status	Specific questions	At present	Parents	Level of education, and current job
Symptom status	Symptom status	Specific question	Past week	Children	Recently been in a hospital or have a long disease
Functional status	Development status	WET	At present	Parents and Children	Put on the shoes, assists in housework
Characteristics of the individual	Individual Behavior	VBV 3–6 scale	Past four weeks	Kindergarten Teacher	Shows feelings spontaneously

physiological factors' were not obtainable from our data. Symptom status was collected using the information concerning hospital visits or having a chronic disease. In the case of functional status, we used the overall developmental score of the WET that was the sum of the six subscales: visual, motor, learning/memory, cognitive stage, language, and socio-emotional development. As a characteristic of the individual behavior we used the social-emotional behavior score of the VBV 3–6 scale. We also included the socioeconomic status of the family's main sustainer as well as the area of education as a measure of the environment. We tested the model with general HRQoL, since most of instruments that evaluate HRQoL measure general HRQoL and we tested a predominantly healthy group. The same relationships (arrows) that Wilson and Cleary model suggested (Figure 2) were hypothesized.

Statistical Analyses

Structural equation modeling was used to assess the measurement structure of the model [15,16]. Model fit was evaluated using $\chi 2$, and Standardized Root Mean Square Residual (SRMR) [17]. The values to accept the model should be non-significant in the $\chi 2$, and be lower than 0.07 in the SRMR. We divided the variable that measures HRQoL (Kiddy-KINDL) by 10 to obtain similar range of values across all variables, since it had a wide range scale (0–100), whereas the other instruments had ranges of 0–10 and 0–9. The socioeconomic variable and the area of education were introduced in the model with dummy coding. The reference category for the socioeconomic variable was unemployment. Modification indices were explored. For 214 children sufficient information was collected to be included in the analyses. Missing data were imputed by substituting for the missing value the scale mean rounded to an integer. Means for all instruments used in the analysis were calculated if up to 33% of responses were missing. The analyses were performed using maximum likelihood in M-Plus.

Results

50.5% of the participants were boys. They reported a score of 66.70 (SD 17.33) in HRQoL, and girls 72.39 (SD 15.94). Regarding socioeconomic status,15% of the main sustainers of the children families were skilled manual workers, and 13.2% of them were unemployed. The 6.5% of the sample declared to have a chronic disease or having been hospitalized the last week. Developmental status overall score for boys was 4.27 (SD 1.00), while for girls was 4.71 (SD 1.26). In the case of individual behavior, the score for boys was 4.14 (SD 2.08) and 5.03 (SD 2.41) for girls. 214 children presented sufficient information to be included in the present analysis (Table 2).

Figure 3 shows the model factors that were hypothesized to affect HRQoL in children. Model fit was $\chi 2 = 5.5$; df = 6; p = 0.48;

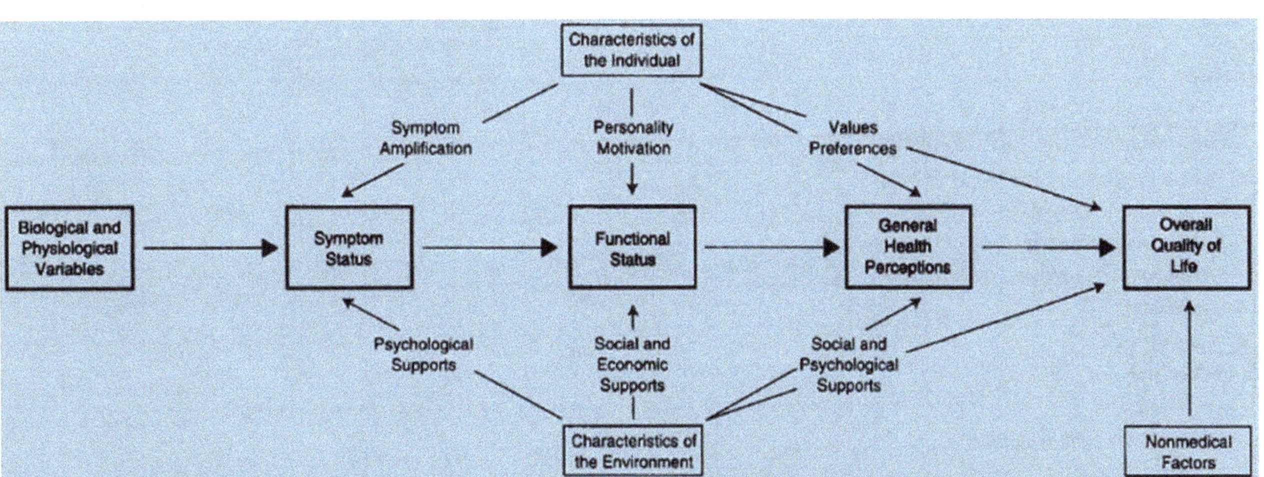

Figure 1. Wilson and Cleary theoretical framework.

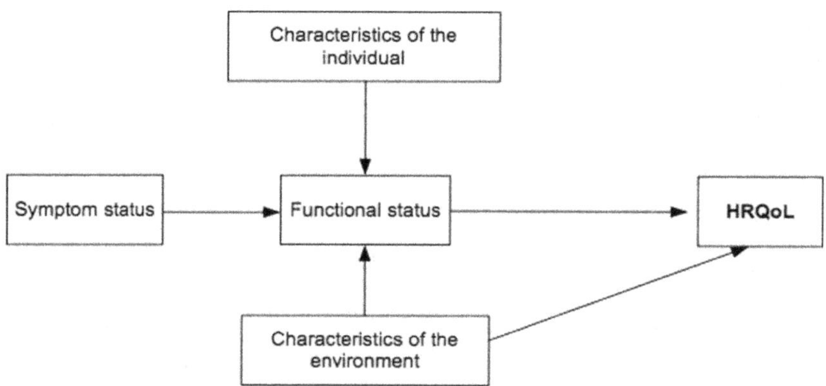

Figure 2. Structural model to test contributions to HRQoL in children. Adapted from the Wilson and Cleary theoretical framework.

SRMR = 0.01. The overall variance of HRQoL explained by the model was 15%. Socioeconomic status had a significant positive effect on children's functional status. Those children that were in households where the main sustainer of the family was categorized as professional or professional with advanced qualifications, which was the 28.3% of the sample, had respectively 0.59 and 0.43 higher standard deviations on children's functional status compared to the unemployed, indicating the protective effect of better socioeconomic status. Four areas of education had a significant decrement on HRQoL. The most important of these effects was of −1.05 ($p = 0.00$). Modification indices suggested the areas of education would have an effect on the developmental status. We included the path into the model after revision of its theoretical implications. This path was significant in one area of education, and indicated a significant negative effect of −0.44 ($p = 0.20$), and contributed to a better goodness of fit of the model. Symptoms did not have an effect on the developmental status. Regarding symptoms, despite the hypothesis, we considered the result normal, since only 6.5% of children suffered from a chronic disease or were hospitalized the week before the test. However, the variable remained in the model to maintain all the factors related to HRQoL in the hypothesized model. Individual behaviors showed a positive significant effect on the developmental status of 0.37 ($p = 0.00$). Then, an increment of one SD in individual behavior implies an increment of 0.37 SD in development status. And development status had a positive significant effect on HRQoL of 0.18 ($p = 0.00$). Then, an increment in one SD in development status implies an increment in 0.18 SD in HRQoL.

Discussion

The goodness of fit of the model was good, indicating that our adaptation of the Wilson and Cleary theoretical framework can be used in children. Compared with previous studies that measured general HRQoL in children with adverse health conditions and diseases [18,19], the variance explained of HRQoL was acceptable. However, the amount of variance explained suggests that factors that contribute to HRQoL in children are lacking in our model.

Table 2. Descriptive statistics of the study sample.

	Overall N = 214	Boys N = 108	Girls N = 106
	Mean (SD) Percentage	**Mean (SD) Percentage**	**Mean (SD) Percentage**
Age	4.28 (1.47)	4.25 (1.57)	4.31 (1.37)
HRQoL	69.54 (16.63)	66.70 (17.33)	72.39 (15.94)
Area of education(kindergarten 1 = St Gallus)	29.0%	26.9%	31.1%
Area of education (kindergarten 2 = St Pius)	19.5%	23.1%	16.0%
Area of education(kindergarten 3 = St Fidelis)	19.6%	19.4%	19.8%
Area of education(kindergarten 4 = St Martin)	14.7%	13.5%	16.0%
Area of education(kindergarten 5 = St Michael)	16.8%	16.7%	17.0%
Professionals with advanced qualifications	17.2%	15.6%	18.8%
Professionals	11.1%	10.4%	11.8%
Skilled workers	43.5%	45.8%	41.2%
Unskilled workers	15.0%	13.5%	16.5%
Unemployed	13.2%	14.6%	11.8%
Symptom status (with symptoms)	6.5%	4.6%	8.5%
Development status	4.49 (1.13)	4.27 (1.00)	4.71 (1.26)
Individual behavior	4.58 (2.24)	4.14 (2.08)	5.03 (2.41)

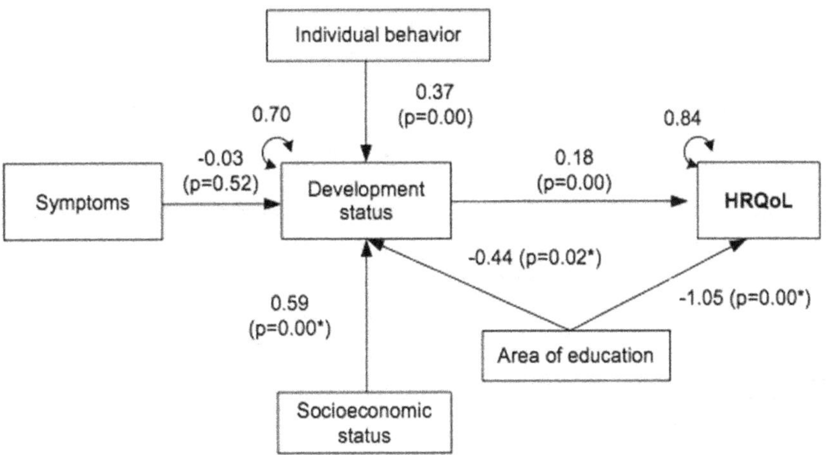

Figure 3. Measurement of variables and standardized estimates (β, ρ values and residual variances) of the test of the Wilson and Cleary theoretical framework using pediatric data. (Note: $\chi 2 = 5.5$; df = 6; p = 0.48; SRMR = 0.01. Standardized coefficients are given. *P value and coefficients with the highest effect in categories of the dummy variables socioeconomic status and area of education.

Our results confirm the relevance of developmental status and environmental factors as influences on HRQoL among kindergarten children from predominantly migrant backgrounds.

As we hypothesized, developmental status is an important variable directly associated with HRQoL [20]. Our test also supports the notion that individual behavior has an important effect on developmental status. It suggests that children's behaviors such as communication with peers, and social interactions in the kindergarten, among others, affect their development positively. Additional contextual and socioeconomic variables, viz., socioeconomic status and school-areas may also play an important role in child development. In the case of the contextual variables, these play an important role in different ways. First, higher socioeconomic position acts as a protective factor in our study. The relationship between the socioeconomic position of individuals and their health is well established – the socioeconomically better off perform better on most measures of health status, including HRQoL. The general pattern of better health among those who are socioeconomically better off is found across time periods, demographic groups, most measures of health and disease, as well as different measures of socioeconomic position [21,22]. Second, the association between school-areas with HRQoL can be explained by several mechanisms. A contextual explanation posits that there are differences in the quality of the social or physical environment associated with different neighborhoods that influence the health of those exposed to them. More affluent neighborhoods are more likely to be associated with the provision of decent housing, safe playing areas, transport, green spaces and street lighting – all of which generate positive feelings about the community and leads to greater levels of social interaction and community participation; and consequently, better health related outcomes. Conversely when there is a lack of these characteristics, the impacts on health are correspondingly bad. Environmental design and layout can influence social interactions and the level of social cohesion [22,23].

Sousa et al. performed one of the few studies that validated the Wilson and Cleary theoretical framework in a general adult population. To our knowledge, this is the unique report that uses structural equation modeling to do so [7,24]. Despite the differences in population and methodology used in these studies, we believe that a comparison is illustrative in terms of the constructs that are missing with respect to the instruments used to measure HRQoL. The authors obtained good results in the model fit and explained 83% of the variance of overall HRQoL. The differences in results between this and our study can have several explanations. First, we performed our analyses including environmental factors and characteristics of the individual, while Sousa et al. did not include indicators of these concepts, but information about general health perceptions of adults was included. Second, the indicators used to test each construct differed strongly, as expected. For example, a specific scale to measure symptoms, as well as a disability index to assess functional status were included in the model of Sousa et al [7]. Interestingly, symptom status explained almost 49% of the variance in functional status in the Sousa et al. study. While in our study, the variance explained of functional status in our model was 31% and the contribution of symptoms was low. However, in children, the assessment had some differences. The sample was homogeneous. This means that in our sample, only the 6.5% of children reported having a chronic disease or having being recently hospitalized. Even though we consider this result is normal in pediatric populations, we probably lacked sufficient variation to observe the relationship between symptom status and functional status and a better indicator as it was assessed in the test with adult populations. In addition, our analysis was performed using comprehensive generic HRQoL measurement, and the test with the adult population investigated overall HRQoL and it comprised a disease specific population. It is also possible that fewer variables would explain more variance of overall HRQoL in a specific population than using generic HRQoL in general population. The questionnaire administered to quantify functional status had some variations. We included an indicator of functioning based on development, since the main difference of childhood is the rapid development in a physical, sensory-motor, mental, emotional and social dimension [9]. Sousa et al. assessed functioning based on the ICF suggesting that disability should be considering the level of functioning of a person [4]. However, our measure did not include an indicator of physical health or social functioning [9].

Apart from the differences we have enumerated between the Sousa et al. model test and ours, we consider there are essential differences between pediatric and adult questionnaires that can have had an influence in our results. During the development of the original theoretical framework, Wilson and Cleary stated that they were presenting a conceptual model, a taxonomy of patient

Table 3. Mapping the Kiddy-KINDL into SF-36 dimensions of HRQoL.

Underlying health domains of the SF-36	SF-36 dimensions	Kiddy-KINDL dimensions
Behavioral functioning	Physical functioning	Physical well-being
Social and role disability	Role physical	
Social and role disability Perceived well-being	Bodily pain	Partially related with Physical well-being items
Personal evaluations and health in general	General health	
Perceived well-being	Vitality*	Everyday functioning at the kindergarten, family, friends*
Social and role disability	Social functioning	Everyday functioning at the kindergarten, family, friends
Social and role disability	Role emotional*	Self-esteem*
Perceived well-beingBehavioral functioning	Mental health	Psychological well-being

Note: *The dimensions are not extremely connected.

outcomes, that categorizes measures of patient outcomes according to the underlying health concepts they represent and proposed specific causal relationships between the different health concepts. They then said that there is a conceptual distinction between identifying the dimensions of health that are necessary to comprehensively and validly describe health, versus specifying a series of critical concepts on a causal pathway [9], and that the latter was their main goal. Following these statements, in the literature there have been different attempts using the Wilson and Cleary theoretical framework: to test HRQoL itself, as opposed to identifying the contributing factors that are affecting HRQoL [25]. For example, in some cases, factors such as social well-being have been suggested to be contributing factors, predictors that would affect HRQoL, instead of being part of HRQoL itself. Whereas, on the contrary, social well-being has been part of HRQoL too. This means that, in the current debate, there could be some factors that exist both inside and outside the concept.

There are two examples that clearly reflect the mixed approaches in the measurement of HRQoL in children. Pediatric questionnaires that assess general HRQoL include "resilience" and "bullying" as part of HRQoL, and these are included as dimensions of general HRQoL [26,27]. Yet resilience would also seem to be a determinant of HRQoL that is part of the characteristics of an individual, rather than a constituent dimension of HRQoL. Nevertheless, it has been targeted as a component of HRQoL. Bullying is another example of a factor that can clearly be a determinant of HRQoL which is part of the social context; however, it too has been used as a component of HRQoL [28]. This confusion between the concept and its determinants can lead to problems not only in assessing the model we test, but also in identifying outcomes and treatment [25]. A review of the literature reveals substantial heterogeneity in instruments for measuring HRQoL in children [29], which has been attributed to the paucity of theoretical grounding during the construction of these instruments. It has also been attributed to the lack of a common definition of HRQoL [29].

One of the most widely used measures to assess generic subjective health status in adults is the SF-36 which has been validated extensively. It is based on a multidimensional model of health and represents eight of the most important health domains, included in the Medical Outcomes Study and other commonly used health surveys [20,30,31]. The SF-36 captures dimensions with indicators that have a strong relationship with the Wilson and Cleary theoretical framework. Hence, multiple categories of operational definitions were chosen to investigate each health domain when the SF-36 was developed: behavioral functioning, perceived well-being, social and role disability, and personal evaluations and health in general.

To test the conceptual unity between the SF-36 and the KK, we mapped the dimensions of the KK onto the SF-36 dimensions considering the underlying concepts the SF-36 includes. Taking into account our previous premise that HRQoL components should have in common underlying concepts in adults and children measures, we suggest there should not be a lot of differences between the dimensions measured by the SF-36 and pediatric measures that assess general HRQoL.

This mapping however revealed some conceptual problems (Table 3). The indicators for HRQoL in both instruments are clearly different, because age determines the indicators that should be included to represent each concept, which are different in children compared to adults. However, not all the dimensions that are captured by the SF-36 are clearly reflected in the instrument we used. The mapping results indicate that general health is not reflected in the KK instrument, and that vitality and bodily pain are only partially reflected. However, these dimensions can be key points for children too. Children are normally healthy and report good general health and good levels of vitality, so it is especially important to detect those that have low levels of negative outcomes.

Parts of the underlying concepts "personal evaluations and health in general", and "social role and disability" are lacking in the questionnaire we used to test HRQoL. We have used the short version of the KINDL, the Kiddy-KINDL, which is more in accordance with the age of the kids of our sample; however the concepts are only partly reflected in the Kiddy-KINDL. Considering other measures of generic HRQoL for pediatric population, like the CHIP, the KIDSCREEN-52 or the GHQ, these underlying concepts are more represented in the dimension "self-perception" of the KIDSCREEN-52, and "satisfaction and diseases" of the CHIP questionnaire, and the CHQ has a wide relationship with the SF-36 underlying concepts [26,27,32–34]. Thus, caution is needed when generic HRQoL is under investigation in children, since several components have been related to it, and these vary considerably between questionnaires. Furthermore, the inclusion of "economic resources" as a dimension in a questionnaire that measures HRQoL like the KIDSCREEN-52 demonstrates again that some factors exist both inside and outside the concept. All this indicates substantial heterogeneity in the instruments for measuring HRQoL in children [29].

Some further limitations of our study deserve comment. First, our results are based on a kindergarten-based sample and results cannot be generalized. But we are confident that the results have high internal validity, and the relationships we have tested do not need participants be representative to drive our conclusions [35,36]. Second, we only used cross-sectional baseline data, while longitudinal data are more appropriate to test a model using Structural Equation Modeling. Nevertheless, the variables included in the model followed the temporal sequence of the variables. Third, the sample size was small, and limited our statistical power, and the indicators we selected to test the model were those that we had available in our study and had some limitations, above all because we did not have indicators of each factor available in our study and because some indicators were poor, as in case of symptoms. However, we were able to include some indicators that were not included in previous validations of the theoretical framework and we have seen that despite this limitation, a number of relationships in the model are statistically significant and the variance explained of HRQoL is high.

The study also has several strengths. To our knowledge, this is the first study that investigates HRQoL in young kindergarten children via self-report; it also presents the first validation attempt of the Wilson and Cleary theoretical framework to use structural equation modeling in a pediatric population. And we used multiple informants considering the content of the measures we wanted to test.

In conclusion, the analysis implies that the relations depicted in the figures we present were supported by the data. This can be seen as an initial step in comprehensive testing of the Wilson and Cleary theoretical framework in a pediatric population and it suggests the framework can be largely used to test the contributors to HRQoL in children. However, our findings also underscore the need to study the influence of other factors to HRQoL, and to assess whether the variance explained increases. Our investigation suggests a conceptual gap between adult and children measures, and a great variation in the assessments of children's HRQoL. There is a common view of the multidimensionality of HRQoL, and that the construct of health is viewed differently by children in comparison to adults [1]. But it appears that instruments of generic HRQoL in children are based on distinct definitions. We suggest that pediatric measures need to add indicators, determinants or predictors that are more related to a common definition of HRQoL. Hence, given how difficult is to conceptualize HRQoL in children, we recommend that pediatric HRQoL researchers invest more time developing a common perspective of which are the basic dimensions that should be tested in pediatric populations.

Acknowledgments

The authors would like to thank Donald Halstead (from Harvard School of Public Health) for his useful comments on the paper.

Author Contributions

Analyzed the data: EVO JA CW BL. Wrote the paper: EVO IK JA CKH NV.

References

1. Ravens-Sieberer U, Bullinger M (1998) Assessing health-related quality of life in chronically ill children with the German KINDL: first psychometric and content analytical results. Qual Life Res 7: 399–407.
2. Simon AE, Chan KS, Forrest CB (2008) Assessment of children's health-related quality of life in the United States with a multidimensional index. Pediatrics 121: e118–126. doi:10.1542/peds.2007-0480.
3. Heo S, Moser DK, Riegel B, Hall LA, Christman N (2005) Testing a published model of health-related quality of life in heart failure. J Card Fail 11: 372–379.
4. World Health Organization (2007) International Classification of Functioning, Disability, and Health (ICF-CY): Children and Youth Version. Geneva: World Health Organization. 352 p.
5. Seid M, Varni JW, Kurtin PS (2000) Measuring quality of care for vulnerable children: challenges and conceptualization of a pediatric outcome measure of quality. Am J Med Qual 15: 182–188.
6. Bakas T, McLennon SM, Carpenter JS, Buelow JM, Otte JL, et al. (2012) Systematic review of health-related quality of life models. Health Qual Life Outcomes 10: 134. doi:10.1186/1477-7525-10-134.
7. Sousa KH, Kwok O-M (2006) Putting Wilson and Cleary to the test: analysis of a HRQOL conceptual model using structural equation modeling. Qual Life Res 15: 725–737. doi:10.1007/s11136-005-3975-4.
8. Valderas JM, Alonso J (2008) Patient reported outcome measures: a model-based classification system for research and clinical practice. Qual Life Res 17: 1125–1135. doi:10.1007/s11136-008-9396-4.
9. Wilson IB, Cleary PD (1995) Linking clinical variables with health-related quality of life. A conceptual model of patient outcomes. JAMA 273: 59–65.
10. Eurostat's Metadata Server. Available: http://ec.europa.eu/eurostat/ramon/index.cfm?TargetUrl=DSP_PUB_WELC. Accessed 9 January 2014.
11. Ravens-Sieberer U, Ellert U, Erhart M (2007) [Health-related quality of life of children and adolescents in Germany. Norm data from the German Health Interview and Examination Survey (KiGGS)]. Bundesgesundheitsblatt Gesundheitsforschung Gesundheitsschutz 50: 810–818. doi:10.1007/s00103-007-0244-4.
12. Kastner-Koller U, Deimann P (2002) Wiener Entwicklungstest (WET). Göttingen: Hogrefe.
13. Döpfner M, Berner W, Fleischmann T, Schmidt M (1993) Verhaltensbeurteilungsbogen für Vorschulkinder (VBV 3–6). Weinheim: Beltz Test.
14. Elliott P, Wartenberg D (2004) Spatial epidemiology: current approaches and future challenges. Environ Health Perspect 112: 998–1006.
15. Musil CM, Jones SL, Warner CD (1998) Structural equation modeling and its relationship to multiple regression and factor analysis. Res Nurs Health 21: 271–281.
16. Hays RD, Revicki D, Coyne KS (2005) Application of structural equation modeling to health outcomes research. Eval Health Prof 28: 295–309. doi:10.1177/0163278705278277.
17. Hu L, Bentler PM (1999) Cutoff criteria for fit indexes in covariance structure analysis: Conventional criteria versus new alternatives. Struct Equ Model Multidiscip J 6: 1–55. doi:10.1080/10705519909540118.
18. Maurice-Stam H, Oort FJ, Last BF, Brons PPT, Caron HN, et al. (2008) Longitudinal assessment of health-related quality of life in preschool children with non-CNS cancer after the end of successful treatment. Pediatr Blood Cancer 50: 1047–1051. doi:10.1002/pbc.21374.
19. Matterne U, Schmitt J, Diepgen TL, Apfelbacher C (2011) Children and adolescents' health-related quality of life in relation to eczema, asthma and hay fever: results from a population-based cross-sectional study. Qual Life Res 20: 1295–1305. doi:10.1007/s11136-011-9868-9.
20. Ware JE, Kosinski M, Gandek B (1993) SF-36 Health Survey: Manual and Interpretation Guide. Boston: The Health Institute, New England Medical Center.
21. Berkman LF, Kawachi I (2000) Social epidemiology. New York: Oxford University Press. 391 p.
22. Berkman LF, Kawachi I, Glymour MM, editors (2014) Social epidemiology. Second edition. New York: Oxford University Press. 640 p.
23. Kawachi I, Berkman LF (2003) Neighborhoods and Health. New York: Oxford University Press. 370 p.
24. Ferrans CE, Zerwic JJ, Wilbur JE, Larson JL (2005) Conceptual model of health-related quality of life. J Nurs Scholarsh 37: 336–342.
25. Marie-Christine Taillefer, GD, Marie-Anne Roberge SLM(2003) Health-Related Quality of Life Models: Systematic Review of the Literature. Soc Indic Res 64: 293–323.
26. Ravens-Sieberer U, Gosch A, Rajmil L, Erhart M, Bruil J, et al. (2008) The KIDSCREEN-52 quality of life measure for children and adolescents: psychometric results from a cross-cultural survey in 13 European countries. Value Health 11: 645–658. doi:10.1111/j.1524-4733.2007.00291.x.
27. Riley AW, Forrest CB, Starfield B, Rebok GW, Robertson JA, et al. (2004) The Parent Report Form of the CHIP-Child Edition: reliability and validity. Med Care 42: 210–220.
28. Analitis F, Velderman MK, Ravens-Sieberer U, Detmar S, Erhart M, et al. (2009) Being bullied: associated factors in children and adolescents 8 to 18 years old in 11 European countries. Pediatrics 123: 569–577. doi:10.1542/peds.2008-0323.
29. Davis E, Waters E, Mackinnon A, Reddihough D, Graham HK, et al. (2006) Paediatric quality of life instruments: a review of the impact of the conceptual framework on outcomes. Dev Med Child Neurol 48: 311–318. doi:10.1017/S0012162206000673.
30. Ware JE Jr, Gandek B (1998) Overview of the SF-36 Health Survey and the International Quality of Life Assessment (IQOLA) Project. J Clin Epidemiol 51: 903–912.

31. Ware JE Jr, Gandek B (1998) Methods for testing data quality, scaling assumptions, and reliability: the IQOLA Project approach. International Quality of Life Assessment. J Clin Epidemiol 51: 945–952.
32. Starfield B, Riley AW, Green BF, Ensminger ME, Ryan SA, et al. (1995) The adolescent child health and illness profile. A population-based measure of health. Med Care 33: 553–566.
33. Ashing-Giwa KT (2005) The contextual model of HRQoL: a paradigm for expanding the HRQoL framework. Qual Life Res 14: 297–307.
34. Landgraf JM, Maunsell E, Speechley KN, Bullinger M, Campbell S, et al. (1998) Canadian-French, German and UK versions of the Child Health Questionnaire: methodology and preliminary item scaling results. Qual Life Res 7: 433–445.
35. Rothman KJ, Gallacher JEJ, Hatch EE (2013) Why representativeness should be avoided. Int J Epidemiol 42: 1012–1014. doi:10.1093/ije/dys223.
36. Elwood JM (2013) Commentary: On representativeness. Int J Epidemiol 42: 1014–1015. doi:10.1093/ije/dyt101.

16

Entrenched Geographical and Socioeconomic Disparities in Child Mortality: Trends in Absolute and Relative Inequalities in Cambodia

Eliana Jimenez-Soto, Jo Durham, Andrew Hodge*

The University of Queensland, School of Population Health, Brisbane, Queensland, Australia

Abstract

Background: Cambodia has made considerable improvements in mortality rates for children under the age of five and neonates. These improvements may, however, mask considerable disparities between subnational populations. In this paper, we examine the extent of the country's child mortality inequalities.

Methods: Mortality rates for children under-five and neonates were directly estimated using the 2000, 2005 and 2010 waves of the Cambodian Demographic Health Survey. Disparities were measured on both absolute and relative scales using rate differences and ratios, and where applicable, slope and relative indices of inequality by levels of rural/urban location, regions and household wealth.

Findings: Since 2000, considerable reductions in under-five and to a lesser extent in neonatal mortality rates have been observed. This mortality decline has, however, been accompanied by an increase in relative inequality in both rates of child mortality for geography-related stratifying markers. For absolute inequality amongst regions, most trends are increasing, particularly for neonatal mortality, but are not statistically significant. The only exception to this general pattern is the statistically significant positive trend in absolute inequality for under-five mortality in the Coastal region. For wealth, some evidence for increases in both relative and absolute inequality for neonates is observed.

Conclusion: Despite considerable gains in reducing under-five and neonatal mortality at a national level, entrenched and increased geographical and wealth-based inequality in mortality, at least on a relative scale, remain. As expected, national progress seems to be associated with the period of political and macroeconomic stability that started in the early 2000s. However, issues of quality of care and potential non-inclusive economic growth might explain remaining disparities, particularly across wealth and geography markers. A focus on further addressing key supply and demand side barriers to accessing maternal and child health care and on the social determinants of health will be essential in narrowing inequalities.

Editor: David O. Carpenter, Institute for Health & the Environment, United States of America

Funding: The research described in this paper is made possible through the Department of Foreign Affairs and Trade, Australia, grant ID 47734. The funders of the study had no role in the study design, data collection, the analysis or the interpretation of the results, or the writing of this paper.

* Email: a.hodge@uq.edu.au

Introduction

The Millennium Development Goal 4 (MDG 4) targets a two-thirds reduction in under-five mortality and has prompted increased international efforts to reduce child mortality and measure progress. Evidence at the national level suggests that globally under-five mortality is declining. Nevertheless, despite global gains in reducing child mortality, disparities remain between countries and within-countries [1–3]. Consideration of inequalities in access to health services and health outcomes has become an issue of increasing attention in the public health arena by scholars and policy makers [1,4]. The post-MDG agenda with its focus on universal health coverage has also drawn attention to the degree of equity in the distribution of improved health outcomes [4,5]. Most of the research to date has focussed on urban/rural disparities and socioeconomic disadvantage. There is increasing recognition, however, of the importance of other dimensions, such as ethnicity and geography in determining health outcomes [2,6,7].

Cambodia is a low-income country in South East Asia with a large rural population [8]. Both the demographic and epidemiological transitions are underway and the country is experiencing rapid economic growth [8]. Recent assessments show an impressive decline in the under-five mortality rate per 1,000 live births (U5MR) from approximately 124 in 2000 to 54 in 2010 [9]. The neonatal mortality rate (NMR) has also noticeably reduced between the years 2000 and 2005, from 37 to 28, but since 2005 has stagnated with a rate of 27 in 2010 [9]. According to the recent

2010 Global Burden of Disease estimates, the main causes of under-five mortality are lower respiratory infections, preterm birth complications, congenital anomalies, neonatal encephalopathy and diarrhoeal diseases [10]. Undernutrition and micronutrient deficiency are high and are the most significant risk factors for under-five mortality [10]. Most under-five deaths occur in early infancy and neonatal mortality contributes to over a third of all under-five mortality in Cambodia [11], The leading causes of neonatal mortality are preterm birth, birth asphyxia, sepsis and pneumonia [11].

Regional inequalities, differences between rural and urban populations and disparities associated with the wealth gradient have also been observed [4,5,9,12]. Over the last ten years, Cambodia has prioritised addressing health disparities particularly in relation to maternal and child health. Demand-side policies and programs have focussed on improving access to health services for the poor through a number of social protection measures. These have included user fee exemptions, health equity funds, vouchers and community-based health insurance [13–16]. Supply-side interventions have included the training of midwives, a midwifery financial incentive scheme, banning the use of untrained traditional birth attendants, increasing coverage of reproductive and maternal health services [4,17] and increasing immunization coverage [18].

The policy and program focus on decreasing maternal and child health disparities warrants further analysis. While research has revealed that inequity in a range of maternal and child health service use by wealth quintile has generally decreased over time [4], to date there has been no analysis of changes in equity in neonatal health mortality. To the best of our knowledge this is the first comprehensive study of levels, trends and inequalities – both absolute and relative – of under-five and neonatal mortality in Cambodia across regions, wealth and rural/urban residence markers.

Methods

Ethics

This study is based on the Cambodian Demographic Health Surveys (DHS) [9]. The DHS is undertaken by the National Institute of Statistics who were responsible for the management and review of the survey, with technical assistance from international advisors. Full review of this study from an institutional review board was not sought as the datasets were anonymous, with no identifiable information on the survey participants.

Data

The data source was the DHS series conducted in Cambodia in 2000, 2005 and 2010 as part of the global MEASURE DHS. The DHS is a nationally representative household survey, with a women's module of females aged 15 to 49 years [9]. In each of the three surveys households were sampled from 14 individual provinces and five groups of provinces resulting in 19 sampling domains, stratified into urban and rural areas. Details of the sampling design are provided elsewhere [9]. All women interviewed were asked to give a detailed history of all her live births in chronological order. Information collected included: whether a birth was single or multiple; sex of the child; date of birth; survival status; age of the child on the date of interview or age at death of each live birth.

In the present study rural/urban place of residence, region and household wealth were used as stratifying variables across which disparities in child mortality were estimated. Provinces were categorised into five agro-ecological regions commonly used in socioeconomic assessments in Cambodia. These provinces were grouped into areas with broadly similar terrain, accessibility, climate and economic activity. These regions are the Plains, Tonle Sap, Plateau/Mountain, Phnom Penh (the base group) and Coastal [19]. Household wealth was gauged through an asset index, which provides a reliable proxy measure of wealth in the absence of household income or consumption that is not contained within the DHS [20,21]. The survey-provided asset index was constructed for each survey round using principal component analysis (PCA), incorporating three categories of assets: durable consumer goods (e.g. ownership of a refrigerator, television, motorbike, etc.), quality of the dwelling (e.g. roof material, floor material etc.) and access to utilities and infrastructure (e.g. main source of drinking water, type of toilet facility). Using the factor scores from the first principal component, socioeconomic categorisation was obtained by ranking, then classifying households within the distribution into three groupings. Thus the derived indices are relative measures of socioeconomic status and not measures of absolute poverty [22,23].

Analysis and Measures of Disparities

The outcome measures were under-five and neonatal mortality. These rates were estimated directly following the methods of Rajaratnam and colleagues [24]. The estimation procedure is identical at both national and sub-national levels, with rates estimated biennially due to the relative rarity of child deaths. We assembled mortality records for each child detailing the life or death in each month of the first five years of each child's life, which we denote person-months data. For each two-year time period, survival rates for the following age groups were calculated: 0 to 1; 1 to 11; 12 to 23; 24 to 35; 36 to 47; and 48 to 59 months. The mortality rate is computed as one minus the survival rate. The biennial survival rates (i.e. mean survival probability) for the aforementioned age groups were directly estimated by dividing the total number of person-months where children were alive by the total number of person-months in the time period of interest, accounting for sample weights. The survival rates for each age group are then used to obtain the desired child mortality indicator by amalgamating the correct age groups: that is, under-five mortality is one minus the survival rates from all the age groups multiplied together, while neonatal mortality is one minus the survival rate from birth to 1 month. Confidence intervals were constructed using 1,000 simulations, with the survival probability generated assuming a binomial distribution and the lower and upper confidence bounds extracted from the 2.5^{th} and 97.5^{th} percentiles [24,25]. This standard simulation method captures both sampling and model uncertainty [24,26].

In context of declining mortality rates, it is well known that different conclusions about inequalities can be drawn depending on the scale used [27]. Hence, both absolute and relative measures of inequalities were computed, namely: rate difference (RD) and the slope index of inequality (SII) on the absolute scale and rate ratio (RR) and the relative index of inequality (RII) on the relative scale [27–29]. These measures were computed using the biennial mortality rates. Further details on the computation of these measures are provided in Box S1 in File S1. The main advantage of the RIIs and SIIs over the RDs and RRs is that the former accounts for changes in the distribution of the equity marker. The RII and SII are computed via weighted linear regression [30] and the need for ordinal social groups to rank the population implies that the RIIs and SIIs can only feasibly be computed using wealth. For the non-wealth equity markers, RDs and RRs are computed for each sub-population in reference to a base group, which is chosen as the group with the lowest average under-five mortality rate over the sample period. Confidence intervals for the RIIs and SIIs were calculated using standard methods outlined by Hayes and Berry [31]; and for the RDs and RRs were computed using the simulation process utilised for the mortality estimates. Comparisons over time were gauged by comparing the mortality rates and measures of inequalities over the sample period and considering 95% confidence intervals and *p*-values for tests of the statistical significance of a linear trend in these estimates [29]. In the cases of RRs and RIIs, we used the natural logarithm of these measures in the regressions. We used Newey-West standard errors (using one lag) in these regressions, which are robust to both heteroskedasticity and serial correlation.

All statistical analyses were conducted using the two software programs, *Stata* and *R*.

Results

National estimates derived using the above outlined methodology confirms the general pattern reported elsewhere. Figure 1 presents national estimates. The U5MR remained constant during the 1990s, hovering around approximately 121 deaths per 1,000 live births, with 120 (95% CI 111 to 128) in 1989–90 and 123 (95% CI 115 to 133) in 1999–2000. During the 2000s, U5MR declined dramatically, with the most recent estimate suggesting mortality rates have more than halved to 48 (95% CI 40 to 60) in 2009–10. The pattern of reduction in the NMR was similar, with the exception of possible stagnation since 2005 at approximately 25 deaths per 1,000 live births. Despite these reductions at the national level, closer examination of trends in disparities showed significant within-country inequalities.

As to be expected, high income households experience lower rates of under-five and neonatal mortality compared to households with poorer socioeconomic status. With the observed reductions in under-five mortality rates by wealth (see Figure 2), we find the well-known pattern of reducing absolute but rising relative inequalities as reported in Table 1. However, with respect to U5MR none of the trends are statistically significant at conventional levels. The results show increasing trends in both relative and absolute inequality for neonates. For example, the RDs for neonatal mortality have increased from 10.9 (95% CI −1.6 to 23.9) in 1989–90 to 11.26 (95% CI −5.3 to 30.7) in 2009–10 for low income households and from 9.3 (95% CI −2.6 to 20.1) in 1989–90 to 13.4 (95% CI −5.3 to 33.9) in 2009–10 for middle income households. Similarly, the SII was found to have increased from 16.18 (95% CI −69.2 to 101.6) to 16.70 (95% CI −151 to 184.4) over the same period. Note, however, when different assumptions (i.e. the standard variance estimator and Huber-White sandwich estimator) with respect to the standard errors are used (results not reported), the positive trends in absolute inequalities are statistically significant only in a few cases. Positive trends in RRs and RIIs are associated with greater statistical significance than the trends in absolute inequalities, and are robust to changes in the assumptions underlying the standard errors.

As shown in Table 2, similar patterns are observed pertaining to the disparities in child mortality across rural-urban locations and regions. Absolute disparities in under-five mortality were found to have reduced over time while the opposite was estimated for neonatal mortality. However, most trends were not statistically significant. On the other hand, rising relative inequalities were statistically significant at conventional levels for both under-five and neonatal mortality. For example, RRs by rural-urban location for under-five children increased from 1.56 (95% CI 1.2 to 2) in 1989–90 to 2.41 (95% CI 1.1 to 3.6) in 2009–10, with an average biennial increase of 7.8%. Across the regions, this average increase ranged from 11.2% to 18.2% for under-five mortality and 16% to 17.9% for neonatal mortality.

Contrary to the general pattern, the estimates for two regions showed patterns of widening inequalities on both relative and absolute scales for under-five mortality. The upward trajectories, however, are only statistically significant for the trend in the Coastal region, with a *p*-value less than 0.01 associated with the positive trend. Full estimates of mortality, inequalities and trends are available in Tables S1–S4 in File S1.

Discussion

Notwithstanding Cambodia's recent history of genocide under the Khmer Rouge (1975–1979) and internal conflict until the 1997 coup, this study confirms the noteworthy national reduction in under-five and neonatal mortality since 2000 [9]. These improvements are consistent with improvements in the maternal mortality ratio which decreased from 472 per 100,000 live births in 2000–2005 to 206 in 2006–2010 [9]. While it is not possible to make causal inferences from the available data, improvements are likely to be due to more than a decade of relative political and macroeconomic stability and high economic growth, increased female participation in the waged workforce and improved access to communications, transport infrastructure, education and potable water and sanitation [17,32,33]. These factors, particularly those related to the social determinants of health, are likely to have influenced health-related behaviours including changes in traditional birthing and feeding practices [4,9,12,17,19]. The government has also taken deliberate steps through its National Strategy for Reproductive and Sexual Health (2006–2010) [34] to address supply and demand side barriers in accessing maternal and child health services, which have also contributed to the observed reductions in under-five and neonatal mortality. Strategies have included demand-side financing policies, midwifery training and incentive schemes [17,33,35]. They have also been accompanied by strong malaria control and eradication strategies which have led to a decrease in the incidence of malaria including *Plasmodium falciparum*, which previously was one of the leading risk factors for under-five mortality [36].

Parallel to the observed national progress in U5MR, absolute inequalities by socioeconomic status show a decreasing, though not statistically significant trend, suggesting some gains in mortality across the wealth spectrum. This can be partly related to the observed reductions in disparities in access to family planning, safe abortion and immunization coverage among children across wealth groups [4,9]. However, these gains have been tempered by stagnating chronic malnutrition, which has disproportionately affected the poor [9,19,37] and a widening equity gap for prevalence of under-five diarrhoea and coverage of postnatal care [4,38].

Despite improvements in U5MR, the declines in the NMR seem to have stagnated since 2005 suggesting the need for increased investment in the more complex aspects of health system strengthening. Of concern are the persistent, and sometimes increasing, relative inequalities by socioeconomic status. The results show increasing trends in both relative and absolute inequality for neonates. These findings are consistent with the results from other studies [6,12,39] and reflect the general trend in Cambodia of increasing inequality across a number of socioeconomic markers [19] including a decreased concentration of landholding amongst the poor. We should note that increases in inequality for neonatal outcomes have been observed notwithstanding reductions in the equity gap for services like skilled birth

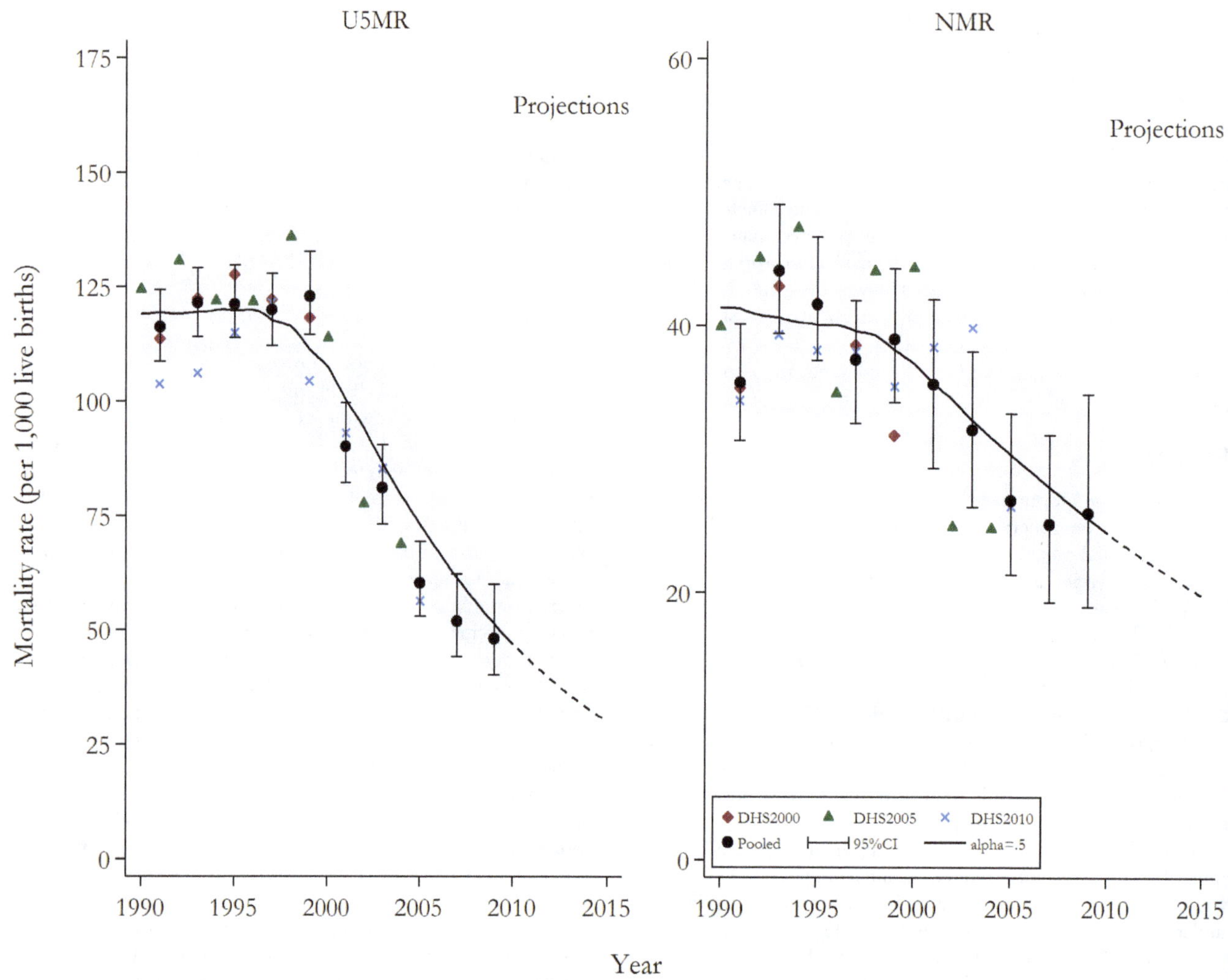

Figure 1. Under-five and neonatal mortality rates (per 1,000 live births) at the national level: actual 1990–2010; projected to 2015. *Notes*: National estimates by source and the pooled data are displayed. The solid represent the continuous mortality estimates calculated from the two-year estimates and loess regression with a smoothing parameter of 0.5 [43]. semi-broken lines are projections computed using the last set of parameter estimates for the Loess regression [44]. The shaded area signifies the corresponding 95% confidence intervals. U5MR, under-five mortality rate; NMR, neonatal mortality rate; DHS, Demographic Health Survey; CI, confidence intervals.

attendant and antenatal care. This seems to suggest that similar to other settings, increases in coverage for disadvantaged populations might lack adequate levels of quality of care [40]. Therefore, more attention and resources should be devoted to measures targeting quality beyond extending coverage of critical interventions.

Across rural-urban locations similar patterns in child mortality inequality were observed as those seen by socioeconomic groups, which is not surprising since both equity markers show substantial overlap. For example, the distribution of households from the most recent DHS wave are such that over 90% of the households in the bottom two quintiles reside in rural areas, while approximately 75% of households in the top quintile dwell in urban areas. Interestingly, our results suggest that since Cambodia started experiencing increased economic growth (post-2000), relative urban/rural disparities have increased. This is also reflected in most other socioeconomic indicators [19]. This suggests that similar to many other low and middle income countries, economic growth has been accompanied by increased inequalities [41]. The observed increase in relative inequality across both wealth and rural/urban location of residence further points to the need for inclusive economic growth strategies as well as substantial political and financial investments in addressing important health system constraints in the provision of quality antennal and post-natal care, skilled birth attendants and intrapartum obstetric services to rural and other disadvantaged populations [4,17,19].

This study also revealed increasing relative and stable absolute inequalities amongst regions when compared with Phnom Penh. Given most of the urban population reside in Phnom Penh this is likely to be linked to rural/urban disparities discussed above. Households living in the regions, particularly in rural areas, may face persistent difficulties that relate to the social determinants of health and work against further under-five and neonatal mortality reduction.

An unexpected finding was the statistically significant sharp increase in absolute inequality for under-five mortality for coastal areas. The Coastal region has a thriving tourist industry and is neither the poorest nor the most remote of the regions. It is possible that this is due to systematic poverty and health

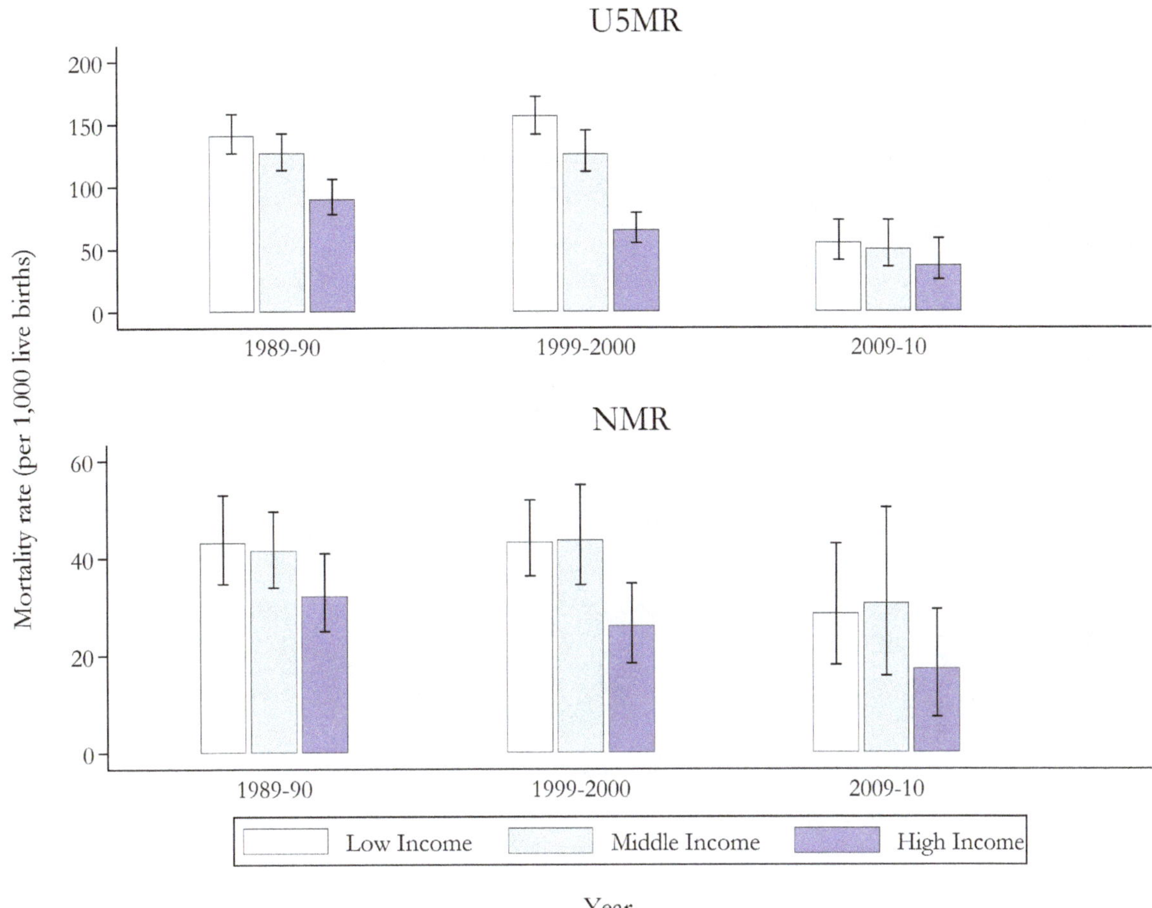

Figure 2. Under-five and neonatal mortality rates (per 1,000 live births) by wealth groups for selected two-year periods, with 95% confidence intervals. *Notes*: See File S1 for full results. The population was divided into thirds using the wealth index. U5MR, under-five mortality rate; NMR, neonatal mortality rate.

disadvantage in some districts where local capacity is weak. The available data, however, did not allow us to explore this further with a reasonable level of robustness. The finding does warrant further quantitative and qualitative examination and suggests the need for disaggregated measures of health outcomes at the district level. Since the mountainous/plateau region has high poverty rates, undernutrition, low density of trained health workers and health services, future research should investigate whether several sources of potential biases exist in the DHS data. For example, it is possible that under-reporting occurs in the poorer and more remote mountainous/plateau region where 90% of births are estimated to take place at home. Under-reporting may be due to a number of issues including shame and stigma of reporting neonatal mortality especially if the birth was attended by a traditional birth attendant.

As with all similar mortality trend studies our analysis is subject to some limitations. First, a household asset index was used as a proxy measure for household wealth. This is a common measure in low-income settings where measures of income are often hard to obtain as many people work in informal labour markets with highly variable incomes often engaging in a mix of cash and non-monetary forms of trade. Similarly, accurate estimates of expenditure and consumption are often hard to obtain [42]. Nevertheless, there is some debate regarding the reliability and validity of the asset index as a proxy measure of household wealth [20,21]. Second, as the DHS is a cross-sectional survey there may be disparity between reported household assets at the time of the survey, as opposed to the time of the reported child death [4]. Third, our analysis does not allow for examination of intra-region disparities. Finally, while pooling the data for various waves helps to reduce recall bias for overlapping periods and provides larger sub-national sample sizes, caution should be exercised when asserting the magnitude of inequalities and any small changes in mortality. Hence, we have emphasised the consistently observed trends in disparities, which are likely to be most valid.

To conclude, the trends revealed in this study suggest that across socioeconomic and geography markers under-five and neonatal mortality have improved in Cambodia although neo-natal mortality has stagnated. Geographical markers suggest entrenched and increased relative inequality in mortality. A number of factors have been discussed which may explain these geographical inequalities. The present study has helped highlight the importance of monitoring equity when evaluating child-health interventions. Cambodia's reliance on periodic household surveys to measure progress in under-five and neonatal mortality and health equity outcomes makes the quality of those surveys and subsequent analysis of particular importance. To meaningfully inform policy

Table 1. Inequalities in under-five and neonatal mortality by wealth for selected years, with 95% confidence intervals and p-values for trend.

Measure	U5MR				NMR			
	1989–90	1999–2000	2009–10	Trend	1989–90	1999–2000	2009–10	Trend
Relative Inequalities								
RR								
Low income	1.57	2.40	1.50	1.037	1.34	1.65	1.65	1.070
	(1.29 to 1.91)	(1.93 to 2.93)	(0.87 to 2.39)	[0.142]	(0.96 to 1.88)	(1.19 to 2.49)	(0.82 to 4.58)	[0.019]
Middle income	1.42	1.93	1.35	1.024	1.29	1.67	1.77	1.064
	(1.16 to 1.71)	(1.56 to 2.43)	(0.77 to 2.36)	[0.186]	(0.93 to 1.77)	(1.16 to 2.61)	(0.79 to 4.8)	[0.003]
RII	1.93	3.43	1.84	1.078	1.52	1.87	1.98	1.114
	(−2.92 to 6.78)	(−14.22 to 21.09)	(−1.99 to 5.67)	[0.096]	(−1.98 to 5.02)	(−9.48 to 13.21)	(−12.87 to 16.83)	[0.057]
Absolute Inequalities								
RD								
Low income	51.19	91.43	18.28	−2.648	10.93	17.12	11.26	0.791
	(29.89 to 73.1)	(72.5 to 110.46)	(−6.98 to 38.44)	[0.177]	(−1.59 to 23.89)	(6.28 to 29.13)	(−5.27 to 30.26)	[0.078]
Middle income	37.38	60.92	12.97	−2.130	9.27	17.50	13.36	0.649
	(16.31 to 56.58)	(42.38 to 82.78)	(−12.24 to 38.13)	[0.154]	(−2.63 to 20.05)	(4.9 to 31.58)	(−5.25 to 33.87)	[0.049]
SII	75.91	133.32	28.08	−3.685	16.18	16.70	16.70	1.189
	(−190.53 to 342.34)	(−285.28 to 551.93)	(−61.23 to 117.39)	[0.180]	(−69.24 to 101.59)	(−186.85 to 233.6)	(−150.98 to 184.37)	[0.091]

Notes: See File S1 for full results. U5MR, under-five mortality rate; NMR, neonatal mortality rate; CI, confidence interval; RR, rate ratio; RD, rate difference; RII, relative index of inequality; SII, slope index of inequality. 95% confidence intervals are reported in parentheses and p-values in brackets. The small number of observations and possible non-linear relationships implies that the trend estimates should be treated with caution. Additionally, since the bounds of the CI depend on the mean of mortality, comparisons over time must be treated cautiously.

Table 2. Inequalities in under-five and neonatal mortality (per 1,000 live births) by rural-urban and regions for selected years, with 95% confidence intervals and *p*-values for trend.

Equity Marker	U5MR				NMR			
	RR	95% CI	RD	95% CI	RR	95% CI	RD	95% CI
Urban/Rural (base = Urban)								
Rural								
1989–90	1.56	(1.18 to 2.04)	44.9	(18.68 to 66.73)	2.00	(1.31 to 3.28)	21.0	(9.62 to 31)
1999–2000	1.56	(1.23 to 1.86)	46.4	(22.8 to 62.34)	1.40	(1.01 to 2.04)	11.7	(0.22 to 22.02)
2009–10	2.41	(1.12 to 3.64)	31.1	(5.4 to 43.48)	2.91	(1.21 to 7.93)	19.1	(4.25 to 29.48)
Trend [*p*-value]	1.078	[0.012]	−0.562	[0.454]	1.066	[0.050]	0.109	[0.782]
Island Division (base = Phnom Penh)								
Plain								
1989–90	1.42	(0.9 to 2.24)	38.1	(−13.6 to 75)	1.61	(0.87 to 4.26)	17.8	(−6.73 to 38.64)
1999–2000	2.14	(1.22 to 3.52)	71.5	(23.1 to 102.4)	1.50	(0.64 to 4.62)	14.6	(−22.89 to 38.21)
2009–10	5.55	(0.61 to 10.04)	39.0	(−27.8 to 57.8)	6.10	(0.93 to 95.01)	29.4	(2.01 to 50.64)
Trend [*p*-value]	1.112	[0.001]	−1.187	[0.497]	1.160	[0.000]	0.673	[0.150]
Tonle Sap								
1989–90	1.25	(0.8 to 1.96)	23.0	(−28 to 59.3)	0.99	(0.54 to 2.62)	−0.4	(−23.02 to 18.65)
1999–2000	1.92	(1.1 to 3.1)	57.3	(10.9 to 83.1)	1.14	(0.52 to 3.45)	4.0	(−31.35 to 26.04)
2009–10	5.69	(0.65 to 9.58)	40.2	(−24.4 to 55.7)	4.33	(0.67 to 66.08)	19.2	(−5.32 to 36.45)
Trend [*p*-value]	1.113	[0.000]	−0.770	[0.655]	1.163	[0.004]	1.100	[0.180]
Coastal								
1989–90	0.97	(0.61 to 1.66)	−2.3	(−52.9 to 41)	1.20	(0.61 to 3.5)	6.0	(−17.92 to 30.24)
1999–2000	1.86	(1.06 to 3.2)	53.8	(6 to 90.5)	1.34	(0.56 to 4.41)	10.1	(−26.44 to 37.13)
2009–10	7.75	(0.86 to 17.1)	57.9	(−8 to 111.4)	3.75	(0.31 to 55.07)	15.9	(−10.39 to 45.99)
Trend [*p*-value]	1.182	[0.000]	4.103	[0.006]	1.179	[0.007]	1.464	[0.116]
Plateau/Mountain								
1989–90	1.45	(0.93 to 2.34)	41.3	(−10.4 to 84.1)	1.50	(0.8 to 4.01)	14.6	(−9.31 to 36.46)
1999–2000	2.06	(1.17 to 3.36)	66.3	(17.8 to 96)	1.42	(0.59 to 4.32)	12.2	(−25.33 to 35.3)
2009–10	7.21	(0.85 to 12.62)	53.2	(−8.8 to 81)	3.33	(0.44 to 40.02)	13.4	(−10.75 to 33.87)
Trend [*p*-value]	1.144	[0.000]	0.056	[0.977]	1.162	[0.006]	0.993	[0.189]

Notes: See File S1 for full results. U5MR, under-five mortality rate; NMR, neonatal mortality rate; RR, rate ratio; RD, rate difference; CI, confidence interval. The small number of observations and possible non-linear relationships implies that the trend estimates should be treated with caution.

and planning decisions, data must be available at a disaggregated district level that complements the decentralised governance arrangements of the health system. This also requires improving survey quality to allow such analysis. Concurrently strengthening routine health information systems including birth and death registers is vital. Finally, concerted efforts are required to ensure that traditionally disadvantaged populations, start narrowing the inequality gap. This will be dependent on substantial health system investments to ensure the necessary services are accessible to all.

Acknowledgments

The authors thank project staff at School of Population Health, The University of Queensland for their assistance in the development of this paper.

Supporting Information

File S1 Combined Supporting Information file containing: Box S1. Measures of Inequality. **Table S1.** Inequalities in under-five and neonatal mortality (per 1,000 live births) by wealth for all years, with 95% confidence intervals and *p*-values for trend. **Table S2.** Inequalities in under-five and neonatal mortality (per 1,000 live births) by rural/urban location and regions for all years, with 95% confidence intervals and *p*-values for trend. **Table S3.** Under-five mortality rates per 1,000 live births. **Table S4.** Neonatal mortality rates per 1,000 live births.

Author Contributions

Conceived and designed the experiments: EJS AH. Performed the experiments: AH. Analyzed the data: EJS JD AH. Contributed reagents/materials/analysis tools: EJS JD AH. Wrote the paper: EJS JD AH.

References

1. Ahmed S, Hill K (2011) Maternal mortality estimation at the subnational level: A model-based method with an application to Bangladesh. Bulletin of the World Health Organisation 89: 12–21.
2. Mulholland E, Smith L, Carneiro I, Becher H, Lehmann D (2008) Equity and child-survival strategies. Bulletin of the World Health Organization 86: 399–407.
3. Wagstaff A (2000) Socioeconomic inequalities in child mortality: Comparisons across nine developing countries. Bulletin of the World Health Organization 78: 19–29.
4. Dingle A, Powell-Jackson T, Goodman C (2013) A decade of improvements in equity of access to reproductive and maternal health services in Cambodia, 2000–2010. Int J Equity Health 12: 51.
5. Boerma JT, Bryce J, Kinfu Y, Axelson H, Victora CG (2008) Mind the gap: equity and trends in coverage of maternal, newborn, and child health services in 54 Countdown countries. Lancet 371: 1259–1267.
6. Bauze AE, Tran LN, Nguyen K-H, Firth S, Eliana J-S, et al. (2012) Equity and geography: The case of child mortality in Papua New Guinea. PLoS ONE 7: e37861.
7. Singh A, Pathak, Chauhan RK, Pan W (2011) Infant and child mortality in India in the last two decades: a geospatial analysis. PLoS ONE 6: e26856.
8. World Bank (2014). World Bank Databank. Available: http://databank.worldbank.org/. Accessed 2014 Apr 5.
9. National Institute of Statistics, Directorate General for Health, Macro I (2011) Cambodia Demographic and Health Survey 2010. Phnom Penh, Cambodia and Calverton, Maryland, USA: National Institute of Statistics, Directorate General for Health, and ICF Macro.
10. Institute for Health Metrics and Evaluation (2013). Global Burden of Disease Estimates 2010. Available: http://www.healthdata.org/gbd. Accessed 2014 Apr 15.
11. MoH Cambodia (2006) Cambodia Child Survival Strategy, 2006–2015. Phnom Penh: Ministry of Health and World Health Organization.
12. Hong R, Mishra V, Michael J (2007) Economic disparity and child survival in Cambodia. Asia Pacific Journal of Public Health 19: 37–44.
13. Hardeman W, Van Damme W, Van Pelt M, Por I, Kimvan H, et al. (2004) Access to health care for all? User fees plus a Health Equity Fund in Sotnikum, Cambodia. Health Policy Plan 19: 22–32.
14. Ir P, Horemans D, Souk N, Van Damme W (2010) Using targeted vouchers and health equity funds to improve access to skilled birth attendants for poor women: a case study in three rural health districts in Cambodia. BMC Pregnancy Childbirth 10: 1.
15. Jacobs B, Price N (2004) The impact of the introduction of user fees at a district hospital in Cambodia. Health Policy Plan 19: 310–321.
16. Jacobs B, Price N (2006) Improving access for the poorest to public sector health services: insights from Kirivong Operational Health District in Cambodia. Health Policy Plan 21: 27–39.
17. Liljestrand J, Sambath MR (2012) Socio-economic improvements and health system strengthening of maternity care are contributing to maternal mortality reduction in Cambodia. Reprod Health Matters 20: 62–72.
18. Hong R, Chhea V (2010) Trend and inequality in immunization dropout among young children in Cambodia. Matern Child Health J 14: 446–452.
19. Asian Development Bank (2012) Cambodia: Country poverty analysis. Mandaluyong City, Philippines: Asian Development Bank.
20. Sahn DE, Stifel D (2003) Exploring alternative measures of welfare in the absence of expenditure data. Rev Incom Wealt 49: 463–489.
21. Wagstaff A, Watanabe N (2003) What difference does the choice of SES make in health inequality measurement? Health Econics 12: 885–890.
22. Vyas S, Kumaranayake L (2006) Constructing socio-economic status indices: How to use principal components analysis. Health Policy and Planning 21: 459–468.
23. Filmer D, Pritchett LH (2001) Estimating wealth effects without expenditure data–or tears: An application to educational enrollments in states of India. Demography 38: 115–132.
24. Rajaratnam JK, Tran LN, Lopez AD, Murray CJL (2010) Measuring under-five mortality: validation of new low-cost methods. PLoS Medicine 7: e1000253.
25. Nguyen K-H, Jimenez-Soto E, Morgan A, Morgan C, Hodge A (2012) How does progress towards the MDG 4 affect inequalities between different sub-populations? Evidence from Nepal. Journal of Epidemiology & Community Health forthcomin.
26. King G, Tomz M, Wittenberg J (2000) Making the most of statistical analyses: Improving interpretation and presentation. American Journal of Political Science 44: 341–355.
27. Harper S, King NB, Young ME (2013) Impact of selective evidence presentation on judgments of health inequality trends: an experimental study. PLoS ONE 8: e63362.
28. Mackenbach J, Kunst A (1997) Measuring the magnitude of socio-economic inequalities in health: an overview of available measures illustrated with two examples from Europe. Social Science & Medicine 44: 757–771.
29. Blakely T, Tobias M, Atkinson J (2008) Inequalities in mortality during and after restructuring of the New Zealand economy: repeated cohort studies. British Medical Journal 336: 371–375.
30. Pamuk ER (1985) Social class inequality in mortality from 1921 to 1972 in England and Wales. Population studies 39: 17–31.
31. Hayes LJ, Berry G (2002) Sampling variability of the Kunst-Mackenbach relative index of inequality. Journal of Epidemiology and Community Health 56: 762–765.
32. Sasaki Y, Ali M, Kakimoto K, Saroeun O, Kanal K, et al. (2010) Predictors of exclusive breast-feeding in early infancy: a survey report from Phnom Penh, Cambodia. J Pediatr Nurs 25: 463–469.
33. Marriott BP, White AJ, Hadden L, Davies JC, Wallingford JC (2010) How well are infant and young child World Health Organization (WHO) feeding indicators associated with growth outcomes? An example from Cambodia. Matern Child Nutr 6: 358–373.
34. Ministry of Health (2006) National strategy for reproductive and sexual health in Cambodia (2006–2010). Phnom Penh, Cambodia: Ministry of Health.
35. Jacobs B, Ir P, Bigdeli M, Annear PL, Van Damme W (2012) Addressing access barriers to health services: an analytical framework for selecting appropriate interventions in low-income Asian countries. Health Policy and Planning 27: 288–300.
36. Cui L, Yan G, Sattabongkot J, Cao Y, Chen B, et al. (2012) Malaria in the Greater Mekong Subregion: Heterogeneity and complexity. Acta Tropica 121: 227–239.
37. Hong R, Mishra V (2006) Effect of wealth inequality on chronic under-nutrition in Cambodian children. J Health Popul Nutr 24: 89–99.
38. Wang W (2013) Assessing Trends in Inequalitieis in Maternal and child Health and Health Care in Cambodia: DHS Further Analysis Reports No. 86. Calverton, Maryland: ICF International.
39. Zimmer Z (2008) Poverty, wealth inequality and health among older adults in rural Cambodia. Soc Sci Med 66: 57–71.
40. Dettrick Z, Jimenez-Soto E, Hodge A (2014) Socioeconomic and geographical disparities in under-five and neonatal mortality in Uttar Pradesh, India. Maternal and child health journal 18: 960–969.
41. Kanbur R, Rhee C, Zhuang J, editors (2014) Inequality in Asia and the Pacific: Trends, drivers and policy implications. London: Asian Development Bank Institute and Routledge.

42. Moser C, Felton A (2007) The construction of an asset index measuring asset accumulation in Ecuador. CPRC Working Paper 87. University of Manchester, UK: Chronic Poverty Research Centre.
43. Cleveland W, Loader C (1996) Smoothing by local regression: principles and methods. In: Haerdle W, Schimek M, editors. Statistical theory and computational aspects of smoothing. New York, USA: Springer.
44. Murray CJL, Laakso T, Shibuya K, Hill K, Lopez AD (2007) Can we achieve Millennium Development Goal 4? New analysis of country trends and forecasts of under-5 mortality to 2015. The Lancet 370: 1040–1054.

17

Risk of Childhood Overweight after Exposure to Tobacco Smoking in Prenatal and Early Postnatal Life

Susanne Eifer Møller[1¶], Teresa Adeltoft Ajslev[2*¶], Camilla Schou Andersen[2], Christine Dalgård[3], Thorkild I. A. Sørensen[2,4]

1 Institute of Public Health, Epidemiology, Biostatistics and Biodemography, University of Southern Denmark, Odense, Denmark, 2 Institute of Preventive Medicine, Bispebjerg and Frederiksberg Hospitals, The Capital Region, Denmark, 3 Institute of Public Health, Environmental Medicine, University of Southern Denmark, Odense, Denmark, 4 Novo Nordisk Foundation Centre for Basic Metabolic Research, Faculty of Health and Medical Sciences, University of Copenhagen, Copenhagen, Denmark

Abstract

Objective: To investigate the association between exposure to mothers smoking during prenatal and early postnatal life and risk of overweight at age 7 years, while taking birth weight into account.

Methods: From the Danish National Birth Cohort a total of 32,747 families were identified with available information on maternal smoking status in child's pre- and postnatal life and child's birth weight, and weight and height at age 7 years. Outcome was overweight according to the International Obesity Task Force gender and age specific body mass index. Smoking exposure was categorized into four groups: no exposure (n = 25,076); exposure only during pregnancy (n = 3,343); exposure only postnatally (n = 140); and exposure during pregnancy and postnatally (n = 4,188). Risk of overweight according to smoking status as well as dose-response relationships were estimated by crude and adjusted odds ratios using logistic regression models.

Results: Exposure to smoking only during pregnancy, or both during pregnancy and postnatally were both significantly associated with overweight at 7 years of age (OR: 1.31, 95% CI: 1.15–1.48, and OR: 1.76, 95% CI: 1.58–1.97, respectively). Analyses excluding children with low birth weight (<2,500 gram) revealed similar results. A significant prenatal dose-response relationship was found. Per one additional cigarette smoked per day an increase in risk of overweight was observed (OR: 1.02, 95% CI: 1.01–1.03). When adjusting for quantity of smoking during pregnancy, prolonged exposure after birth further increased the risk of later overweight in the children (OR 1.28, 95% CI:1.09–1.50) compared with exposure only in the prenatal period.

Conclusions: Mother's perinatal smoking increased child's OR of overweight at age 7 years irrespective of birth weight, and with higher OR if exposed both during pregnancy and in early postnatal life. Clear dose-response relationships were observed, which emphasizes the need for prevention of any tobacco exposure of infants.

Editor: Mohammad Ali, Johns Hopkins Bloomberg School of Public Health, United States of America

Funding: The DNBC has been funded by the Danish National Research Foundation, Pharmacy Foundation, the March of Dimes Birth Defects Foundation, the Augustinus Foundation, and the Health Foundation. TAA received grants from the UNIK Food, Fitness and Pharma program, grant 28a, supported by the Danish Ministry of Science, Technology and Innovation. The funders had no role in study design, data collection and analysis, decision to publish, or preparation of the manuscript.

Competing Interests: The authors have declared that no competing interests exist.

* Email: teresa.ajslev@regionh.dk

¶ These authors are shared first authors on this work.

Introduction

Worldwide, the prevalence of overweight children and adults has increased greatly over the past three decades [1–3]. Although recent research suggests a levelling off in the obesity epidemic, childhood overweight remains an important health problem [4,5].

Smoking during pregnancy is associated with overweight in offspring, which has been demonstrated in a number of studies and confirmed by recent meta-analyses [6–10]. Even though Oken et al's meta-analysis confirmed the association, the analysis was limited by small studies, different definitions of overweight, and by heterogeneity in offspring ages [8]. Maternal smoking during pregnancy may cause intrauterine growth restriction, and is associated with low birth weight (BW) [11]. Limited numbers of studies have looked into the influence of low BW [12] and catch up growth in early childhood on this [13–15]. Catch-up growth refers to accelerated growth in early infancy to compensate for low BW [11,16,17], and has been demonstrated to be an independent risk factor for childhood overweight [9,18]. Other known risk factors are also likely to modify the association between smoking and childhood overweight, such as maternal obesity, maternal gestational weight gain, socio-occupational status, and breastfeeding [7,9,19]. Few studies demonstrate dose-response relationship between maternal smoking during pregnancy and risk of overweight in childhood [10,20–22]. A recent study by Harris et al. revealed that exposure to parental smoking during pregnancy

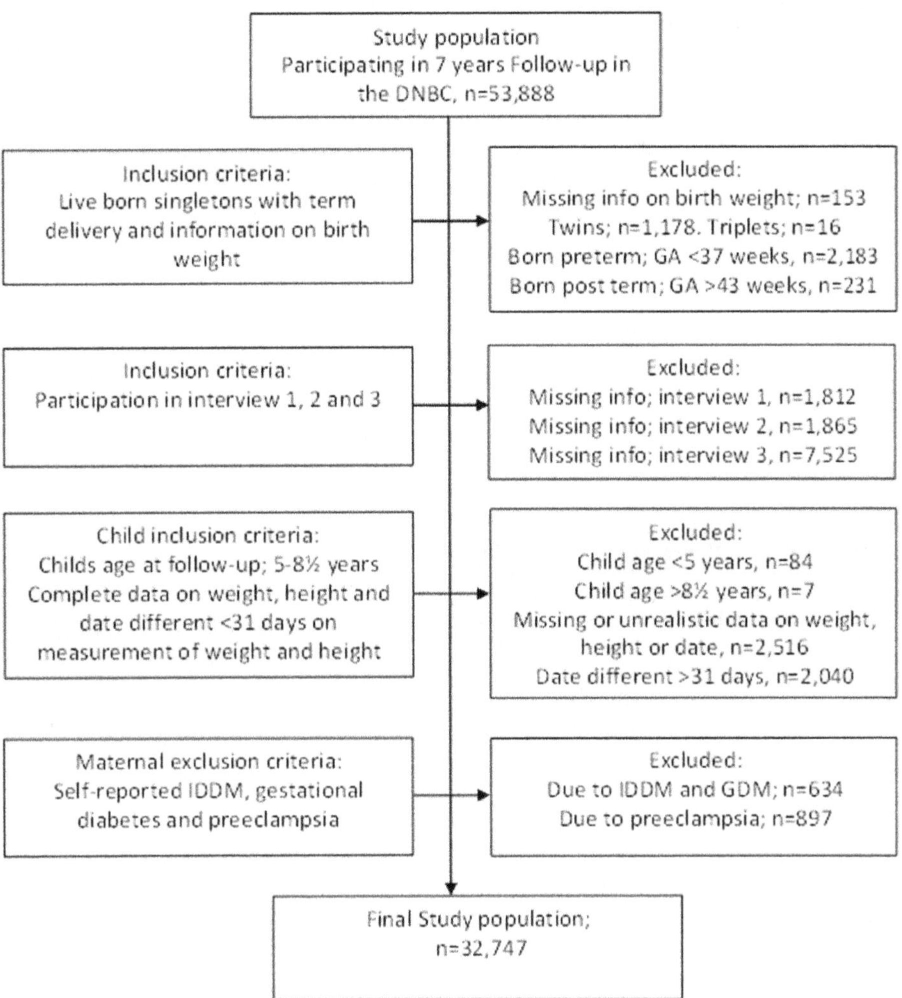

Figure 1. The figure show a flow chart of the study population.

increased the risk of overweight in daughters in adolescence and adulthood in a dose-response manner [23]. Although this was investigated in a very large sample, information on exposure was based on long term recall and limited to exposure of smoking during pregnancy [23].

The child's early postnatal period, while being breastfed, is suggested to be a critical period for mothers smoking exposure [24]. Therefore, we suspected that exposure to maternal smoking also in the early postnatal period throughout lactation might prolong the negative effect on child's health, and may in turn increase the risk of childhood overweight. However, previous studies of the postnatal period are few and the results are not conclusive [24–26]. In a birth cohort study with follow-up at 8 years of 609 children, Florath et al [25] showed that smoking by both mothers and fathers pre- as well as postnatally were associated with increased BMI of their children at 8 years of age. However, they interpreted their findings as indications of confounding by life style, rather than specific intrauterine effects of maternal smoking, which clearly calls for more investigations.

With use of a large cohort, including comprehensive information on mother and child, the objectives were to investigate dose-response relationships of mother's smoking during the child's prenatal period. Furthermore, the aim was to investigate whether mother's prolongation of smoking into the child's early postnatal life while breastfeeding the child, was an independent risk factor, in an otherwise healthy population of mothers and children. Finally, we wanted to investigate whether these relations were independent of the child's BW.

Materials and Methods

Data from The Danish National Birth Cohort (DNBC) were used, which originally included 101,042 pregnant women, who gave birth to a child between 1996 and 2002 [27]. Mothers were interviewed by telephone twice during pregnancy, approximately at week 16 and 30 (Interviews 1 and 2) as well as postnatally, when the child was 6 and 18 month old (Interviews 3 and 4). The 7-year follow-up was carried out from 2005 to 2010 using a mailed questionnaire, where 53,888 mothers and children responded. Mothers were asked to report their child's latest measurement on height and weight at the 7-year follow-up [28,29].

To be included in the present study, the children should be born singleton, alive, and at term (≥37 gestational weeks). Only mother-child pairs, where mothers had participated in Interviews 1, 2 and 3, and with children's complete data on height and weight at the 7-year follow-up were included. Also, child's height and weight should have been measured less than 31 days apart, and the child's age should be between 5 and 8½ year at follow-up. In 31

Maternal and paternal smoking during pregnancy		
Questions asked around gestational week 16 (Interview 1) and 30 (Interview 2)		
Interview 1	•	Did you smoke during pregnancy -please also think back to the beginning of the pregnancy?
	•	Do you smoke now?
	•	How much did you smoke on average?
	•	Does your spouse or partner smoke?
Interview 2	•	Have you smoked since last interveiw?
	•	Do you smoke now?
Maternal smoking postpartum		
Questions asked 6 months after birth		
Interview 3	•	Did you smoke during the period of breastfeeding?

Figure 2. The figure show questions assessing information on maternal and paternal smoking exposure from Interview 1 (obtained around gestational week 16), Interview 2 (obtained around gestational week 32), and Interview 3 (obtained 6 months after child birth).

children, height and weight measures were changed to missing, due to possible errors in the registered measures; being height below 100 cm or above 150 cm, or weight below 15 or above 45 kilos, corresponding to the criteria set by the DNBC, www.dnbc.dk. We excluded mothers with preeclampsia, gestational diabetes and diabetes mellitus. A total of 32,747 mother-child pairs fulfilled these criteria. The inclusions and exclusions are shown in Figure 1.

Ethical statement

The Danish Committee on Biomedical Research Ethics has approved the Danish National Birth Cohort (case no. (KF) 01-471/94). Each participant gave written informed consent at enrollment into the Danish National Birth Cohort. According to the principles stated by the ethics comitees, participants have the right to have their data removed from the cohort at any time. Children born into the cohort participate on their mothers written informed consent until they are able to decide for themselves at age 18 years. The Danish Data Protection Agency has approved the cohort (case no. 2008-54-0431) and the 7-year follow-up (case no. 2004-41-4078). The Danish Data Protection Agency and the Institutional Board Committee of the Danish National Birth Cohort approved the present study.

Exposure variable

Maternal smoking was assessed both at Interview 1 and 2 during pregnancy. Postnatal smoking habits from birth through 6 months during the period of lactation were assessed in Interview 3. The questions assessing maternal smoking are shown in Figure 2. The questions could be answered with yes or no, except the question concerning quantity of smoking during pregnancy. If a woman answered yes in either Interview 1 or in Interview 2, she was categorized as a smoker during pregnancy. The study population was categorized in four groups according to answers from Interviews 1 to 3:1) No smoking 76.6% (n = 25,076); 2) Smoking only during pregnancy 10.2% (n = 3,343); 3) Smoking only postnatally 0.4% (n = 140); and 4) Smoking both during pregnancy and postnatally 12.8% (n = 4,188). Information on quantity of maternal smoking in numbers of cigarettes smoked daily in early pregnancy was obtained from Interview 1, Figure 2. We used quantity of maternal smoking as a continuous variable (1-54 cigarettes) and subsequently categorized it into six groups; 0, <1, 1–4, 5–9, 10–14, 15–19 and ≥20 cigarettes daily, where 0 cigarettes daily were non-smokers.

Outcome variable

The endpoint was overweight at age 7 years. Body Mass Index (BMI = weight (kg)/height (m) ^{2}) was calculated based on the recorded weight and height at the 7-year follow-up. We used the International Obesity Task Force standards to define overweight in children with age- and sex specific cut off points for BMI [30]. Overweight was recorded as a dichotomous variable with obese children included in the overweight group. The reported data on the children's height and weight have been validated previously [31], which showed that they were without any noteworthy random or systematic bias.

Covariates

From Interview 1, information on parity, socio-occupational status, paternal smoking, as well as maternal pre-pregnancy weight and height was obtained. Parity was coded as either primiparous or multiparous. Socio-occupational status was categorized as high, middle, and low, based on the parents combined status. High represented manager position or long/middle long education, middle represented skilled workers or workers with short education, and low represented unskilled workers, with no education, or on special allowance. The question about paternal smoking was coded either smoking or non-smoking, and it was included as a possible confounder influencing the child's odds ratio of overweight independently of the mother's smoking [25,32,33]. Using self-reported pre-pregnancy weight and height, maternal pre-pregnancy BMI was calculated and used as a continuous variable and subsequently categorized in groups for descriptive purpose; <18.5 kg/m^2,18.5–24.9 kg/m^2, 25–29.9 kg/m^2 and ≥30 kg/m^2. From Interview 3, information on maternal gestational weight gain and exclusive breastfeeding was recorded. Both gestational weight gain and breastfeeding were used as continuous variables and categorized into groups; <10 kg, 10–17.99 kg and ≥18 kg and 0 (no breastfeeding), <14 weeks, 14–22 weeks and >22 weeks, respectively. Paternal BMI was calculated from height and weight measures reported at Interview 4, and used as a continuous as well as group variable; <18.5 kg/m^2,18.5–24.9 kg/m^2, 25–29.9 kg/m^2 and ≥30 kg/m. From The Danish Medical Birth Registry information on pregnancy outcome, maternal age, date of birth, gestational age at birth, child sex and BW was obtained. Gestational age was used as a continuous variable. We categorized BW into groups; <2,500 gram, 2,500–4,000 gram and>4,000 g, with low BW defined as a BW <2,500 gram.

Statistical analyses

Between-group differences were tested with Chi-square tests. Risk of overweight, if exposed to maternal smoking during pre- and postnatal life, was estimated by crude and adjusted odds ratios (OR) using univariate and multiple logistic regression analysis with adjustments according to two models, Model 1 and Model 2. Exposure to smoking during and/or after pregnancy was categorized into the described four groups with no smoking as the reference group. We tested for interactions in the association under study and with the following covariates; maternal pre-pregnancy BMI, BW, breastfeeding and child sex. We found no interactions with any of these covariates, except for BW. Thus, maternal pre-pregnancy BMI, and child sex were included as covariates in Model 1 adjusted analyses and breastfeeding was included as a variable contributing to the associations in Model 2 analyses. As low BW modified the effect of maternal smoking on child's risk of overweight additional analyses stratified on BW with adjustment for confounding according to Model 1 were performed. In the first adjusted Model 1, the following pre-specified covariates were entered: Maternal age, maternal pre-pregnancy BMI, gestational weight gain, paternal smoking, socio-occupational status, parity, gestational age, child sex and BW. Model 2 included Model 1 covariates and paternal BMI and breastfeeding. Dose-response relationships were investigated in various ways through multiple logistic regression models to estimate the risk of overweight with increasing quantity of smoking. Analyses were performed for different groups corresponding to either smoke exposure during pregnancy only, or smoke exposure both during pregnancy and postnatally adjusting for prenatal smoke amount. Quantity of maternal smoking was included in groups as described previously, and adjusted for confounding according to Model 1. Moreover, as no interaction with smoking postnatally (yes/no) was observed on risk of overweight with prenatal smoking, another logistic regression model was performed, which included prenatal smoking as a linear variable and smoking postnatally as a categorial variable. In all analyses, a p-value<0.05 was considered statistically significant. Since some mothers (n = 1,233, 4,1%) were entered twice into the cohort, additional regression analyses, using a cluster option taking into account the dependency between the siblings, were carried out for the main results; however, as expected, this did not alter the estimates and widened the confidence intervals only minimally, so the results are presented without this correction. Statistical analyses were performed using: STATA release 11 IC software.

Results

Smoking habits

A total of 76.6% were nonsmokers and 23.4% reported smoking during pregnancy and/or postnatally, Table 1. Mothers who smoked during pregnancy had higher maternal gestational weight gain and were of lower socio-occupational status. They gave birth to children with lower BW and were more likely not breastfed or had "short duration" of breastfeeding than children of nonsmoking mothers (all p-values<0.001), Table 1.

Overweight at 7 years of age

A total of 9.4% (n = 3,085) of the children were overweight. Overweight was more prevalent in girls (10.4%) than in boys (8.5%) (p<0.001), Table 2. Overweight children had higher BW and were more likely not breastfed or had "short duration" of breastfeeding. Their parents were more often overweight or obese and more often of lower socio-occupational status (all p-values <0.001, except for maternal age p = 0.027), Table 2.

Smoking habits and risk of overweight

Figure 3 shows the risk of overweight at age 7 years with different exposure windows during pregnancy and postnatally. Exposure to smoking only during pregnancy or both during pregnancy and postnatally were significantly associated with childhood overweight at age 7 years (OR: 1.31, 95% CI: 1.15–1.48, and OR: 1.76, 95% CI: 1.58–1.97, respectively). A similar tendency was found for the association between exposure to smoking only postnatally and childhood overweight (OR: 1.46, 95% CI: 0.86–2.49). In addition, a significantly higher risk of overweight was observed with exposure to smoking both during pregnancy and postnatally than exposure to smoking only during pregnancy (OR: 1.35, 95% CI: 1.16–1.56). All results were adjusted according to Model 1. None of the included confounders altered the result notably when tested separately, except adjustment for paternal smoking which slightly lowered the risk estimates. In the adjusted model, paternal smoking increased the OR of overweight (OR: 1.27, 95% CI: 1.17–1.39). Additional adjustment (Model 2) for paternal BMI and breastfeeding influenced the risk estimates to a minor degree, Figure 3. Thus, only Model 1 adjustments were carried forward in analyses of pre- and postnatal smoking in which we investigated and adjusted for prenatal quantity of smoking.

Quantity of daily smoking and risk of overweight

Increasing number of cigarettes smoked daily during pregnancy was significantly associated with increased risk of childhood overweight at age 7 years. This pattern appeared for groups of smoking only during pregnancy, as well as smoking both during pregnancy and postnatally, Figure 4. The prenatal dose-response relationship was significant; per one additional cigarette smoked per day an increase in risk of childhood overweight was observed (OR:1.02, 95% CI: 1.01–1.03), Table 3. The risk of overweight increased significantly if exposed to smoking both during pregnancy and in early postnatal life than to exposure only during pregnancy (OR:1.28, 95% CI: 1.09–1.50), Table 3.

Smoking habits, birth weight and risk of overweight

The prevalence of children born with BW <2,500 gram was 0.8% (n = 246) in the study population. Low BW was more frequent in children of smoking than non-smoking mothers. Within the small group of children born with low BW, the risk of overweight was considerably increased if exposed to maternal smoking during pregnancy (Crude OR: 12.60, 95% CI: 2.40–65.55) than in low BW children not exposed to smoking during pregnancy. Hence, adjusted analyses showed that children with BW≥2,500 gram, who were exposed to maternal smoking also had a significantly higher risk of overweight at 7 years of age compared with the unexposed children. This was the case if exposed to maternal smoking only during pregnancy as well as both during pregnancy and postnatally (OR: 1.29, 95% CI: 1.13–1.46 and OR: 1.76, 95% CI: 1.57–1.96, respectively) than in children of non-smoking mothers.

Discussion

This large prospective cohort study showed an increased risk of overweight in children at age 7 years, if exposed to maternal smoking during pregnancy or both during pregnancy and in early postnatal life compared with children of non-smoking mothers. In addition, a clear dose-response relationship was observed between quantity of prenatal smoking exposure and risk of overweight at age 7 years, while taking into account postnatal smoke exposure. Moreover, exposure to smoking both during pregnancy and postnatally lead to a significantly higher risk of overweight compared with smoking exposure only during pregnancy. Thus, maternal smoking either during pregnancy, or postnatally are both independent risk factors for overweight at age 7 years and is independent of BW and breastfeeding.

A growing number of studies have reported maternal smoking during pregnancy as a risk factor for childhood overweight [8,10,19,34–37]. In 2008, Oken et al conducted a meta-analysis on the association between maternal smoking during pregnancy and offspring's risk of overweight, and confirmed that maternal smoking during pregnancy was significantly associated with childhood overweight (OR: 1.50, 95% CI: 1.36–1.65) [8]. The

Table 1. Distribution of covariates in relation to maternal smoking status.

Maternal smoking		No smoking		Smoking only during pregnancy		Smoking only postnatally		Smoking during pregnancy and postnatally		
		n = 25,076		n = 3,343		n = 140		n = 4,188		
		%	±SD	%	±SD	%	±SD	%	±SD	p-value*
		76.6		10.2		0.4		12.8		
Birth weight (g)	Mean	3.688	±486	3.658	±507	3.714	±507	3.456	±494	
	<2,500	0.5		1.1		0.7		1.9		<0.001
	2,500–4,000	73.0		73.5		72.2		83.6		
	>4,000	26.5		25.4		27.1		14.5		
Parity	Primiparous	44.2		57.4		37.9		42.6		<0.001
	Multiparous	55.8		42.6		62.1		57.4		
Sex	Boy	51.6		50.0		49.3		49.5		0.027
	Girl	48.4		50.0		50.7		50.5		
Breast feeding (weeks)	Mean	16.8	±6.8	15.2	±7.7	17.6	±5.7	14.4	±7.3	
	None	4.0		8.3		4.3		3.4		<0.001
	<14	17.1		22.6		9.4		34.1		
	14–22	63.4		56.5		72.6		52.9		
	>22	15.5		12.6		13.7		9.6		
Maternal age (years)	Mean	30.9	±4.1	30.0	±4.2	30.1	±3.7	30.5	±4.6	
	16–25	6.0		11.2		7.2		11.3		<0.001
	25–29.99	38.0		41.7		45.0		35.7		
	30–34.99	39.8		34.9		36.4		35.8		
	≥35	16.2		12.2		11.4		17.2		
Socio-occupational status	High	73.6		66.9		77.2		51.7		<0.001
	Middel	24.2		29.7		22.1		41.5		
	Low	2.2		3.4		0.7		6.8		
Maternal gestational Weight gain (kg)	Mean	14.7	±5.1	17.3	±6.3	16.8	±6.3	15.1	±6.2	
	<10	12.2		7.7		7.9		15.9		<0.001
	10–17.99	61.9		47.0		55.4		51.6		
	≥18	25.9		45.3		36.7		32.5		
Maternal pre-pregnancy BMI (kg/m^2)	Mean	23.4	±4.0	23.3	±4.1	22.8	±3.1	23.3	±4.1	
	<18.5	3.8		4.5		6.4		6.3		<0.001
	18.5–24.9	70.8		70.4		69.8		67.7		
	25–29.9	18.5		18.5		20.9		18.6		
	≥30	6.8		6.5		2.9		7.4		

Table 1. Cont.

Maternal smoking		No smoking		Smoking only during pregnancy		Smoking only postnatally		Smoking during pregnancy and postnatally		
		n = 25,076		n = 3,343		n = 140		n = 4,188		
		%	±SD	%	±SD	%	±SD	%	±SD	p-value*
Paternal BMI (kg/m^2)	Mean	25.0	±3.7	25.3	±3.7	25.8	±4.1	25.3	±3.4	
	<18.5	0.4		0.2		0.0		0.3		<0.001
	18.5–24.9	55.5		52.1		54.2		52.8		
	25–29.9	38.1		40.3		35.0		38.2		
	≥30	6.0		7.4		10.8		8.7		
Paternal smoking	No	79.6		55.1		59.3		38.3		<0.001
	Yes	20.4		44.9		40.7		61.7		

Abbreviations: BMI: Body Mass Index. Missing information on variables; Parity (n = 16), maternal gestational weight gain (n = 284), maternal pre- pregnancy BMI (n = 453), socio-occupational status (n = 91), paternal smoking (n = 500), paternal BMI (n = 6,570) and breastfeeding (n = 8,998). * χ^2-test.

meta-analysis was based on 14 observational studies including in total 84,563 children. However, none of the individual observational studies consisted of more than 8,000 participants, and the meta-analysis was weakened by different definitions of overweight and by heterogenerity in offspring ages (ranging from 3 to 33 years) [8]. The present study, which used a uniform definition of overweight assessed at a well-defined age in a very large population of 32,747 mother-child dyads, could confirm the results from the meta-analysis. Also, we were able to show a very clear dose-response relationship, ie, increasing numbers of cigarettes smoked daily during pregnancy increased the risk of overweight in childhood. This is in agreement with results from another recent study which found a similar dose-response pattern [23]. We were able to expand these findings, by demonstrating that prolonged exposure to smoking both during pregnancy and continuing into the early postnatal period, while adjusting for smoking intensity during pregnancy, further increased the risk of overweight.

We found that low BW modified the association between maternal smoking during pregnancy and risk of overweight at 7 years of age. Indeed, children born at term with low BW had a much higher risk of childhood overweight if they were exposed to maternal smoking during pregnancy than children with low BW not exposed to smoking during pregnancy. This may either be a chance finding or have a yet unknown biological basis, such as a particular susceptibility in low birth weight infants to smoking-induced maternal inflammatory oxidative stress, leading to epigenetic changes and/or programming effects in the child, directly or indirectly related to fat storage and metabolism [38]. When excluding the children born with low BW from the analyses, the risk estimates remained largely unchanged. Thus, our results suggest that children with normal BW (≥2,500 gram) also have an increased risk of overweight if exposed to maternal smoking during pregnancy, revealing that the risk of overweight is independent of low BW, but may be mediated through rapid infant growth. This finding is in agreement with a recent study by Beyerlein et al showing that among 12,383 German children, low BW was unlikely to be the main cause for the association between intrauterine smoking exposure and higher BMI in later life [12]. Adjustment for paternal smoking weakend the strength of the association and father's smoking may be an independent risk factor. In a recent study Florath et al. showed that paternal smoking and smoking of both parents at pre- and postnatal periods increased risk of offspring overweight [25]. Future studies should assess the influence of both maternal and paternal smoking exposures, in which the timing and the possible effects of passive smoking is investigated in more detail both before pregnancy, during pregnancy and postpartum.

Our study sought to address the independent influence of exposure to maternal smoking during the postnatal period only, on risk of overweight. However, the group with exposure to smoking only postnatally was small (n = 140). We found a tendency towards an increased risk of overweight if exposed to maternal smoking only postnatally, but it was not statistically significant. The observation was nevertheless in agreement with a previous study by Raum et al, who found a positive association between exposure to maternal smoking in the child's first year and childhood overweight (OR: 2.08, 95% CI: 1.02–4.24) [24], but others have failed to detect such an association [26]. On the other hand, our study found an increased risk of overweight in children exposed to smoking both during pregnancy and in early postnatal life compared to exposure only during pregnancy, after controlling for the quantity of smoking during pregnancy, which suggest that exposure postnatally is also an important risk factor. Maternal

Table 2. Distribution of covariates according to normal weight and overweight children.

		Normal weight		Overweight*		
		n = 29,662		n = 3,085		
		%	±SD	%	±SD	p-value**
Child weight group at age 7 years		90.6		9.4		
Birth weight (g)	Mean	3.643	±490	3.782	±518	
	<2,500	0.8		0.5		<0.001
	2,500–4,000	75.4		65.3		
	>4,000	23.9		34.2		
Parity	Primiparous	45.7		41.2		<0.001
	Multiparous	54.3		58.8		
Sex	Boy	51.7		46.3		<0.001
	Girl	48.3		53.7		
Breast feeding (weeks)	None	4.1		6.8		<0.001
	<14	19.2		24.2		
	14–22	62.0		56.8		
	>22	14.7		12.2		
Maternal age (years)	Mean	30.7	±4.1	30.7	±4.3	
	<25	7.1		8.5		0.027
	25–29.99	38.2		37.3		
	30–34.99	38.9		37.9		
	≥35	15.8		16.3		
Socio- occupational status	High	71.2		60.0		<0.001
	Middel	26.0		35.7		
	Low	2.8		4.3		
Maternal gestational weight gain (kg)	Mean	15.0	±5.3	15.2	±6.4	
	<10	11.8		15.9		<0.001
	10–17.99	59.9		51.2		
	≥18	28.3		32.9		
Maternal pre- pregnancy BMI (kg/m^2)	Mean	23.2	±3.9	25.6	±5.0	
	<18.5	4.5		1.6		<0.001
	18.5–24.9	72.2		52.6		
	25–29.9	17.4		29.5		
	≥30	5.9		16.3		
Paternal BMI (kg/m^2)	Mean	24.9	±3.1	26.6	±3.7	
	<18.5	0.4		0.0		<0.001
	18.5–24.9	56.6		37.2		
	25–29.9	37.3		48.1		
	≥30	5.7		14.7		
Paternal smoking	No	72.7		63.9		<0.001
	Yes	27.3		36.1		

Abbreviations: BMI: Body Mass Index. Missing information on variables; Parity (n = 16), maternal gestational weight gain (n = 284), maternal pre-pregnancy BMI (n = 453), socio-occupational status (n = 91), paternal smoking (n = 500), paternal BMI (n = 6,570) and breastfeeding (n = 8,998). *Obese children are included in the overweight group. ** χ^2-test.

smoking during lactation establish a route for direct exposure to tobacco components. Hence, if mothers smoke and breastfeed then smoking may impose an even larger effect on the child's health, and may in turn increase the risk of childhood overweight. In contrast, breastfeeding is generally found to have a protective effect on overweight and may therefore be beneficial in spite of the possible transmission of chemicals through the breastmilk [7]. Breastfeeding may act both as an effect-modifier and a mediator of the association between postpartum smoke exposure and overweight and the influence may depend on the timing of smoking while breastfeeding and whether the mother inhale the nicotine. Our study found no interaction with mother's breastfeeding, and inclusion of breastfeeding in our categorical analyses of pre-postpartum smoke exposure suggested marginal influence from

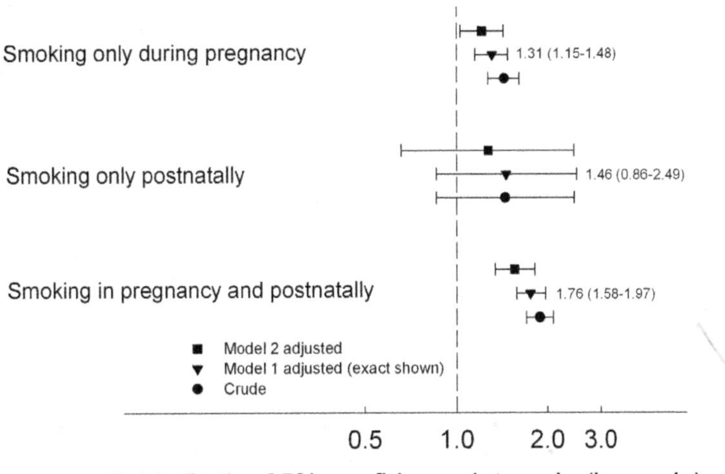

Figure 3. The figure shows the odds ratios with 95% confidence intervals of overweight at age 7 years by different exposure windows of maternal smoking pre- and postnatally. The reference group is children of non-smoking mothers. Model 1 analyses are adjusted for child sex, parity, birth weight, maternal gestational weight gain, maternal age, maternal pre-pregnancy BMI, paternal smoking and socio-occupational status. Exacts estimates with Model 1 adjustments are shown in parentes. Model 2 is adjusted for the same covariates as Model 1, but with additional adjustment for paternal BMI and breastfeeding. Obese children are included in the overweight group.

breastfeeding on the association at interest. Future studies should address the complex influence of mothers smoking while breastfeeding by investigating all beneficial and negative effects. One parameter to measure is the nicotine content of the breastmilk while obtaining information on when mothers smoke while breastfeeding, such as just before or after she breastfeed the child.

In contrast to the conclusions about the observed associations being due to confounding by other life style factors drawn by Florath et al [25], we suggest that the contention that exposure of the fetus and the infant to the chemical content of smoke is a likely

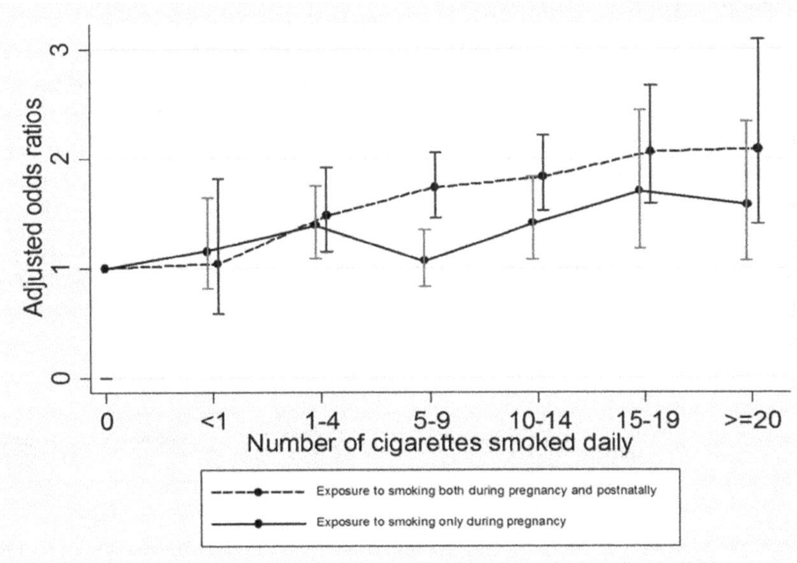

Figure 4. The figure shows the odds ratios of overweight at age 7 years with increasing numbers of cigarettes smoked daily during pregnancy by two different exposure periods, either exposure only during pregnancy, or exposure both during pregnancy and postnatally. The odds ratios were adjusted for child sex, parity, birth weight, gestational age at birth, maternal age at birth, maternal gestational weight gain, maternal pre-pregnancy BMI, paternal smoking and socio-occupational status.

Table 3. The table shows the odds ratios (OR) with 95% confidence intervals (CI) of overweight at age 7 years in children exposed to smoking both during pregnancy and postnatally compared with children exposed only during pregnancy, while adjusting for quantity of prenatal smoking.

Overweight*		Adjusted OR	95% CI	p-value
Smoking during pregnancy and postnatally	vs. smoking exclusively in pregnancy	1.28	1.09–1.50	0.002
One cigarette increase/day during pregnancy		1.02	1.01–1.03	0.003
Maternal age (years)		1.02	0.99–1.03	0.117
Maternal gestational weight gain (kg)		1.02	1.01–1.04	<0.001
Maternal pre- pregnancy BMI (kg/m^2)		1.12	1.11–1.14	<0.001
Paternal smoking	vs. no paternal smoking	1.38	1.18–1.60	<0.001

Odds ratios were additionally adjusted for postnatal smoking, child sex, parity, birth weight, gestational age at birth, and socio-occupational status (not shown). Only mother-child pairs, with information on numbers of cigarettes smoked daily during pregnancy, as well as with information on either smoking during pregnancy only, or smoking both in pregnancy and postnatal, are included in these analyses (n = 6,804). *Obese children are included in the overweight group.
Odds ratios of included covariates i.e. maternal age at birth, maternal gestational weight gain, maternal pre-pregnancy BMI, and paternal smoking are shown as well.

cause of the later overweight may be justified. Moreover, the finding of an even further increased risk of overweight in children who were also exposed to mother's postpartum smoking, and the findings of an increased risk of overweight if fathers smoke as well, suggest that any direct or passive smoking exposure of infants in public or private areas should be avoided, also to avoid other adverse effects [39].

Strength of this study was the prospectively collected information especially on smoking in a large general population based birth cohort which gave us exceptional good opportunities to study the association without the risk of recall bias. However, some limitations have to be kept in mind. Exposure to smoking was based on self-reported smoking habits obtained by interviewer-administrated questionnaires during pregnancy and 6 month postpartum. Loss to follow-up is known to be higher among heavy smokers in this cohort [40,41], and the prevalence of overweight is somewhat lower in the cohort children than in the general population, which may have induced underestimation of the smoking effects. Tobacco smoking, especially during pregnancy and lactation, is not well accepted in many societies. In addition, questions on postnatal smoking were presented along with questions on breastfeeding which may have lead to an underreporting of tobacco use, or in some cases possible misclassification [42,43]. As questions of postpartum smoking in Interview 3 was asked in relation to breastfeeding we may have failed to include some mothers who smoked postpartum, but who reported no breastfeeding. Nevertheless, from the descriptive results (presented in Table 1) we see that at least three per cent of mothers reported smoking without breastfeeding. Moreover, a review and meta-analysis concluded that self-reports of smoking are accurate in most studies [44,45]. The presence of such possible bias may have lowered the observed effect of the postpartum smoke exposure compared with the effect of smoke exposure during pregnancy.

The children were followed up through to age 7 years, and although the outcomes were based on self-reported information, it was concluded in an earlier validation study that the outcome data was valid with no random or systematic bias [31].

Conclusions

Smoking both in the prenatal and early postnatal life, by otherwise healthy mothers increased term delivered childrens risk of overweight at age 7 years, independent of low BW, paternal smoking, and relevant confounders. Prenatal smoking exposure exhibited a clear dose-response relationship. Moreover, if mothers smoking continued into the child's early postnatal life the OR of overweight was significantly higher than for children exposed to smoke only during pregnancy. Findings emphasizes the need for prevention of any tobacco exposure of infants.

Acknowledgments

The authors would like to thank the participating parents for providing detailed health information and the DNBC steering board for allowing the use of data for this study.

Author Contributions

Conceived and designed the experiments: SEM CD TIAS. Analyzed the data: SEM. Contributed reagents/materials/analysis tools: SEM TAA. Wrote the paper: SEM TAA CSA CD TIAS. Generated the figures: SEM TAA.

References

1. Due P, Heitmann BL, Sørensen TIA (2007) Prevalence of obesity in Denmark. Obes Rev 8: 187–189. OBR291 [pii];10.1111/j.1467-789X.2006.00291.x [doi].
2. Han JC, Lawlor DA, Kimm SY (2010) Childhood obesity. Lancet 375: 1737–1748. S0140-6736(10)60171-7 [pii];10.1016/S0140-6736(10)60171-7 [doi].
3. WHO (2000) Obesity: Preventing and managing the global epidemic:Report of a WHO consultation. Geneva:WHO. 894.
4. Rokholm B, Baker JL, Sørensen TIA (2010) The levelling off of the obesity epidemic since the year 1999—a review of evidence and perspectives. Obes Rev 11: 835–846. 10.1111/j.1467-789X.2010.00810.x [doi].
5. Schmidt MC, Rokholm B, Sjoberg BC, Schou AC, Geisler AL, et al. (2013) Trends in prevalence of overweight and obesity in danish infants, children and adolescents—are we still on a plateau? PLoS One 8: e69860. 10.1371/journal.pone.0069860 [doi];PONE-D-13-10725 [pii].
6. Ino T (2010) Maternal smoking during pregnancy and offspring obesity: meta-analysis. Pediatr Int 52: 94–99. PED2883 [pii];10.1111/j.1442-200X.2009.02883.x [doi].
7. Monasta L, Batty GD, Cattaneo A, Lutje V, Ronfani L, et al. (2010) Early-life determinants of overweight and obesity: a review of systematic reviews. Obes Rev 11: 695–708. OBR735 [pii];10.1111/j.1467-789X.2010.00735.x [doi].
8. Oken E, Levitan EB, Gillman MW (2008) Maternal smoking during pregnancy and child overweight: systematic review and meta-analysis. Int J Obes (Lond) 32: 201–210. 0803760 [pii];10.1038/sj.ijo.0803760 [doi].
9. Reilly JJ, Armstrong J, Dorosty AR, Emmett PM, Ness A, et al. (2005) Early life risk factors for obesity in childhood: cohort study. BMJ 330: 1357. bmj.38470.670903.E0 [pii];10.1136/bmj.38470.670903.E0 [doi].
10. von KR, Toschke AM, Koletzko B, Slikker W, Jr. (2002) Maternal smoking during pregnancy and childhood obesity. Am J Epidemiol 156: 954–961.

11. Andersen MR, Simonsen U, Uldbjerg N, Aalkjaer C, Stender S (2009) Smoking cessation early in pregnancy and birth weight, length, head circumference, and endothelial nitric oxide synthase activity in umbilical and chorionic vessels: an observational study of healthy singleton pregnancies. Circulation 119: 857–864. CIRCULATIONAHA.107.755769 [pii];10.1161/CIRCULATIONAHA.107.755769 [doi].
12. Beyerlein A, Ruckinger S, Toschke AM, Schaffrath RA, von KR (2011) Is low birth weight in the causal pathway of the association between maternal smoking in pregnancy and higher BMI in the offspring? Eur J Epidemiol 26: 413–420. 10.1007/s10654-011-9560-y [doi].
13. Ong KK, Ahmed ML, Emmett PM, Preece MA, Dunger DB (2000) Association between postnatal catch-up growth and obesity in childhood: prospective cohort study. BMJ 320: 967–971.
14. Ong KK, Preece MA, Emmett PM, Ahmed ML, Dunger DB (2002) Size at birth and early childhood growth in relation to maternal smoking, parity and infant breast-feeding: longitudinal birth cohort study and analysis. Pediatr Res 52: 863–867. 10.1203/00006450-200212000-00009 [doi].
15. Ong KK (2006) Size at birth, postnatal growth and risk of obesity. Horm Res 65 Suppl 3: 65–69. 91508 [pii];10.1159/000091508 [doi].
16. Horta BL, Victora CG, Menezes AM, Halpern R, Barros FC (1997) Low birthweight, preterm births and intrauterine growth retardation in relation to maternal smoking. Paediatr Perinat Epidemiol 11: 140–151.
17. Ong KK, Dunger DB (2002) Perinatal growth failure: the road to obesity, insulin resistance and cardiovascular disease in adults. Best Pract Res Clin Endocrinol Metab 16: 191–207. 10.1053/beem.2002.0195 [doi];S1521690X02901958 [pii].
18. Monteiro PO, Victora CG (2005) Rapid growth in infancy and childhood and obesity in later life—a systematic review. Obes Rev 6: 143–154. OBR183 [pii];10.1111/j.1467-789X.2005.00183.x [doi].
19. Ino T, Shibuya T, Saito K, Inaba Y (2012) Relationship between body mass index of offspring and maternal smoking during pregnancy. Int J Obes (Lond) 36: 554–558. ijo2011255 [pii];10.1038/ijo.2011.255 [doi].
20. Oken E, Huh SY, Taveras EM, Rich-Edwards JW, Gillman MW (2005) Associations of maternal prenatal smoking with child adiposity and blood pressure. Obes Res 13: 2021–2028. 13/11/2021 [pii];10.1038/oby.2005.248 [doi].
21. Power C, Jefferis BJ (2002) Fetal environment and subsequent obesity: a study of maternal smoking. Int J Epidemiol 31: 413–419.
22. Wideroe M, Vik T, Jacobsen G, Bakketeig LS (2003) Does maternal smoking during pregnancy cause childhood overweight? Paediatr Perinat Epidemiol 17: 171–179. 481 [pii].
23. Harris HR, Willett WC, Michels KB (2013) Parental smoking during pregnancy and risk of overweight and obesity in the daughter. Int J Obes (Lond) 37: 1356–1363. ijo2013101 [pii];10.1038/ijo.2013.101 [doi].
24. Raum E, Kupper-Nybelen J, Lamerz A, Hebebrand J, Herpertz-Dahlmann B, et al. (2011) Tobacco smoke exposure before, during, and after pregnancy and risk of overweight at age 6. Obesity (Silver Spring) 19: 2411–2417. oby2011129 [pii];10.1038/oby.2011.129 [doi].
25. Florath I, Kohler M, Weck MN, Brandt S, Rothenbacher D, et al. (2014) Association of pre- and post-natal parental smoking with offspring body mass index: an 8-year follow-up of a birth cohort. Pediatr Obes 9: 121–134. 10.1111/j.2047-6310.2012.00146.x [doi].
26. Toschke AM, Koletzko B, Slikker W, Jr., Hermann M, von KR (2002) Childhood obesity is associated with maternal smoking in pregnancy. Eur J Pediatr 161: 445–448. 10.1007/s00431-002-0983-z [doi].
27. Olsen J, Melbye M, Olsen SF, Sørensen TIA, Aaby P, et al. (2001) The Danish National Birth Cohort—its background, structure and aim. Scand J Public Health 29: 300–307.
28. [online webpage] (2014) The Danish National Birth Cohort (DNBC), www.dnbc.dk.
29. Andersen AM, Olsen J (2011) The Danish National Birth Cohort: selected scientific contributions within perinatal epidemiology and future perspectives. Scand J Public Health 39: 115-120. 39/7_suppl/115 [pii];10.1177/1403494811407674 [doi].
30. Cole TJ, Bellizzi MC, Flegal KM, Dietz WH (2000) Establishing a standard definition for child overweight and obesity worldwide: international survey. BMJ 320: 1240–1243.
31. Andersen CS (2012) Validation of anthropometric data in the 7-year follow-up.
32. von KR, Bolte G, Baghi L, Toschke AM (2008) Parental smoking and childhood obesity—is maternal smoking in pregnancy the critical exposure? Int J Epidemiol 37: 210–216. dym239 [pii];10.1093/ije/dym239 [doi].
33. Yang S, Decker A, Kramer MS (2013) Exposure to parental smoking and child growth and development: a cohort study. BMC Pediatr 13: 104. 1471-2431-13-104 [pii];10.1186/1471-2431-13-104 [doi].
34. Chen A, Pennell ML, Klebanoff MA, Rogan WJ, Longnecker MP (2006) Maternal smoking during pregnancy in relation to child overweight: follow-up to age 8 years. Int J Epidemiol 35: 121–130. dyi218 [pii];10.1093/ije/dyi218 [doi].
35. Leary SD, Smith GD, Rogers IS, Reilly JJ, Wells JC, Ness AR (2006) Smoking during pregnancy and offspring fat and lean mass in childhood. Obesity (Silver Spring) 14: 2284–2293. 14/12/2284 [pii];10.1038/oby.2006.268 [doi].
36. Mamun AA, O'Callaghan MJ, Williams GM, Najman JM (2012) Maternal smoking during pregnancy predicts adult offspring cardiovascular risk factors - evidence from a community-based large birth cohort study. PLoS One 7: e41106. 10.1371/journal.pone.0041106 [doi];PONE-D-11-25909 [pii].
37. Mizutani T, Suzuki K, Kondo N, Yamagata Z (2007) Association of maternal lifestyles including smoking during pregnancy with childhood obesity. Obesity (Silver Spring) 15: 3133–3139. 15/12/3133 [pii];10.1038/oby.2007.373 [doi].
38. Desai M, Beall M, Ross MG (2013) Developmental origins of obesity: programmed adipogenesis. Curr Diab Rep 13: 27–33. 10.1007/s11892-012-0344-x [doi].
39. Been JV, Nurmatov UB, Cox B, Nawrot TS, van Schayck CP, et al. (2014) Effect of smoke-free legislation on perinatal and child health: a systematic review and meta-analysis. Lancet 383: 1549–1560. S0140-6736(14)60082-9 [pii];10.1016/S0140-6736(14)60082-9 [doi].
40. Greene N, Greenland S, Olsen J, Nohr EA (2011) Estimating bias from loss to follow-up in the Danish National Birth Cohort. Epidemiology 22: 815–822. 10.1097/EDE.0b013e31822939fd [doi].
41. Nohr EA, Frydenberg M, Henriksen TB, Olsen J (2006) Does low participation in cohort studies induce bias? Epidemiology 17: 413–418. 10.1097/01.ede.0000220549.14177.60 [doi].
42. England LJ, Grauman A, Qian C, Wilkins DG, Schisterman EF, et al. (2007) Misclassification of maternal smoking status and its effects on an epidemiologic study of pregnancy outcomes. Nicotine Tob Res 9: 1005–1013. 781797939 [pii];10.1080/14622200701491255 [doi].
43. Russell T, Crawford M, Woodby L (2004) Measurements for active cigarette smoke exposure in prevalence and cessation studies: why simply asking pregnant women isn't enough. Nicotine Tob Res 6 Suppl 2: S141–S151. 10.1080/14622200410001669141 [doi];WPGCAU7ABRULJN8C [pii].
44. Patrick DL, Cheadle A, Thompson DC, Diehr P, Koepsell T, et al. (1994) The validity of self-reported smoking: a review and meta-analysis. Am J Public Health 84: 1086–1093.
45. Wong SL, Shields M, Leatherdale S, Malaison E, Hammond D (2012) Assessment of validity of self-reported smoking status. Health Rep 23: 47–53.

More Evidence on the Impact of India's Conditional Cash Transfer Program, Janani Suraksha Yojana: Quasi-Experimental Evaluation of the Effects on Childhood Immunization and Other Reproductive and Child Health Outcomes

Natalie Carvalho[1,2]*, Naveen Thacker[3], Subodh S. Gupta[4], Joshua A. Salomon[2,5]

1 Global Burden of Disease Group and Center for Health Policy, Melbourne School of Population and Global Health, Melbourne, Australia, **2** Center for Health Decision Sciences, Harvard School of Public Health, Boston, Massachusetts, United States of America, **3** Deep Children Hospital and Research Centre, Gandhidham, Gujarat, India, **4** Department of Community Medicine, Mahatma Gandhi Institute of Medical Sciences, Sewagram, Maharashtra, India, **5** Department of Global Health and Population, Harvard School of Public Health, Boston, Massachusetts, United States of America

Abstract

Background: In 2005, India established a conditional cash transfer program called Janani Suraksha Yojana (JSY), to increase institutional delivery and encourage the use of reproductive and child health-related services.

Objective: To assess the effect of maternal receipt of financial assistance from JSY on childhood immunizations, post-partum care, breastfeeding practices, and care-seeking behaviors.

Methods: We use data from the latest district-level household survey (2007–2008) to conduct a propensity score matching analysis with logistic regression. We conduct the analyses at the national level as well as separately across groups of states classified as high-focus and non-high-focus. We carry out several sensitivity analyses including a subgroup analysis stratified by possession of an immunization card.

Results: Receipt of financial assistance from JSY led to an increase in immunization rates ranging from 3.1 (95%CI 2.2–4.0) percentage points for one dose of polio vaccine to 9.1 (95%CI 7.5–10.7) percentage points in the proportion of fully vaccinated children. Our findings also indicate JSY led to increased post-partum check-up rates and healthy early breastfeeding practices around the time of childbirth. No effect of JSY was found on exclusive breastfeeding practices and care-seeking behaviors. Effect sizes were consistently larger in states identified as being a key focus for the program. In an analysis stratified by possession of an immunization card, there was little to no effect of JSY among those with vaccination cards, while the effect size was much larger than the base case results for those missing vaccination cards, across nearly all immunization outcomes.

Conclusions: Early results suggest the JSY program led to a significant increase in childhood immunization rates and some healthy reproductive health behaviors, but the structuring of financial incentives to pregnant women and health workers warrants further review. Causal interpretation of our results relies on the assumption that propensity scores balance unobservable characteristics.

Editor: Jeremy D. Goldhaber-Fiebert, Stanford University, United States of America

Funding: Natalie Carvalho was supported by the Harvard University Graduate Society Dissertation Completion Fellowship from September 2011 to May 2012. No other sources of funding were received. The funders had no role in study design, data collection and analysis, decision to publish, or preparation of the manuscript.

Competing Interests: The authors have declared that no competing interests exist.

* Email: natalie.carvalho@unimelb.edu.au

Introduction

India has some of the worst maternal and child health indicators in the world, with approximately 18% of global maternal deaths and over 20% of all deaths among children under age five years.[1,2] From 2000 to 2008, India experienced an average annual decline in under-five mortality rate of 3.9%, with highly uneven progress across states, and falling short of the 4.4% reduction per year required to meet the 2015 Millennium Development Goal (MDG) 4 target.[3,4,5] Since 2008, India has experienced a higher rate of decline in under-five mortality,[6] some of which may be attributed to the launch of the national rural health mission in 2005. India now appears much closer to achieving MDG4, which looked distant a few years ago.

Childhood immunizations are critical to safeguarding child health. According to the World Health Organization (WHO), approximately 40% of all under-vaccinated children, defined as children who did not receive 3 doses of diphtheria, tetanus and pertussis (DPT) in their first year of life, live in India.[7] Although immunization rates have increased over time, only slightly more than half of children nationwide are fully vaccinated, with wide variations across geographic and socioeconomic strata.[8] Inadequate rates of childhood immunization persist despite vaccinations being provided free of charge in public health facilities through India's Universal Immunization Program (UIP), which covers 27 million infants and 30 million pregnant women annually.[9,10]

In 2005, India's Ministry of Health and Family Welfare (MOHFW) launched the National Rural Health Mission (NRHM), which aimed to bring in health sector reforms to strengthen public health management and ensure effective health care delivery.[11,12] A key feature of NRHM is a safe motherhood scheme called Janani Suraksha Yojana (JSY). JSY is a conditional cash transfer program that provides financial incentives to pregnant women and female community health workers to encourage the use of health services during the antenatal, intrapartum and post-partum period.[11] With a goal of reducing maternal and childhood mortality, JSY aims to increase safe deliveries among women of low socioeconomic status by promoting institutional deliveries, especially in rural areas. The program operates at the community level through an accredited social health activist (ASHA) who is selected by NRHM to act as the intermediary between the women and the state. ASHAs are responsible for identifying all pregnant women in their community and facilitating their use of reproductive health services offered by the state, including antenatal care visits, facility-based delivery, postnatal checkups, immunization of the newborn, and providing advice and counseling on breastfeeding practices.[13]

Janani Suraksha Yojana is a national program funded exclusively by the federal government and managed at the local level by states.[14,15] Eligibility criteria and financial incentives vary across states, and have been modified over time. In ten Low Performing States (LPS) (Assam, Bihar, Chhattisgarh, Jammu and Kashmir, Jharkhand, Madhya Pradesh, Orissa, Uttarakhand, and Uttar Pradesh) with low rates of institutional deliveries, all women are eligible for the program. These states also tend to have higher fertility rates and worse maternal and child health indicators compared to the rest of the country.[14] Among the other High Performing States (HPS), eligibility is restricted to marginalized women (those with a government-issued below the poverty line (BPL) card or belonging to a scheduled caste or tribe), and only for their first two births.[15] Eligible women receive cash assistance ranging from 600 Indian rupees (Rs.) (~US $10 as of 2014) in urban areas of HPS to 1,400 Rs. (~US $23) in rural areas of LPS upon delivering in an accredited facility.[15] BPL women continue to receive 500 Rs. (~US $8) for deliveries outside of health facilities for their first two births.[16]

Previous studies have shown that JSY led to increased institutional deliveries.[15,17,18] An impact evaluation carried out across all states and union territories (UTs) using three different analytical approaches found a small but significant effect of JSY on increasing antenatal care and reducing perinatal and neonatal mortality among two of three analytic approaches.[17] A more recent impact evaluation, carried out using the same data, found little to no impact of JSY on antenatal care and did not find a significant impact on neonatal and perinatal mortality.[18] Among other methodological differences between the two studies, the latter's differences-in-differences analysis accounts for heterogeneity in timing of the introduction of JSY across districts, in order to control for potential unobserved district-level confounders.[18] Mazumdar and colleagues' preferred estimates were able to statistically rule out a reduction in neonatal mortality of greater than 8.7 deaths per 1,000 live births.[18] In comparison, estimates of the effect of JSY from a matching analysis by Lim et al. indicated a reduction of 2.3 neonatal deaths per 1,000 live births.[17] Lim's district-level differences-in-differences estimates of the effect of JSY on health outcomes showed no statistically significant effect on neonatal or early neonatal mortality.[17] However, Lim and colleagues note that this analysis may not have been powered to detect the reduction in perinatal and neonatal mortality found through their other analytical approaches.[17]

While childhood vaccinations were not the main target of JSY, the program could have had a direct or indirect effect on these outcomes. Early guidelines indicated minimum payments to ASHAs per in-facility delivery of 200 Rs. (~US $3) in urban areas and 600 Rs. in rural areas of LPS, north-east states, and tribal areas, with disbursement provided in two payments, the first upon reaching the institution along with the expectant mother, the second after making a postnatal visit and the child has been immunized with the bacillus Calmette-Guerin vaccine (BCG).[16] More recent government documents indicate financial incentives provided to ASHAs upon (1) motivating women to seek institutional delivery and antenatal care, (2) payment for transport of the pregnant woman to a facility, and (3) escort of the pregnant woman to the institution.[19] Aside from incentives, increased interaction with the health system through institutional deliveries could indirectly lead to an increase in childhood immunizations. Although there is some evidence that immunization rates have increased following the start of JSY, there has been no formal evaluation of the impact of JSY on childhood immunization rates.[15,20] Prior studies evaluating the effect of conditional cash transfers on immunization coverage have generally found minimal improvements in vaccination coverage or non-significant results.[21] The majority of evidence comes from Latin America, and in most study areas, vaccination coverage was high prior to the program's start. A recent study of cluster randomized controlled campaigns in a setting with low immunization coverage in India found that providing small non-financial incentives with improvements in the reliability of services led to a large increase in immunization rates, at a cost of approximately $17.35 per child.[22]

This study evaluates the impact of JSY on childhood immunization rates in India. Using a quasi-experimental analytic design, we compared childhood immunization outcomes among women who had received financial assistance from JSY compared to those who had not, controlling for possible confounders. We also evaluated the impact of the program on a range of secondary outcomes, including receipt of postnatal care, breastfeeding practices, and care-seeking behavior in the post-natal period, using the same approach.

Methods

Study design and participants

We conduct a multivariable logistic regression, with matching to control for confounding, to compute the average effect of JSY on reproductive and childhood outcomes. Many of the analyses were modeled after the matching analytical approach used by Lim et al.[17]

Data used were from the most recent round of the District Level Household Survey (DLHS-3), one of the largest demographic and health surveys conducted in India. The DLHS-3 is a nation-wide survey designed primarily to provide estimates of reproductive and child health indicators.[8] The survey was carried out across 34 states and union territories in India (excluding Nagaland) from December 2007 to December 2008. Using a multi-stage stratified sampling design, interviewers collected data from 720,320 households across urban and rural areas of 601 districts in the country.[8] For households in rural areas, a village-level questionnaire covering 22,825 villages was used to gather information on village characteristics. We used responses from currently married women aged 15–44 years who reported having had a live birth within the period covered by the survey (from January 1, 2004 onwards).

In analyses on postnatal care, breastfeeding practices, and care-seeking behaviors, data were restricted to children born within the last 12 months before the survey, to obtain the most recent sample, and to reduce the effect of varying fertility rates and differential introduction and scale-up of JSY, on study results.[17,18] For analyses on immunizations, data were restricted to children 12-23 months of age who were alive at the time of the interview to prevent premature censuring of vaccine outcomes among children under 12 months of age.[23]

This study was approved by the Population and Global Health Human Ethics Advisory Group at the Melbourne School of Population and Global Health, University of Melbourne.

Study measures

Women were asked whether they had received financial assistance from JSY for their most recent delivery; those who responded "yes" to this question were coded as JSY = 1, and those who responded "no" were coded as JSY = 0. Because women were only asked about their most recent pregnancy, only data on women's most recent live birth could be used to investigate the effect of JSY on post-delivery indicators and immunization rates.

Childhood immunization outcomes considered include receiving the following vaccines: polio at birth (or "polio zero"), one dose of BCG, at least one dose of DPT, three doses of DPT, at least one dose of polio, three doses of polio, measles, and any hepatitis B.[24] We also considered the proportion of fully vaccinated children and children who did not receive any vaccination. In line with WHO guidelines we defined a fully vaccinated child as one who had received one dose of BCG vaccine, 3 doses of DPT and polio vaccines (not including polio at birth), and one dose of measles vaccine by the age of 12 months.[8,25]

Vaccination status was determined from immunization cards, supplemented by mothers' reports where immunization cards were incomplete or missing. While there are important limitations to using this type of data, household surveys are regularly used for estimating childhood immunization rates.[23] For polio at birth, we include children who had an immunization date for polio zero in their immunization cards, and those whose mothers reported them having their first polio vaccine within 2 weeks of birth. Information on hepatitis B was not included in the immunization card data; it was the only immunization outcome that relied solely on maternal reporting. Furthermore, although three doses of hepatitis B are recommended (similar to DPT and polio),[24] only one survey question was asked about any hepatitis B vaccination.

Children with missing data (<0.5% of observations) or with a response of "don't know" reported for one or more vaccines were treated as missing observations, and these children were not included in the denominator. We also considered a more conservative definition for all vaccines, counting children with missing vaccination data or "don't know" responses as not having been vaccinated; this more conservative definition matched immunization means reported in the DLHS-3.[8]

Other reproductive and child health indicators included prompt post-natal check-ups for the mother (within 48 hours of delivery) and baby (within 24 hours of delivery), three breastfeeding behavior outcomes (early initiation of breastfeeding within the first hour of birth, child breastfed colostrum, exclusively breastfed for 6 months or continuing to be breastfed), and care-seeking behaviors for symptoms of childhood diarrhea and pneumonia (sought advice or treatment).

Other measures available from the household survey and included as covariates in the analysis were measures of household assets, maternal age and education, information on birth history, gender of the child, caste or tribe, religion, below-the-poverty-line card ownership, urban or rural residence, and distance to the nearest health facility.

Statistical Analysis

We used factor analysis to construct a household wealth index based on the following categorical household characteristics and assets: access to an improved drinking water source; access to improved sanitation; type of house (3 categories, with pucca of highest quality, kaccha of lowest quality); type of cooking fuel; access to an electricity connection; presence of other household assets including fan, television, telephone, scooter and car. Household wealth quintiles and deciles were generated from this wealth index.

To investigate the effect of maternal receipt of financial assistance from JSY on childhood immunization rates and other reproductive and child health indicators, we conducted a propensity-score matching (PSM) analysis with logistic regression to control for potentially confounding differences between the JSY and non-JSY groups. PSM is a widely used method in impact evaluation literature when experimental data are not available. This method can correct for biases in treatment effect due to observed covariates, that result from confounding due to non-random assignment of the treatment.[26] Matching allows for the "treated" group to be made as similar to the "untreated" group as possible based on observed pre-treatment matching covariates, to reduce the link between the treatment variable (receipt of JSY) and background characteristics of the participant.[27] In order to draw causal inferences, this method relies on the assumption that balancing observables also balances unobservables.

We used a logit model to estimate propensity scores and 1:1 nearest neighbor matching algorithm without replacement to generate matched groups. Matching covariates included maternal age, number of live births, birth interval, whether the birth was part of a multiple birth, maternal education category, household wealth decile, BPL-card ownership, caste or tribe, religion, location of residence with respect to distance to the nearest health facility, and state of residence. We defined categorical variables to be consistent with the Lim et al. analysis,[17] to facilitate comparison to prior findings. We performed several PSM diagnostics including visual inspection of propensity scores in the treated and control group pre- and post- matching and comparison of background characteristics between groups pre- and post-matching. (**Figure S1** and **Table S1**)

The main analysis to identify 'treatment effects' for JSY used logistic regression with state-level fixed effects and robust, clustered standard errors at the district level. We included the same regression covariates as in the PSM step. The estimated treatment effect for a given outcome was obtained using fitted probabilities, by computing the difference between the probability of the outcome of interest for the treated group (JSY = 1) and the control group (JSY = 0), which results in the interpretation of the findings as average effects across all JSY recipients. We repeated analyses separately for LPS and HPS. Following prior guidance suggesting that survey weights are not needed for matched analyses if the model is correctly specified,[28] we did not include survey weights in the main analysis, but we conducted a sensitivity analysis that did include survey weights. The propensity score matching was done in R (version 2.12.1) and all other analyses were conducted in Stata (version 12).

Sensitivity analyses

We tested various alternative model specifications such as including child's gender and an indicator for LPS (alone and interacted with the treatment effect) as covariates, running the analysis with district-level fixed effects, and accounting for calendar time heterogeneity. We carried out an analysis including ever-married women 45–49 years of age. For immunization outcomes, we replicated the coarsened-exact matching analysis carried out by Lim and colleagues using the same coarsened matching covariates as the authors.[17] For these outcomes, we also re-ran the analyses restricted to children born within the last 12 months before the survey. In addition, we reran the analyses separately for individuals with immunization cards and those missing immunization cards, to investigate any potential differences in the effect of JSY between the two groups. Roughly 43% of individuals had immunization cards for their children that they were able to produce to the interviewers. Of the remaining 57% of the sample, just over half (54%) reported having an immunization card but were unable to show it to the interviewers, and the remaining group did not have a card. We grouped together all families that were unable to show an immunization card to the survey interviewers (and thus relied on parental recall) and considered them as those with missing immunization cards. Finally, we re-ran the propensity score matching and logistic regressions separately for women who delivered in a health facility, and women who delivered elsewhere. While susceptible to endogeneity bias, this stratified analysis allows for the control of unobserved heterogeneity between women who delivered in facilities and those who didn't, and corrects for biases related to the potential reverse causality between institutional delivery and receipt of the cash transfer.[18]

Results

Mean immunization rates among our sample population (children aged 12 to 23 months that were the most recent births of women 15 to 44 years of age) are shown in **Table 1**. Nearly 95% of children had been vaccinated at least once against polio, while only 71% of children had received a measles vaccine. Large drops in coverage rates between the first and third recommended doses were seen for both polio (23 percentage point drop) and DPT (18 percentage point drop) vaccines. At the national level, 54% of children aged 12 to 23 months were fully vaccinated; less than 5% of children had received no vaccine.

National-level means mask substantial variation in immunization rates across geographic and socioeconomic strata of the country. **Figure 1** shows district-level variations in the proportion of children aged 12 to 23 months who are fully vaccinated. States with bolded outlines are LPS. As can be seen from this figure, these LPS, along with the Northeast states, both of which were priorities of JSY, have consistently lower immunization rates compared to HPS. (**Figure 1**)

Selected results from the multivariate logistic regression on matched samples are shown in **Table 2**. (Full regression results in **Table S2**) Computed predicted probabilities show that receipt of financial assistance from JSY led to a significant increase in immunization rates of several percentage points among children aged 12–23 months, across all vaccines considered. (**Table 3**) With the exception of hepatitis B, which was borderline significant at the 95% confidence level in the base case analysis, the smallest effect of JSY (3.1 percentage points) was on the first dose of polio vaccine, which also had the highest national coverage rate (94%). (**Table 1**) The largest effect sizes (7.8 percentage points) were seen on the coverage of polio zero and DPT3, which have much lower national level coverage rates. (**Table 1**) For most vaccines, JSY payments resulted in a 3 to 8 percentage point increase in coverage. Maternal receipt of cash payments from JSY led to an increase in 9.1 percentage points in the proportion of fully vaccinated children, and a reduction of 3.2 percentage points in the proportion of children who had not received a single vaccine.

A conservative definition of vaccine status, which considered children with missing or "Don't know" responses as not having been vaccinated, produced the same results across all vaccines, with the exception of polio at birth. For this outcome, which had high proportion (8%) of "Don't know" responses, particularly from caregivers asked whether their child had received their first polio vaccine within 2 weeks of birth, the estimated JSY treatment effect was lower than that found using the base case vaccine status definitions.

National-level means for all other reproductive and child health indicators, including postnatal check-up rates, breastfeeding behavior, and IMCI-related indicators are shown **Table 4**. Nearly half of all mothers and their newborns received a postnatal check-up following delivery. While the majority of mothers (82%) breastfed colostrum to their baby, less than half (41%) started breastfeeding within one hour of birth. Only 37% of infants born within the last 12 months prior to the survey were exclusively breastfed for 6 months (or were still currently being breastfed). The majority of caregivers sought advice or treatment if their children had diarrhea, fever, or symptoms of pneumonia.

Receipt of financial assistance from JSY had a large and significant positive effect of 26–27 percentage points on postnatal check-ups among mothers and newborns. (**Table 5**) JSY also had a positive effect on breastfeeding behaviors immediately following childbirth. Of 100 women who received cash assistance from JSY, an additional 7 women began breastfeeding within an hour after delivery, and an additional 4 women breastfed their baby colostrum. No significant effect was found from maternal receipt of financial assistance from JSY on exclusive breastfeeding or care-seeking behaviors for sick children.

Results were consistent across an array of different model specifications. Hepatitis B was the only exception, for which the treatment effect ceased to remain significant across several robustness checks. Effect estimates were insensitive to the use of survey weights and calendar time of interview fixed effects. Child's gender was found to have a small but significant association with postnatal check-ups, seeking advice or treatment for diarrhea or pneumonia, and some vaccination outcomes, with male children slightly more likely to be involved in these healthy behaviors. Being a LPS was negatively associated with all reproductive and child health indicators considered, controlling for individual-level covariates, and this association was significant across all outcomes except care-seeking behaviors. When including interaction effects between LPS and JSY, the treatment effect of JSY ceased to remain significant for some immunization outcomes (polio zero, first dose of polio, no vaccine) and the early breastfeeding outcomes. For these outcomes, the differential effect of the program in LPS remained significant. Similarly to findings by

Table 1. National level immunization coverage estimates, most recent births 12–23 months prior to survey to women 15–44 years.

	Mean	95% CI, upper	95% CI, lower
BCG	87.5%	87.2%	87.8%
Polio at birth	58.1%	57.6%	58.5%
Polio 1	93.8%	93.5%	94.0%
Polio 3	70.9%	70.4%	71.3%
DPT 1	83.9%	83.6%	84.2%
DPT 3	66.0%	65.6%	66.4%
Measles	70.9%	70.5%	71.3%
Hepatitis B	29.6%	29.2%	30.1%
Fully vaccinated child*	54.1%	53.7%	54.6%
No vaccine	4.6%	4.5%	4.8%

*A fully vaccinated child was defined as a child who had received one dose of BCG vaccine, 3 doses of DPT and polio vaccines (not including polio at birth), and one dose of measles vaccine. [IIPS 2010]

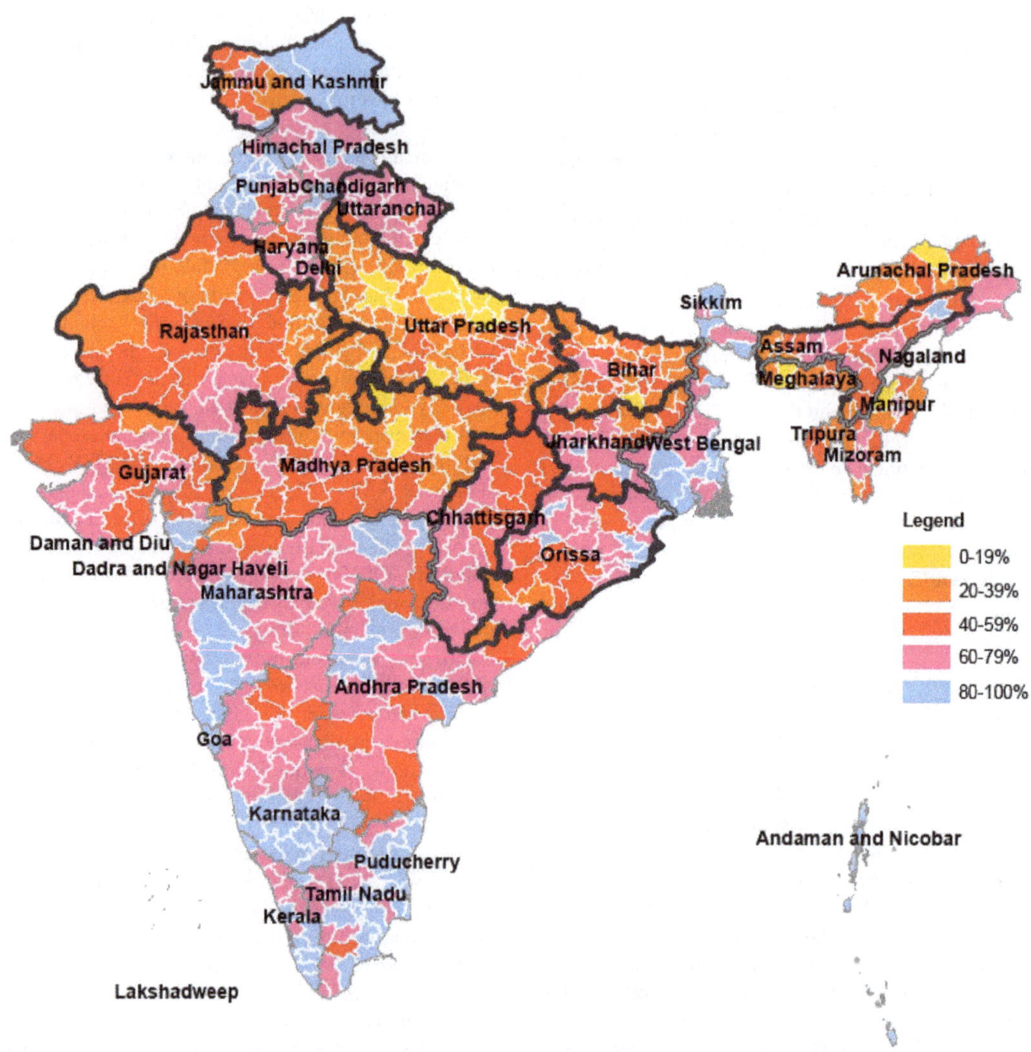

Figure 1. Percent of children 12-23 months at the time of the survey who were fully vaccinated by district, for high and low performing states, 2007-08.* *Among most recent births for women ages 15–44 years of age. A fully vaccinated child was defined as a child who had received one dose of BCG vaccine, 3 doses of DPT and polio vaccines (not including polio at birth), and one dose of measles vaccine. [IIPS 2010] Dark (bolded) outlines represent the ten low-performing states (LPS): Uttar Pradesh, Uttarakhand, Bihar, Jharkhand, Madhya Pradesh, Chhattisgarh, Assam, Rajasthan, Orissa, and Jammu and Kashmir. Districts with no data are in white.

Table 2. Abbreviated regression results for selected immunization outcomes, run on sample of children 12–23 months of age.

		BCG n = 12,520			Fully vaccinated* n = 12,592			Not Vaccinated n = 12,177		
		OR	**SE**	**p-value**	**OR**	**SE**	**p-value**	**OR**	**SE**	**p-value**
	JSY	**2.57**	**0.22**	**<0.01**	**1.58**	**0.06**	**<0.01**	**0.36**	**0.04**	**<0.01**
Maternal age (years)	15–19	0.65	0.13	0.04	0.72	0.08	<0.01	2.11	0.64	0.01
	20–24	0.74	0.12	0.06	0.78	0.06	<0.01	2.62	0.59	<0.01
	25–29	0.95	0.14	0.70	0.89	0.07	0.11	1.98	0.43	<0.01
	30–34	1.00	–	–	1.00	–	–	1.00	–	–
	35–39	0.87	0.19	0.53	0.85	0.11	0.21	1.57	0.48	0.14
	40–44	1.47	0.51	0.27	0.86	0.20	0.51	0.35	0.25	0.14
Number of live births	1 birth	1.00	–	–	1.00	–	–	1.00	–	–
	2 births	0.98	0.11	0.89	0.86	0.05	<0.01	1.09	0.15	0.55
	3–4 births	0.74	0.09	0.01	0.72	0.05	<0.01	1.55	0.25	0.01
	5 or more	0.54	0.12	<0.01	0.47	0.06	<0.01	2.33	0.65	<0.01
Maternal education	No education	1.00	–	–	1.00	–	–	1.00	–	–
	1–5 years	1.41	0.16	<0.01	1.35	0.08	<0.01	0.71	0.10	0.02
	6–11 years	2.34	0.27	<0.01	1.73	0.09	<0.01	0.45	0.07	<0.01
	12 or more	2.72	0.76	<0.01	1.77	0.17	<0.01	0.37	0.15	0.02
Household wealth	Poorest decile	1.00	–	–	1.00	–	–	1.00	–	–
	Decile 2	0.93	0.13	0.60	1.12	0.10	0.21	0.82	0.17	0.34
	Decile 3	1.24	0.19	0.15	1.14	0.10	0.13	0.89	0.16	0.54
	Decile 4	1.08	0.16	0.62	1.23	0.11	0.02	0.89	0.18	0.56
	Decile 5	1.36	0.22	0.06	1.27	0.11	0.01	0.69	0.14	0.08
	Decile 6	1.47	0.26	0.03	1.27	0.12	0.01	0.63	0.14	0.04
	Decile 7	1.49	0.28	0.03	1.48	0.14	<0.01	0.35	0.10	<0.01
	Decile 8	1.97	0.42	<0.01	1.74	0.18	<0.01	0.33	0.10	<0.01
	Decile 9	2.98	0.86	<0.01	1.91	0.23	<0.01	0.29	0.12	<0.01
	Richest decile	14.25	9.04	<0.01	2.27	0.35	<0.01	0.14	0.09	<0.01

* A fully vaccinated child was defined as a child who had received one dose of BCG vaccine, 3 doses of DPT and polio vaccines (not including polio at birth), and one dose of measles vaccine. [IIPS 2010]

Table 3. National level results from logistic regression of JSY effects on immunization outcomes among most recent births 12–23 months prior to survey to women 15–44 years.

	Estimated JSY treatment effect			N
	Point est.	95% CI, lower	95% CI, upper	
BCG	4.9%	4.0%	5.8%	12,520
Polio at birth	7.8%	6.1%	9.4%	12,303
Polio 1	3.1%	2.2%	4.0%	12,526
Polio 3	6.3%	5.0%	7.6%	12,026
DPT1	5.6%	4.6%	6.6%	12,436
DPT3	7.8%	6.3%	9.3%	12,188
Measles	5.9%	4.4%	7.3%	12,438
Hepatitis B	1.8%	0.3%	3.3%	11,907
Fully Vaccinated*	9.1%	7.5%	10.7%	12,592
No vaccine	−3.2%	−4.0%	−2.4%	12,177

*A fully vaccinated child was defined as a child who had received one dose of BCG vaccine, 3 doses of DPT and polio vaccines (not including polio at birth), and one dose of measles vaccine. [IIPS 2010]

Lim et al., the treatment effect of JSY was larger in LPS across all immunization outcomes (**Figure 2**) and all check-up and breastfeeding behavior outcomes considered.[17] Including district-level fixed effects had minimal impact on results for most vaccine outcomes. The estimated treatment effect had overlapping 95% confidence intervals for all but the "no vaccine" outcome, for which the effect size was larger (−6.9% vs −3.2%) compared to the base case. Results from the coarsened exact matching method were similar to the base case findings. (**Figure S2**)

In the sensitivity analysis restricted to most recent births within the last 12 months prior to the survey, larger effects of JSY were found among vaccine outcomes that occur close to the time of birth (including no vaccine), while smaller effects were found for measles and the proportion of fully vaccinated children. (**Figure 3**) Because most children in this sample population are under 12 months of age, their vaccine status would be subject to a censoring effect. This effect would be greatest for vaccine outcomes that occur closer to 1 year of age (measles, third dose of polio and DPT, fully vaccinated). Results from the analysis stratified by possession of an immunization card showed important differences in the effect of JSY across both groups. Receipt of financial incentives from JSY had a small (≤ 3%) or no effect among those with vaccination cards while the effect size was much larger than the base case results for the group missing vaccination cards, for nearly all immunization outcomes. (**Figure 4**) For all outcomes, mean immunization levels were consistently higher in the group with vaccination cards. (**Table S3**) Finally, a stratified analysis by delivery location generally resulted in lower treatment effect sizes, particularly among analyses restricted to women delivering in a health facility. (**Figure 5**) Most results remained significant at the 95% confidence level despite much wider confidence intervals, especially among out-of-facility deliveries that involved smaller sample sizes.

Table 4. National level child health outcomes relating to the most recent births to women 15–44 years born within the last 12 months prior to the survey.

	Mean	95% CI, upper	95% CI, lower
Post-natal care			
Woman, within 48 hr after delivery	49.9%	49.4%	50.3%
Newborn, within 24 hr after birth	50.6%	50.1%	51.0%
Breastfeeding behavior			
Early initiation of breastfeeding*	41.1%	40.7%	41.5%
Breastfed colostrum to child	81.2%	80.9%	81.5%
Excl. breastfed for 6 months or continuing	37.0%	36.6%	37.4%
*IMCI** indicators*			
Sought advice or treatment for diarrhea	68.5%	67.5%	69.5%
Sought advice or treatment for symptoms of pneumonia*** or fever	73.1%	72.3%	73.8%

*Defined as started breastfeeding within 1 hour of birth.
**Integrated management of childhood illnesses (IMCI).
***Pneumonia defined as cough plus fast breathing.

Table 5. National level results from logistic regression of JSY effects on child health outcomes among most recent births to women 15–44 years born within the last 12 months prior to the survey.

	Estimated JSY treatment effect			N
	Point est.	95% CI, lower	95% CI, upper	
Post-natal care				
Woman, within 48 hr after delivery	24.8%	22.9%	26.7%	24,258
Newborn, within 24 hr after birth	25.7%	23.9%	27.4%	23,924
Breastfeeding behavior				
Early initiation of breastfeeding*	6.8%	5.3%	8.3%	23,923
Breastfed colostrum to child	4.1%	3.0%	5.2%	23,917
Excl. breastfed for 6 months or continuing	−1.0%	−2.5%	0.4%	23,316
*IMCI** indicators*				
Sought advice or treatment for diarrhea	3.7%	0.6%	6.9%	3,754
Sought advice or treatment for symptoms of pneumonia*** or fever	2.0%	−0.2%	4.3%	5,799

*Defined as started breastfeeding within 1 hour of birth.
**Integrated management of childhood illnesses (IMCI).

Discussion

Our results indicate that India's conditional cash transfer program led to improvements in reproductive and child health indicators in India, in particular childhood immunization outcomes. Receipt of cash assistance for delivery resulted in increased immunization rates, by several percentage points, across the full range of vaccines considered. The smallest effect was seen in a single dose of polio vaccine, which had a coverage rate of nearly 95%. Vaccines with the lowest coverage rates (polio at birth, three doses of DPT and polio, and measles) had higher treatment effects, ranging from six to eight percentage points increase. The treatment effect of JSY on the proportion of children 12 to 23 months of age who were fully vaccinated was an increase of nine percentage points. In other words, for every 100 children whose mother received financial assistance from JSY for delivery, nine additional children were fully vaccinated. The effect size for hepatitis B immunization was small, and ceased to remain significant across robustness checks. It is worth noting that hepatitis B vaccine was introduced into select states and districts as a pilot in 2002–03, and only expanded to the rest of the country in 2010–11.[9] Although women received cash assistance from JSY at the time of delivery, as opposed to when their child was vaccinated, the effects on immunizations were still found to be

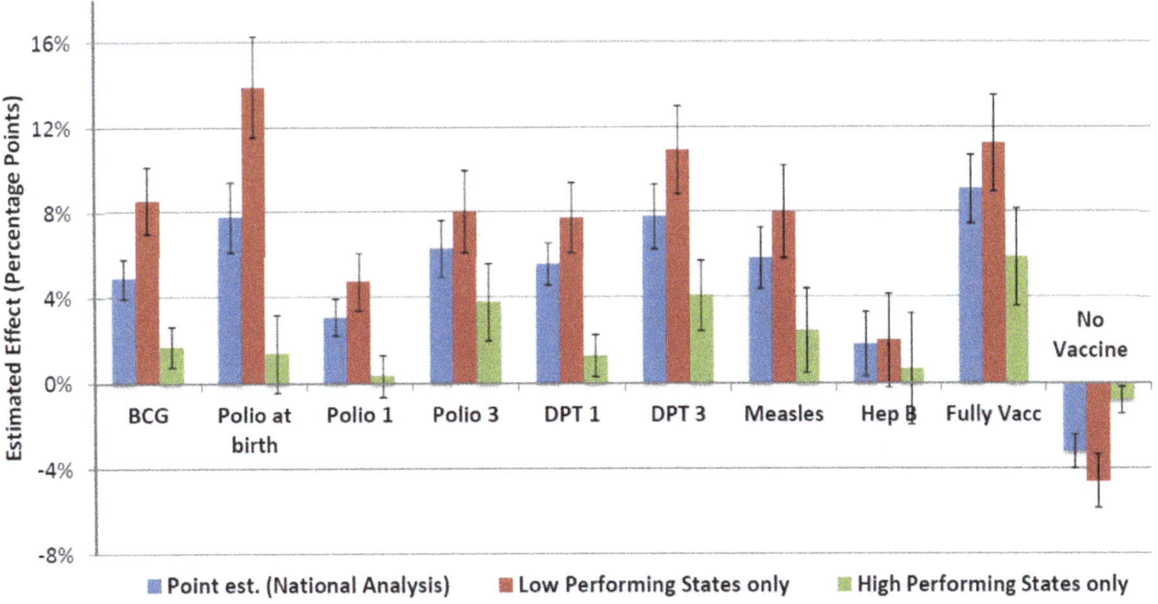

Figure 2. Estimated JSY treatment effect on childhood immunization outcomes among children 12 to 23 months of age, stratified by LPS and HPS compared to national level results. Error bars represent 95% confidence intervals from regression estimates. * A fully vaccinated child was defined as a child who had received one dose of BCG vaccine, 3 doses of DPT and polio vaccines (not including polio at birth), and one dose of measles vaccine. [IIPS 2010]

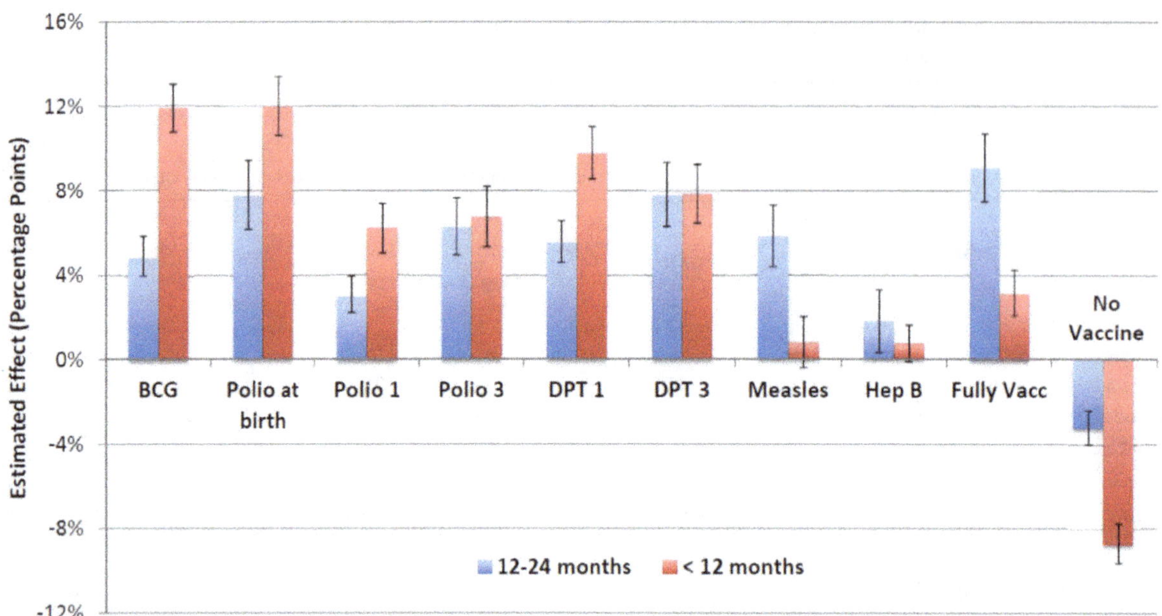

Figure 3. Estimated JSY treatment effect on childhood immunization outcomes: among children 12 to 23 months of age and children under 12 months of age. Error bars represent 95% confidence intervals from regression estimates. * A fully vaccinated child was defined as a child who had received one dose of BCG vaccine, 3 doses of DPT and polio vaccines (not including polio at birth), and one dose of measles vaccine. [IIPS 2010]

significant, and for some vaccines, quite large. Similarly, Lim et al. had noted a significant effect of JSY on increasing antenatal care, for which payment was not directly linked.[17]

There are several mechanisms through which cash transfers for safe deliveries could impact on post-delivery reproductive and child health indicators. One hypothesis is that increased interaction with the health system as a result of JSY could have add-on effects on health-related behaviors, particularly in the early post-partum period. Although some have hypothesized that childhood vaccinations occur too far after delivery for JSY to have an impact,[18] several vaccinations, such as polio at birth and BCG, take place at the time of childbirth or soon afterward. In addition, the role of ASHAs involves promoting healthy reproductive behaviors in the postpartum period including immunizations. In a qualitative assessment carried out in eight LPS states, it was found that although ASHAs were not provided additional incentives for

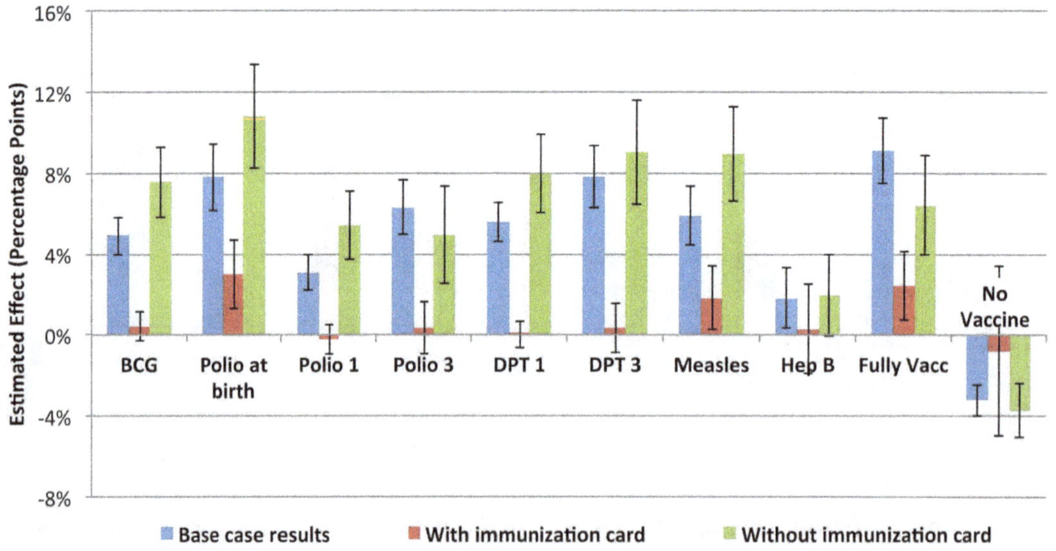

Figure 4. Estimated JSY treatment effect on childhood immunization outcomes among children 12 to 23 months of age: stratified by possession of an immunization card. Error bars represent 95% confidence intervals from regression estimates. * A fully vaccinated child was defined as a child who had received one dose of BCG vaccine, 3 doses of DPT and polio vaccines (not including polio at birth), and one dose of measles vaccine. [IIPS 2010]

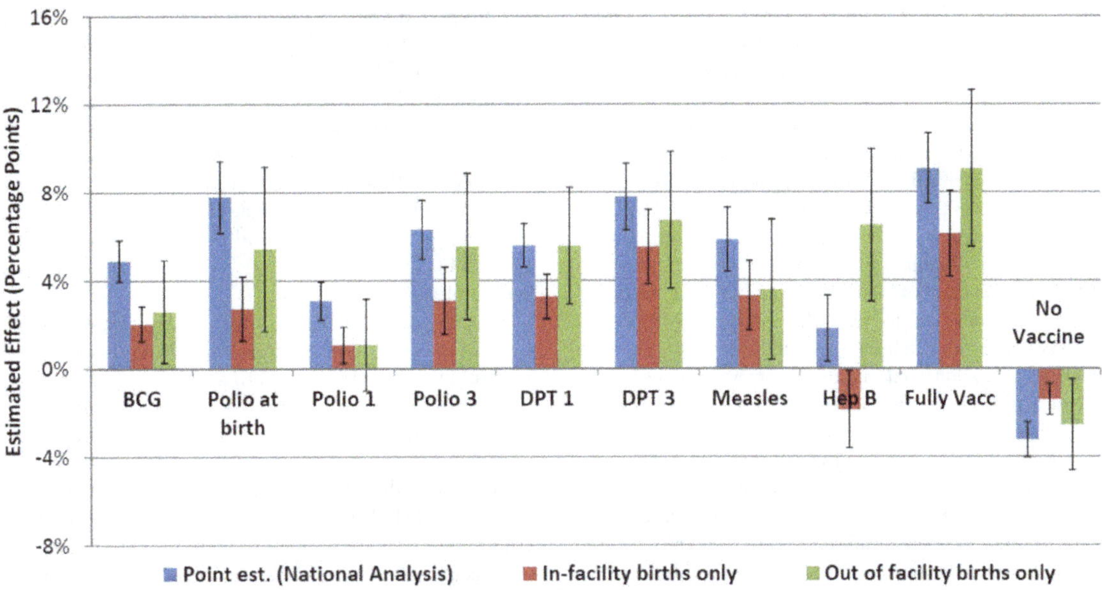

Figure 5. Estimated JSY treatment effect on childhood immunization outcomes among children 12 to 23 months of age: nationally and stratified by delivery location. Error bars represent 95% confidence intervals from regression estimates. * A fully vaccinated child was defined as a child who had received one dose of BCG vaccine, 3 doses of DPT and polio vaccines (not including polio at birth), and one dose of measles vaccine. [IIPS 2010]

postnatal visits, they made more home visits than any other grassroots functionary.[19] In assessments carried out in 5 LPS, the majority of ASHAs surveyed responded that they had provided help or advice regarding breastfeeding practices and had recommended childhood vaccinations to pregnant women and recently delivered mothers.[15,29] A small study using records from a tertiary level health center in the state of Orissa found that 'at birth' immunization (within 7 days of birth) increased significantly following the implementation of JSY at the health center.[30] In this study, ASHAs were cited by parents as the primary motivator for immunization.

Still, it remains unclear just how much influence ASHAs have on women's behavior, especially decisions outside of choosing an institutional delivery.[31] A few schemes started in the last two years are expected to create more opportunities for ASHAs to reach families during the postnatal period. In a scheme launched in 2011 to strengthen home-based newborn care (HBNC), ASHAs will be given incentives for providing home visits, with incentives tied to BCG at birth and DPT and polio vaccines at 6 weeks.[32] Another scheme exists for home delivery of contraceptives through ASHAs, which will also help to increase contact during the postnatal period.[33] Although incentives are not tied with breastfeeding under this scheme, early breastfeeding is an indicator for monitoring the HBNC scheme. Also, the training package for ASHAs incorporates knowledge on immunization and child nutrition. These approaches create more opportunities for postnatal home visits by ASHAs, and may help to increase immunization coverage and improve breastfeeding and complementary feeding practices in India.

The large impact of JSY on postnatal check-ups was expected given JSY has previously been found to have led to a considerable increase in institutional deliveries, but offers a useful validation of the model and analysis. Perhaps more surprising was the minimal effect on breastfeeding behaviors. Although an increase in several percentage points was seen for early initiation of breastfeeding and among children breastfed colostrum, no effect of cash assistance for delivery was found on exclusive breastfeeding rates, even though the proportion of children who were exclusively breastfed for 6 months or currently being breastfed was well under 50%. Qualitative evidence from surveys conducted in five LPS showed that while ASHAs responded similarly to questions asking about type of support or advice provided to pregnant women or recently delivered mothers regarding immunizations and breastfeeding behaviors, responses from recently-delivered women indicated less advice received from ASHAs regarding breastfeeding behaviors compared to immunizations.[15,29]

Results remained consistent across a range of model robustness checks and sensitivity analyses. However, there are several important limitations to consider. First, this analysis uses propensity score matching on non-experimental data to make causal claims. Doing so relies on the assumption that balancing observations based on observable characteristics also balances unobservables. This is a strong assumption that we were unable to test. Although we have matched observations on a number of individual and household level covariates that are likely to affect receipt of financial assistance from JSY and the outcomes of interest, our results are not robust against bias arising from unobservable characteristics that are correlated with uptake of JSY and study outcomes. Another main limitation of this analysis concerns the differential timing and scale-up of JSY across the country. While the program was officially established by the federal government in April 2005, it took months (and in some cases over a year) for JSY to be implemented and operationalized across all states and UTs. During implementation of JSY, priority was given to low performing states and the scheme was launched early, while in several high performing states, ASHA recruitment was slow and did not cover all areas during the first few years of the scheme. Furthermore, differences in how the scheme was institutionalized, including the way JSY was advertised, the effectiveness of ASHAs, and the paperwork required for eligibility, could have led to important differences in the effectiveness of JSY across states and districts.

The survey data used for this analysis cover the period soon after JSY was established, and thus the effects may differ compared to when implementation is complete and awareness of the scheme is high across all states. Restricting the analysis to most recent births in the last 12 months reduces issues related to the differential introduction of JSY across districts and states: the earliest births included in analyses restricted to this sample population occurred in December 2006, over 1.5 years after JSY was established. To avoid censored observations as a result of partially immunized children, analyses on vaccination outcomes were restricted to children 12 to 24 months of age. This sample thus included children born seven months to over 2.5 years after JSY was established. We explored including an indicator for LPS to potentially reduce any additional bias due to heterogeneous timing in the implementation of JSY across the country. While this was only a partial remedy, any bias in the treatment effect of JSY will be towards the null, and the estimates obtained will likely underestimate the true effect of JSY. As an additional check, our breastfeeding results are similar to those found by Mazumdar and colleagues of a statistically significant effect of JSY of 7.4 percentage points on breastfeeding in the first hour, but no effect on breastfeeding behavior within 24 hours.[18] Their analysis controlled for time invariant district-level unobservables and accounted for heterogeneity in the timing of the introduction of JSY across the country.[18]

The validity of our results is limited by the quality of the household survey data, in particular the reliability of immunization card data and maternal recall and self-reporting on their child's vaccination status. The subsample analysis shows that these two groups differ significantly with respect to the effect of JSY on childhood immunization outcomes. Maternal receipt of financial incentives from JSY had little to no effect among the group with immunization cards. There are several possible explanations for this. First, it is likely that these two groups are systematically different from each other in ways that are not controlled for in the analysis. Second, immunization rates among the group relying on maternal recall may be over- or underestimated. It is also possible that those relying on maternal recall may be more likely to report receiving specific vaccinations linked to the JSY program even if their child had not received the vaccine. In this case, the effect of the program would be overestimated. On the other hand, childhood immunization rates are much higher among those with immunization cards, with little room for increased coverage for some vaccine outcomes.

We also did not consider the timing of vaccines and whether vaccines were received at the appropriate time to ensure full protection against disease.[34] Interestingly, restricting the sample to children born in the last 12 months prior to the survey generally resulted in larger treatment effects among immunization outcomes that occur early in life, possibly indicating improved timing of vaccines with JSY.

In an analysis stratified by in-facility delivery, we attempted to control for unobserved heterogeneity between women who delivered in facilities and those who did not. While treatment effects are lower in both stratified analyses, we still find significant effects of financial receipt of JSY on immunization outcomes. The biggest drops in effect size were among women delivering in a health facility, as would be expected, given the pathway of increased immunization as a result of interaction with a health facility is not being captured.

The evolution of JSY post 2008 was rapid. The program has expanded considerably since it began in 2005, reaching over 10 million beneficiaries in 2011-2012 (up from 3 million in 2006–2007, and 7 million in 2007–2008).[35] Our results must therefore be interpreted in light of the current shape of the program, as well as other related programs that have more recently been implemented. With over 870,000 ASHAs currently engaged in communities in all states, and along with the recent home based newborn care scheme, an even bigger emphasis may be placed on childhood immunizations. Another new initiative launched in 2011, Janani Shishu Suraksha Karyakaram (JSSK), provides free and cashless services for delivery care in public institutions, including cesarean section, and postnatal care for sick newborns, and is being further expanded to include free antenatal and postnatal care for all infants.[36]

Despite the limitations, our findings have a number of promising implications. Increased childhood vaccination coverage as a result of JSY translates into protection from disease, disability and death among many children who would not have previously been immunized. Further insights gained from this analysis are the existence of untapped opportunities to piggyback additional benefits on to this program, such as improvements in breastfeeding behaviors, IMCI indicators, and nutrition and sanitation outcomes.

Vaccination is one of the most cost-effective ways to prevent disease and disability and improve childhood survival. However from an operational standpoint, increasing the coverage of immunizations can be difficult and costly. A pilot project conducted in Moradabad district of Uttar Pradesh from mid-2006 to early 2007 that sought to identify and vaccinate all newborns with oral polio vaccine within 72 hours of birth had disappointing results.[37] Researchers found the program to have high expansion costs and marginal impacts. One of the major insights from that study was that no mechanism was in place to routinely identify newborns, especially for deliveries that occur outside of health facilities.[37]

Janani Suraksha Yojana is one of the largest cash transfer programs in the world,[36] and offers a potential new opportunity to reach newborns and infants that previously would not have had much interaction with the health system. At an expenditure that increased from 383 million Rs. (~\$6.3 million) in the 2004–2005 financial year to 16 billion Rs. (~\$266 million in 2011–2012),[38] policy makers must be aware of the financial implications of the program. Although we have not attempted to estimate the cost-effectiveness of India's JSY program here, this is an important area of further research.[21]

The structuring of financial incentives also requires careful consideration. Early assessments of JSY point to delays in receipt of payments by mothers and ASHAs, and in some cases, informal payments were required to receive the cash.[15,39] Grievances by ASHAs regarding the uneven balance between expected workload and payment received for some services (including immunizations) could indicate the need for a revision of the payment structure.[40] The home-based newborn care and home delivery of contraceptives schemes will help to increase the incentives ASHAs receive every month and could help allay the grievances of ASHAs. Recent evidence of corruption in India's most populous state, Uttar Pradesh, which has some of the worst health indicators and therefore was also the state allocated the largest budget for JSY, warns of the need for systems in place to monitor and evaluate the scheme carefully at all levels of administration.[41]

There are important health systems issues that could jeopardize the success of the program. Shortages of human resources and absence of health personnel in facilities are problematic, as these workers are needed to administer vaccines. There is also substantial evidence of poor quality of infrastructure, including limited cold chain capacity of many states for accommodating even routine UIP vaccines, and limited awareness in some areas about safe injection practices and waste management.[42] Further monitoring of vaccine coverage is critical, and additional health systems research to identify and target poor management, and lack of human resources, infrastructure and supplies is necessary. Behavioral research into the role of ASHAs and their influence on reproductive health behaviors is also a priority. Finally, given the persistent health and coverage inequalities across geographic areas socioeconomic groups in India, it will be essential to ensure the program reaches population groups that were initially targeted as having the highest need.

In December 2010, a Decade of Vaccines Collaboration was declared by a partnership of international agencies working in immunization.[7] While India is still far off from achieving 90% coverage of DPT3, one of the goals of the Global Immunization Vision and Strategy, it is evidently progressing in the right direction.[7] With one fifth of all children under-five in the world,[43] even a few percentage points increase in childhood immunization rates could be of global health significance. India has achieved success in its polio eradication efforts, with 2011 being the first year India was declared polio free; policy makers must sustain efforts to preserve these successes.

Supporting Information

Table S1 Background characteristics* of women, pre- and post-matching. * Shown for the Fully-vaccinated child outcome only; restricted to women with children aged 12 to 24 months.

Table S2 Regression results for immunization outcomes, run on sample of children 12-23 months of age.

Table S3 Immunization coverage estimates by immunization card possession, most recent births 12-23 months prior to survey to women 15-44 years. *A fully vaccinated child was defined as a child who had received one dose of BCG vaccine, 3 doses of DPT and polio vaccines (not including polio at birth), and one dose of measles vaccine. [IIPS 2010]

Figure S1 Histograms* of propensity scores. * Shown for the fully vaccinated child outcome only.

Figure S2 Estimated JSY treatment effect on childhood immunization outcomes among children 12 to 23 months of age: Propensity Score Matching compared with Coarsened Exact Matching. Error bars represent 95% confidence intervals from regression estimates. * A fully vaccinated child was defined as a child who had received one dose of BCG vaccine, 3 doses of DPT and polio vaccines (not including polio at birth), and one dose of measles vaccine. [IIPS 2010]

Acknowledgments

We are grateful to the authors of the Lim et al. (2010) paper, in particular Joseph Hoisington and Spencer James, who shared their programming code for a replication exercise and willingly answered questions, along with Natalie Carvalho's colleagues Slawa Rokicki and Sorapop Kiatpongsan, who were partners on this replication project. We also thank Stephen Resch, Sue Goldie, and Peter Berman for their insightful comments and helpful feedback as this analysis progressed. Finally, we are grateful to our nominated discussant from the 4th Australasian Health Economics and Econometrics Workshop, Peter Siminski, as well as PLOS ONE's academic editor, Jeremy Goldhaber-Fiebert, for both of their constructive suggestions on ways to improve the methods of our analysis.

Author Contributions

Conceived and designed the experiments: NC JAS. Analyzed the data: NC. Wrote the paper: NC. Contributed to interpretation of results: NC JAS. Contributed to interpretation of policy context and results: NT SSG. Contributed to redrafting: NC NT SSG JAS.

References

1. Lozano R, Wang H, Foreman KJ, Rajaratnam JK, Naghavi M, et al. (2011) Progress towards Millennium Development Goals 4 and 5 on maternal and child mortality: an updated systematic analysis. Lancet 378: 1139–1165.
2. Black RE, Cousens S, Johnson HL, Lawn JE, Rudan I, et al. (2010) Global, regional, and national causes of child mortality in 2008: a systematic analysis. Lancet 375: 1969–1987.
3. Bhutta ZA, Chopra M, Axelson H, Berman P, Boerma T, et al. (2010) Countdown to 2015 decade report (2000–10): taking stock of maternal, newborn, and child survival. Lancet 375: 2032–2044.
4. Rajaratnam JK, Marcus JR, Flaxman AD, Wang H, Levin-Rector A, et al. (2010) Neonatal, postneonatal, childhood, and under-5 mortality for 187 countries, 1970-2010: a systematic analysis of progress towards Millennium Development Goal 4. Lancet 375: 1988–2008.
5. Reddy H, Pradhan MR, Ghosh R, Khan AG (2012) India's progress towards the Millennium Development Goals 4 and 5 on infant and maternal mortality. WHO South-East Asia Journal of Public Health 1: 279–289.
6. India Office of the Registrar General and Census Commissioner (2014) Census of India. SRS Bulletins for years 2008, 2009, 2010, and 2011. New Delhi, India: Office of the Registrar General & Census Commissioner (India). Available: http://www.censusindia.gov.in/vital_statistics/SRS_Bulletins/Bulletins.html. Accessed: 30 September 2013.
7. World Health Organization (2011) Global routine vaccination coverage 2010. Weekly epidemiological record 86: 509–520.
8. International Institute for Population Sciences (IIPS) (2010) District Level Household and Facility Survey (DLHS-3), 2007–08: India. Mumbai: IIPS. Available: http://www.rchiips.org. Accessed: 17 November 2010.
9. India Ministry of Health and Family Welfare (2011) Annual Report 2010–2011. Available: http://mohfw.nic.in/WriteReadData/l892s/9028879081Annual report part-1.pdf. Accessed: 13 April 2013.
10. India Ministry of Health and Family Welfare (2011) National Vaccine Policy. New Delhi. Available: http://mohfw.nic.in/WriteReadData/l892s/1084811197NATIONAL VACCINE POLICY BOOK.pdf. Accessed: 30 September 2013.
11. Results-Based Financing for Health (2012) Bredenkamp C India: The Janani Suraksha Yojana Program. Available: http://www.rbfhealth.org. Accessed: 28 February 2012.
12. Planning Commission of India (2011) Report of the Working Group on National Rural Health Mission (NRHM) for the Twelfth Five Year Plan (2012–2017). Available: http://planningcommission.nic.in/aboutus/committee/wrkgrp12/health/WG_1NRHM.pdf. Accessed: 13 April 2013.
13. India Ministry of Health and Family Welfare (2013) ASHA: Accredited Social Health Activist. National Rural Health Mission. Available: http://www.mohfw.nic.in/NRHM/asha.htm Accessed: 17 April 2013.
14. Vora KS, Mavalankar DV, Ramani KV, Upadhyaya M, Sharma B, et al. (2009) Maternal health situation in India: a case study. J Health Popul Nutr 27: 184–201.
15. UNFPA (2009) Concurrent assessment of Janani Suraksha Yojana in selected states: Bihar, Madyha Pradesh, Orissa, Rajasthan, Uttar Pradesh. New Delhi: UNFPA - India. Available: http://india.unfpa.org/drive/JSYConcurrentAssessment.pdf. Accessed: 17 April 2013.
16. India Ministry of Health and Family Welfare (2006) Janani Suraksha Yojana: Features and frequently asked questions and answers. New Delhi: Government of India. Available: http://jknrhm.com/PDF/JSR.pdf Accessed: 28 February 2012.
17. Lim SS, Dandona L, Hoisington JA, James SL, Hogan MC, et al. (2010) India's Janani Suraksha Yojana, a conditional cash transfer program to increase births in health facilities: an impact evaluation. Lancet 375.
18. Mazumdar S, Mills A, Powell-Jackson T (2011) Financial incentives in health: New evidence from India's Janani Suraksha Yojana. Social Science Research Network. Available: http://www.researchgate.net/publication/255707981_Financial_Incentives_in_Health_New_Evidence_from_India's_Janani_Suraksha_Yojana?ev=srch_pub. Accessed: 28 February 2012.
19. India Ministry of Health and Family Welfare (2011) Program Evaluation of the Janani Suraksha Yojana. Report by National Health Systems Resource Centre for National Rural Health Mission. New Delhi: National Health Systems Resource Centre.

20. Rajan VS (2011) India Reproductive and Child Health Second Phase (Implementation Status & Results Report). World Bank. Available: http://documents.worldbank.org/curated/en/2011/02/13735166/india-reproductive-p075060-implementation-status-results-report-sequence-10 Accessed: 28 February 2012.
21. Lagarde M, Haines A, Palmer N (2009) The impact of conditional cash transfers on health outcomes and use of health services in low and middle income countries. Cochrane Database Syst Rev: CD008137.
22. Banerjee AV, Duflo E, Glennerster R, Kothari D (2010) Improving immunisation coverage in rural India: clustered randomised controlled evaluation of immunisation campaigns with and without incentives. BMJ 340: c2220.
23. Lim SS, Stein DB, Charrow A, Murray CJ (2008) Tracking progress towards universal childhood immunisation and the impact of global initiatives: a systematic analysis of three-dose diphtheria, tetanus, and pertussis immunisation coverage. Lancet 372: 2031–2046.
24. India Ministry of Health and Family Welfare (2008) Immunization handbook for medical officers. Government of India. Available: http://nihfw.org/pdf/NCHRC-Publications/ImmuniHandbook.pdf. Accessed: 17 April 2013.
25. Arokiasamy P, Pradhan J (2011) Measuring wealth-based health inequality among Indian children: the importance of equity vs efficiency. Health Policy Plan 26: 429–440.
26. Rosenbaum PR, Rubin DB (1983) The central role of the propensity score in observational studies for causal effects. Biometrika 70: 41–55.
27. Ho D, Imai K, King G, Stuart E (2007) Matching as nonparametric preprocessing for reducing model dependence in parametric causal inference. Polit Anal 15: 199–236.
28. Gelman A (2007) Struggles with Survey Weighting and Regression Modeling. Statist Sci 22: 153–164.
29. Khan ME, Hazra A, Bhatnagar I (2010) Impact of Janani Suraksha Yojana on selected family health behaviors in rural Uttar Pradesh. Journal of Family Welfare 56.
30. Satapathy D, Malini DS, Behera T, Reddy S, Tripathy R (2009) Janani surakhya yojana and 'at birth' immunization: a study in a tertiary level health center. Indian J Community Med 34: 351–353.
31. Sydney K, Diwan V, El Khatib Z, De Costa A (2012) India's JSY cash transfer program for maternal health: Who participates and who doesn't - a report from Ujjain district. Reproductive health 9.
32. India Ministry of Health and Family Welfare (2011) Home-based Newborn Care Operational Guidelines. Available: http://nrhm.gov.in/images/pdf/programs/child-health/guidelines/deworming_guidelines.zip. Accessed: 13 April 2013.
33. India Ministry of Health and Family Welfare (2011) Home delivery of contraceptives (Condoms, OCPs, ECPs) by the ASHA at the doorstep of beneficiaries. Available: http://mohfw.nic.in/WriteReadData/l892s/1318292396Home Delivery of Condems.pdf. Accessed: 13 April 2013.
34. Prinja S, Gupta M, Singh A, Kumar R (2010) Effectiveness of planning and management interventions for improving age-appropriate immunization in rural India. Bulletin of the World Health Organization 88: 97–103.
35. India Ministry of Health and Family Welfare (2013) Annual Report 2012–13. Executive Summary. Available: http://mohfw.nic.in/WriteReadData/l892s/4 Executive Summary-20688879.pdf. Accessed: 22 July 2014.
36. India Ministry of Health and Family Welfare (2014) Janani-Shishu Suraksha Karyakram: Background. Available: http://nrhm.gov.in/nrhm-components/rmnch-a/maternal-health/janani-shishu-suraksha-karyakram/background.html. Accessed: 22 July 2014.
37. Rainey JJ, Bhatnagar P, Estivariz CF, Durrani S, Galway M, et al. (2009) Providing monovalent oral polio vaccine type 1 to newborns: findings from a pilot birth-dose project in Moradabad district, India. Bull World Health Organ 87: 955–959.
38. India Ministry of Health and Family Welfare (2013) Annual Report 2012–13. Chapter 4: Maternal Health Program. Available: http://mohfw.nic.in/WriteReadData/l892s/CHAPTER 4.pdf. Accessed: 22 July 2014.
39. Devadasan N, Elias M, John D, Grahacharya S, Ralte L (2008) A conditional cash assistance program for promoting institutional deliveries among the poor in India: process evaluation results Studies in HSO&P 24: 257–273.
40. UNFPA (2007) Assessment of ASHA and Janani Suraksha Yojana in Rajasthan. New Delhi: UNFPA - India. Available: http://www.cortindia.in/RP%5CRP-2007-0302.pdf. Accessed: 17 April 2013.
41. Shukla S (2012) India probes corruption in flagship health program. Lancet 379: 698.
42. India Ministry of Health and Family Welfare (2005) India Universal Immunization Program Review 2004 New Delhi: Ministry of Health & Family Welfare.
43. United Nations Department of Economic and Social Affairs Populations Division (2011) World Population Prospects: The 2010 Revision. Available: http://esa.un.org/wpp/. Accessed: 30 September 2013.

19

Poor Clinical Outcomes for HIV Infected Children on Antiretroviral Therapy in Rural Mozambique: Need for Program Quality Improvement and Community Engagement

Sten H. Vermund[1,2,6]*, Meridith Blevins[1,3], Troy D. Moon[1,2,6], Eurico José[6], Linda Moiane[6], José A. Tique[1,6], Mohsin Sidat[7], Philip J. Ciampa[1,5], Bryan E. Shepherd[1,3], Lara M. E. Vaz[1,4,6¤]

1 Vanderbilt Institute for Global Health, Vanderbilt University School of Medicine, Nashville, Tennessee, United States of America, 2 Department of Pediatrics, Vanderbilt University School of Medicine, Nashville, Tennessee, United States of America, 3 Department of Biostatistics, Vanderbilt University School of Medicine, Nashville, Tennessee, United States of America, 4 Department of Preventive Medicine, Vanderbilt University School of Medicine, Nashville, Tennessee, United States of America, 5 Department of Medicine, Vanderbilt University School of Medicine, Nashville, Tennessee, United States of America, 6 Friends in Global Health, Quelimane and Maputo, Mozambique, 7 School of Medicine, Universidade Eduardo Mondlane, Maputo, Mozambique

Abstract

Introduction: Residents of Zambézia Province, Mozambique live from rural subsistence farming and fishing. The 2009 provincial HIV prevalence for adults 15–49 years was 12.6%, higher among women (15.3%) than men (8.9%). We reviewed clinical data to assess outcomes for HIV-infected children on combination antiretroviral therapy (cART) in a highly resource-limited setting.

Methods: We studied rates of 2-year mortality and loss to follow-up (LTFU) for children <15 years of age initiating cART between June 2006–July 2011 in 10 rural districts. National guidelines define LTFU as >60 days following last-scheduled medication pickup. Kaplan-Meier estimates to compute mortality assumed non-informative censoring. Cumulative LTFU incidence calculations treated death as a competing risk.

Results: Of 753 children, 29.0% (95% CI: 24.5, 33.2) were confirmed dead by 2 years and 39.0% (95% CI: 34.8, 42.9) were LTFU with unknown clinical outcomes. The cohort mortality rate was 8.4% (95% CI: 6.3, 10.4) after 90 days on cART and 19.2% (95% CI: 16.0, 22.3) after 365 days. Higher hemoglobin at cART initiation was associated with being alive and on cART at 2 years (alive: 9.3 g/dL vs. dead or LTFU: 8.3–8.4 g/dL, p<0.01). Cotrimoxazole use within 90 days of ART initiation was associated with improved 2-year outcomes Treatment was initiated late (WHO stage III/IV) among 48% of the children with WHO stage recorded in their records. Marked heterogeneity in outcomes by district was noted (p<0.001).

Conclusions: We found poor clinical and programmatic outcomes among children taking cART in rural Mozambique. Expanded testing, early infant diagnosis, counseling/support services, case finding, and outreach are insufficiently implemented. Our quality improvement efforts seek to better link pregnancy and HIV services, expand coverage and timeliness of infant diagnosis and treatment, and increase follow-up and adherence.

Editor: David W. Dowdy, Johns Hopkins Bloomberg School of Public Health, United States of America

Funding: This research was supported by the President's Emergency Plan for AIDS Relief (PEPFAR) through the Centers for Disease Control and Prevention (grant #U2GPS000631). The findings and conclusions in this report are those of the authors and do not necessarily represent the official position of the CDC. Dr. Tique was supported by the Fogarty AIDS International Training and Research Program, National Institutes of Health #D43TW001035. The funders had no role in study design, data collection and analysis, decision to publish, or preparation of the manuscript.

* Email: sten.vermund@vanderbilt.edu

¤ Current address: Save the Children, Washington DC, United States of America

Introduction

Mozambique is one of the most HIV-affected countries with an estimated national HIV prevalence in 2009 of 11.5%, translating into approximately 1.4 million adults living with HIV. [1,2] Because of its heavy HIV burden, Mozambique is a priority nation for support from the U.S. President's Emergency Plan for AIDS Relief (PEPFAR). [3] National combination antiretroviral therapy (cART) coverage is low; only an estimated 52% of adults and 20% of children in need of cART were believed to be receiving it as of the end of 2011. [4] In 2010, an estimated 70.8% of pregnant women in their first antenatal care appointment received HIV counseling and testing and 40.2% of HIV-infected pregnant women received ARV prophylaxis for the prevention of mother-to-child transmission (PMTCT), typically single-dose nevirapine [5].

Under 5 (U5) mortality rates have been falling rapidly in Mozambique with 2011 national U5 mortality estimated at 135/1000 live births compared to 219/1000 live births in 1990, in large part because of improvements in vaccination coverage and efforts to manage childhood diarrheal and acute respiratory illnesses. [6] The most recent national estimate is 97/1000 live births, from the latest Demographic Health Survey [7], still shy of the 2015 Millennium Development Goal of 73 deaths per 1000 live births. HIV/AIDS contributes 10% to the U5 mortality nationally [6].

Zambézia Province is a very low-income region of 4.2 million persons in north-central Mozambique whose majority of residents are rural subsistence farmers and fishermen. Zambézia has the nation's second largest provincial population, representing ≈20% of Mozambique's total. [1,8] Provincial HIV prevalence among adults 15–49 years in 2009 was estimated at 12.6% overall, 15.3% among women and 8.9% among men, all higher than national averages, e.g., 13.1% for women 15–49 nationally. [1] Current U5 mortality estimates show Zambézia as having the worst U5 mortality of all provinces, with deaths estimated at 142/1000 live births. [9] Leading causes of U5 deaths in Zambézia in 2009 include neonatal deaths (26.1%), malaria (27.7%) and acute lower respiratory infection (13.7%). HIV/AIDS-related deaths account for 11.5% of U5 deaths in the province [9,10].

Children with HIV are not in care at as high a proportion as adults with HIV in Africa, and their outcomes are not as good in most programs. [11–71] To assess mortality for HIV-infected children on cART, we reviewed data from PEPFAR-supported clinics run by the Zambézia Provincial Health Directorate (Direcção Provincial de Saúde, DPS) in 10 districts where a Vanderbilt University non-governmental organization (NGO) provides technical assistance.

Methods

Both the Mozambican National Bioethics Committee for Health (*Comité Nacional de Bioética em Saúde* [CNBS]) and the Institutional Review Board of Vanderbilt University approved this analysis. Analysis was performed on routinely collected, de-identified, aggregate patient level data and no individual informed consent was obtained. The CNBS and the Vanderbilt Institutional Review Board explicitly waived the need for written informed consent from the participants.

We analyzed data from a cohort of HIV-infected children <15 years of age initiating cART between June 2006–July 2011 in 10 of 17 rural districts in Zambézia Province. Details of our Friends in Global Health NGO clinical program with the DPS and the Ministry of Health (Ministério de Saúde [MISAU]) have been reported previously. [72] Two districts for which we were responsible did not have electronic medical records at the time of analysis and so were excluded;[73] five additional districts were supported by another NGO in this time period. [74] Patients who transferred from another facility after starting cART were not included in this analysis as data on their care history was incomplete (N = 156).

Patient characteristics at treatment initiation of those alive, lost, and dead at the end of 2 years' follow-up were compared using rank sum and chi-square tests. Deaths were ascertained from both clinical records and from parental testimonials. Mozambican national guidelines define loss to follow-up (LTFU) as no effective clinical contact within 60 days after the last scheduled medication pickup. [75] Two additional definitions of LTFU from the literature were also applied for the purpose of cross-cohort comparisons. The 'universal' definition classifies patients as LTFU if there is no effective clinical contact within 180 days of database closure. [76] The 'reference' definition assigns 1 day of follow-up to any individual who does not return following treatment initiation, includes only individuals initiating ART 6 months prior to the database closure, and classifies patients as LTFU if there is no effective clinical contact within 180 days of database closure. [77] All three LTFU definitions deem the patient lost at the date of last contact as opposed to the date of missed visit. Kaplan-Meier estimates were used to compute mortality and the combined endpoint of mortality and LTFU. Cumulative incidence of LTFU was calculated by treating death as a competing risk. Mortality estimates assumed non-informative censoring, i.e., patients LTFU were assumed to have rates of death similar to patients not LTFU. This likely implies that our mortality calculations are under-estimates of true mortality.

Our study did not include children enrolled in HIV care who never initiated treatment. [78] Cotrimoxazole (CTX) data were treated as a tick box for "yes", collected each visit for the corresponding visit date. If a patient was on CTX anywhere from 0 to 365 days before ART initiation, we considered the patient as "CTX use prior to cART". If a patient was on CTX anywhere from 90 days before to 90 days after ART initiation, we considered the patient as "current CTX use".

Results

During five years of PEPFAR support, 753 HIV-infected children <15 years of age initiated cART. Of these children, 678 (90.0%) were <8 years of age at cART initiation, 397 (52.7%) were <2 years, and 191 (25.4%) were <1 years. Girls represented 57% of the pediatric cART patients. Median CD4+ T-lymphocyte cell count (CD4 counts) and percentage (CD4 percentage) at cART initiation were 497 and 15, respectively, although these quantities were missing for 62% and 70% of patients. Nearly half (48%) of children initiated cART very late in their disease progression (WHO stage III or IV), although WHO stage was missing for 58% of patients.

Two years after cART initiation, 152 patients had died and 240 were LTFU. At two years, the estimated probability of death was 29.0% (95% confidence interval [CI] 24.5–33.2), the cumulative incidence of LTFU was 38.7 (95% CI 34.8–42.9), and the probability of either death or LTFU was 62.0% (95% CI 57.6–65.9). We observed substantial heterogeneity between districts in two-year outcomes (Figure 1). Two year LTFU ranged from a district low of 25% to a high of 70% (Fig. 1A; $p<0.001$), mortality ranged from 16–34% (Fig. 1B; $p = 0.19$), and death or LTFU ranged from 51.1–88.1% (Fig. 1C; $p<0.001$). The association between treatment duration and mortality rate did not suggest a marked decline in mortality over time. At 90 days on cART, the mortality rate was 8.4% (95% CI: 6.3, 10.4). At 365 days on cART, the mortality rate was 19.2% (95% CI: 16.0, 22.3) and at 730 days (two years) on cART, the mortality rate was 29.0% (95% CI: 24.5%, 33.2%). Cumulative incidence of LTFU was lower when applying two definitions from the literature. [75] The cumulative incidence of LTFU using the 'universal' definition was 26.0% (95% CI 22.6–29.9) at 2 years. [76] The cumulative incidence of LTFU using the 'reference' definition was 26.4% (95% CI 22.9–30.2) at 2 years [77].

Table 1 compares patient characteristics at cART initiation between those who were alive, dead, and lost after two years. We did not detect any difference in CD4 counts or percentage at cART initiation in children who were alive and on treatment at 2 years compared to those who were either not alive or not in care at

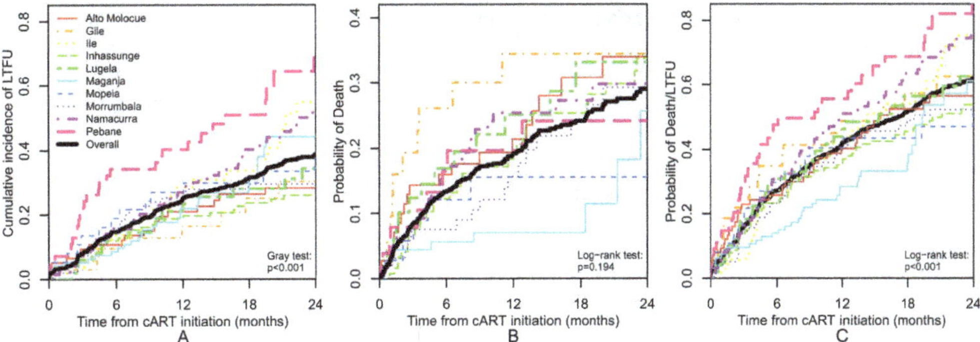

Figure 1. Variation by district in pediatric loss to follow up (LTFU), death, and death or LTFU for 2 years following combination antiretroviral therapy initiation, 10 districts of Zambézia Province, Mozambique, 2006–2011.

that time (p = 0.6), though we had high rates of missing data. We observed higher hemoglobin at the time of cART initiation among those children alive and on treatment at 2 years (alive: median 9.3 g/dL; 8.3 for dead; 8.4 g/dL for LTFU, p<0.01 for alive vs. dead or LTFU). Any cotrimoxazole use in the year prior to ART initiation was associated with improved 2-year outcomes (alive: 76%, dead: 49%, lost: 55%). Cotrimoxazole use within 90 days of ART initiation was associated with improved 2-year outcomes (alive: 69%, dead: 58%, lost: 59%).

Discussion

The experience from our PEPFAR cART program found that 29% of children initiating cART were dead within two years. It is likely that many of the 39% LTFU are at high risk of death or have already died. HIV care for children is not yet optimized in this impoverished setting with a backdrop of health workforce shortages, poor health care infrastructures, challenging transportation, poor maternal and child health outcomes, high rates of tuberculosis and malaria infections, high levels of malnutrition, low adult and pediatric cART and maternal ARV prophylaxis coverage rates, and limited formal counseling/social support programs. Similar challenges are reported elsewhere, particularly where cART is initiated late and co-infections are already extant. [20,79,80] Considerably better outcomes are reported from LMIC outside of Africa. [81–92] While a number of pediatric cART programs have reported much better success, we do not know the extent to which there is a reporting bias in the literature, i.e., overrepresentation in the literature of more favorable program outcomes. [11,44,60,64,65,68,69,85,93–110] Challenges we face have been reported from many low and middle-income nations, though we think our results are especially worrisome [25,111–117].

We observed a wide range of LTFU in different districts, suggesting possible inconsistent fidelity across sites to the active case-finding (*busca activa*) program that is in place, as well as variations in the quality of care, system infrastructure and/or community engagement. [118] In PMTCT work in Zambia and subsequently in the multinational PEARL study, similar clinic-by-clinic diversity has been seen, documenting that the specific component of the continuum of care that is "broken" in lower functioning clinics may differ by clinic [119–123].

In a poorly functioning clinic in Mozambique, we may find health providers who are able to speak only Portuguese with clients, rather than the local language. We have learned from pediatric and obstetric quality improvement work that mothers frequently do not understand complex instructions in Portuguese from health providers who often come from other provinces and may not speak one of the local languages spoken in this ethnically diverse province. [8,118,124] On aggregate, Zambézia residents have low health literacy and numeracy rates, likely contributing to patient/caregiver-provider miscommunication and, possibly to LTFU and suboptimal adherence [125].

Another common occurrence in a poorly functioning clinic generally is the failure of pyschosocial services to effectively engage caregivers fully in chronic pediatric care services, as well as HIV services for themselves. Prior to HIV services, long-term follow-up of chronic diseases was not something with which residents of Zambézia Province were familiar. It is common, especially in rural Africa, that asymptomatic or improving children, parents or guardians do not recognize the need for ongoing services. [126–132] The same applies to parents themselves; they may be LTFU once they feel better. [72,78] We have also had anecdotal reports of parents in our program avoiding care for their children (or themselves) due to stigma and fear of persons learning of the HIV infections in their children. These are daunting challenges that call for more effective counseling and trust-building between providers and clients, and potentially for earlier engagement of children in their health care. The active case-finding approach (*busca active*) of the DPS/MISAU needs serious review and improvement in the face of high mortality and LTFU data in children. It is also possible that traditional active case-finding efforts need to be tailored for special populations, such as children. Improved counseling and family-centered treatment approaches need further exploration. Any innovation in engaging HIV-infected women in their own care can be expected to improve follow-up for their children as well. [133–135] A recent review found that although there is evidence of effectiveness of interventions to improve access and adherence to cART, there is less known about major barriers and ways to address them among vulnerable groups such as women, children and adolescents [136].

There is little tradition of long-term pediatric care in rural Zambézia Province. Mothers take children for vaccines and acute illnesses, but only a tuberculosis diagnosis results in chronic care involving long-term drug administration that can reasonably be expected to be available (such medications as insulin and oncology drugs are not available in the rural clinics). In fact, loss to follow-up rates for children with HIV are high throughout southern Africa. [137] Mothers have told us that they and/or their fathers do not want the stigma of having them take the child for HIV care, that they live too far away and cannot afford the time or money for care, they do not know the health workers due to high turnover rates, and that health workers often mistreat them and violate their confidentiality and their privacy [124,138,139].

Table 1. Characteristics of children at initiation of combination antiretroviral therapy by 2 year outcome in 10 districts of Zambézia Province, Mozambique, 2006–2011 (PITC = Provider-initiated testing and counseling; PMTCT = Prevention of mother-to-child HIV transmission; BMI = Body Mass Index or weight in kg divided by height squared).

	Alive	Dead	Lost	Combined	P-value
	(n = 361)	(n = 152)	(n = 240)	(n = 753)	
Female, n(%)	204 (57%)	73 (48%)	118 (49%)	395 (52%)	0.1
Age (years), median (IQR)	2 (1, 4)	1 (0, 2)	1 (1, 3)	1 (0, 4)	<0.001
District, n(%)					0.002
Alto Molócuè	38 (11%)	19 (12%)	19 (8%)	76 (10%)	
Gilé	15 (4%)	10 (7%)	8 (3%)	33 (4%)	
Ile	23 (6%)	10 (7%)	22 (9%)	55 (7%)	
Inhassunge	69 (19%)	31 (20%)	30 (12%)	130 (17%)	
Lugela	22 (6%)	13 (9%)	15 (6%)	50 (7%)	
Maganja	58 (16%)	9 (6%)	28 (12%)	95 (13%)	
Mopeia	19 (5%)	5 (3%)	13 (5%)	37 (5%)	
Morrumbala	52 (14%)	18 (12%)	26 (11%)	96 (13%)	
Namacurra	47 (13%)	28 (18%)	50 (21%)	125 (17%)	
Pebane	18 (5%)	9 (6%)	29 (12%)	56 (7%)	
Referral site[4], n(%)					0.7
Missing	297 (83%)	134 (88%)	193 (80%)	624 (83%)	
External consultation (PITC)	10 (16%)	4 (22%)	6 (13%)	20 (16%)	
Medical inpatient (PITC)	2 (3%)	0 (0%)	4 (9%)	6 (5%)	
Tuberculosis care (PITC)	1 (2%)	0 (0%)	0 (0%)	1 (<1%)	
PMTCT site	7 (11%)	3 (17%)	8 (17%)	18 (14%)	
Voluntary counseling and testing site	44 (69%)	11 (61%)	29 (62%)	84 (65%)	
Height (cm), median (IQR)[1]	85 (67, 109)	70 (63, 84.2)	72 (66, 81.8)	75 (66, 103.5)	0.04
Missing	206 (57%)	118 (78%)	174 (72%)	498 (66%)	
Weight (kg), median (IQR)[1]	8.5 (6.3, 14)	6.7 (5, 9.5)	7 (5.8, 10)	7.5 (6, 12.4)	<0.001
Missing	4 (1%)	10 (7%)	24 (10%)	38 (5%)	
BMI (kg/m^2), median (IQR)[1]	15.2 (14.1, 16.6)	14.4 (13.8, 17.4)	14.9 (14.2, 16.6)	15.1 (14.1, 16.8)	1
Missing	274 (76%)	132 (87%)	197 (82%)	603 (80%)	
CD4+ cell count/μL, median (IQR)[2]	458 (248, 760)	595 (164, 734)	513 (314, 841)	497 (237, 774)	0.7
Missing	222 (61%)	90 (59%)	149 (62%)	461 (61%)	
CD4 percentage, median (IQR)[2]	15 (10, 21)	15 (12, 22)	15 (8, 21)	15 (10, 21)	0.6
Missing	251 (70%)	107 (70%)	171 (71%)	529 (70%)	
Hemoglobin (g/dL), median (IQR)[2]	9.3 (8, 10.4)	8.3 (7, 9.3)	8.4 (7.4, 9.4)	8.9 (7.6, 9.9)	<0.001
Missing	237 (66%)	100 (66%)	163 (68%)	500 (66%)	
WHO stage, n(%)[2]					0.1
Missing	224 (62%)	75 (49%)	130 (54%)	429 (57%)	
I	47 (34%)	18 (23%)	32 (29%)	97 (30%)	
II	30 (22%)	11 (14%)	29 (26%)	70 (22%)	
III	43 (31%)	39 (51%)	37 (34%)	119 (37%)	
IV	17 (12%)	9 (12%)	12 (11%)	38 (12%)	
Cotrimoxazole use (prior to ART), n(%)[3]	273 (76%)	75 (49%)	132 (55%)	480 (64%)	<0.001
Cotrimoxazole use (current), n(%)[3]	249 (69%)	88 (58%)	142 (59%)	479 (64%)	0.01

Percentages are computed using the number of patients with a non-missing value.
[1]Weight, height, and BMI are collected at enrollment. [2]Collected within 90 days before and 14 days after ART initiation. [3]Prior to ART means any cotrimoxazole (CTX) use recorded in 365 days prior to ART initiation. Current means any CTX use in 90 days before or 90 days after ART initiation. CTX use is recorded along with the visit date; data is not collected on non-users so we are unable to assess missing data. [4]When PITC referral sites are grouped: p = 0.9.

There is evidence from this study and elsewhere that early infant diagnosis, provider initiated testing and counseling, case finding of older children, and family support and outreach are not sufficiently developed in rural Mozambique.

[8,73,78,118,124,125,134,135,140–152] As of 2011, all HIV-infected children <2 years of age should be started on cART as per Mozambican national guidelines, based on results of the South African CHER trial. [79] As of May 2013, Mozambican guidelines changed further to mandate cART for all infected children <5 years of age, independent of clinical status or CD4+ cell count. Yet our study suggests that poor adherence by health workers to standards of screening and HIV staging and subsequent CD4 monitoring impairs pediatric outcomes by delaying recognition of children in need of cART and prophylaxis for opportunistic infections (OI). OI prophylaxis with cotrimoxazole was a protective factor for adverse outcomes in our study. We do not believe that co-trimoxazole benefits are explained by urban-rural differences, as all our sites were rural, nor by family income or assets. All HIV-related services provided by the Ministry, which includes all of the services in this study, are available free of cost, including provision of cotrimoxazole. Family income is not recorded on the clinical record, only patient (or parent) profession; we are thus unable to distinguish subsistence farmers from those who sell their crops, small merchants from larger ones. Over 80 percent of the overall population in the province subsists on less than USD 2 per day as we have documented in a baseline USAID report (Vergara, AE, Blevins M, Vaz LME, et al (2011). Baseline survey report: Improving livelihoods and health of children, women and families in the Province of Zambézia, Republic of Mozambique (available at [http://globalhealth.vanderbilt.edu/programs/scip/]).

Since many children are not diagnosed early or begun on cART early and/or fail to stay in (or adhere to) cART-based care, adverse events are high. [118] We believe that poor interpretation of the guidelines by providers and an overall reluctance to place young children on cART is playing a major role. Quality improvement efforts are essential [148] and are underway to improve infant diagnosis and treatment initiation. [124,135] Linkages across MCH services are being forged to improve treatment outcomes.

Health worker shortages contribute to poor quality of pediatric care. Given severe health care worker shortages and structural impediments to effective long-term care services, we believe that international support, such as that available from PEPFAR and the Global Fund to Fight AIDS, Tuberculosis and Malaria, will be needed for many years to come. [153–157] Whether traditional healers, far more numerous than allopathic practitioners, can be engaged in a productive way for early referral and for assistance in adherence and follow up is unknown. [158,159] More effective community engagement is essential and some success has been had with church-based outreach. [159,160] It is also unknown the extent to which efforts such as the Medical Education Partnership Initiative,[161] the Royal Society-DFID Africa Capacity Building Initiative,[162] or the Consortium of New Southern African Medical Schools [163] will make a major difference over the next 5–10 years in addressing chronic health worker shortages in rural Africa. [164–167] Task-shifting would be a reasonable approach, but nursing and medical assistants (*técnicos de medicina* in Mozambique) are also in very short supply. [8] Creative approaches to patient-to-patient adherence and retention show promise [168–170].

Our data have limitations that affect the completeness of our study. Missing data were frequent, particularly CD4 counts, CD4%, and WHO stage, limiting our ability to examine delays in initiation of treatment. Multivariable analyses were not performed to estimate independent associations with clinical outcomes due to large amounts of missing data and potential for misclassification among those LTFU. We only ask age (in years) of the child such that age subgroups are less reliable, particularly for younger ages, than if we had reliable birthdate; however, rural populations often do not know specific birthdates. Information on cotrimoxazole use was recorded; however, the nature of the documentation is to record use and thus we are unable to differentiate between non-users and missing data. If data are not missing completely at random, there would be bias in the summary statistics of non-missing data. Generalizability of findings to the whole province was limited because data were available for 10 of the total 17 districts. Our database does not collect information on risk factors for poor clinical outcomes external to the patient visit; prospective data collection on such factors (e.g., health facility staffing, drug stock-outs, family support) would permit more robust risk assessment. Nonetheless, we believe that our data clearly indicate a seriously underperforming pediatric care program in need of aggressive quality improvement; despite limitations, we have found these real-world data to be adequate to guide programmatic improvement and community engagement. These efforts are beginning to bear fruit [124,135,148].

There are many challenges not likely to be resolved soon: health care worker shortages and high turnover rates, particularly in remote rural settings, drug and supply stockouts, language barriers, gender-power distortions, literacy and numeracy challenges, poor attitudes of health care workers towards patients, lack of appreciation of the germ theory of disease, crushing rural poverty, poor transportation infrastructures, and structural barriers within the clinical care setting. [73,78,146,148,153,171–173] Co-infections prevalent in the tropics and food shortages are recurring challenges that are far less prevalent in higher income nations. [174–177] Drug resistance has not been studied widely in Mozambique [178].

Even in the face of these obstacles, we and others are having some success in pediatric care HIV quality improvement. [124,135,179–181] That our real-world findings of co-trimoxazole benefit to children in HIV care reinforces clinical trial results suggesting that HIV-infected children benefit from continued co-trimoxazole (protecting against both malaria and non-malarial disease), even when they are on cART. [182] To better retain children on cART and co-trimoxazole, more comprehensive quality improvement efforts are needed to identify staff, structural, cultural, social and policy challenges and to craft solutions for support to pediatric patients, their caregivers, and health care providers.

Acknowledgments

The authors thank Megan Pask, Wilson Silva, Tito Jequicene, Jairzinho Tereso, Carlos Castel-Branco, Ferreira Ferreira, Kulssum Faque, and Deidra Parrish for their help with this work.

Disclosures: This research was supported by the President's Emergency Plan for AIDS Relief (PEPFAR) through the Centers for Disease Control and Prevention (grant #U2GPS000631). The findings and conclusions in this report are those of the authors and do not necessarily represent the official position of the CDC. Dr. Tique was supported by the Fogarty AIDS International Training and Research Program, National Institutes of Health #D43TW001035).

Author Contributions

Conceived and designed the experiments: SHV MB TDM EJ BES LMEV. Performed the experiments: MB TDM EJ LM JAT MS LMEV. Analyzed the data: SHV MB BES LMEV. Contributed reagents/materials/analysis tools: SHV MB TDM EJ LM LMEV. Wrote the paper: SHV MB TDM BES LMEV. Edited and improved the paper: SHV MB TDM EJ LM JAT MS PJC BES LMEV.

References

1. Ministério da Saúde Instituto Nacional de Saúde (INS), Instituto Nacional de Estatística (INE), ICF Macro (2010) Inquérito Nacional de Prevalência, Riscos Comportamentais e Informação sobre o HIV e SIDA (INSIDA) em Moçambique 2009. Calverton, Maryland, EUA: INS, INE, e ICF Macro.
2. Auld AF, Mbofana F, Shiraishi RW, Sanchez M, Alfredo C, et al. (2011) Four-year treatment outcomes of adult patients enrolled in Mozambique's rapidly expanding antiretroviral therapy program. PLoS One 6: e18453.
3. U.S. State Department (2011) The United States President's Emergency Plan for AIDS Relief.
4. Republic of Mozambique, National AIDS Council, CNCS (2012) 2012 Global AIDS Response Progress Report for the Period 2010–2011. Mozambique: Ministério da Saúde Instituto Nacional de Saúde (INS).
5. National Public Health Directorate MoH, Republic of Mozambique (2011) Preliminary Report of the National Evaluation of the Prevention of Mother-to-Child Transmission Program.
6. WHO (2012) Partnership for Maternal, Newborn & Child Health, World Health Organization. Countdown to 2015: Building a Future for Women and Children, Mozambique Country Reports.
7. Instituto Nacional de Estastistica, Ministerio da Saude, US AID (2013) Moçambique Inquérito Demográfico e de Saúde 2011. Calverton, Maryland, USA.
8. Audet CM, Burlison J, Moon TD, Sidat M, Vergara AE, et al. (2010) Sociocultural and epidemiological aspects of HIV/AIDS in Mozambique. BMC Int Health Hum Rights 10: 15.
9. Institute NS (2009) Preliminary Report on the Multiple Indicator Cluster Survey, 2008. Maputo, Mozambique.
10. Republic of Mozambique, Ministry of Health, National Institute of Health (2009) Mozambique National Child Mortality Study 2009 Summary.
11. Bolton-Moore C, Mubiana-Mbewe M, Cantrell RA, Chintu N, Stringer EM, et al. (2007) Clinical outcomes and CD4 cell response in children receiving antiretroviral therapy at primary health care facilities in Zambia. JAMA 298: 1888–1899.
12. Bland RM, Ndirangu J, Newell ML (2013) Maximising opportunities for increased antiretroviral treatment in children in an existing HIV programme in rural South Africa. BMJ 346: f550.
13. Patel SD, Larson E, Mbengashe T, O'Bra H, Brown JW, et al. (2012) Increases in pediatric antiretroviral treatment, South Africa 2005–2010. PLoS One 7: e44914.
14. Munyagwa M, Baisley K, Levin J, Brian M, Grosskurth H, et al. (2012) Mortality of HIV-infected and uninfected children in a longitudinal cohort in rural south-west Uganda during 8 years of follow-up. Trop Med Int Health 17: 836–843.
15. Meyers T, Dramowski A, Schneider H, Gardiner N, Kuhn L, et al. (2012) Changes in pediatric HIV-related hospital admissions and mortality in Soweto, South Africa, 1996–2011: light at the end of the tunnel? J Acquir Immune Defic Syndr 60: 503–510.
16. Johnson LF, Davies MA, Moultrie H, Sherman GG, Bland RM, et al. (2012) The effect of early initiation of antiretroviral treatment in infants on pediatric AIDS mortality in South Africa: a model-based analysis. Pediatr Infect Dis J 31: 474–480.
17. Bland RM (2011) Management of HIV-infected children in Africa: progress and challenges. Arch Dis Child 96: 911–915.
18. Eley B (2006) Addressing the paediatric HIV epidemic: a perspective from the Western Cape Region of South Africa. Trans R Soc Trop Med Hyg 100: 19–23.
19. De Baets AJ, Bulterys M, Abrams EJ, Kankassa C, Pazvakavambwa IE (2007) Care and treatment of HIV-infected children in Africa: issues and challenges at the district hospital level. Pediatr Infect Dis J 26: 163–173.
20. Braitstein P, Nyandiko W, Vreeman R, Wools-Kaloustian K, Sang E, et al. (2009) The clinical burden of tuberculosis among human immunodeficiency virus-infected children in Western Kenya and the impact of combination antiretroviral treatment. Pediatr Infect Dis J 28: 626–632.
21. Nicoll A, Timaeus I, Kigadye RM, Walraven G, Killewo J (1994) The impact of HIV-1 infection on mortality in children under 5 years of age in sub-Saharan Africa: a demographic and epidemiologic analysis. AIDS 8: 995–1005.
22. Martinson NA, Moultrie H, van Niekerk R, Barry G, Coovadia A, et al. (2009) HAART and risk of tuberculosis in HIV-infected South African children: a multi-site retrospective cohort. Int J Tuberc Lung Dis 13: 862–867.
23. Sutcliffe CG, van Dijk JH, Bolton-Moore C, Cotham M, Tambatamba B, et al. (2010) Differences in presentation, treatment initiation, and response among children infected with human immunodeficiency virus in urban and rural Zambia. Pediatr Infect Dis J 29: 849–854.
24. Sutcliffe CG, van Dijk JH, Bolton C, Persaud D, Moss WJ (2008) Effectiveness of antiretroviral therapy among HIV-infected children in sub-Saharan Africa. Lancet Infect Dis 8: 477–489.
25. van Dijk JH, Sutcliffe CG, Munsanje B, Hamangaba F, Thuma PE, et al. (2009) Barriers to the care of HIV-infected children in rural Zambia: a cross-sectional analysis. BMC Infect Dis 9: 169.
26. Feucht UD, Kinzer M, Kruger M (2007) Reasons for delay in initiation of antiretroviral therapy in a population of HIV-infected South African children. J Trop Pediatr 53: 398–402.
27. Thomas TA, Shenoi SV, Heysell SK, Eksteen FJ, Sunkari VB, et al. (2010) Extensively drug-resistant tuberculosis in children with human immunodeficiency virus in rural South Africa. Int J Tuberc Lung Dis 14: 1244–1251.
28. Adjorlolo-Johnson G, Wahl Uheling A, Ramachandran S, Strasser S, Kouakou J, et al. (2013) Scaling up pediatric HIV care and treatment in Africa: clinical site characteristics associated with favorable service utilization. J Acquir Immune Defic Syndr 62: e7–e13.
29. Kabue MM, Buck WC, Wanless SR, Cox CM, McCollum ED, et al. (2012) Mortality and clinical outcomes in HIV-infected children on antiretroviral therapy in Malawi, Lesotho, and Swaziland. Pediatrics 130: e591–599.
30. Okomo U, Togun T, Oko F, Peterson K, Townend J, et al. (2012) Treatment outcomes among HIV-1 and HIV-2 infected children initiating antiretroviral therapy in a concentrated low prevalence setting in West Africa. BMC Pediatr 12: 95.
31. Grimwood A, Fatti G, Mothibi E, Malahlela M, Shea J, et al. (2012) Community adherence support improves programme retention in children on antiretroviral treatment: a multicentre cohort study in South Africa. J Int AIDS Soc 15: 17381.
32. Chhagan MK, Kauchali S, Van den Broeck J (2012) Clinical and contextual determinants of anthropometric failure at baseline and longitudinal improvements after starting antiretroviral treatment among South African children. Trop Med Int Health 17: 1092–1099.
33. Satti H, McLaughlin MM, Omotayo DB, Keshavjee S, Becerra MC, et al. (2012) Outcomes of comprehensive care for children empirically treated for multidrug-resistant tuberculosis in a setting of high HIV prevalence. PLoS One 7: e37114.
34. Laughton B, Cornell M, Grove D, Kidd M, Springer PE, et al. (2012) Early antiretroviral therapy improves neurodevelopmental outcomes in infants. AIDS 26: 1685–1690.
35. Haberer JE, Kiwanuka J, Nansera D, Ragland K, Mellins C, et al. (2012) Multiple measures reveal antiretroviral adherence successes and challenges in HIV-infected Ugandan children. PLoS One 7: e36737.
36. Kekitiinwa A, Asiimwe AR, Kasirye P, Korutaro V, Kitaka S, et al. (2012) Prospective long-term outcomes of a cohort of Ugandan children with laboratory monitoring during antiretroviral therapy. Pediatr Infect Dis J 31: e117–125.
37. Musiime V, Kayiwa J, Kiconco M, Tamale W, Alima H, et al. (2012) Response to antiretroviral therapy of HIV type 1-infected children in urban and rural settings of Uganda. AIDS Res Hum Retroviruses 28: 1647–1657.
38. Workneh G, Scherzer L, Kirk B, Draper HR, Anabwani G, et al. (2013) Evaluation of the effectiveness of an outreach clinical mentoring programme in support of paediatric HIV care scale-up in Botswana. AIDS Care 25: 11–19.
39. Heidari S, Mofenson LM, Hobbs CV, Cotton MF, Marlink R, et al. (2012) Unresolved antiretroviral treatment management issues in HIV-infected children. J Acquir Immune Defic Syndr 59: 161–169.
40. Kim MH, Cox C, Dave A, Draper HR, Kabue M, et al. (2012) Prompt initiation of ART With therapeutic food is associated with improved outcomes in HIV-infected Malawian children with malnutrition. J Acquir Immune Defic Syndr 59: 173–176.
41. Zyl GU, Rabie H, Nuttall JJ, Cotton MF (2011) It is time to consider third-line options in antiretroviral-experienced paediatric patients? J Int AIDS Soc 14: 55.
42. Reubenson G (2011) Pediatric drug-resistant tuberculosis: a global perspective: a global perspective. Paediatr Drugs 13: 349–355.
43. Geddes R, Giddy J, Butler LM, Van Wyk E, Crankshaw T, et al. (2011) Dual and triple therapy to prevent mother-to-child transmission of HIV in a resource-limited setting - lessons from a South African programme. S Afr Med J 101: 651–654.
44. Fatti G, Bock P, Eley B, Mothibi E, Grimwood A (2011) Temporal trends in baseline characteristics and treatment outcomes of children starting antiretroviral treatment: an analysis in four provinces in South Africa, 2004–2009. J Acquir Immune Defic Syndr 58: e60–67.
45. Ahoua L, Guenther G, Rouzioux C, Pinoges L, Anguzu P, et al. (2011) Immunovirological response to combined antiretroviral therapy and drug resistance patterns in children: 1- and 2-year outcomes in rural Uganda. BMC Pediatr 11: 67.
46. Desmonde S, Coffie P, Aka E, Amani-Bosse C, Messou E, et al. (2011) Severe morbidity and mortality in untreated HIV-infected children in a paediatric care programme in Abidjan, Cote d'Ivoire, 2004–2009. BMC Infect Dis 11: 182.
47. Ciaranello AL, Perez F, Maruva M, Chu J, Engelsmann B, et al. (2011) WHO 2010 guidelines for prevention of mother-to-child HIV transmission in Zimbabwe: modeling clinical outcomes in infants and mothers. PLoS One 6: e20224.
48. Bakanda C, Birungi J, Mwesigwa R, Nachega JB, Chan K, et al. (2011) Survival of HIV-infected adolescents on antiretroviral therapy in Uganda: findings from a nationally representative cohort in Uganda. PLoS One 6: e19261.
49. Schneider K, Puthanakit T, Kerr S, Law MG, Cooper DA, et al. (2011) Economic evaluation of monitoring virologic responses to antiretroviral therapy in HIV-infected children in resource-limited settings. AIDS 25: 1143–1151.

50. Frohoff C, Moodley M, Fairlie L, Coovadia A, Moultrie H, et al. (2011) Antiretroviral therapy outcomes in HIV-infected children after adjusting protease inhibitor dosing during tuberculosis treatment. PLoS One 6: e17273.
51. De Maayer T, Saloojee H (2011) Clinical outcomes of severe malnutrition in a high tuberculosis and HIV setting. Arch Dis Child 96: 560–564.
52. McCollum ED, Preidis GA, Golitko CL, Siwande LD, Mwansambo C, et al. (2011) Routine inpatient human immunodeficiency virus testing system increases access to pediatric human immunodeficiency virus care in sub-Saharan Africa. Pediatr Infect Dis J 30: e75–81.
53. Ndondoki C, Dabis F, Namale L, Becquet R, Ekouevi D, et al. (2011) [Survival, clinical and biological outcomes of HIV-infected children treated by antiretroviral therapy in Africa: systematic review, 2004–2009]. Presse Med 40: e338–357.
54. Peacock-Villada E, Richardson BA, John-Stewart GC (2011) Post-HAART outcomes in pediatric populations: comparison of resource-limited and developed countries. Pediatrics 127: e423–441.
55. Fatti G, Bock P, Grimwood A, Eley B (2010) Increased vulnerability of rural children on antiretroviral therapy attending public health facilities in South Africa: a retrospective cohort study. J Int AIDS Soc 13: 46.
56. Buck WC, Kabue MM, Kazembe PN, Kline MW (2010) Discontinuation of standard first-line antiretroviral therapy in a cohort of 1434 Malawian children. J Int AIDS Soc 13: 31.
57. Musoke PM, Mudiope P, Barlow-Mosha LN, Ajuna P, Bagenda D, et al. (2010) Growth, immune and viral responses in HIV infected African children receiving highly active antiretroviral therapy: a prospective cohort study. BMC Pediatr 10: 56.
58. Sutcliffe CG, Bolton-Moore C, van Dijk JH, Cotham M, Tambatamba B, et al. (2010) Secular trends in pediatric antiretroviral treatment programs in rural and urban Zambia: a retrospective cohort study. BMC Pediatr 10: 54.
59. Nyandiko WM, Mwangi A, Ayaya SO, Nabakwe EC, Tenge CN, et al. (2009) Characteristics of HIV-infected children seen in Western Kenya. East Afr Med J 86: 364–373.
60. Sauvageot D, Schaefer M, Olson D, Pujades-Rodriguez M, O'Brien DP (2010) Antiretroviral therapy outcomes in resource-limited settings for HIV-infected children <5 years of age. Pediatrics 125: e1039–1047.
61. Davies MA, Keiser O, Technau K, Eley B, Rabie H, et al. (2009) Outcomes of the South African National Antiretroviral Treatment Programme for children: the IeDEA Southern Africa collaboration. S Afr Med J 99: 730–737.
62. Leyenaar JK, Novosad PM, Ferrer KT, Thahane LK, Mohapi EQ, et al. (2010) Early clinical outcomes in children enrolled in human immunodeficiency virus infection care and treatment in lesotho. Pediatr Infect Dis J 29: 340–345.
63. Ciaranello AL, Chang Y, Margulis AV, Bernstein A, Bassett IV, et al. (2009) Effectiveness of pediatric antiretroviral therapy in resource-limited settings: a systematic review and meta-analysis. Clin Infect Dis 49: 1915–1927.
64. Janssen N, Ndirangu J, Newell ML, Bland RM (2010) Successful paediatric HIV treatment in rural primary care in Africa. Arch Dis Child 95: 414–421.
65. Memirie ST (2009) Clinical outcome of children on HAART at police referral hospital, Addis Ababa, Ethiopia. Ethiop Med J 47: 159–164.
66. Ntanda H, Olupot-Olupot P, Mugyenyi P, Kityo C, Lowes R, et al. (2009) Orphanhood predicts delayed access to care in Ugandan children. Pediatr Infect Dis J 28: 153–155.
67. Van Winghem J, Telfer B, Reid T, Ouko J, Mutunga A, et al. (2008) Implementation of a comprehensive program including psycho-social and treatment literacy activities to improve adherence to HIV care and treatment for a pediatric population in Kenya. BMC Pediatr 8: 52.
68. Kiboneka A, Wangisi J, Nabiryo C, Tembe J, Kusemererwa S, et al. (2008) Clinical and immunological outcomes of a national paediatric cohort receiving combination antiretroviral therapy in Uganda. AIDS 22: 2493–2499.
69. Jaspan HB, Berrisford AE, Boulle AM (2008) Two-year outcomes of children on non-nucleoside reverse transcriptase inhibitor and protease inhibitor regimens in a South African pediatric antiretroviral program. Pediatr Infect Dis J 27: 993–998.
70. Bock P, Boulle A, White C, Osler M, Eley B (2008) Provision of antiretroviral therapy to children within the public sector of South Africa. Trans R Soc Trop Med Hyg 102: 905–911.
71. Walker AS, Ford D, Mulenga V, Thomason MJ, Nunn A, et al. (2009) Adherence to both cotrimoxazole and placebo is associated with improved survival among HIV-infected Zambian children. AIDS Behav 13: 33–41.
72. Moon TD, Burlison JR, Sidat M, Pires P, Silva W, et al. (2010) Lessons Learned while Implementing an HIV/AIDs Care and Treatment Program in Rural Mozambique. Retrovirology: Research and Treatment 3: 1.
73. Manders EJ, Jose E, Solis M, Burlison J, Nhampossa JL, et al. (2010) Implementing OpenMRS for patient monitoring in an HIV/AIDS care and treatment program in rural Mozambique. Stud Health Technol Inform 160: 411–415.
74. Lahuerta M, Lima J, Elul B, Okamura M, Alvim MF, et al. (2011) Patients enrolled in HIV care in Mozambique: baseline characteristics and follow-up outcomes. J Acquir Immune Defic Syndr 58: e75–86.
75. Shepherd BE, Blevins M, Vaz LM, Moon TD, Kipp AM, et al. (2013) Impact of Definitions of Loss to Follow-up on Estimates of Retention, Disease Progression, and Mortality: Application to an HIV Program in Mozambique. Am J Epidemiol.
76. Chi BH, Yiannoutsos CT, Westfall AO, Newman JE, Zhou J, et al. (2011) Universal definition of loss to follow-up in HIV treatment programs: a statistical analysis of 111 facilities in Africa, Asia, and Latin America. PLoS Med 8: e1001111.
77. Grimsrud AT, Cornell M, Egger M, Boulle A, Myer L (2013) Impact of definitions of loss to follow-up (LTFU) in antiretroviral therapy program evaluation: variation in the definition can have an appreciable impact on estimated proportions of LTFU. J Clin Epidemiol.
78. Moon TD, Burlison JR, Blevins M, Shepherd BE, Baptista A, et al. (2011) Enrolment and programmatic trends and predictors of antiretroviral therapy initiation from president's emergency plan for AIDS Relief (PEPFAR)-supported public HIV care and treatment sites in rural Mozambique. Int J STD AIDS 22: 621–627.
79. Violari A, Cotton MF, Gibb DM, Babiker AG, Steyn J, et al. (2008) Early antiretroviral therapy and mortality among HIV-infected infants. N Engl J Med 359: 2233–2244.
80. Ylitalo N, Brogly S, Hughes MD, Nachman S, Dankner W, et al. (2006) Risk factors for opportunistic illnesses in children with human immunodeficiency virus in the era of highly active antiretroviral therapy. Arch Pediatr Adolesc Med 160: 778–787.
81. Rath BA, von Kleist M, Castillo ME, Kolevic L, Caballero P, et al. (2013) Antiviral resistance and correlates of virologic failure in the first cohort of HIV-infected children gaining access to structured antiretroviral therapy in Lima, Peru: a cross-sectional analysis. BMC Infect Dis 13: 1.
82. Christie CD, Pierre RB (2012) Eliminating vertically-transmitted HIV/AIDS while improving access to treatment and care for women, children and adolescents in Jamaica. West Indian Med J 61: 396–404.
83. Hansudewechakul R, Naiwatanakul T, Katana A, Faikratok W, Lolekha R, et al. (2012) Successful clinical outcomes following decentralization of tertiary paediatric HIV care to a community-based paediatric antiretroviral treatment network, Chiangrai, Thailand, 2002 to 2008. J Int AIDS Soc 15: 17358.
84. Diniz LM, Maia MM, Camargos LS, Amaral LC, Goulart EM, et al. (2011) Impact of HAART on growth and hospitalization rates among HIV-infected children. J Pediatr (Rio J) 87: 131–137.
85. Lumbiganon P, Kariminia A, Aurpibul L, Hansudewechakul R, Puthanakit T, et al. (2011) Survival of HIV-infected children: a cohort study from the Asia-Pacific region. J Acquir Immune Defic Syndr 56: 365–371.
86. Oliveira R, Krauss M, Essama-Bibi S, Hofer C, Robert Harris D, et al. (2010) Viral load predicts new world health organization stage 3 and 4 events in HIV-infected children receiving highly active antiretroviral therapy, independent of CD4 T lymphocyte value. Clin Infect Dis 51: 1325–1333.
87. Rodriguez de Schiavi MS, Scrigni A, Garcia Arrigoni P, Bologna R, Barboni G, et al. (2009) [Highly active antiretroviral therapy in HIV sero-positive children. Disease progression by baseline clinical, immunological and virological status]. Arch Argent Pediatr 107: 212–220.
88. Prasitsuebsai W, Bowen AC, Pang J, Hesp C, Kariminia A, et al. (2010) Pediatric HIV clinical care resources and management practices in Asia: a regional survey of the TREAT Asia pediatric network. AIDS Patient Care STDS 24: 127–131.
89. McConnell MS, Chasombat S, Siangphoe U, Yuktanont P, Lolekha R, et al. (2010) National program scale-up and patient outcomes in a pediatric antiretroviral treatment program, Thailand, 2000–2007. J Acquir Immune Defic Syndr 54: 423–429.
90. Souza E, Santos N, Valentini S, Silva G, Falbo A (2010) Long-term follow-up outcomes of perinatally HIV-infected adolescents: infection control but school failure. J Trop Pediatr 56: 421–426.
91. Kumarasamy N, Venkatesh KK, Devaleenol B, Poongulali S, Mothi SN, et al. (2009) Safety, tolerability and effectiveness of generic HAART in HIV-infected children in South India. J Trop Pediatr 55: 155–159.
92. Noel F, Mehta S, Zhu Y, Rouzier Pde M, Marcelin A, et al. (2008) Improving outcomes in infants of HIV-infected women in a developing country setting. PLoS One 3: e3723.
93. Reddi A, Leeper SC, Grobler AC, Geddes R, France KH, et al. (2007) Preliminary outcomes of a paediatric highly active antiretroviral therapy cohort from KwaZulu-Natal, South Africa. BMC Pediatr 7: 13.
94. Puthanakit T, Aurpibul L, Oberdorfer P, Akarathum N, Kanjananit S, et al. (2007) Hospitalization and mortality among HIV-infected children after receiving highly active antiretroviral therapy. Clin Infect Dis 44: 599–604.
95. Puthanakit T, Oberdorfer A, Akarathum N, Kanjanavanit S, Wannarit P, et al. (2005) Efficacy of highly active antiretroviral therapy in HIV-infected children participating in Thailand's National Access to Antiretroviral Program. Clin Infect Dis 41: 100–107.
96. Janssens B, Raleigh B, Soeung S, Akao K, Te V, et al. (2007) Effectiveness of highly active antiretroviral therapy in HIV-positive children: evaluation at 12 months in a routine program in Cambodia. Pediatrics 120: e1134–1140.
97. Nyandiko WM, Ayaya S, Nabakwe E, Tenge C, Sidle JE, et al. (2006) Outcomes of HIV-infected orphaned and non-orphaned children on antiretroviral therapy in western Kenya. J Acquir Immune Defic Syndr 43: 418–425.
98. Wamalwa DC, Obimbo EM, Farquhar C, Richardson BA, Mbori-Ngacha DA, et al. (2010) Predictors of mortality in HIV-1 infected children on antiretroviral therapy in Kenya: a prospective cohort. BMC Pediatr 10: 33.
99. O'Brien DP, Sauvageot D, Zachariah R, Humblet P, Medecins Sans F (2006) In resource-limited settings good early outcomes can be achieved in children

using adult fixed-dose combination antiretroviral therapy. AIDS 20: 1955–1960.

100. Adje-Toure C, Hanson DL, Talla-Nzussouo N, Borget MY, Kouadio LY, et al. (2008) Virologic and immunologic response to antiretroviral therapy and predictors of HIV type 1 drug resistance in children receiving treatment in Abidjan, Cote d'Ivoire. AIDS Res Hum Retroviruses 24: 911–917.
101. Song R, Jelagat J, Dzombo D, Mwalimu M, Mandaliya K, et al. (2007) Efficacy of highly active antiretroviral therapy in HIV-1 infected children in Kenya. Pediatrics 120: e856–861.
102. Kline MW, Matusa RF, Copaciu L, Calles NR, Kline NE, et al. (2004) Comprehensive pediatric human immunodeficiency virus care and treatment in Constanta, Romania: implementation of a program of highly active antiretroviral therapy in a resource-poor setting. Pediatr Infect Dis J 23: 695–700.
103. Kabue MM, Kekitiinwa A, Maganda A, Risser JM, Chan W, et al. (2008) Growth in HIV-infected children receiving antiretroviral therapy at a pediatric infectious diseases clinic in Uganda. AIDS Patient Care STDS 22: 245–251.
104. Kline MW, Rugina S, Ilie M, Matusa RF, Schweitzer AM, et al. (2007) Long-term follow-up of 414 HIV-infected Romanian children and adolescents receiving lopinavir/ritonavir-containing highly active antiretroviral therapy. Pediatrics 119: e1116–1120.
105. Evans-Gilbert T, Pierre R, Steel-Duncan JC, Rodriguez B, Whorms S, et al. (2004) Antiretroviral drug therapy in HIV-infected Jamaican children. West Indian Med J 53: 322–326.
106. Pierre RB, Steel-Duncan JC, Evans-Gilbert T, Rodriguez B, Moore J, et al. (2008) Effectiveness of antiretroviral therapy in treating paediatric HIV/AIDS in Jamaica. West Indian Med J 57: 223–230.
107. Eley B, Davies MA, Apolles P, Cowburn C, Buys H, et al. (2006) Antiretroviral treatment for children. S Afr Med J 96: 988–993.
108. Collins IJ, Jourdain G, Hansudewechakul R, Kanjanavanit S, Hongsiriwon S, et al. (2010) Long-term survival of HIV-infected children receiving antiretroviral therapy in Thailand: a 5-year observational cohort study. Clin Infect Dis 51: 1449–1457.
109. Meyers TM, Yotebieng M, Kuhn L, Moultrie H (2011) Antiretroviral therapy responses among children attending a large public clinic in Soweto, South Africa. Pediatr Infect Dis J 30: 974–979.
110. van Kooten Niekerk NK, Knies MM, Howard J, Rabie H, Zeier M, et al. (2006) The first 5 years of the family clinic for HIV at Tygerberg Hospital: family demographics, survival of children and early impact of antiretroviral therapy. J Trop Pediatr 52: 3–11.
111. Kamya MR, Mayanja-Kizza H, Kambugu A, Bakeera-Kitaka S, Semitala F, et al. (2007) Predictors of long-term viral failure among ugandan children and adults treated with antiretroviral therapy. J Acquir Immune Defic Syndr 46: 187–193.
112. Zanoni BC, Phungula T, Zanoni HM, France H, Feeney ME (2011) Risk factors associated with increased mortality among HIV infected children initiating antiretroviral therapy (ART) in South Africa. PLoS One 6: e22706.
113. Bong CN, Yu JK, Chiang HC, Huang WL, Hsieh TC, et al. (2007) Risk factors for early mortality in children on adult fixed-dose combination antiretroviral treatment in a central hospital in Malawi. AIDS 21: 1805–1810.
114. Callens SF, Shabani N, Lusiama J, Lelo P, Kitetele F, et al. (2009) Mortality and associated factors after initiation of pediatric antiretroviral treatment in the Democratic Republic of the Congo. Pediatr Infect Dis J 28: 35–40.
115. Raguenaud ME, Isaakidis P, Zachariah R, Te V, Soeung S, et al. (2009) Excellent outcomes among HIV+ children on ART, but unacceptably high pre-ART mortality and losses to follow-up: a cohort study from Cambodia. BMC Pediatr 9: 54.
116. Taye B, Shiferaw S, Enquselassie F (2010) The impact of malnutrition in survival of HIV infected children after initiation of antiretroviral treatment (ART). Ethiop Med J 48: 1–10.
117. Anaky MF, Duvignac J, Wemin L, Kouakoussui A, Karcher S, et al. (2010) Scaling up antiretroviral therapy for HIV-infected children in Cote d'Ivoire: determinants of survival and loss to programme. Bull World Health Organ 88: 490–499.
118. Groh K, Audet CM, Baptista A, Sidat M, Vergara A, et al. (2011) Barriers to antiretroviral therapy adherence in rural Mozambique. BMC Public Health 11: 650.
119. Stringer EM, Sinkala M, Stringer JS, Mzyece E, Makuka I, et al. (2003) Prevention of mother-to-child transmission of HIV in Africa: successes and challenges in scaling-up a nevirapine-based program in Lusaka, Zambia. AIDS 17: 1377–1382.
120. Stringer JS, Sinkala M, Maclean CC, Levy J, Kankasa C, et al. (2005) Effectiveness of a city-wide program to prevent mother-to-child HIV transmission in Lusaka, Zambia. AIDS 19: 1309–1315.
121. Reithinger R, Megazzini K, Durako SJ, Harris DR, Vermund SH (2007) Monitoring and evaluation of programmes to prevent mother to child transmission of HIV in Africa. BMJ 334: 1143–1146.
122. Stringer EM, Ekouevi DK, Coetzee D, Tih PM, Creek TL, et al. (2010) Coverage of nevirapine-based services to prevent mother-to-child HIV transmission in 4 African countries. JAMA 304: 293–302.
123. Stringer EM, Chintu NT, Levy JW, Sinkala M, Chi BH, et al. (2008) Declining HIV prevalence among young pregnant women in Lusaka, Zambia. Bull World Health Organ 86: 697–702.
124. Ciampa PJ, Burlison JR, Blevins M, Sidat M, Moon TD, et al. (2011) Improving retention in the early infant diagnosis of HIV program in rural Mozambique by better service integration. J Acquir Immune Defic Syndr 58: 115–119.
125. Ciampa PJ, Vaz LM, Blevins M, Sidat M, Rothman RL, et al. (2012) The association among literacy, numeracy, HIV knowledge and health-seeking behavior: a population-based survey of women in rural Mozambique. PLoS One 7: e39391.
126. Nyandiko W, Vreeman R, Liu H, Shangani S, Sang E, et al. (2013) Nonadherence to clinic appointments among HIV-infected children in an ambulatory care program in western Kenya. J Acquir Immune Defic Syndr 63: e49–55.
127. Sengayi M, Dwane N, Marinda E, Sipambo N, Fairlie L, et al. (2013) Predictors of loss to follow-up among children in the first and second years of antiretroviral treatment in Johannesburg, South Africa. Glob Health Action 6: 19248.
128. Wachira J, Middlestadt SE, Vreeman R, Braitstein P (2012) Factors underlying taking a child to HIV care: implications for reducing loss to follow-up among HIV-infected and -exposed children. SAHARA J 9: 20–29.
129. Langat NT, Odero W, Gatongi P (2012) Antiretroviral drug adherence by HIV infected children attending Kericho District Hospital, Kenya. East Afr J Public Health 9: 101–104.
130. McNairy ML, Lamb MR, Carter RJ, Fayorsey R, Tene G, et al. (2012) Retention of HIV-infected children on antiretroviral treatment in HIV care and treatment programs in Kenya, Mozambique, Rwanda and Tanzania. J Acquir Immune Defic Syndr.
131. Okomo U, Togun T, Oko F, Peterson K, Jaye A (2012) Mortality and loss to programme before antiretroviral therapy among HIV-infected children eligible for treatment in The Gambia, West Africa. AIDS Res Ther 9: 28.
132. Chetty T, Knight S, Giddy J, Crankshaw TL, Butler LM, et al. (2012) A retrospective study of Human Immunodeficiency Virus transmission, mortality and loss to follow-up among infants in the first 18 months of life in a prevention of mother-to-child transmission programme in an urban hospital in KwaZulu-Natal, South Africa. BMC Pediatr 12: 146.
133. Audet CM, Silva Matos C, Blevins M, Cardoso A, Moon TD, et al. (2012) Acceptability of cervical cancer screening in rural Mozambique. Health Educ Res 27: 544–551.
134. Moon TD, Silva-Matos C, Cordoso A, Baptista AJ, Sidat M, et al. (2012) Implementation of cervical cancer screening using visual inspection with acetic acid in rural Mozambique: successes and challenges using HIV care and treatment programme investments in Zambezia Province. J Int AIDS Soc 15: 17406.
135. Ciampa PJ, Tique JA, Juma N, Sidat M, Moon TD, et al. (2012) Addressing poor retention of infants exposed to HIV: a quality improvement study in rural Mozambique. J Acquir Immune Defic Syndr 60: e46–52.
136. Scanlon ML, Vreeman RC (2013) Current strategies for improving access and adherence to antiretroviral therapies in resource-limited settings. HIV AIDS (Auckl) 5: 1–17.
137. Fenner L, Brinkhof MW, Keiser O, Weigel R, Cornell M, et al. (2010) Early mortality and loss to follow-up in HIV-infected children starting antiretroviral therapy in Southern Africa. Journal of acquired immune deficiency syndromes (1999) 54: 524.
138. Groh K, Audet C, Baptista A, Sidat M, Vergara A, et al. (2011) Barriers to antiretroviral therapy adherence in rural Mozambique. BMC public health 11: 650.
139. Audet CM, Groh K, Moon TD, Vermund SH, Sidat M (2012) Poor-quality health services and lack of programme support leads to low uptake of HIV testing in rural Mozambique. African Journal of AIDS Research 11: 327–335.
140. Geelhoed D, Lafort Y, Chissale E, Candrinho B, Degomme O (2013) Integrated maternal and child health services in Mozambique: structural health system limitations overshadow its effect on follow-up of HIV-exposed infants. BMC Health Serv Res 13: 207.
141. Lambdin BH, Micek MA, Sherr K, Gimbel S, Karagianis M, et al. (2013) Integration of HIV care and treatment in primary health care centers and patient retention in central Mozambique: a retrospective cohort study. J Acquir Immune Defic Syndr 62: e146–152.
142. Audet CM, Sidat M, Blevins M, Moon TD, Vergara A, et al. (2012) HIV knowledge and health-seeking behavior in Zambezia Province, Mozambique. SAHARA J 9: 41–46.
143. Ciampa PJ, Skinner SL, Patricio SR, Rothman RL, Vermund SH, et al. (2012) Comprehensive knowledge of HIV among women in rural Mozambique: development and validation of the HIV knowledge 27 scale. PLoS One 7: e48676.
144. Lehe JD, Sitoe NE, Tobaiwa O, Loquiha O, Quevedo JI, et al. (2012) Evaluating operational specifications of point-of-care diagnostic tests: a standardized scorecard. PLoS One 7: e47459.
145. Bandali S (2013) HIV Risk Assessment and Risk Reduction Strategies in the Context of Prevailing Gender Norms in Rural Areas of Cabo Delgado, Mozambique. J Int Assoc Provid AIDS Care 12: 50–54.
146. Yao J, Murray AT, Agadjanian V, Hayford SR (2012) Geographic influences on sexual and reproductive health service utilization in rural Mozambique. Appl Geogr 32: 601–607.

147. Wandeler G, Keiser O, Pfeiffer K, Pestilli S, Fritz C, et al. (2012) Outcomes of antiretroviral treatment programs in rural Southern Africa. J Acquir Immune Defic Syndr 59: e9–16.
148. Cook RE, Ciampa PJ, Sidat M, Blevins M, Burlison J, et al. (2011) Predictors of successful early infant diagnosis of HIV in a rural district hospital in Zambezia, Mozambique. J Acquir Immune Defic Syndr 56: e104–109.
149. Noden BH, Gomes A, Ferreira A (2010) Influence of religious affiliation and education on HIV knowledge and HIV-related sexual behaviors among unmarried youth in rural central Mozambique. AIDS Care 22: 1285–1294.
150. Posse M, Baltussen R (2009) Barriers to access to antiretroviral treatment in Mozambique, as perceived by patients and health workers in urban and rural settings. AIDS Patient Care STDS 23: 867–875.
151. Agadjanian V, Sen S (2007) Promises and challenges of faith-based AIDS care and support in Mozambique. Am J Public Health 97: 362–366.
152. Vuylsteke B, Bastos R, Barreto J, Crucitti T, Folgosa E, et al. (1993) High prevalence of sexually transmitted diseases in a rural area in Mozambique. Genitourin Med 69: 427–430.
153. Vermund SH, Sidat M, Weil LF, Tique JA, Moon TD, et al. (2012) Transitioning HIV care and treatment programs in southern Africa to full local management. AIDS 26: 1303–1310.
154. Gormley W, McCaffery J, Quain EE (2011) Moving forward on human resources for health: next steps for scaling up toward universal access to HIV/AIDS prevention, treatment, and care. J Acquir Immune Defic Syndr 57 Suppl 2: S113–115.
155. Lambdin BH, Micek MA, Koepsell TD, Hughes JP, Sherr K, et al. (2011) Patient volume, human resource levels, and attrition from HIV treatment programs in central Mozambique. J Acquir Immune Defic Syndr 57: e33–39.
156. Fulton BD, Scheffler RM, Sparkes SP, Auh EY, Vujicic M, et al. (2011) Health workforce skill mix and task shifting in low income countries: a review of recent evidence. Hum Resour Health 9: 1.
157. Adjorlolo-Johnson G, Wahl A, Ramachandran S, Strasser S, Kouakou J, et al. (2012) Scaling up Pediatric HIV Care and Treatment in Africa: Clinical Site Characteristics Associated with Favorable Service Utilization. J Acquir Immune Defic Syndr.
158. Audet CM, Blevins M, Moon TD, Shepherd BE, Vergara A, et al. (2012) Knowledge and Treatment of HIV/AIDS by traditional healers in central Mozambique. J Altern Comlement Med [In Press].
159. Audet CM, Blevins M, Moon TD, Sidat M, Shepherd BE, et al. (2012) Traditional healers in rural Mozambique: Qualitative survey of HIV/AIDS-related attitudes and practices. Journal of Social Aspects of HIV/AIDS [In Press].
160. Agadjanian V, Menjivar C (2011) Fighting down the scourge, building up the church: organisational constraints in religious involvement with HIV/AIDS in Mozambique. Glob Public Health 6 Suppl 2: S148–162.
161. MEPI (Medical Education Partnership Initiative) (2010)Medical Education Partnership Initiative.
162. The Africa Capacity Building Initiative (1991) The Africa Capacity Building Initiative.
163. CONSAMS (Consortium of New Southern African Medical Schools) (2011) Consortium of New Southern African Medical Schools.
164. Eichbaum Q, Nyarango P, Bowa K, Odonkor P, Ferrao J, et al. (2012) "Global networks, alliances and consortia" in global health education - The case for south-to-south partnerships. J Acquir Immune Defic Syndr.
165. Chen C, Buch E, Wassermann T, Frehywot S, Mullan F, et al. (2012) A survey of Sub-Saharan African medical schools. Hum Resour Health 10: 4.
166. Mullan F, Frehywot S, Omaswa F, Sewankambo N, Talib Z, et al. (2012) The Medical Education Partnership Initiative: PEPFAR's effort to boost health worker education to strengthen health systems. Health Aff (Millwood) 31: 1561–1572.
167. Mullan F, Frehywot S, Omaswa F, Buch E, Chen C, et al. (2011) Medical schools in sub-Saharan Africa. Lancet 377: 1113–1121.
168. Decroo T, Telfer B, Biot M, Maikere J, Dezembro S, et al. (2011) Distribution of antiretroviral treatment through self-forming groups of patients in Tete Province, Mozambique. J Acquir Immune Defic Syndr 56: e39–44.
169. Decroo T, Panunzi I, das Dores C, Maldonado F, Biot M, et al. (2009) Lessons learned during down referral of antiretroviral treatment in Tete, Mozambique. J Int AIDS Soc 12: 6.
170. Decroo T, Van Damme W, Kegels G, Remartinez D, Rasschaert F (2012) Are Expert Patients an Untapped Resource for ART Provision in Sub-Saharan Africa? AIDS Res Treat 2012: 749718.
171. Bandali S (2012) HIV Risk Assessment and Risk Reduction Strategies in the Context of Prevailing Gender Norms in Rural Areas of Cabo Delgado, Mozambique. J Int Assoc Physicians AIDS Care (Chic).
172. Bandali S (2011) Norms and practices within marriage which shape gender roles, HIV/AIDS risk and risk reduction strategies in Cabo Delgado, Mozambique. AIDS Care 23: 1171–1176.
173. Lahuerta M, Lima J, Nuwagaba-Biribonwoha H, Okamura M, Alvim MF, et al. (2012) Factors associated with late antiretroviral therapy initiation among adults in Mozambique. PLoS One 7: e37125.
174. Hendriksen IC, Ferro J, Montoya P, Chhaganlal KD, Seni A, et al. (2012) Diagnosis, Clinical Presentation, and In-Hospital Mortality of Severe Malaria in HIV-Coinfected Children and Adults in Mozambique. Clin Infect Dis 55: 1144–1153.
175. Naniche D, Letang E, Nhampossa T, David C, Menendez C, et al. (2011) Alterations in T cell subsets in human immunodeficiency virus-infected adults with co-infections in southern Mozambique. Am J Trop Med Hyg 85: 776–781.
176. Modjarrad K, Vermund SH (2010) Effect of treating co-infections on HIV-1 viral load: a systematic review. Lancet Infect Dis 10: 455–463.
177. Modjarrad K, Vermund SH (2011) An addition to the effect of treating co-infections on HIV-1 viral load. Lancet Infect Dis 11: 81.
178. Vaz P, Augusto O, Bila D, Macassa E, Vubil A, et al. (2012) Surveillance of HIV drug resistance in children receiving antiretroviral therapy: a pilot study of the World Health Organization's generic protocol in Maputo, Mozambique. Clin Infect Dis 54 Suppl 4: S369–374.
179. Holmes CB, Blandford JM, Sangrujee N, Stewart SR, DuBois A, et al. (2012) PEPFAR's past and future efforts to cut costs, improve efficiency, and increase the impact of global HIV programs. Health Aff (Millwood) 31: 1553–1560.
180. Jani IV, Sabatier J, Vubil A, Subbarao S, Bila D, et al. (2012) Evaluation of a high-throughput diagnostic system for detection of HIV-1 in dried blood spot samples from infants in Mozambique. J Clin Microbiol 50: 1458–1460.
181. Jani IV, Sitoe NE, Alfai ER, Chongo PL, Quevedo JI, et al. (2011) Effect of point-of-care CD4 cell count tests on retention of patients and rates of antiretroviral therapy initiation in primary health clinics: an observational cohort study. Lancet 378: 1572–1579.
182. Bwakura-Dangarembizi M, Kendall L, Bakeera-Kitaka S, Nahirya-Ntege P, Keishanyu R, et al. (2014) A Randomized Trial of Prolonged Co-trimoxazole in HIV-Infected Children in Africa. New England Journal of Medicine 370: 41–53.

Novel Respiratory Syncytial Virus (RSV) Genotype ON1 Predominates in Germany during Winter Season 2012–13

Julia Tabatabai[1,2], Christiane Prifert[3], Johannes Pfeil[4,5], Jürgen Grulich-Henn[4], Paul Schnitzler[1]*

1 Department of Infectious Diseases, Virology, University of Heidelberg, Heidelberg, Germany, **2** London School of Hygiene and Tropical Medicine, London, United Kingdom, **3** Institute of Virology and Immunobiology, University of Würzburg, Würzburg, Germany, **4** Department of Pediatrics, University of Heidelberg, Heidelberg, Germany, **5** German Centre for Infectious Diseases (DZIF), Heidelberg, Germany

Abstract

Respiratory syncytial virus (RSV) is the leading cause of hospitalization especially in young children with respiratory tract infections (RTI). Patterns of circulating RSV genotypes can provide a better understanding of the molecular epidemiology of RSV infection. We retrospectively analyzed the genetic diversity of RSV infection in hospitalized children with acute RTI admitted to University Hospital Heidelberg/Germany between October 2012 and April 2013. Nasopharyngeal aspirates (NPA) were routinely obtained in 240 children younger than 2 years of age who presented with clinical symptoms of upper or lower RTI. We analyzed NPAs via PCR and sequence analysis of the second variable region of the RSV G gene coding for the attachment glycoprotein. We obtained medical records reviewing routine clinical data. RSV was detected in 134/240 children. In RSV-positive patients the most common diagnosis was bronchitis/bronchiolitis (75.4%). The mean duration of hospitalization was longer in RSV-positive compared to RSV-negative patients (3.5 vs. 5.1 days; $p<0.01$). RSV-A was detected in 82.1%, RSV-B in 17.9% of all samples. Phylogenetic analysis of 112 isolates revealed that the majority of RSV-A strains (65%) belonged to the novel ON1 genotype containing a 72-nucleotide duplication. However, genotype ON1 was not associated with a more severe course of illness when taking basic clinical/laboratory parameters into account. Molecular characterization of RSV confirms the co-circulation of multiple genotypes of subtype RSV-A and RSV-B. The duplication in the G gene of genotype ON1 might have an effect on the rapid spread of this emerging RSV strain.

Editor: Steven M. Varga, University of Iowa, United States of America

Funding: The authors have no support or funding to report.

Competing Interests: The authors have declared that no competing interests exist.

* Email: Paul_Schnitzler@med.uni-heidelberg.de

Introduction

Respiratory syncytial virus (RSV) is the major pathogen of lower respiratory tract infections (RTI) in infants and young children. By the age of 2 years, virtually all children have been infected at least once with RSV [1]. Re-infections are common throughout life; in older children and adults infections are associated with milder disease indicating that RSV induces only partial immunity [2]. Strain variation is thought to contribute to its ability to cause frequent re-infections [3] enabling RSV to remain present at high levels in the population [4]. Viral strains are separated into two major groups based on its genetic and antigenic variability. Several lineages within the subtypes RSV-A and RSV-B co-circulate simultaneously in the population [5] and their relative proportions may differ between epidemics, although RSV-A viruses tend to predominate [6]. The main differences between RSV-A and RSV-B are found in the attachment (G) glycoprotein [7]. The G protein is a type II surface glycoprotein of about 300 amino acids in length, consisting of a cytoplasmic domain, a transmembrane domain and an ectodomain. The G protein is heavily glycosylated with N-linked and O-linked sugars. However, the amino acid sequence positions of potential glycosylation sites are poorly conserved [8].

This protein is able to accommodate drastic changes with the emergence of new variants. Diversity occurs mainly in the two hypervariable regions of the ectodomain which are separated by a highly conserved 13-amino acid (aa) length domain [9]. Sequencing of the second hypervariable region at the C-terminal end of the G gene has been widely used to further subdivide RSV-A and RSV-B into genotypes and facilitated differentiation between RSV isolates. To date, 11 RSV-A genotypes, GA1-GA7, SAA1, NA1-NA2, and ON1 [10–12], and 23 RSV-B genotypes, GB1-GB4, SAB1-SAB3, SAB4, URU1, URU2, BAI - BAXII, and THB [10,13–21] have been described based on nucleotide sequence analysis.

RSV strains show an accumulation of translated amino acid changes over the years, suggesting antigenic drift-based immunity-mediated selection [22]. In 1999, a new RSV-B genotype BA emerged in Buenos Aires, Argentina, containing a 60-nucleotide (nt) duplication in the second hypervariable region of the G gene [23]. In the following ten years, the BA genotype spread worldwide and largely replaced previous described RSV-B genotypes [24]. During the 2010–11 winter season, a novel

RSV-A genotype ON1 with a 72-nt duplication has been reported in Canada [14]. In line with the gradual spread of the BA genotype making it the dominant circulating RSV-B genotype today, the nucleotide duplication of the ON1 genotype might likewise result in a similar selection advantage [25]. There is an increasing number of reports from across the world describing this novel genotype and the following seasons will show its impact on the evolution of RSV-A [6].

In Germany, there is only limited information regarding the molecular epidemiology of RSV, the emergence of novel viral strains and their impact on the course of RSV infection. In the present study, we evaluated hospitalized children below the age of 2 years presenting with acute RTI in the Pediatric Department in Heidelberg, Germany during the winter season 2012–13. We investigated the genetic diversity and patterns of the co-circulating genotypes of Heidelberg RSV-A and RSV-B strains in comparison with other RSV strains circulating worldwide. Furthermore we explored a possible association between individual RSV genotypes and the course of RSV infection by retrospectively analyzing basic clinical and laboratory data.

Materials and Methods

Patients and clinical samples

We retrospectively analyzed children under the age of 2 years admitted to the Pediatric Department at the Heidelberg University Hospital between October 2012 and April 2013 with clinical symptoms of upper or lower respiratory tract infection (RTI) as part of their admission diagnosis or as concomitant symptom. Prior to the transfer to the inpatient unit, nasopharyngeal aspirates (NPA) are obtained and these children are routinely screened for RSV infection using a rapid antigen test in order to inform for isolation strategies. All obtained NPAs (242 samples from 240 children) were collected and stored frozen for further molecular analysis by RSV PCR and phylogenetic analysis. Medical records were reviewed from all children to obtain routine clinical and laboratory data. Patient records were anonymized and de-identified prior to analysis. The Ethical Committee of the University of Heidelberg has approved this study (S-166/2014).

PCR and sequencing

For PCR analysis, RNA was extracted from NPAs using the QIAamp viral RNA mini kit (Qiagen, Hilden, Germany) according to the manufacturer's protocol. Amplification and detection of viral RNA was performed with the RealStar RSV real-time PCR kit (altona Diagnostics, Hamburg, Germany) on a LightCycler 480 instrument II (Roche, Mannheim, Germany). This assay differentiated RSV into subtypes A and B. For sequencing and identification of RSV genotypes, extracted RNA was initially reverse transcribed and cDNA was synthesized using random hexamer primers. Subsequently, PCR targeting the second hypervariable region of the G gene was performed using primer pairs as previously described by Peret et al. [11]. PCR products were sequenced with the same primer pairs previously used for amplification. Overlapping sequences were assembled and edited using the SEQMAN II software of the Lasergene package (DNAstar, Madsion, WI). Nucleotide sequences of the second hypervariable region of the G gene retrieved in this study were deposited in GenBank under accession numbers [KJ710364-KJ710420].

Phylogenetic and deduced amino acid sequence analysis

Multiple sequence alignments and phylogenetic analysis of the second hypervariable region of the G gene were conducted using the Clustal W 1.6 method of MEGA software version 6 [26]. Phylogenetic trees were generated using the maximum-likelihood method and bootstrap values with 1,000 replicates were calculated to evaluate confidence estimates. Reference strains representing known genotypes were retrieved from GenBank (http://www.ncbi.lm.nih.gov) and included in the tree. Pairwise nucleotide distances were calculated to compare the differences within and between genotypes of subgroup RSV-A and RSV-B using MEGA software version 6. Positive selected sites were estimated by use of the Datamonkey Web server (http://www.datamonkey.org) identifying the rates of non-synonymous and synonymous substitutions [27].

Deduced amino acid sequences were translated with the standard genetic code using MEGA software version 6. Alignments of the second hypervariable region of the G protein of Heidelberg RSV-A and RSV-B strains were compared to references strains from GenBank to identify amino acid substitutions. Putative N-glycosylation sites were predicted if the encoded amino acid sequence was Asn-Xaa-Thr/Ser, where Xaa was not a proline and accepted if the glycosylation potential was $\geq$0.5 in NetNGlyc 1.0 server [28]. O-glycosylation was determined using the NetOGlyc 3.1 server and sites were predicted using a G-score $\geq$0.5 [29].

Statistical analysis of epidemiological factors

To describe the temporal distribution of admitted RSV cases, we aggregated RSV results as obtained by PCR by calendar month and week. Demographic and clinical data in our study population was summarized. Group comparisons were performed using $\chi 2$ or Fisher's exact test for categorical variables and by Student's t-test or analysis of variance (ANOVA) for continuous variables, as appropriate. P-values <0.05 were considered statistically significant. Stata/IC13.0 (StataCorp. LP, College Station, TX, USA) was used for all statistical analysis.

Results

Detection of RSV

Between October 2012 and April 2013, a total of 242 samples from hospitalized infants and children were analyzed for RSV infection by PCR resulting in 134 (55.4%) RSV-positive samples. Among these RSV-positive samples, 110 (82.1%) were subgrouped as RSV-A and 24 (17.9%) as RSV-B, respectively. No co-infection for RSV-A and RSV-B was detected. Two children presented twice and were tested RSV-positive at their first admission and RSV-negative at the consecutive admission few weeks later. The distribution of RSV-A and RSV-B per calendar week and month is shown in Fig. 1.

Sequence alignments and phylogenetic analysis

Sequences of the second hypervariable region of the G gene from 97 (72.4%) RSV-A and 15 (11.2%) RSV-B samples were successfully obtained and aligned with representative GenBank sequences of previously published genotypes. Due to a low viral load some RSV-positive samples (n = 22; 16.4%) could not be sequenced. The phylogenetic trees of RSV-A and RSV-B sequences are shown in Figure 2. Heidelberg RSV_A and RSV-B strains clustered into three genotypes for RSV-A and two genotypes for RSV-B, respectively.

The majority of RSV-A strains (n = 73, 75.3%) clustered with strains that were previously assigned to the novel ON1 genotype with a 72-nt duplication, followed by strains clustering with genotype NA1 (n = 23, 31.5%) and one strain clustering with GA5 (Fig. 2A). Sequence homology between Heidelberg sequences and

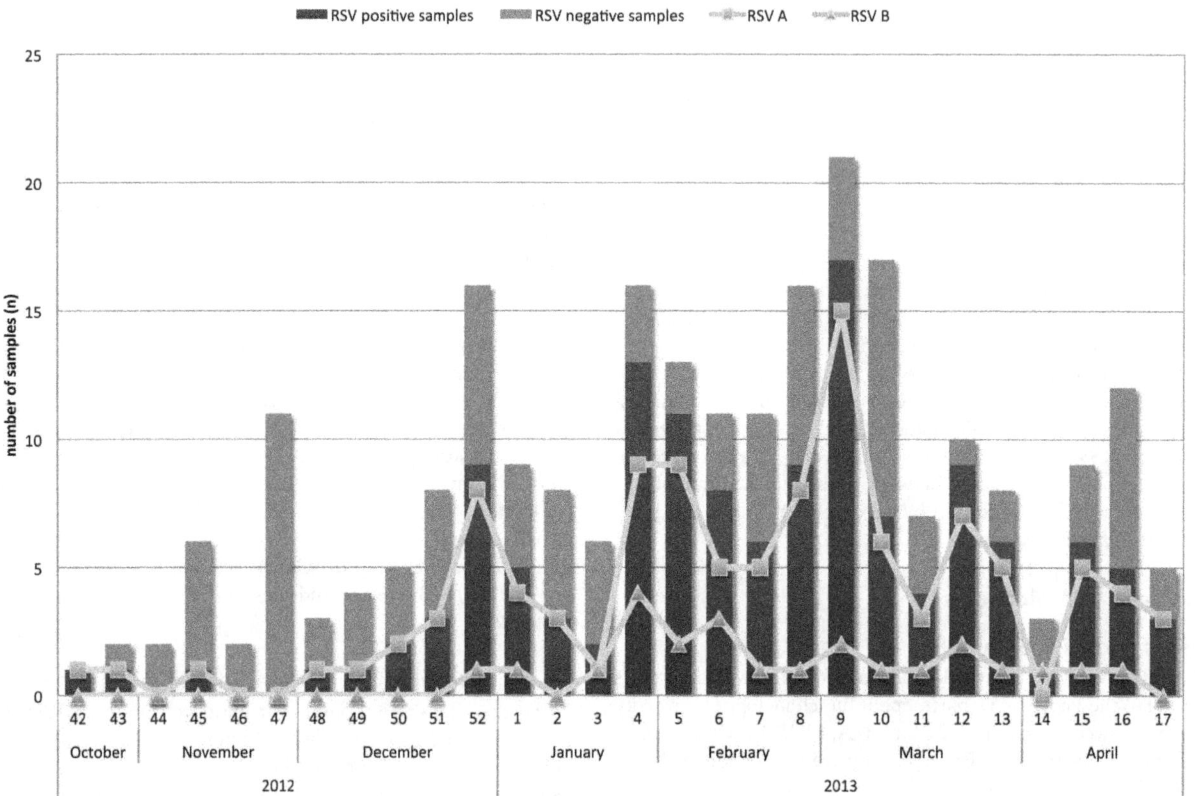

Figure 1. Weekly/monthly distribution of subgroup RSV A/RSV B in children ≤2 years with acute RTI in Heidelberg/Germany, winter season 2012/13.

the ON1 reference strain [JN257693] was ≥96.9% at the nucleotide level and ≥94.1% at the amino acid level. The intragenotypic p-distance was 1.9% for ON1 and 6.2% for NA1 for Heidelberg sequences. The intergenotypic p-distance for ON1 and NA1 was not comparable because of the 72-nt duplication.

All RSV-B strains (n = 15) clustered with strains that were previously assigned to the BA genotype with a 60-nt duplication. In addition, BA strains could be further differentiated into the previously designated genotypes BAIX (n = 10, 66.7%) and BAX (n = 5, 33.3%) (Fig. 2B). Sequence homology between Heidelberg sequences and the BA reference strain (AY333364) was 94.3%–96.6% at the nucleotide level and 87%–95% at the amino acid level. The intergenotypic p-distance for BAIX and BAX was 4.7% for Heidelberg sequences, with an intragenotypic p-distance of 3% for BAIX and 0.8% for BAX.

Deduced amino acid sequence analysis

We aligned and compared Heidelberg RSV-A genotype NA1 and GA5 strains with the A2 reference strain (M11486) (Fig. 3A). The majority of NA1 strains had three predicted N-glycosylation sites at amino acid (aa) positions 237, 251 and 294. However, HD12262 had an additional predicted N-glycosylation site at aa position 242 and HD12188 at aa position 273. A group of 11 isolates lost the N-glycosylation site at aa positions 237 due to a N237D/H substitution. Strain HD12055 lost all N-glycosylation site but the aa position 294. The N-glycosylation site at aa position 250 is characteristic for the GA5 genotype as found in one of the Heidelberg isolates. O-glycosylation patterns varied between Heidelberg isolates with 32±3 sites potentially O-glycosylated (G-score ≥0.5) in NA1 isolates and 23 sites in the one GA5 isolate.

As a consequence of the insertion in the G gene, ON1 genotype strains translate into a polypeptide with a length of 321 amino acids and are thereby lengthened by 24 aa when compared to the A2 reference strain (Fig. 3B). The insertion contains a 23 aa duplicated region. The comparison of Heidelberg ON1 strains with ON1 strains from other countries with reference to the original strain from Canada (JN257693) revealed that Heidelberg isolates can be divided into three sub-clusters: The first sub-cluster (n = 12) comprises isolates closely related to the primary Canadian strain (JN257693) with few mixed substitutions. This sub-cluster also includes one strain with an E308K substitution as previously described in South African strains [JX885730]. The second sub-cluster (n = 28) contained three characteristic substitutions, L274P, L298P and Y304H as previously described in strains from Wuerzburg, Germany [JX912364, JX12364], as well as in strains from Italy and Japan [KC858245, KC587959; AB808774, AB808757]. Furthermore, on group of 13 identical isolates showed a E287K substitution which was unique for Heidelberg strains. The third sub-cluster consists of 28 isolates with a L310P substitution in addition to the three substitutions found in the second sub-cluster and aligned with isolates from Japan, India and Kenya [AB808774, AB808757; KF246641, KF246640; KF587959]. A group of 19 identical strains additionally showed a V303A substitution, which was also seen in strains from Italy, Croatia and India [KC858245, KC587959; KF057865;

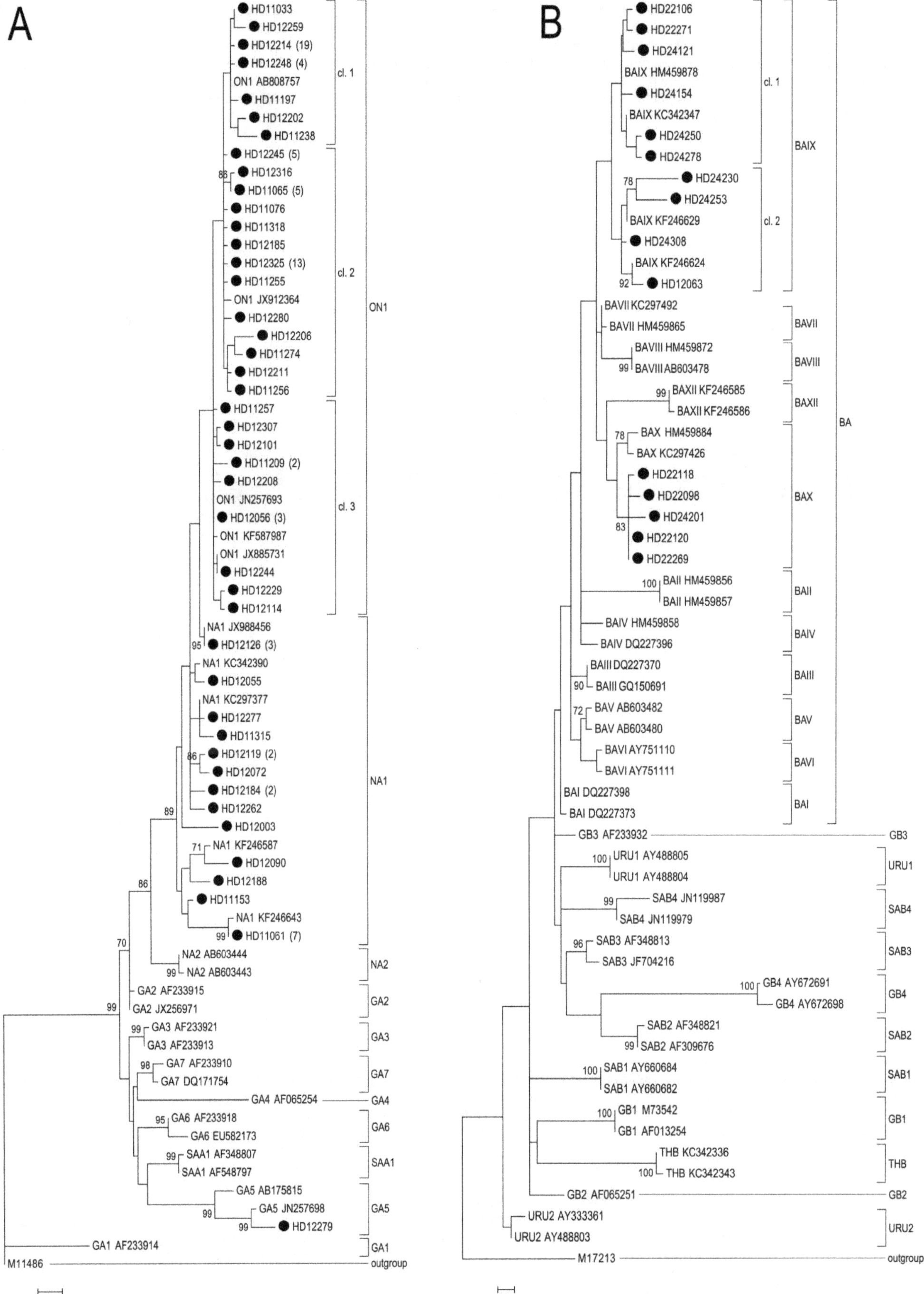
A
HD11033
HD12259
HD12214 (19)
HD12248 (4)
ON1 AB808757
HD11197
HD12202
HD11238
cl. 1
HD12245 (5)
86
HD12316
HD11065 (5)
HD11076
HD11318
HD12185
HD12325 (13)
HD11255
ON1 JX912364
HD12280
HD12206
HD11274
HD12211
HD11256
cl. 2
HD11257
HD12307
HD12101
HD11209 (2)
HD12208
ON1 JN257693
HD12056 (3)
ON1 KF587987
ON1 JX885731
HD12244
HD12229
HD12114
cl. 3
ON1
NA1 JX988456
95
HD12126 (3)
NA1 KC342390
HD12055
NA1 KC297377
HD12277
HD11315
86
HD12119 (2)
HD12072
HD12184 (2)
HD12262
89
HD12003
71
NA1 KF246587
HD12090
HD12188
86
HD11153
NA1 KF246643
99
HD11061 (7)
NA1
70
NA2 AB603444
99
NA2 AB603443
NA2
GA2 AF233915
99
GA2 JX256971
GA2
99
GA3 AF233921
GA3 AF233913
GA3
98
GA7 AF233910
GA7 DQ171754
GA7
GA4 AF065254
GA4
95
GA6 AF233918
GA6 EU582173
GA6
99
SAA1 AF348807
SAA1 AF548797
SAA1
GA5 AB175815
99
GA5 JN257698
99
HD12279
GA5
GA1 AF233914
GA1
M11486
outgroup
0.02
B
HD22106
HD22271
HD24121
BAIX HM459878
HD24154
BAIX KC342347
HD24250
HD24278
cl. 1
78
HD24230
HD24253
BAIX KF246629
HD24308
BAIX KF246624
92
HD12063
cl. 2
BAIX
BAVII KC297492
BAVII HM459865
BAVII
BAVIII HM459872
99
BAVIII AB603478
BAVIII
99
BAXII KF246585
BAXII KF246586
BAXII
78
BAX HM459884
BAX KC297426
HD22118
HD22098
HD24201
83
HD22120
HD22269
BAX
BA
100
BAII HM459856
BAII HM459857
BAII
BAIV HM459858
BAIV DQ227396
BAIV
BAIII DQ227370
90
BAIII GQ150691
BAIII
72
BAV AB603482
BAV AB603480
BAV
BAVI AY751110
BAVI AY751111
BAVI
BAI DQ227398
BAI DQ227373
BAI
GB3 AF233932
GB3
100
URU1 AY488805
URU1 AY488804
URU1
99
SAB4 JN119987
SAB4 JN119979
SAB4
96
SAB3 AF348813
SAB3 JF704216
SAB3
100
GB4 AY672691
GB4 AY672698
GB4
SAB2 AF348821
99
SAB2 AF309676
SAB2
100
SAB1 AY660684
SAB1 AY660682
SAB1
100
GB1 M73542
GB1 AF013254
GB1
THB KC342336
100
THB KC342343
THB
GB2 AF065251
GB2
URU2 AY333361
URU2 AY488803
URU2
M17213
outgroup
0.01

Figure 2. Phylogenetic tree of RSV A/RSV B strains and reference sequences of identified genotypes. Phylogenetic trees for RSV A (A) and RSV B (B) strains were constructed with maximum-likelihood method with 1,000 bootstrap replicates using MEGA 6 software. RSV strains from Heidelberg/Germany are indicated by "●HD" followed by their strain identification number. Number of identical strains is indicated in brackets after the strain identifier. Reference strains representing known genotypes were retrieved from GenBank and included in the tree (labels include accession number). The genotype assignment is shown on the right by brackets. Prototype strains (M11486 for subgroup A and M17213 for subgroup B) were used as an outgroup. Bootstrap values greater than 70% are indicated at the branch nodes. The scale bar represents the number of nucleotide substitutions per site. cl. = cluster.

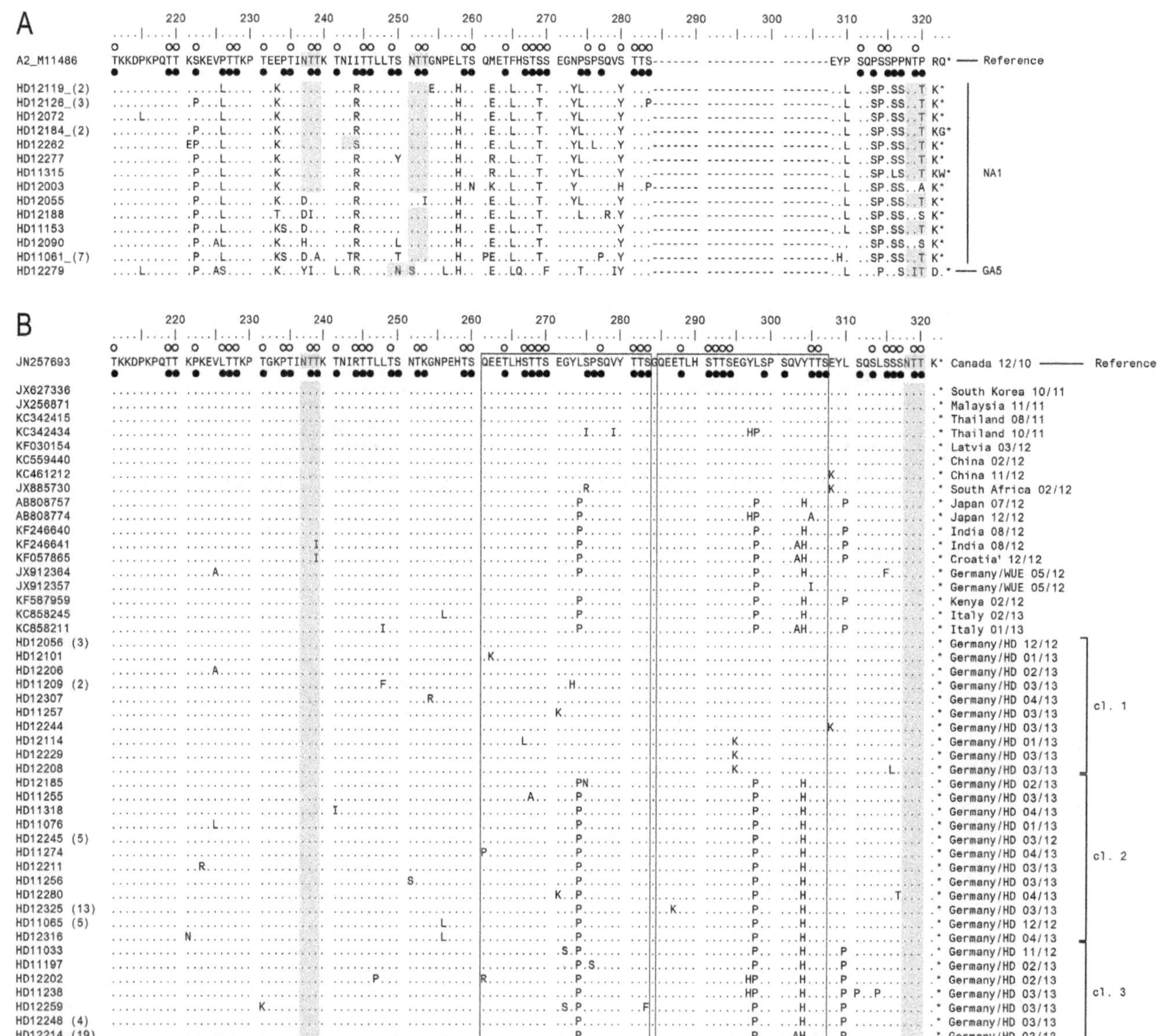

Figure 3. Alignment of deduced amino acid sequences of RSV-A strains. A) Alignment of RSV-A genotype NA1 and GA5 are shown relative to the sequence of prototype strain A2 (GenBank accession number M11486). Alignment of sequences was performed using the Clustal W 1.6 method via MEGA 6 software. The amino acid positions correspond to positions 210 to 298 of the G protein of strain A2. Identical residues are indicated by dots, asterisks indicate the position of stop codons. Number of identical strains is indicated in brackets after the strain identifier in the left column. Gray shading highlights predicted N-glycosylation sites. Unfilled circles indicate predicted O-glycosylation sites of the prototype strain A2; potential O-glycosylation sites of Heidelberg strains are indicated by black dots. The genotype assignment is shown on the right by brackets. B) Alignments are shown relative to the sequence of ON1 strain first described in Canada (GenBank accession number JN257693). Alignment of sequences was performed using the Clustal W 1.6 method via MEGA 6 software. The amino acid positions correspond to positions 210 to 298 of the G protein of the prototype strain A2. Identical residues are indicated by dots, asterisks indicate the position of stop codons. Boxes frame the 23 amino acid duplicated region of the 24 amino acid insertion. Gray shading highlights predicted N-glycosylation sites. Unfilled circles indicate predicted O-glycosylation sites of the Canadian reference ON1 strain; potential O-glycosylation sites of Heidelberg strains are indicated by black dots. On the right hand site, GenBank and Heidelberg strains are labeled with the country and time of occurrence (month/year).

[1] Sequences were published in GenBank only.

HD= Heidelberg; WUE= Wuerzburg, cl.= cluster.

KF246641, KF246640]. However, positive selection analysis of ON1 strains revealed no positive selected site.

All Heidelberg ON1 strains had two predicted N-glycosylation sites at aa positions 237 and 318 and lost the N-glycosylation sites at aa position 251 due to a T251K substitution. ON1 strains showed different patterns of O-glycosylation sites with 31 to 44 predicted sites and showed some new sites when compared to the Ontario reference strain. The 23-aa duplicated region contained a maximum of 10 glycosylation sites as observed in 17 ON1 isolates from Heidelberg.

Heidelberg RSV-B genotype BA strains were compared to BA reference strain from Buenos Aires [AF33364] (Fig. 4). Stop codons were either at aa position 320 for HD24308, HD24250 and HD24278 or at aa position 313 for the remaining BA strains. All BA strains had a K218P, L223P and S247P substitution. The BAIX genotype had a H287Y and a V271A substitution. Furthermore some BAIX strains (sub-cluster 1) had a P291L substitution whereas other BAIX strains (sub-cluster 2) had an I281T substitution. The BAX strains had a P291G substitution.

All Heidelberg RSV B strains had a predicted N-glycosylation site at aa positions 296. However the N-glycosylation site at aa position 310 only fulfilled the typical amino acid patterns but the glycosylation potential calculated by NetOGlyc 3.1 server was below 0.5 in isolates with a stop codon at aa position 313. HD24253 had an additional potential N-glycosylation site at aa position 230. O-glycosylation of BA strains varied between 40 and 47 predicted sites and showed an additional predicted site at aa position 317 in longer strains with a stop codon at aa position 320.

Basic and clinical characteristics of the study cohort

The mean age of the all screened children was 7.9 months and ranged in line with the inclusion criteria between 11 days and 23.8 months. RSV-positive patients were significantly younger compared to RSV-negative patients (t-test; $p<0.001$). The age group distribution showed that 62.7% RSV-positive children were below 6 months of age. All children had at least a concomitant acute RTI at time of admission; however, in some patients the main clinical diagnosis was non-respiratory (total 12.4%, RSV positive 4.5%). In RSV-positive patients the most common diagnosis was bronchitis/bronchiolitis (75.4%). The mean duration of hospitalization was longer in RSV-positive patients (3.5 vs. 5.1 days; $p<0.01$).

We performed a group comparison of the main three genotypes (RSV-A: ON1 and NA1; RSV-B: BA) using basic and clinical characteristics of RSV-positive infants and children (Table 1). There were no risk factors for one of the three groups of genotypes identified when looking at the demographic characteristics (age, gender, weight). Furthermore, we could not identify any association between a specific genotype and a more severe course of illness when taking the retrospectively available clinical and laboratory parameters into account.

Discussion

RSV accounts for a significant burden of acute respiratory tract infections particularly in infants and young children in need for hospital care [30]. Patterns of circulating RSV genotypes can provide a better understanding of the molecular epidemiology of RSV infection. In our study, we analyzed the genetic diversity and patterns of co-circulating genotypes of both, subtypes RSV-A and RSV-B, during the winter season 2012–13 in Heidelberg/Germany. RSV was detected in 134 out of 242 samples of which 110 (82.1%) were sub-grouped as RSV-A and 24 (17.9%) as RSV-B, respectively. Phylogenetic analysis revealed that the majority of RSV-A strains (n = 73, 75.3%) clustered with strains of the novel ON1 genotype with a 72-nt duplication first described by Eshaghi et al. in Ontario, Canada in 2010 [14]. In Germany, circulation of this genotype was reported for the first time in Wuerzburg in winter 2011–12 [31]. In line with another study in Europe, this study reports ON1 as the predominant genotype during the RSV epidemic season 2012–13, suggesting a rapid spread of this emerging RSV strain [32,33].

Most RSV cases were detected between December 2012 and April 2013, which is in line with the previously described seasonality of RSV infection in Germany [30]. However, the core season with more than half of all RSV-positive cases was from end-January to mid-March, which can be considered a late pattern of a RSV epidemic season in Germany [22]. Within our study population RSV was detectable in 55.4% of hospitalized children below the age of 2 years emphasizing the need for RSV screening on admission to assure proper management and to prevent nosocomial infections [34].

In our cohort, age group analysis revealed that infants below 6 months of age had the highest infection rates, as expected. Primary RSV infection commonly occurs within the first year of life [13]

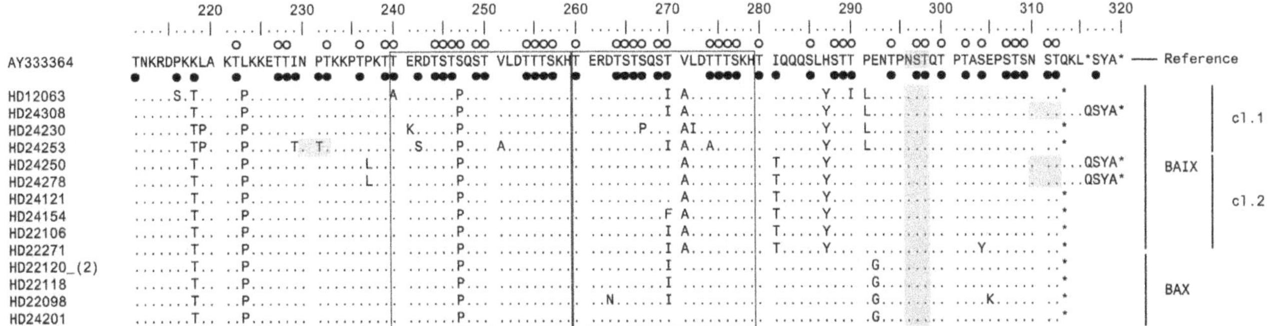

Figure 4. Alignment of deduced amino acid sequences of the second variable region of the G protein of RSV-B strains isolated in Heidelberg/Germany during 2012–2013 winter season. Alignments are shown relative to the sequence of a prototype BA strain (GenBank accession number AY333364). Alignment of sequences was performed using the Clustal W 1.6 method via MEGA 6 software. The amino acid positions correspond to positions 210 to 315 of the G protein of the BA strain. Identical residues are indicated by dots, asterisks indicate the position of stop codons. Number of identical strains is indicated in brackets after the strain identifier in the left column. Boxes frame the 20 amino acid duplication. Gray shading highlights predicted N-glycosylation sites. Open circles indicate predicted O-glycosylation sites of the prototype BA strain; potential O-glycosylation sites of Heidelberg strains are indicated by black dots. Genotypes are shown on the right by brackets.

Table 1. Basic and clinical characteristics of RSV positive children by genotype.

		RSV A*		RSV B	
	RSV positive	ON1	NA1	BA	p-value
	n = 134	n = 73	n = 23	n = 15	
Demographic characteristics					
Age in months, mean ±SD	6.5±6.2	6.4±6.2	5.7±5.6	4.8±5.1	0.63
Age group, n (%)					
0–6 months	84 (62.7)	48 (65.8)	15 (65.2)	10 (66.7)	0.18
>6–12 months	20 (14.9)	7 (9.6)	6 (26.1)	3 (20.0)	
>12–18 months	20 (14.9)	13(17.8)	0 (0.0)	2 (13.3)	
>18–24 months	10 (7.5)	15 (6.9)	2 (8.7)	0 (0.0)	
Gender, n (%)					
Male	83 (61.9)	44 (60.3)	18 (78.3)	9 (60.0)	0.28
Female	51 (38.1)	29 (39.7)	5 (21.7)	6 (40.0)	
Weight in kg, mean ±SD	6.2±2.3	5.9±2.1	7.0±2.7	5.8±2.3	0.11
Leading clinical diagnosis, n (%)					
Non-respiratory	6 (4.5)	4 (5.5)	0 (0.0)	1 (6.7)	0.49
Respiratory	128 (95.5)	69 (94.5)	23 (100.0)	14 (93.3)	
Upper RTI	4 (3.0)	1 (1.4)	1 (4.4)	0 (0.0)	0.61
Bronchitis/Bronchiolitis	101 (75.4)	54 (74.0)	20 (87.0)	12 (80.0)	
Pneumonia	23 (17.2)	14 (19.2)	2 (8.7)	2 (6.7)	
Course of disease					
Symptoms prior to hospitalization in days, mean ±SD	4.2±3.6	3.9±3.1	3.9±2.9	3.8±5.0	0.98
Hospital stay in days, mean ±SD#	5.3±3.9	5.3±3.8	5.5±2.8	4.5±2.1	0.68
Need for intensive care, n (%)	6 (4.5)	4 (5.5)	0 (0.0)	1 (6.7)	0.49
Laboratory parameters on admission					
Hemoglobin in g/dl, mean ±SD	11.7±1.7	11.4±1.5	11.9±1.9	11.7±2.0	0.45
Leucocytes/nl, mean ±SD	11.5±4.7	11.0±4.5	10.1±3.6	10.4±3.8	0.64
Thrombocytes/nl, mean ±SD	434.2±120.5	435.8±130.9	391.5±84.6	467.9±117.4	0.17
C-reactive protein in mg/L, mean ±SD	22.5±37.0	20.1±26.7	22.4±24.5	17.5±17.7	0.88
pCO2 in mmHg, mean ±SD	41.5±8.8	41.6±9.4	42.1±8.4	45.6±8.9	0.44

*RSV A genotype GA5 was not included in this table as this genotype was only present in one patient. In total, 112 of 134 RSV positive patients could be sequenced and a genotype could be determined.
#Hospital stay was only calculated for patients who stayed at least 24 hours in hospital.
SD = standard deviation; RTI = respiratory tract infection, RSV = Respiratory Syncytial Virus.

and the risk of RSV infection decreases with increasing age [22]. The majority of RSV-positive children presented with bronchitis/bronchiolitis followed by pneumonia and the duration of hospitalization was significantly longer compared to RSV-negative patients. However, the median duration of hospital stay of 5 days in RSV-positive patients in this study was shorter compared to previous findings of 7 days [30].

Molecular analysis of RSV-positive samples demonstrated that RSV-A was the predominant subtype which is in line with previous findings of multiple-season studies from Europe and other geographical areas [21,22]. Phylogenetic analysis revealed that the majority of RSV-A strains (n = 73, 75.3%) clustered with strains of the novel ON1 genotype with a 72-nt duplication. Phylogenetic analysis of Tsukagoshi et al. estimated that genotype ON1 evolved from genotype NA1 [35]. Recent estimates place the time of the ON1 emergence around 2008/09 [36,37].

Over the past three epidemic seasons (2010–2013) the prevalence of ON1 strains among all circulating strains varied between the different reports, but there seems to be a trend towards ON1 as the predominating RSV-A strain. In its first description in Ontario/Canada, the genotype ON1 accounted for 10% of RSV-positive samples in the season 2010-11 [14]. In the same season in Thailand, the majority of RSV isolates belonged to NA1, only few isolates belonged to ON1 [20]. One season later in 2011–12, RSV-A genotype ON1 was reported in different studies from Asia, Africa and Europe suggesting a worldwide emergence of the novel RSV-A strain. However, ON1 was only sporadically detected during that time and some countries like Pakistan did not report ON1 among circulating genotypes in 2011–12 [34]. A study from Heidelberg/Germany evaluating the genetic diversity of RSV in an outbreak in a haematology unit in 2012 also did not describe any ON1 strains [38]. In a study from Bejing, China, only one sample from February 2012 out of about 250 sequenced RSV-positive samples between 2007 and 2012 was characterized as ON1 genotype [39]. One report from Wuerzburg/Germany, assigned 10% of the identified strains to genotype ON1 in 2011–

12 [31]. In the past months an increasing number of reports about circulating genotypes in the season 2012–13 were published. In line with the findings in this study, reports from Cyprus, Italy, Kenya and South Korea described ON1 as the predominating genotype in the epidemic season 2012–13 [32,33,36,37]. Our study therefore describes a further cohort in Europe with ON1 as the predominating genotype in 2012–13 suggesting a rapid emergence of this novel strain. Further surveillance of circulating genotypes will be needed to observe the future global distribution of the ON1 strain and its trend to diversify.

The comparison of Heidelberg ON1 strains with ON1 strains from other countries revealed that Heidelberg isolates could be divided into three sub-clusters with characteristic substitutions as previously described in different countries and continents. Similar to the subdivision of RSV-B genotype BA into several sub-genotypes (BA-I – BAXII), this could be a first trend to a diversification of the ON1 genotype. However, none of the sub-clusters had bootstrap values ≥70%. Furthermore, positive selection analysis did not reveal any positively selective sites among ON1 isolates. This is also reflected by two groups of identical isolates (n = 13 and n = 18) of the ON1 genotype, suggesting the absence of selective pressure among the newly emerging strains.

Although the majority of strains was subtyped as RSV-A, 13.4% of all Heidelberg trains were subtyped as RSV-B. All RSV-B strains clustered with strains of the BA genotype with a 60-nt duplication, first described by Trento et al. in Buenos Aires, Argentina in 1999 [23], further differentiating into the genotypes BAIX (n = 10, 66.7%) and BAX (n = 5, 33.3%). Genotype BAIX separated into two sub-clusters: one including the BAIX reference sequence from Japan designated by Dapat et al. [18] who first described this genotype in 2007, and the second including the BAIX reference sequence from India described by Choudhary et al. in 2010 [40]. However, none of the two sub-clusters had bootstrap values ≥70%.

Similar to genotype BA, the nucleotide duplication of the ON1 genotype seems to result in a selection advantage compared to other RSV-A genotypes. Interestingly, despite the emergence of the ON1 virus there is conflicting data concerning the virulence in terms of disease severity [31–33]. In our cohort, retrospective analysis of basic clinical and laboratory parameters such as the duration of hospital stay, the need for intensive care as well as pCO_2 levels on admission did not reveal any association between a specific genotype and disease severity. Further surveillance of circulating RSV genotypes and corresponding clinical data is needed to understand the evolution, transmission and pathogenicity of genotype ON1 RSV infections.

Our study is subject to several limitations: We report the genetic diversity of RSV during one season in winter 2012–13 and a comparison of proportions of circulating genotypes is therefore restricted to other reports from Germany as well as worldwide. Our analysis included hospitalized children with community acquired RSV infection and therefore cannot draw conclusions for the overall population of community acquired RSV infections. However, the cohort of hospitalized children is of particular clinical relevance. Due to the retrospective study design, the evaluation of the association between pathogenicity of RSV infection and genotypes was limited to the available data. Furthermore, we did not include an analysis of further co-infections, which might also have an effect on disease severity in the evaluated study cohort. Further surveillance of the molecular epidemiology for several seasons in combination with prospectively complied clinical data is needed to directly compare the emergence of new variants and their transmissibility and virulence.

In summary, molecular characterization of RSV in Heidelberg, Germany during winter season 2012–13 confirmed the co-circulation of multiple genotypes of subtype RSV-A and RSV-B and the predominance of the novel genotype ON1. In line with the emergence of the BA genotype, it can be hypothesized that genotype ON1 could spread in a similar way and several branches might subdivide into further sub-genotypes. However, we could not find any association between disease severity and this newly emerging RSV-A genotype ON1. Continuing and long-term molecular epidemiological surveys for early detection of circulating and newly emerging genotypes in combination with clinical data are necessary to gain a better understanding of underlying genetic and antigenic mechanisms of RSV infection.

Acknowledgments

We would like to thank all nurses in the Department of Pediatrics, Heidelberg, Germany for collecting respiratory samples and all technicians in the virology diagnostic laboratory Heidelberg, Germany and Benedikt Weissbrich from the virology diagnostic laboratory at the University of Wuerzburg, Germany for excellent technical assistance. Furthermore, we cordially thank our colleague Steffen Geis from the virology diagnostic laboratory Heidelberg for the support in developing the methodology, critical reading of the manuscript as well as for his statistical advice.

Author Contributions

Conceived and designed the experiments: JT CP JGH PS. Performed the experiments: JT CP. Analyzed the data: JT CP JP. Wrote the paper: JT PS.

References

1. Glezen WP, Taber LH, Frank AL, Kasel JA (1986) Risk of primary infection and reinfection with respiratory syncytial virus. Am J Dis Child 140: 543–546.
2. Henderson FW, Collier AM, Clyde WA, Denny FW (1979) Respiratory-syncytial-virus infections, reinfections and immunity. A prospective, longitudinal study in young children. N Engl J Med 300: 530–534. doi: 10.1056/NEJM197903083001004
3. García O, Martín M, Dopazo J, Arbiza J, Frabasile S, et al. (1994) Evolutionary pattern of human respiratory syncytial virus (subgroup A): cocirculating lineages and correlation of genetic and antigenic changes in the G glycoprotein. J Virol 68: 5448–5459.
4. Hall CB, Walsh EE, Long CE, Schnabel KC (1991) Immunity to and frequency of reinfection with respiratory syncytial virus. J Infect Dis163: 693–698.
5. Storch GA, Anderson LJ, Park CS, Tsou C, Dohner DE (1991) Antigenic and genomic diversity within group A respiratory syncytial virus. 163: 858–861.
6. Pretorius MA, van Niekerk S, Tempia S, Moyes J, Cohen C, et al. (2013) Replacement and Positive Evolution of Subtype A and B Respiratory Syncytial Virus G-Protein Genotypes From 1997–2012 in South Africa. J Infect Dis 208: S227–S237. doi: 10.1093/infdis/jit477
7. Anderson LJ, Hierholzer JC, Tsou C, Hendry RM, Fernie BF, et al. (1985) Antigenic characterization of respiratory syncytial virus strains with monoclonal antibodies. J Infect Dis 151: 626–633.
8. Wertz GW, Krieger M, Ball LA (1989) Structure and cell surface maturation of the attachment glycoprotein of human respiratory syncytial virus in a cell line deficient in O glycosylation. J Virol 63: 4767–4776.
9. Johnson PR, Spriggs MK, Olmsted RA, Collins PL (1987) The G glycoprotein of human respiratory syncytial viruses of subgroups A and B: extensive sequence divergence between antigenically related proteins. Proc Natl Acad Sci USA 84: 5625–5629.
10. Peret TC, Hall CB, Schnabel KC, Golub JA, Anderson LJ (1998) Circulation patterns of genetically distinct group A and B strains of human respiratory syncytial virus in a community. J Gen Virol 79 (Pt 9): 2221–2229.
11. Peret TCT, Hall CB, Hammond GW, Piedra PA, Storch GA, et al. (2000) Circulation patterns of group A and B human respiratory syncytial virus genotypes in 5 communities in North America. J Infect Dis 181: 1891–1896. doi: 10.1086/315508
12. Venter M, Madhi SA, Tiemessen CT, Schoub BD (2001) Genetic diversity and molecular epidemiology of respiratory syncytial virus over four consecutive

seasons in South Africa: identification of new subgroup A and B genotypes. J Gen Virol 82: 2117–2124.
13. Shobugawa Y, Saito R, Sano Y, Zaraket H, Suzuki Y, et al. (2009) Emerging Genotypes of Human Respiratory Syncytial Virus Subgroup A among Patients in Japan. J Clin Microbiol 47: 2475–2482. doi: 10.1128/JCM.00115-09
14. Eshaghi A, Duvvuri VR, Lai R, Nadarajah JT, Li A, et al. (2012) Genetic variability of human respiratory syncytial virus A strains circulating in Ontario: a novel genotype with a 72 nucleotide G gene duplication. PLoS ONE 7: e32807. doi: 10.1371/journal.pone.0032807
15. Arnott A, Vong S, Mardy S, Chu S, Naughtin M, et al. (2011) A study of the genetic variability of human respiratory syncytial virus (HRSV) in Cambodia reveals the existence of a new HRSV group B genotype. J Clin Microbiol 49: 3504–3513. doi: 10.1128/JCM.01131-11
16. Blanc A, Delfraro A, Frabasile S, Arbiza J (2005) Genotypes of respiratory syncytial virus group B identified in Uruguay. Arch Virol 150: 603–609. doi: 10.1007/s00705-004-0412-x
17. Trento A, Viegas M, Galiano M, Videla C, Carballal G, et al. (2006) Natural history of human respiratory syncytial virus inferred from phylogenetic analysis of the attachment (G) glycoprotein with a 60-nucleotide duplication. J Virol 80: 975–984. doi: 10.1128/JVI.80.2.975-984.2006
18. Dapat IC, Shobugawa Y, Sano Y, Saito R, Sasaki A, et al. (2010) New Genotypes within Respiratory Syncytial Virus Group B Genotype BA in Niigata, Japan. J Clin Microbiol 48: 3423–3427. doi: 10.1128/JCM.00646-10
19. Baek YH, Choi EH, Song M-S, Pascua PNQ, Kwon H-I, et al. (2012) Prevalence and genetic characterization of respiratory syncytial virus (RSV) in hospitalized children in Korea. Arch Virol 157: 1039–1050. doi: 10.1007/s00705-012-1267-1
20. Khor C-S, Sam I-C, Hooi P-S, Chan Y-F (2013) Displacement of predominant respiratory syncytial virus genotypes in Malaysia between 1989 and 2011. Infect Genet Evol 14: 357–360. doi: 10.1016/j.meegid.2012.12.017
21. Auksornkitti V, Kamprasert N, Thongkomplew S, Suwannakarn K, Theamboonlers A, et al. (2014) Molecular characterization of human respiratory syncytial virus, 2010–2011: identification of genotype ON1 and a new subgroup B genotype in Thailand. Arch Virol 159: 499–507. doi: 10.1007/s00705-013-1773-9
22. Reiche J, Schweiger B (2009) Genetic variability of group A human respiratory syncytial virus strains circulating in Germany from 1998 to 2007. J Clin Microbiol 47: 1800–1810. doi: 10.1128/JCM.02286-08
23. Melero JA, Trento A, Videla C, Galiano M, Carballal G, et al. (2003) Major changes in the G protein of human respiratory syncytial virus isolates introduced by a duplication of 60 nucleotides. J Gen Virol 84: 3115–3120. doi: 10.1099/vir.0.19357-0
24. Trento A, Casas I, Calderón A, Garcia-Garcia ML, Calvo C, et al. (2010) Ten years of global evolution of the human respiratory syncytial virus BA genotype with a 60-nucleotide duplication in the G protein gene. J Virol 84: 7500–7512. doi: 10.1128/JVI.00345-10
25. Valley-Omar Z, Muloiwa R, Hu N-C, Eley B, Hsiao N-Y (2013) Novel respiratory syncytial virus subtype ON1 among children, Cape Town, South Africa, 2012. Emerging Infect Dis 19: 668–670. doi: 10.3201/eid1904.121465
26. Tamura K, Stecher G, Peterson D, Filipski A, Kumar S (2013) MEGA6: Molecular Evolutionary Genetics Analysis version 6.0. Mol Biol Evol 30: 2725–2729. doi: 10.1093/molbev/mst197
27. Delport W, Poon AFY, Frost SDW, Kosakovsky Pond SL (2010) Datamonkey 2010: a suite of phylogenetic analysis tools for evolutionary biology. Bioinformatics 26: 2455–2457. doi: 10.1093/bioinformatics/btq429
28. Gupta R, Jung E, Brunak S (2004) Prediction of N-glycosylation sites in human proteins. NetNGlycServer. Available: http://www.cbs.dtu.dk/services/NetNGlyc/. Accessed: 2014 Apr 6.
29. Julenius K, Mølgaard A, Gupta R, Brunak S (2005) Prediction, conservation analysis, and structural characterization of mammalian mucin-type O-glycosylation sites. Glycobiology 15: 153–164. doi: 10.1093/glycob/cwh151
30. Berner R, Schwoerer F, Schumacher RF, Meder M, Forster J (2001) Community and nosocomially acquired respiratory syncytial virus infection in a German paediatric hospital from 1988 to 1999. Eur J Pediatr 160: 541–547.
31. Prifert C, Streng A, Krempl CD, Liese J, Weissbrich B (2013) Novel respiratory syncytial virus a genotype, Germany, 2011–2012. Emerging Infect Dis 19: 1029–1030. doi: 10.3201/eid1906.121582
32. Panayiotou C, Richter J, Koliou M, Kalogirou N, Georgiou E, et al. (2014) Epidemiology of respiratory syncytial virus in children in Cyprus during three consecutive winter seasons (2010–2013): age distribution, seasonality and association between prevalent genotypes and disease severity. Epidemiol Infect: 1–6. doi: 10.1017/S0950268814000028
33. Pierangeli A, Trotta D, Scagnolari C, Ferreri ML, Nicolai A, et al. (2014) Rapid spread of the novel respiratory syncytial virus A ON1 genotype, central Italy, 2011 to 2013. Euro Surveill 19.
34. Aamir UB, Alam MM, Sadia H, Zaidi SSZ, Kazi BM (2013) Molecular Characterization of Circulating Respiratory Syncytial Virus (RSV) Genotypes in Gilgit Baltistan Province of Pakistan during 2011–2012 Winter Season. PLoS ONE 8: e74018. doi: 10.1371/journal.pone.0074018
35. Tsukagoshi H, Yokoi H, Kobayashi M, Kushibuchi I, Okamoto-Nakagawa R, et al. (2013) Genetic analysis of attachment glycoprotein (G) gene in new genotype ON1 of human respiratory syncytial virus detected in Japan. Microbiol Immunol 57: 655–659. doi: 10.1111/1348-0421.12075
36. Agoti CN, Otieno JR, Gitahi CW, Cane PA, Nokes DJ (2014) Rapid spread and diversification of respiratory syncytial virus genotype ON1, Kenya. Emerging Infect Dis 20: 950–959. doi: 10.3201/eid2006.131438
37. Kim Y-J, Kim D-W, Lee W-J, Yun M-R, Lee HY, et al. (2014) Rapid replacement of human respiratory syncytial virus A with the ON1 genotype having 72 nucleotide duplication in G gene. Infect Genet Evol 26C: 103–112. doi: 10.1016/j.meegid.2014.05.007
38. Geis S, Prifert C, Weissbrich B, Lehners N, Egerer G, et al. (2013). Molecular characterization of a respiratory syncytial virus (RSV) outbreak in a haematology unit, Heidelberg, Germany. J Clin Microbiol 51: 155–162.
39. Cui G, Qian Y, Zhu R, Deng J, Zhao L, et al. (2013) Emerging human respiratory syncytial virus genotype ON1 found in infants with pneumonia in Beijing, China. Emerg Microbes Infect 2: e22. doi: 10.1038/emi.2013.19
40. Choudhary ML, Anand SP, Wadhwa BS, Chadha MS (2013) Genetic variability of human respiratory syncytial virus in Pune, Western India. Infect Genet Evol 20C: 369–377. doi: 10.1016/j.meegid.2013.09.025

21

Rapid Antigen Group A Streptococcus Test to Diagnose Pharyngitis

Emily H. Stewart[1¶], Brian Davis[2¶], B. Lee Clemans-Taylor[3], Benjamin Littenberg[4], Carlos A. Estrada[5,6*], Robert M. Centor[3]

1 Walter Reed National Military Medical Center, Bethesda, Maryland, United States of America, **2** University of Texas Southwestern Medical Center, Dallas, Texas, United States of America, **3** The University of Alabama at Birmingham, Huntsville Campus, Huntsville, Alabama, United States of America, **4** University of Vermont, Burlington, Vermont, United States of America, **5** University of Alabama at Birmingham, Birmingham, Alabama, United States of America, **6** Birmingham Veterans Affairs Medical Center and Veterans Affairs Quality Scholar Program, Birmingham, Alabama, United States of America

Abstract

Background: Pharyngitis management guidelines include estimates of the test characteristics of rapid antigen streptococcus tests (RAST) using a non-systematic approach.

Objective: To examine the sensitivity and specificity, and sources of variability, of RAST for diagnosing group A streptococcal (GAS) pharyngitis.

Data Sources: MEDLINE, Cochrane Reviews, Centre for Reviews and Dissemination, Scopus, SciELO, CINAHL, guidelines, 2000–2012.

Study Selection: Culture as reference standard, all languages.

Data Extraction and Synthesis: Study characteristics, quality.

Main Outcome(s) and Measure(s): Sensitivity, specificity.

Results: We included 59 studies encompassing 55,766 patients. Forty three studies (18,464 patients) fulfilled the higher quality definition (at least 50 patients, prospective data collection, and no significant biases) and 16 (35,634 patients) did not. For the higher quality immunochromatographic methods in children (10,325 patients), heterogeneity was high for sensitivity (inconsistency [I^2] 88%) and specificity (I^2 86%). For enzyme immunoassay in children (342 patients), the pooled sensitivity was 86% (95% CI, 79–92%) and the pooled specificity was 92% (95% CI, 88–95%). For the higher quality immunochromatographic methods in the adult population (1,216 patients), the pooled sensitivity was 91% (95% CI, 87 to 94%) and the pooled specificity was 93% (95% CI, 92 to 95%); however, heterogeneity was modest for sensitivity (I^2 61%) and specificity (I^2 72%). For enzyme immunoassay in the adult population (333 patients), the pooled sensitivity was 86% (95% CI, 81–91%) and the pooled specificity was 97% (95% CI, 96 to 99%); however, heterogeneity was high for sensitivity and specificity (both, I^2 88%).

Conclusions: RAST immunochromatographic methods appear to be very sensitive and highly specific to diagnose group A streptococcal pharyngitis among adults but not in children. We could not identify sources of variability among higher quality studies. The present systematic review provides the best evidence for the wide range of sensitivity included in current guidelines.

Editor: Sean D. Reid, Wake Forest University School of Medicine, United States of America

Funding: RMC received funding from Justin Rogers Foundation. The funders had no role in study design, data collection and analysis, decision to publish, or preparation of the manuscript.

Competing Interests: RMC has received funding from the Justin Rogers Foundation.

* Email: cestrada@uab.edu

¶ These authors are co-first authors on this work.

Introduction

Rapid antigen testing to detect group A Streptococcal (GAS) infection provides important information for the antibiotic decision making for patients presenting with acute pharyngitis. Pharyngitis accounts for over 13 million office visits annually in the United States [1], highlighting the importance of these decisions. Patients with GAS pharyngitis can develop either suppurative or non-suppurative complications. Given the importance of chronic rheumatic fever in the 1950s, preventing acute rheumatic fever became the main focus of treating pharyngitis at the time. While the incidence of acute rheumatic fever has decreased, the focus in patients with acute pharyngitis is on treating GAS infections to decrease suppurative complications (especially peritonsillar abscess), decrease person-to-person spread, and to shorten symptom duration.

The Infectious Diseases Society of America (IDSA) guideline [2] on streptococcal pharyngitis recommends using a rapid test in patients with a modest probability of GAS infection, treating those with a positive rapid test and withholding antibiotics in rapid test negative patients. The guideline recommends culturing rapid test negative children and treating patients having positive cultures; the guideline does not recommend culturing the rapid test negative adults given the lower prevalence and significantly reduced chance of non-suppurative complications of the disease in the adult population [2], unless the clinician wishes to increase diagnostic sensitivity.

The IDSA guidelines and reviews have documented excellent specificity of rapid antigen streptococcal testing; however, the sensitivity estimate varies from 70% to 95% [3–6]. These reports did not apply a systematic approach to make these estimates. A systematic review published in Spanish [7] did not examine potential sources of heterogeneity.

The present study explores the variability of sensitivity and specificity using a systematic approach; the goal of this systematic review was to identify accurate, unbiased estimates of rapid antigen streptococcus test (RAST) characteristics for children, adults, and RAST variety.

Materials and Methods

We performed a systemic review and meta-analysis of the performance of various rapid antigen streptococcus tests to diagnose Group A streptococcal pharyngitis in adult and pediatric populations using standard guidelines for diagnostic studies [8]. We also used the Preferred Reporting Items for Systematic reviews and Meta-Analyses for reporting [9]. We limited our study to more recent publications because the technology of rapid antigen testing has improved over the years and to exclude tests no longer used.

Data Sources and Searches

In preparation for identifying search terms, a professional medical librarian (BLCT) searched the National Library of Medicine's MEDLINE electronic database from January 2000 to April 2012 using PubMed, limiting the search to the English language only and meta-analyses or systematic reviews. We then ran preliminary test searches to identify all possible terms necessary to design a comprehensive and systematic search strategy. Finally, we used medical subject headings (MeSH terms) and text words to search for three main concept areas: target condition, index test, and test characteristics (see Methods S1). The three main concepts were combined using AND as the Boolean operator. In addition, we supplemented the search with the PubMed/MEDLINE's Clinical Queries feature to combine the target condition with the diagnosis/broad automatic filter. We completed the first search on April 11, 2012 and repeated the same search strategy on October 26, 2012 to update the search and expand the scope by including non-English citations.

We also checked online through PubMed/MEDLINE and hand searched several major infectious disease, clinical microbiology, and pediatric textbooks for updates to current guidelines on the use of rapid antigen detection tests in the diagnosis of group a beta-hemolytic streptococcus including the Infectious Diseases Society of America (IDSA), American Heart Association, American Academy of Pediatrics, the American College of Physicians (ACP), the Centers for Disease Control, and the American Academy of Family Physicians. In addition, we searched the electronic sources Cochrane Reviews, Centre for Reviews and Dissemination [10], UpToDate, DynaMed, and Essential Evidence Plus; we also reviewed references from personal files (RMC, one of the authors). We also reviewed references from cost-effectiveness studies.

We did not include data from package inserts of commercially available RAST as study characteristics were not included [11]. Finally, we searched the electronic sources Scopus [12], SciELO (Scientific Electronic Library Online) [13], and CINAHL (Cumulative Index to Nursing and Allied Health Literature) on December 6, 2012 for studies published after 2000 without language limits.

Study Selection

Two of the authors independently reviewed the titles of the initial search results and excluded titles that were not relevant, non-English, lacking a RAST, review articles, studies that lacked culture as reference standard, or other reasons (ex: duplicate publications, non-human studies, case reports, letters to the editor, no data reported). Discrepancies were included in the second review. A third author reviewed all excluded titles (CAE). In the second review, two authors independently read the titles and abstracts for the same exclusion criteria; a third author resolved conflicts. In the third review, one author read the articles and another confirmed the excluded articles (a third author resolved conflicts during this step). We excluded articles that did not use a culture reference standard.

Data Extraction and Quality Assessment

We recorded country of study, funding source, index test location (point-of-care or laboratory), number of swabs for the reference test (one or two), culture medium, age of population, setting (outpatient clinic, student health, emergency room), inclusion and exclusion criteria, and study design (prospective, retrospective). We constructed 2×2 contingency tables (true positives, false positives, false negatives, true negatives) from the published data for the main study results and for any subgroups reported. We excluded articles where a 2×2 contingency table could not be calculated from the published data. We used the Quality Assessment of Diagnostic Accuracy Studies (QUADAS) checklist to assess methodological quality of the studies [14]. Each of two authors abstracted data for half of the studies selected; at the end, the other author reviewed the abstracted data for independent verification.

Data Synthesis and Analysis

Based on the 2×2 contingency table, we computed prevalence, sensitivity, and specificity for each study and each subgroup.

We examined heterogeneity with graphical methods using coupled forest plots of sensitivity and specificity and hierarchical summary receiver-operating characteristic (HSROC) curves [8,15–17]. The HSROC uses a random-effects model and accounts for the relationship between sensitivity and specificity in each study. The HSROC analyses provide estimates of uncertainty that includes a 95% confidence region (for the summary estimate) and a 95% prediction region (for a forecast of the sensitivity and specificity in a future study) [18]. Wider prediction regions suggest significant heterogeneity [8,17]. The summary ROC may also identify a threshold effect, suggested by a shoulder-like appearance of the curve, that could explain heterogeneity between studies [8].

We also used the inconsistency (I^2) value to examine heterogeneity and regarded values as low, moderate, or high heterogeneity for values of 25%, 50%, or 75% (respectively). However, a recent review noted limitations of the I^2 as it does not account for the correlation between sensitivity and specificity, does not account for variation explained by threshold effects, and overestimates heterogeneity [17]. We include pooled estimates of sensitivity and specificity in the results section when values were deemed homogeneous enough or for illustration purposes.

We explored heterogeneity, a-priori, by examining studies of highest quality, defined as those with at least 50 patients, prospective data collection, and three items of the QUADAS methodological quality criteria [14]: "Did the whole sample or a random selection of the sample, receive verification using a reference standard for diagnosis?" (partial verification avoided), "Did patients receive the same reference standard regardless of the index test results?" (differential verification avoided), and "Was the reference standard independent of the index test (i.e.: the index test did not form part of the reference standard)?" (incorporation bias avoided). We did not require blinding of the reference standard or the index test to define a study as high quality.

We examined publication bias with the Deeks' funnel plots and tested asymmetry with linear regression of log diagnostic odds ratios (DOR) on the inverse root of the effective sample size [19]. In the absence of publication bias, studies of smaller sample size would have a wider distribution of results (in diagnostic test studies, DOR) due to random variation as compared to studies with larger sample size that would have a narrower distribution of results. A non-vertical line with a p value<0.10 for the slope of the coefficient indicates asymmetry and suggests publication bias. The Deeks' funnel plot method [19] overcomes limitations of other methodologies.

We also explored heterogeneity post-hoc. The purpose of these analyses was to identify study sub-groups with sufficient clinical and statistical homogeneity to calculate summary estimates of sensitivity and specificity. We limited the exploratory analyses to the highest quality studies as defined above. We analyzed age groups separately, exclusive pediatric population vs. other, as the clinical features and epidemiology are different. We also analyzed separately by index test methodology (immuno-chromatographic, enzyme immunoassay, optical immune-assay). Finally, we explored sponsorship (commercial vs. none or none reported), location of performance of the index test (laboratory vs. point-of-care or not reported), risk score (Centor or McIassac), location of care (outpatient vs. emergency room), publication year (2000–2005 vs. 2006–2012), prevalence (by tertiles), and region (USA/Canada vs. Europe vs. other). We also performed meta-regression to estimate the independent contribution of the variables listed above that may explain heterogeneity [20].

We used STATA 11.2 software (College Station, Texas, USA) and the midas [20] and metandi [18] modules for statistical analyses.

Results

Study selection

Figure 1 displays the overall summary of the evidence search; we could not retrieve three studies for full article review [21–23]. Our searches identified all 24 studies included in the systematic review published in Spanish [7]. We included 58 studies that examined 55,766 patients [24–81]. One study [28] utilized two designs, hence 59 studies are mentioned in the rest of the manuscript. The overall prevalence of GAS infection was 28.2% (15,254/54,098 patients) (range 3.7% to 66.6%); we did not include one study [28] in the prevalence calculation as only patients with positive cultures were reported (n = 1,688).

Characteristics of Included Studies

The Table S1 in File S1 displays the overall study characteristics. The study design was prospective in all but eight (11.9%) studies [39,40,50–52,55,63,66], most were in the pediatric population (n = 35, 59.3%). The setting was solely in outpatient areas (n = 37, 62.7%) or emergency room settings (n = 19, 32.2%). Point of care testing was done in 27 studies (45.6%). Commercial funding was acknowledged in 16 studies (27.2%) [33,36,41,48,49,57–61,64,68,70,71,78,80]. The Table S2 in File S1 displays the main study characteristics for each study.

Quality of Included Studies (Risk of Bias)

The overall quality of the studies using the QUADAS criteria is shown in Figure 2; in 48 (81.4%) studies partial verification bias was avoided, in 47 (79.7%) studies differential verification bias was avoided, and in 47 (79.7%) studies incorporation bias was avoided (Figure 2). The quality assessment for each study is shown in the Table S3 in File S1. The funnel plot shown in Figure S1 in File S2 was asymmetric and the regression line was not vertical, suggesting the presence of publication bias (p<0.001). In the absence of publication bias, studies of smaller sample size would have a wider distribution of results due to random variation as compared to studies with larger sample size.

Analyses – Quantitative, Qualitative, and Heterogeneity

The operating test characteristics of the studies are shown in the Table S4 in File S1. The sensitivity ranged from 44% to 100%. The specificity ranged from 69% to 100%.

We explored heterogeneity a-priori by examining studies of highest quality (those with at least 50 patients, prospective data collection, and no verification or differential verification or incorporation biases). Of the 59 studies, 43 (72.9%; 18,464 patients) fulfilled the higher quality definition [24–29,31–34,36–38,41–46,48,49,53,54,56,57,59–62,64,65,67–71,73,75–79,81] and 16 (27.1%; 35,634 patients) did not [28,30,35,39,40,47,50,51,58,63,66,72,74,80]. The coupled forest plots for sensitivity and specificity and HSROC are shown for higher quality studies (Figure S2 in File S2, Figure S4 in File S2) and lower quality studies (Figure S3 in File S2, Figure S4 in File S2). Both, higher and lower quality studies were highly heterogeneous as demonstrated by high inconsistency values and confidence intervals in the forest plots and wide prediction regions in the HSROC. Also, the summary ROCs have a shoulder-like appearance, suggesting a threshold effect for both higher and lower quality studies.

Exploratory Analyses- Higher Quality Studies – Pediatrics and Adults Strata

Among the higher quality studies, immunochromatographic methods were described in 34 strata (28 pediatric, six adults), in five enzyme immunoassay strata (three pediatric, two adults), and in four optical immunoassay methods (three pediatric, one adult). The summary of diagnostic accuracy estimates for studies of higher methodological quality is shown in Table 1.

Pediatrics -Immunochromatographic Methods

The prevalence of GAS infection in the 28 pediatrics strata was 29.7% (3,062/10,325 patients) (range 11.0% to 66.6%). The studies were of high methodological quality, four studies met all 14

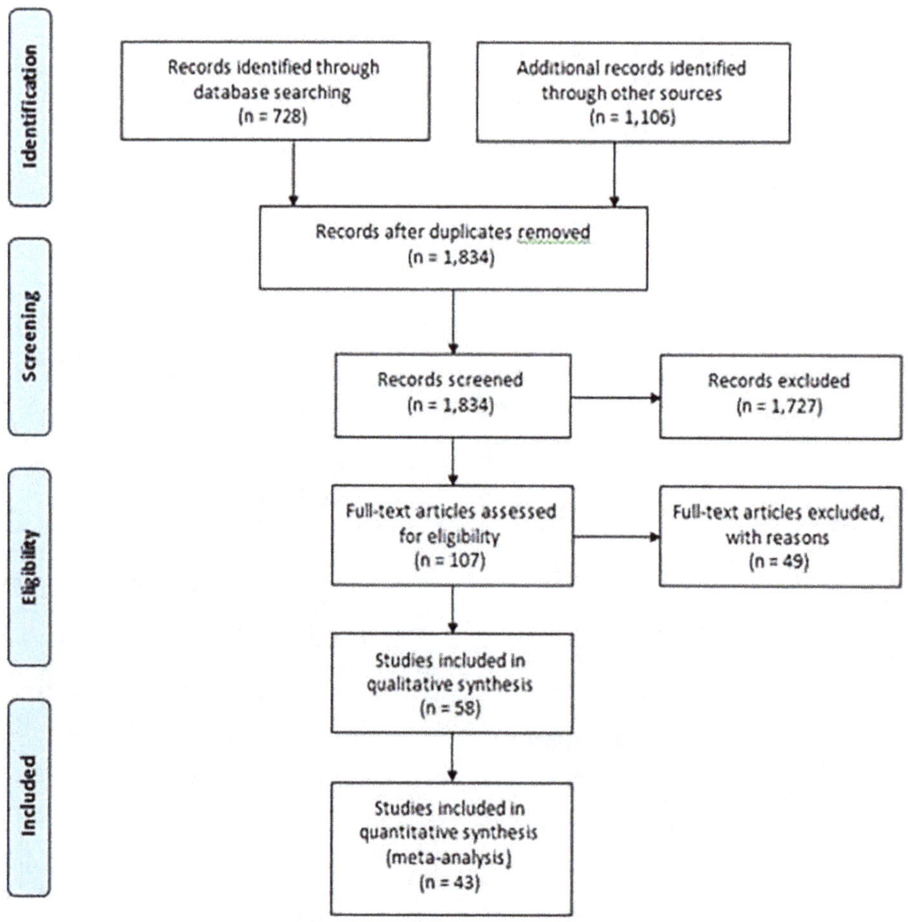

Figure 1. PRISMA Flow Diagram.

criteria [36,48,49,78], nine met 13 criteria [26,31,34,37,38,41, 43,46,65], three met 12 criteria [25,32,71], and two met 10 criteria [24,57] (Table S3 in File S1).

The coupled forest plots for sensitivity and specificity shows high heterogeneity (I^2 = 88% for sensitivity and I^2 = 86% for specificity; Figure 3, Table 1). As mentioned in the Methods section, we explored additional variables that may explain heterogeneity. In three of the 28 strata, the testing was performed in the laboratory. None of the 28 strata reported Centor or McIssac score. Supplementary figures show HSROC subgroups, no single variable yielded homogenous groups, sponsorship (Figure S5 in File S2), location of care (Figure S6 in File S2), publication year (Figure S7 in File S2), prevalence (Figure S8 in File S2), and region (Figure S9 in File S2). The sensitivity and specificity of the studies remained heterogeneous (large prediction regions) regardless of sponsorship, studies conducted in emergency rooms, studies published more contemporarily, studies with higher GAS infection prevalence, and studies conducted in North America and Europe. Meta-regression showed that in the univariate analyses all strata mentioned above but prevalence of GAS infection by tertile were significant predictors for heterogeneity for both sensitivity and specificity. However, in the joint model, outpatient setting (p = 0.03) and prevalence of GAS infection by tertile prevalence of GAS (p = 0.05) were the only significant variables (data not shown).

Among the 28 high quality studies in the pediatrics strata and immunochromatographic methods, the sensitivity was over 90% in 14 strata (n = 3,362 patients; prevalence of GAS infection, median 32% [Q1–Q3, 28–33%]) [34,37,38,43,46,48,57,65,71], between 80–90% in eight strata (n = 4,277 patients; prevalence of GAS infection, median 25% [Q1–Q3, 24–36%]) [24,25,32,34,36,49], and less than 80% in six strata (n = 2,685 patients; prevalence of GAS infection, median 25% [Q1–Q3, 21–29%]) [26,31,36,41,78].

Among the 28 high quality studies in the pediatrics strata and immunochromatographic methods, the specificity was over 95% in 17 strata (n = 7,451 patients; prevalence of GAS infection, median 29% [Q1–Q3, 25–33%]) [25,26,32,34,36,37,41,49,65, 71,78], >90–95% in eight strata (n = 2,340 patients; prevalence of GAS infection, median 32% [Q1–Q3, 22–36%]) [26,34,36,38, 46,48,57], 80–90% in two strata (n = 323 patients; prevalence of GAS, 25–26%) [24,31], and less than 80% in one strata (n = 211 patients; prevalence of GAS infection, 34%) [43].

Pediatrics - Enzyme Immunoassay and Optical Immunoassay Methods

The prevalence of GAS infection in the 3 enzyme immunoassay pediatric strata was 36.3% (124/342 patients) (range 33.3% to 38.5%). The coupled forest plots for sensitivity and specificity shows no or little heterogeneity (I^2 = 0% for sensitivity and I^2 = 55% for specificity; Figure 4, top panels; Table 1). The pooled sensitivity was 86% (95% CI, 79–92%) and the pooled specificity was 92% (95% CI, 88–95%).

The prevalence of GAS infection in the 3 optical immunoassay pediatric strata was 29.7% (977/3,294 patients) (range 28.7% to

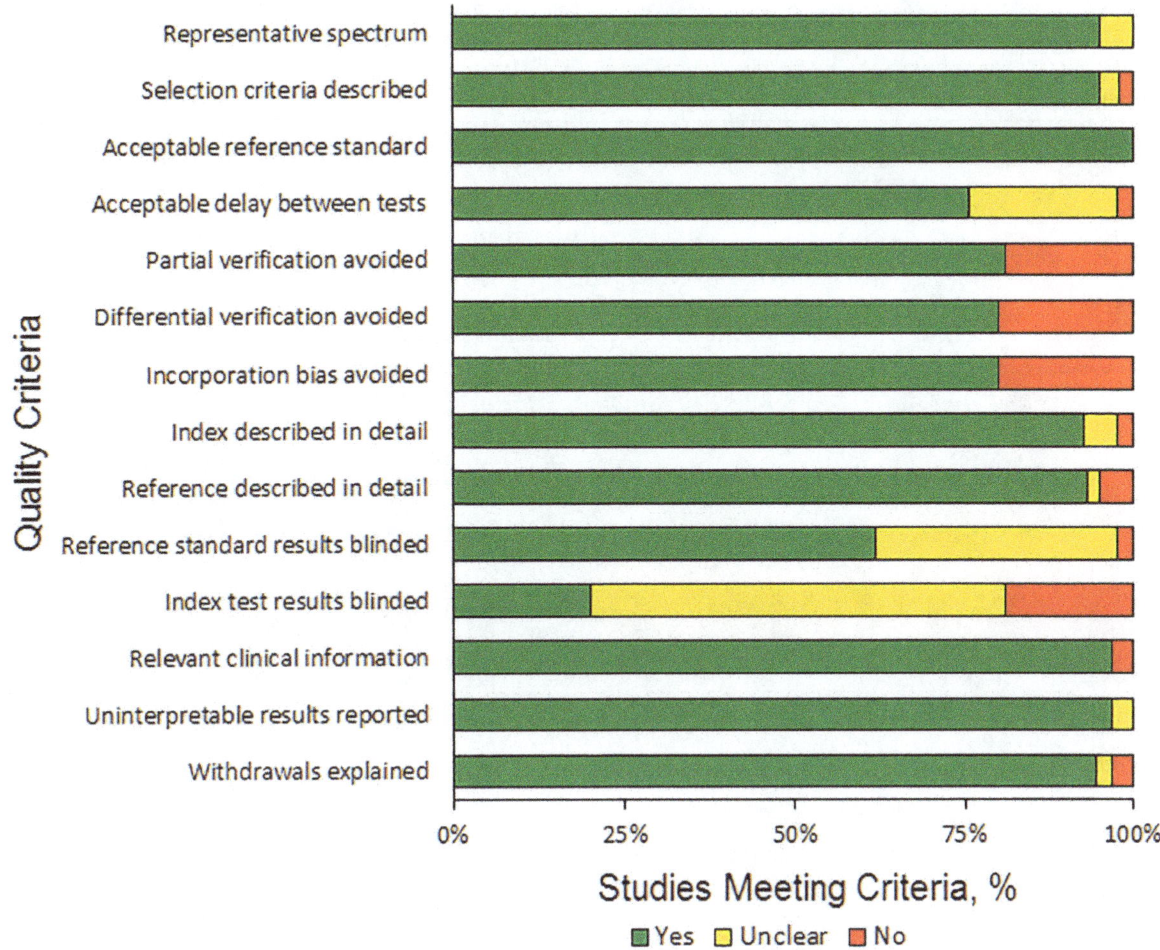

Figure 2. Quality Assessment of Diagnostic Accuracy Studies (QUADAS) assessments of the quality of included studies.

33.3%). The coupled forest plots for sensitivity and specificity shows moderate to high heterogeneity ($I^2 = 67\%$ for sensitivity and $I^2 = 90\%$ for specificity; Figure 4; bottom panels, Table 1). The pooled sensitivity was 80% (95% CI, 77–82%) and the pooled specificity was 93% (95% CI, 92–94%).

Adults - Immunochromatographic Methods

The prevalence of GAS infection in the 6 adults strata was 21.3% (259/1,216 patients) (range 16.1% to 25.7%). The coupled forest plots for sensitivity and specificity shows modest heterogeneity ($I^2 = 61\%$ for sensitivity and $I^2 = 72\%$ for specificity; Figure 5; top panels, Table 1). The pooled sensitivity was 91% (95% CI, 87–94%) and the pooled specificity was 93% (95% CI, 92 to 95%). One outlier study [75] met 12 quality criteria (Table S3 in File S1) and enrolled 100 patients presenting to an emergency room in Istanbul [75]. Another outlier study, [29] met nine quality criteria (Table S3 in File S1) and enrolled 148 patients presenting to two primary care settings in Boston (Massachusetts).

Adults - Enzyme immunoassay and Optical Immunoassay Methods

The prevalence of GAS infection in the 2 EIA adult strata was 21.9% (73/333 patients). The coupled forest plots for sensitivity and specificity shows high heterogeneity ($I^2 = 88\%$ for sensitivity and $I^2 = 88\%$ for specificity; Figure 5; bottom panels, Table 1). The pooled sensitivity was 86% (95% CI, 81–91%) and the pooled specificity was 97% (95% CI, 96 to 99%).

The prevalence of GAS infection in the single OIA adult strata was 40.7% (33/81 patients), Table 1.

Discussion

In this systematic review of rapid antigen strep testing, the number of patients included in studies that met high methodological quality criteria was significantly smaller than the number of patients included in lower quality studies (18,464 vs. 35,634, respectively). We also observed publication bias. We could not identify important sources of the high heterogeneity of sensitivity and specificity estimates among higher quality studies using immunochromatographic methods in children (10,325 patients). For higher quality studies using enzyme immunoassay in children (342 patients), the pooled sensitivity was 86% and the pooled specificity was 92% (studies had no or little heterogeneity). In children, immunochromatographic and enzyme immunoassay methods outperform optical immunoassay methods. For the higher quality immunochromatographic methods in the adult population (1,216 patients), the pooled sensitivity was 91% and the pooled specificity was 93%; however, heterogeneity was modest for sensitivity and specificity.

Table 1. Summary of diagnostic accuracy estimates, higher study methodological quality*.

Type of test	Pediatrics	Adults
Immunochromatographic		
Number of patients	10,325	1,216
Number of strata	28	6
Sensitivity, %	86 (85–87)	91 (87–94)
Specificity, %	96 (95–96)	93 (92–95)
Inconsistency (I^2)		
- Sensitivity	88%	61%
- Specificity	86%	72%
Enzyme Immunoassay (EIA)		
Number of patients	342	333
Number of strata	3	2
Sensitivity, %	86 (79–92)	86 (81–91)
Specificity, %	92 (88–95)	97 (96–99)
Inconsistency (I^2)		
- Sensitivity	0%	88%
- Specificity	55%	88%
Optical immunoassay (OIA)		
Number of patients	3,294	81
Number of strata	3	1
Sensitivity, %	80 (77–82)	94 (80–99)
Specificity, %	93 (92–94)	69 (54–81)
Inconsistency (I^2)		
- Sensitivity	67%	-
- Specificity	90%	-

*Numbers in parenthesis are 95% confidence intervals.

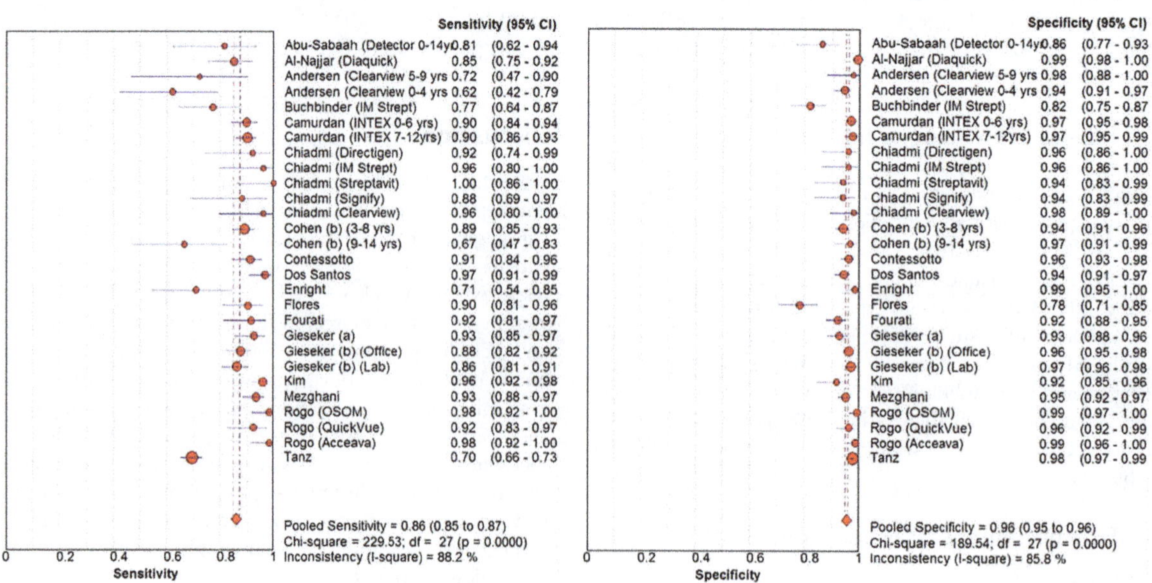

Figure 3. Pediatric strata, forest plots for immunochromatographic methods, higher study methodological quality.

Enzyme immunoassay

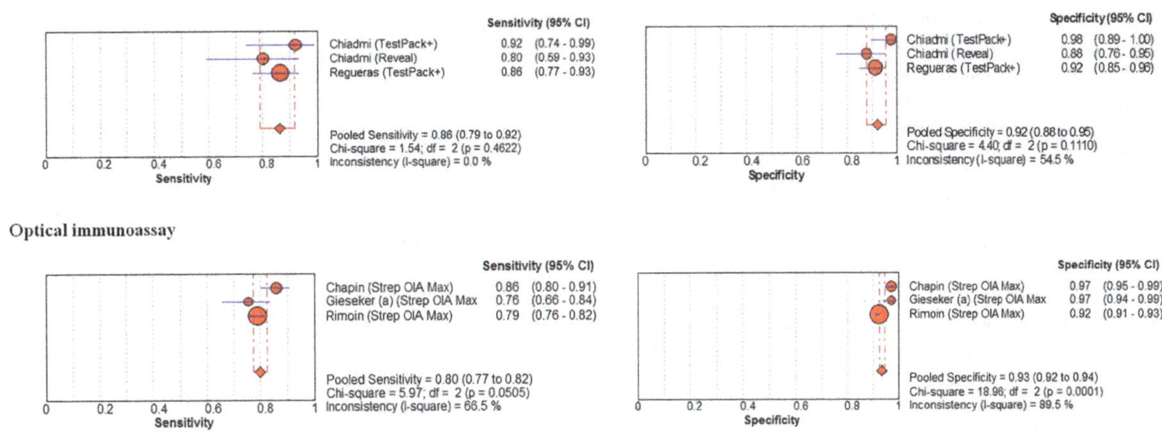

Figure 4. Pediatric strata, forest plots for enzyme immunoassay (EIA, top panels) and optical immunoassay (OIA, bottom panels) methods to diagnose group A streptococcal pharyngitis, higher study methodological quality.

The appropriate diagnosis and management of pharyngitis patients continues to provoke controversy. The controversy exists not just between "experts" but also between guideline panels. Matthys and colleagues reviewed 10 guidelines from both North America and Europe [82]. These guidelines took three different approaches to pharyngitis patients. Some European countries consider pharyngitis a self-limited problem with only rare complications. They eschew testing or antibiotic treatment.

Some guidelines recommend either rapid antigen strep testing or empiric treatment of patients more likely to have GAS pharyngitis, with neither testing nor treatment for patients very unlikely to have GAS infection [82]. Other guidelines aim to limit antibiotic use, and "require" a positive rapid antigen strep test prior to prescribing antibiotics [2].

The debate between the first strategy and the other two strategies rests on a disagreement over the benefits of treating GAS pharyngitis. The debate between the remaining two strategies depends on our estimates of the sensitivity of rapid antigen strep testing and the implications of not treating patients with false negative rapid strep tests.

The profound heterogeneity of the test characteristics among the most studied method, immunochromatographic, represents the major finding of our analysis. When an analysis reveals this degree of heterogeneity then one cannot reliably assign a point estimate to either sensitivity or specificity. Although the pooled estimate of sensitivity (85%; 95% CI 84 to 87%) reported in the systematic review published in Spanish [7] is remarkably similar to the one provided for immunochromatographic methods shown in Table 1 of our study, none can be used as a reliable point estimate given the large heterogeneity observed. While we observed no or little heterogeneity of enzyme immunoassay methods in children,

Immunochromatographic

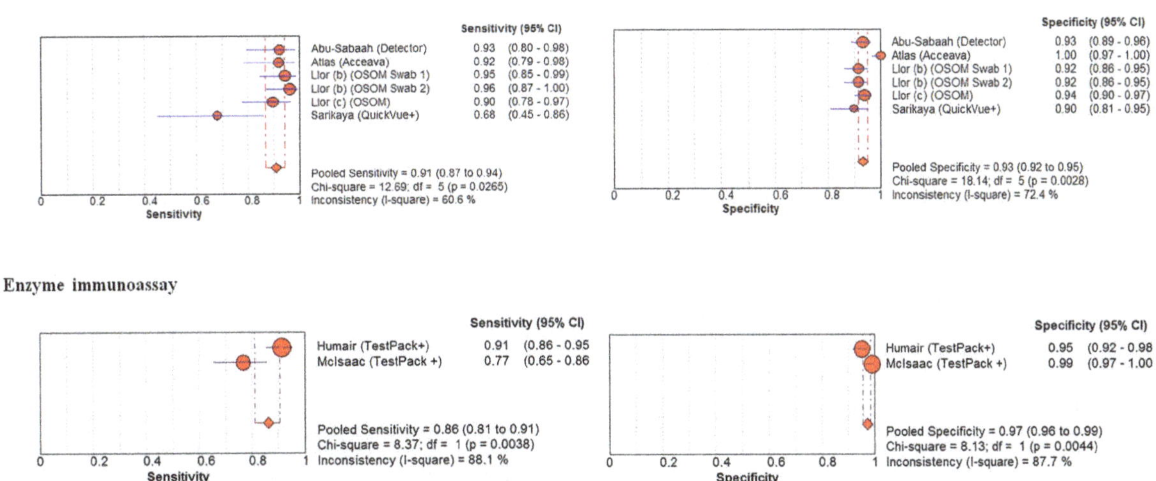

Figure 5. Adult strata, forest plots for immunochromatographic (top panels), enzyme immunoassay (EIA, middle panels) and optical immunoassay (OIA, bottom panels) methods to diagnose group A streptococcal pharyngitis, higher study methodological quality.

we caution the reader given the relatively small sample size in this group.

Why do these studies show such great heterogeneity for most of the groups? We can only speculate that several factors influence this finding. First, we have a mixture of practical studies in routine clinical settings and research studies with specially trained study personnel. Second, the tests have significant technical variances, as they use different methods to determine the presence of the group A antigen; hence, we could not examine a threshold effect. Finally, evidence suggests the high variability in sensitivity based on clinical spectrum, inoculum size, technical training, and personnel conducting the tests [83–85]; the nature of reporting of the studies reviewed precluded further exploration. In our pre-specified approach, we were not able to identify the source of such heterogeneity. Standardization of tests across manufacturers would better define the sensitivity of the RAST. Our finding of great heterogeneity means that we do not have strong confidence in the estimate of sensitivity.

We do not expect this analysis to resolve the ongoing debates about relying on rapid antigen strep testing to make treatment decisions. However, physician decision makers would appreciate accurate estimates of the test characteristics of any test that we use. This study provides estimates of the test characteristics; however, the consistency of performance leaves a broad range of confidence.

Our study has limitations. We could not retrieve three studies for full article review [21–23] and we observed publication bias.

Conclusion

In conclusion, RAST immunochromatographic methods appear to be very sensitive and highly specific to diagnose group A streptococcal pharyngitis among adults but not in children. Using the best evidence, we could not identify important sources of variability of sensitivity and specificity. The present systematic review provides the best evidence for the wide range of sensitivity included in current guidelines.

Supporting Information

File S1 Contains the following files: **Table S1.** Study Characteristics, Overall (n = 59). **Table S2.** Study Characteristics. **Table S3.** Quality assessment using QUADAS criteria. **Table S4.** Operating Test Characteristics.

File S2 Contains the following files: **Figure S1.** Funnel plot for rapid antigen tests diagnostic odds ratio. EES = Effective Sample Size. The non-vertical regression line suggests publication bias. The non-vertical regression line suggests publication bias (the results of the studies do not fall into the "funnel" depicted in blue). In the absence of publication bias, studies of smaller sample size would have a wider distribution of Diagnostic Odds Ratios; represented as a wider distribution at the base, which is absent from the plot. **Figure S2.** Forest plots sensitivities and specificities from test accuracy studies of rapid antigen tests to diagnose group A streptococcal pharyngitis for higher study methodological quality. Study test characteristics are sensitivity (left panel) and specificity (right panel). Circles represent the sensitivity or specificity and are proportional to study sample size. Blue lines represent 95% confidence intervals. Diamonds represent pooled estimates of sensitivity or specificity, red lines correspond to their respective 95% confidence intervals. **Figure S3.** Forest plots sensitivities and specificities from test accuracy studies of rapid antigen tests to diagnose group A streptococcal pharyngitis for lower study methodological quality. Study test characteristics are sensitivity (left panel) and specificity (right panel). Circles represent the sensitivity or specificity and are proportional to study sample size. Blue lines represent 95% confidence intervals. Diamonds represent pooled estimates of sensitivity or specificity, red lines correspond to their respective 95% confidence intervals. **Figure S4.** Hierarchical summary receiver-operating characteristic curve plots of rapid antigen tests to diagnose group A streptococcal pharyngitis by study methodological quality. **Figure S5.** Pediatric strata, immunochromatographic methods, higher quality studies. HSROC by sponsorship. **Figure S6.** Pediatric strata, immunochromatographic methods, higher quality studies. HSROC by location of care. **Figure S7.** Pediatric strata, immunochromatographic methods, higher quality studies. HSROC by publication year. **Figure S8.** Pediatric strata, immunochromatographic methods, higher quality studies. HSROC by prevalence. **Figure S9.** Pediatric strata, immunochromatographic methods, higher quality studies. HSROC by region.

Acknowledgments

Drs. Stewart and Davis contributed equally to the study conception, design, and overall conduction of the study and both qualify as first authors. Drs. Stewart and Davis were medical students at the time of the study and now are at Walter Reed National Military Medical Center (Dr. Stewart) and University of Texas Southwestern Medical Center (Dr. Davis).

The contents of this article are solely the responsibility of the authors and do not necessarily represent the official views of the Department of Veterans Affairs. Presented in part at the Southern Society of General Internal Medicine, New Orleans, February 22–23, 2013, and at the Society of General Internal Medicine National Meeting, Denver, Colorado, April 24–27, 2013.

Author Contributions

Conceived and designed the experiments: EHS BD BLCT RMC BL CAE. Performed the experiments: EHS BD. Analyzed the data: RMC BL CAE. Contributed reagents/materials/analysis tools: EHS BD BLCT RMC BL CAE. Contributed to the writing of the manuscript: EHS BD BLCT RMC BL CAE.

References

1. Ambulatory Health Care Data (2010) National Ambulatory Medical Care Survey: Summary Tables. Centers for Disease Control and Prevention. Available at: http://www.cdc.gov/nchs/ahcd/web_tables.htm#2010. Accessed October 13, 2014.
2. Shulman ST, Bisno AL, Clegg HW, Gerber MA, Kaplan EL, et al. (2012) Clinical practice guideline for the diagnosis and management of group A streptococcal pharyngitis: 2012 update by the Infectious Diseases Society of America. Clin Infect Dis 55: 1279–1282.
3. Gerber MA, Shulman ST (2004) Rapid diagnosis of pharyngitis caused by group A streptococci. Clin Microbiol Rev 17: 571–580.
4. Hillner BE, Centor RM (1987) What a difference a day makes: a decision analysis of adult streptococcal pharyngitis. J Gen Intern Med 2: 244–250.
5. Neuner JM, Hamel MB, Phillips RS, Bona K, Aronson MD (2003) Diagnosis and management of adults with pharyngitis. A cost-effectiveness analysis. Ann Intern Med 139: 113–122.
6. Wessels MR (2011) Clinical practice. Streptococcal pharyngitis. N Engl J Med 364: 648–655.
7. Ruiz-Aragon J, Rodriguez Lopez R, Molina Linde JM (2010) [Evaluation of rapid methods for detecting Streptococcus pyogenes. Systematic review and meta-analysis]. An Pediatr (Barc) 72: 391–402.

8. Leeflang MM, Deeks JJ, Gatsonis C, Bossuyt PM, Cochrane Diagnostic Test Accuracy Working G (2008) Systematic reviews of diagnostic test accuracy. Ann Intern Med 149: 889–897.
9. Moher D, Liberati A, Tetzlaff J, Altman DG, Group P (2009) Preferred reporting items for systematic reviews and meta-analyses: the PRISMA statement. PLoS Med 6: e1000097.
10. Centre for Reviews and Dissemination. University of York. National Institute for Health Research (NHS). Available at: http://www.crd.york.ac.uk/CRDWeb/. Accessed October 13, 2014.
11. Patel T, Brown E, Davis B, Clemans-Taylor BL, Centor RM, et al. (2014) What does industry tell us about test characteristics? The rapid antigen streptococcus test. J Invest Med 62: 584–585.
12. Scopus. Elsevier B.V. Available at URL: http://www.info.sciverse.com/scopus. Accessed October 13, 2014.
13. Scientific Electronic Library Online (SciELO). Available at URL: http://www.scielo.org/php/index.php. Accessed October 13, 2014.
14. Whiting P, Rutjes AW, Dinnes J, Reitsma J, Bossuyt PM, et al. (2004) Development and validation of methods for assessing the quality of diagnostic accuracy studies. Health Technol Assess 8: iii, 1–234.
15. Rutter CM, Gatsonis CA (2001) A hierarchical regression approach to meta-analysis of diagnostic test accuracy evaluations. Stat Med 20: 2865–2884.
16. Macaskill P (2004) Empirical Bayes estimates generated in a hierarchical summary ROC analysis agreed closely with those of a full Bayesian analysis. J Clin Epidemiol 57: 925–932.
17. Bossuyt P, Davenport C, Deeks J, Hyde C, Leeflang M, et al. (2013) Chapter 11:Interpreting results and drawing conclusions. In: Deeks JJ, Bossuyt PM, Gatsonis C (editors), Cochrane Handbook for Systematic Reviews of Diagnostic Test Accuracy Version 0.9. The Cochrane Collaboration, 2013. Available at URL: http://srdta.cochrane.org/. Accessed October 13, 2014.
18. Harbord RM, Whiting P (2009) metandi: Meta-analysis of diagnostic accuracy using hierarchical logistic regression. Stata Journal 9: 211–229.
19. Deeks JJ, Macaskill P, Irwig L (2005) The performance of tests of publication bias and other sample size effects in systematic reviews of diagnostic test accuracy was assessed. J Clin Epidemiol 58: 882–893.
20. Dwamena B (2007) MIDAS: Stata module for meta-analytical integration of diagnostic test accuracy studies. Boston College Department of Economics, 2007. Available at: http://ideas.repec.org/c/boc/bocode/s456880.html. Accessed October 13, 2014.
21. Shaheen BH, Hamdan AT (2006) Rapid identification of streptococcal pharyngitis Qatar Med J 15: 37–39.
22. Faverge B, Marie-Cosenza S, Bietrix M, Attou D, Bensekhria S, et al. (2004) [Use in hospital of a rapid diagnosis test of group A streptococcal pharyngotonsillitis in children]. Arch Pediatr 11: 862–863.
23. Bischoff A (2007) [Diagnosis of streptococcal tonsillitis. Rapid test prevents treatment error]. MMW Fortschritte der Medizin 149: 17.
24. Abu-Sabaah AH, Ghazi HO (2006) Better diagnosis and treatment of throat infections caused by group A beta-haemolytic streptococci. Br J Biomed Sci 63: 155–158.
25. Al-Najjar FY, Uduman SA (2008) Clinical utility of a new rapid test for the detection of group A Streptococcus and discriminate use of antibiotics for bacterial pharyngitis in an outpatient setting. Int J Infect Dis 12: 308–311.
26. Andersen JB, Dahm TL, Nielsen CT, Frimodt-Moller N (2003) [Diagnosis of streptococcal tonsillitis in the pediatric department with the help of antigen detection test]. Ugeskr Laeger 165: 2291–2295.
27. Araujo Filho BC, Imamura R, Sennes LU, Sakae FA (2005) Role of rapid antigen detection test for the diagnosis of group A beta-hemolytic streptococcus in patients with pharyngotonsillitis. Braz J Otorhinolaryngol 71: 168–171.
28. Armengol CE, Schlager TA, Hendley JO (2004) Sensitivity of a rapid antigen detection test for group A streptococci in a private pediatric office setting: answering the Red Book's request for validation. Pediatrics 113: 924–926.
29. Atlas SJ, McDermott SM, Mannone C, Barry MJ (2005) The role of point of care testing for patients with acute pharyngitis. J Gen Intern Med 20: 759–761.
30. Ayanruoh S, Waseem M, Quee F, Humphrey A, Reynolds T (2009) Impact of rapid streptococcal test on antibiotic use in a pediatric emergency department. Pediatr Emerg Care 25: 748–750.
31. Buchbinder N, Benzdira A, Belgaid A, Dufour D, Paon JC, et al. (2007) [Streptococcal pharyngitis in the pediatric emergency department: value and impact of rapid antigen detection test]. Arch Pediatr 14: 1057–1061.
32. Camurdan AD, Camurdan OM, Ok I, Sahin F, Ilhan MN, et al. (2008) Diagnostic value of rapid antigen detection test for streptococcal pharyngitis in a pediatric population. Int J Pediatr Otorhinolaryngol 72: 1203–1206.
33. Chapin KC, Blake P, Wilson CD (2002) Performance characteristics and utilization of rapid antigen test, DNA probe, and culture for detection of group a streptococci in an acute care clinic. J Clin Microbiol 40: 4207–4210.
34. Chiadmi F, Schlatter J, Mounkassa B, Ovetchkine P, Vermerie N (2004) [Fast diagnostic tests in the management of group A beta-heamolytic streptococcal pharyngitis]. Ann Biol Clin (Paris) 62: 573–577.
35. Cohen R, Levy C, Ovetchkine P, Boucherat M, Weil-Olivier C, et al. (2004) Evaluation of streptococcal clinical scores, rapid antigen detection tests and cultures for childhood pharyngitis. Eur J Pediatr 163: 281–282.
36. Cohen JF, Chalumeau M, Levy C, Bidet P, Thollot F, et al. (2012) Spectrum and inoculum size effect of a rapid antigen detection test for group A streptococcus in children with pharyngitis. PLoS One 7: e39085.
37. Contessotto Spadetto C, Camara Simon M, Aviles Ingles MJ, Ojeda Escuriet JM, Cascales Barcelo I, et al. (2000) [Rational use of antibiotics in pediatrics: impact of a rapid test for detection of beta-haemolytic group A streptococci in acute pharyngotonsillitis]. An Esp Pediatr 52: 212–219.
38. dos Santos AG, Berezin EN (2005) [Comparative analysis of clinical and laboratory methods for diagnosing streptococcal sore throat]. J Pediatr (Rio J) 81: 23–28.
39. Dimatteo LA, Lowenstein SR, Brimhall B, Reiquam W, Gonzales R (2001) The relationship between the clinical features of pharyngitis and the sensitivity of a rapid antigen test: evidence of spectrum bias. Ann Emerg Med 38: 648–652.
40. Edmonson MB, Farwell KR (2005) Relationship between the clinical likelihood of group a streptococcal pharyngitis and the sensitivity of a rapid antigen-detection test in a pediatric practice. Pediatrics 115: 280–285.
41. Enright K, Kalima P, Taheri S (2011) Should a near-patient test be part of the management of pharyngitis in the pediatric emergency department? Pediatr Emerg Care 27: 1148–1150.
42. Ezike EN, Rongkavilit C, Fairfax MR, Thomas RL, Asmar BI (2005) Effect of using 2 throat swabs vs 1 throat swab on detection of group A streptococcus by a rapid antigen detection test. Arch Pediatr Adolesc Med 159: 486–490.
43. Flores Mateo G, Conejero J, Grenzner Martinel E, Baba Z, Dicono S, et al. (2010) [Early diagnosis of streptococcal pharyngitis in paediatric practice: Validity of a rapid antigen detection test]. Aten Primaria 42: 356–361.
44. Fontes MJ, Bottrel FB, Fonseca MT, Lasmar LB, Diamante R, et al. (2007) Early diagnosis of streptococcal pharyngotonsillitis: assessment by latex particle agglutination test. J Pediatr (Rio J) 83: 465–470.
45. Forward KR, Haldane D, Webster D, Mills C, Brine C, et al. (2006) A comparison between the Strep A Rapid Test Device and conventional culture for the diagnosis of streptococcal pharyngitis. Can J Infect Dis Med Microbiol 17: 221–223.
46. Fourati S, Smaoui H, Jegiurim H, Berriche I, Taghorti R, et al. (2009) [Use of the rapid antigen detection test in group A streptococci pharyngitis diagnosis in Tunis, Tunisia]. Bull Soc Pathol Exot 102: 175–176.
47. Fox JW, Marcon MJ, Bonsu BK (2006) Diagnosis of streptococcal pharyngitis by detection of Streptococcus pyogenes in posterior pharyngeal versus oral cavity specimens. J Clin Microbiol 44: 2593–2594.
48. Gieseker KE, Mackenzie T, Roe MH, Todd JK (2002) Comparison of two rapid Streptococcus pyogenes diagnostic tests with a rigorous culture standard. Pediatr Infect Dis J 21: 922–927.
49. Gieseker KE, Roe MH, MacKenzie T, Todd JK (2003) Evaluating the American Academy of Pediatrics diagnostic standard for Streptococcus pyogenes pharyngitis: backup culture versus repeat rapid antigen testing. Pediatrics 111: e666–670.
50. Gurol Y, Akan H, Izbirak G, Tekkanat ZT, Gunduz TS, et al. (2010) The sensitivity and the specifity of rapid antigen test in streptococcal upper respiratory tract infections. Int J Pediatr Otorhinolaryngol 74: 591–593.
51. Hall MC, Kieke B, Gonzales R, Belongia EA (2004) Spectrum bias of a rapid antigen detection test for group A beta-hemolytic streptococcal pharyngitis in a pediatric population. Pediatrics 114: 182–186.
52. Hinfey P, Nicholls BH, Garcia F, Ripper J, Cameron Y, et al. (2010) Sensitivity of a rapid antigen detection test for the diagnosis of group a streptoccal pharyngitis in the emergency department. J Emerg Med 56: S132.
53. Humair JP, Revaz SA, Bovier P, Stalder H (2006) Management of acute pharyngitis in adults: reliability of rapid streptococcal tests and clinical findings. Arch Intern Med 166: 640–644.
54. Johansson L, Mansson NO (2003) Rapid test, throat culture and clinical assessment in the diagnosis of tonsillitis. Fam Pract 20: 108–111.
55. Kawakami S, Ono Y, Yanagawa Y, Miyazawa Y (2003) [Basic and clinical evaluation of the new rapid diagnostic kit for detecting group A streptococci with the immunochromatographical method]. Rinsho Biseibutshu Jinsoku Shindan Kenkyukai Shi 14: 9–16.
56. Keahey L, Bulloch B, Jacobson R, Tenenbein M, Kabani A (2002) Diagnostic accuracy of a rapid antigen test for GABHS performed by nurses in a pediatric ED. Am J Emerg Med 20: 128–130.
57. Kim S (2009) The evaluation of SD Bioline Strep A rapid antigen test in acute pharyngitis in pediatric clinics. Korean J Lab Med 29: 320–323.
58. Lindbaek M, Hoiby EA, Lermark G, Steinsholt IM, Hjortdahl P (2004) Which is the best method to trace group A streptococci in sore throat patients: culture or GAS antigen test? Scand J Prim Health Care 22: 233–238.
59. Llor C, Hernandez Anadon S, Gomez Bertomeu FF, Santamaria Puig JM, Calvino Dominguez O, et al. (2008) [Validation of a rapid antigenic test in the diagnosis of pharyngitis caused by group a beta-haemolytic Streptococcus]. Aten Primaria 40: 489–494.
60. Llor C, Calvino O, Hernandez S, Crispi S, Perez-Bauer M, et al. (2009) Repetition of the rapid antigen test in initially negative supposed streptococcal pharyngitis is not necessary in adults. Int J Clin Pract 63: 1340–1344.
61. Llor C, Madurell J, Balague-Corbella M, Gomez M, Cots JM (2011) Impact on antibiotic prescription of rapid antigen detection testing in acute pharyngitis in adults: a randomised clinical trial. Br J Gen Pract 61: e244–251.
62. Maltezou HC, Tsagris V, Antoniadou A, Galani L, Douros C, et al. (2008) Evaluation of a rapid antigen detection test in the diagnosis of streptococcal pharyngitis in children and its impact on antibiotic prescription. J Antimicrob Chemother 62: 1407–1412.

63. Mayes T, Pichichero ME (2001) Are follow-up throat cultures necessary when rapid antigen detection tests are negative for group A streptococci? Clin Pediatr (Phila) 40: 191–195.
64. McIsaac WJ, Kellner JD, Aufricht P, Vanjaka A, Low DE (2004) Empirical validation of guidelines for the management of pharyngitis in children and adults. JAMA 291: 1587–1595.
65. Mezghani Maalej S, Rekik M, Boudaouara M, Jardak N, Turki S, et al. (2010) [Childhood pharyngitis in Sfax (Tunisia): epidemiology and utility of a rapid streptococcal test]. Med Mal Infect 40: 226–231.
66. Mirza A, Wludyka P, Chiu TT, Rathore MH (2007) Throat culture is necessary after negative rapid antigen detection tests. Clin Pediatr (Phila) 46: 241–246.
67. Nerbrand C, Jasir A, Schalen C (2002) Are current rapid detection tests for Group A Streptococci sensitive enough? Evaluation of 2 commercial kits. Scand J Infect Dis 34: 797–799.
68. Parviainen M, Koskela M, Ikäheimo I, Kelo E, Sirola H, et al. (2011) A novel strep A test for a rapid test reader compared with standard culture method and a commercial antigen assay. Eur Infect Dis 5: 143–145.
69. Regueras De Lorenzo G, Santos Rodriguez PM, Villa Bajo L, Perez Guirado A, Arbesu Fernandez E, et al. (2012) [Use of the rapid antigen technique in the diagnosis of Streptococcus pyogenes pharyngotonsillitis]. An Pediatr (Barc) 77: 193–199.
70. Rimoin AW, Walker CL, Hamza HS, Elminawi N, Ghafar HA, et al. (2010) The utility of rapid antigen detection testing for the diagnosis of streptococcal pharyngitis in low-resource settings. Int J Infect Dis 14: e1048–1053.
71. Rogo T, Schwartz RH, Ascher DP (2011) Comparison of the Inverness Medical Acceava Strep A test with the Genzyme OSOM and Quidel QuickVue Strep A tests. Clin Pediatr (Phila) 50: 294–296.
72. Roosevelt GE, Kulkarni MS, Shulman ST (2001) Critical evaluation of a CLIA-waived streptococcal antigen detection test in the emergency department. Ann Emerg Med 37: 377–381.
73. Rosenberg P, McIsaac W, Macintosh D, Kroll M (2002) Diagnosing streptococcal pharyngitis in the emergency department: Is a sore throat score approach better than rapid streptococcal antigen testing? Cjem 4: 178–184.
74. Santos O, Weckx LL, Pignatari AC, Pignatari SS (2003) Detection of Group A beta-hemolytic Streptococcus employing three different detection methods: culture, rapid antigen detecting test, and molecular assay. Braz J Infect Dis 7: 297–300.
75. Sarikaya S, Aktas C, Ay D, Cetin A, Celikmen F (2010) Sensitivity and specificity of rapid antigen detection testing for diagnosing pharyngitis in the emergency department. Ear Nose Throat J 89: 180–182.
76. Schmuziger N, Schneider S, Frei R (2003) [Reliability and general practice value of 2 rapid Streptococcus A tests]. HNO 51: 806–812.
77. Sheeler RD, Houston MS, Radke S, Dale JC, Adamson SC (2002) Accuracy of rapid strep testing in patients who have had recent streptococcal pharyngitis. J Am Board Fam Pract 15: 261–265.
78. Tanz RR, Gerber MA, Kabat W, Rippe J, Seshadri R, et al. (2009) Performance of a rapid antigen-detection test and throat culture in community pediatric offices: implications for management of pharyngitis. Pediatrics 123: 437–444.
79. Uhl JR, Adamson SC, Vetter EA, Schleck CD, Harmsen WS, et al. (2003) Comparison of LightCycler PCR, rapid antigen immunoassay, and culture for detection of group A streptococci from throat swabs. J Clin Microbiol 41: 242–249.
80. Van Limbergen J, Kalima P, Taheri S, Beattie TF (2006) Streptococcus A in paediatric accident and emergency: are rapid streptococcal tests and clinical examination of any help? Emerg Med J 23: 32–34.
81. Wong MC, Chung CH (2002) Group A streptococcal infection in patients presenting with a sore throat at an accident and emergency department: prospective observational study. Hong Kong Med J 8: 92–98.
82. Matthys J, De Meyere M, van Driel ML, De Sutter A (2007) Differences among international pharyngitis guidelines: not just academic. Ann Fam Med 5: 436–443.
83. Cohen JF, Chalumeau M, Levy C, Bidet P, Benani M, et al. (2013) Effect of clinical spectrum, inoculum size and physician characteristics on sensitivity of a rapid antigen detection test for group A streptococcal pharyngitis. Eur J Clin Microbiol Infect Dis 32: 787–793.
84. Fox JW, Cohen DM, Marcon MJ, Cotton WH, Bonsu BK (2006) Performance of rapid streptococcal antigen testing varies by personnel. J Clin Microbiol 44: 3918–3922.
85. Toepfner N, Henneke P, Berner R, Hufnagel M (2013) Impact of technical training on rapid antigen detection tests (RADT) in group A streptococcal tonsillopharyngitis. Eur J Clin Microbiol Infect Dis 32: 609–611.

22

Whole Exome Sequencing Identifies Novel Genes for Fetal Hemoglobin Response to Hydroxyurea in Children with Sickle Cell Anemia

Vivien A. Sheehan[1]*, Jacy R. Crosby[2,3], Aniko Sabo[4], Nicole A. Mortier[5], Thad A. Howard[5], Donna M. Muzny[4], Shannon Dugan-Perez[4], Banu Aygun[6], Kerri A. Nottage[7], Eric Boerwinkle[3,4], Richard A. Gibbs[4], Russell E. Ware[5], Jonathan M. Flanagan[1]

1 Hematology Center, Department of Pediatrics, Baylor College of Medicine, Houston, Texas, United States of America, **2** The University of Texas Graduate School of Biomedical Sciences at Houston, Department of Biostatistics, Bioinformatics, and Systems Biology, University of Texas, Houston, Texas, United States of America, **3** Human Genetics Center, University of Texas, Houston, Texas, United States of America, **4** Human Genome Sequencing Center, Baylor College of Medicine, Houston, Texas, United States of America, **5** Division of Hematology, Cincinnati Children's Hospital Medical Center, Cincinnati, Ohio, United States of America, **6** Steven and Alexandra Cohen Children's Medical Center of New York, New Hyde Park, New York, United States of America, **7** Department of Hematology, St. Jude Children's Research Hospital, Memphis, Tennessee, United States of America

Abstract

Hydroxyurea has proven efficacy in children and adults with sickle cell anemia (SCA), but with considerable inter-individual variability in the amount of fetal hemoglobin (HbF) produced. Sibling and twin studies indicate that some of that drug response variation is heritable. To test the hypothesis that genetic modifiers influence pharmacological induction of HbF, we investigated phenotype-genotype associations using whole exome sequencing of children with SCA treated prospectively with hydroxyurea to maximum tolerated dose (MTD). We analyzed 171 unrelated patients enrolled in two prospective clinical trials, all treated with dose escalation to MTD. We examined two MTD drug response phenotypes: HbF (final %HbF minus baseline %HbF), and final %HbF. Analyzing individual genetic variants, we identified multiple low frequency and common variants associated with HbF induction by hydroxyurea. A validation cohort of 130 pediatric sickle cell patients treated to MTD with hydroxyurea was genotyped for 13 non-synonymous variants with the strongest association with HbF response to hydroxyurea in the discovery cohort. A coding variant in *Spalt-like transcription factor*, or *SALL2*, was associated with higher final HbF in this second independent replication sample and *SALL2* represents an outstanding novel candidate gene for further investigation. These findings may help focus future functional studies and provide new insights into the pharmacological HbF upregulation by hydroxyurea in patients with SCA.

Editor: Wilbur Lam, Emory University/Georgia Insititute of Technology, United States of America

Funding: This work was supported by the National Human Genome Research Institute (U54-HGOO3273)(EB, RAG), National Heart, Lung and Blood Institute (U01-HL078787, R01-HL090941)(REW), Doris Duke Charitable Foundation (2010036)(REW), and the Russell and Diana Hawkins Family Foundation Discovery Fellowship (JRC). The funders had no role in study design, data collection and analysis, decision to publish, or preparation of the manuscript.

Competing Interests: The authors have declared that no competing interests exist.

* Email: vsheehan@bcm.edu

Introduction

Sickle cell anemia (SCA) is an inherited blood disorder, affecting 1 in 400 African Americans, causing significant morbidity and mortality. Although a monogenic disease, individuals with SCA (usually homozygous HbSS) exhibit wide variability in their laboratory and clinical phenotypes. One of the most powerful and reproducible modifiers of disease severity is an individual's endogenous level of fetal hemoglobin (HbF) [1]. If produced in sufficient amounts, HbF is able to prevent the intracellular polymerization of deoxygenated sickle hemoglobin (HbS), which is the nidus of the clinical disease process [2,3]. Pharmacologic induction of HbF is clinically beneficial, and the most widely used and safest method for increasing HbF levels in patients with SCA is treatment with hydroxyurea. Currently, it is the only FDA-approved pharmacologic treatment for induction of HbF in adult patients with SCA, and is approved by the European Medicines Agency for both children and adults with SCA. Hydroxyurea significantly reduces pain and acute chest episodes, the need for blood transfusions and hospitalizations, and most importantly, reduces mortality [4–6]. While hydroxyurea has suspected disease modulating effects outside of HbF induction, the majority of its benefit is directly related to the amount of HbF produced in response to the drug [7,8]. There is an inverse relationship between levels of drug-induced HbF and number of pain episodes, hospitalizations, and overall mortality [9,10].

Several clinical studies have shown that individual hematological responses to hydroxyurea treatment are highly variable, with induced HbF levels ranging from 10% to greater than 30% HbF even for compliant patients on similar dosing regimens [11–14].

Previous efforts to identify predictors associated with final HbF produced in response to hydroxyurea have identified higher baseline HbF values, higher white blood cell count (WBC), and absolute reticulocyte count (ARC) as important factors [13,15,16]. However, none of these parameters can accurately predict the degree of HbF induction by hydroxyurea in an individual patient. From analysis of sibling pairs, it is known that the degree of HbF induction by hydroxyurea has a strong heritable component [17], indicating that genetic modifiers may have a large effect on drug response. Identification of specific genetic variants associated with HbF induction may elucidate reasons for this phenotypic variability and provide new insights into the drug's mechanisms of action related to HbF induction.

The aim of this study was to use a whole exome sequencing (WES) pharmacogenomics approach to identify genetic predictors of HbF response to hydroxyurea. Using two prospective pediatric cohorts with robust HbF phenotype data and standardized dose escalation regimen to MTD as a discovery cohort, we undertook a novel unbiased screen to test the entire exome for variants that are associated with hydroxyurea-induced HbF response levels (as measured by maximum %HbF at MTD [final HbF] or the change in %HbF from baseline to final [ΔHbF]). We focused on genetic variants with predicted functional effects on protein coding regions and identified several non-synonymous mutations that may influence the HbF response to hydroxyurea in children with SCA. We then validated a coding variant in *SALL2* in an unrelated, "real-world" cohort of children treated with hydroxyurea.

Results

Patient characteristics

Overall, both cohorts showed robust response to hydroxyurea with evidence of substantial individual variability in drug response (Table 1). All discovery cohort samples were genotyped for variants in *BCL11A* (rs1427407, rs4671393, rs11886868, rs7599488) and *HBSIL-MYB* (rs9399137, rs9402686); we found an association with baseline HbF for all *BCL11A* variants tested other than rs7599488. There was no significant association between the *BCL11A* variants tested and final HbF. No association with baseline, final or HbF was seen for either *HBSIL-MYB* variants tested. Linear association was performed with *BCL11A* variants as a covariate, without a significant change in associations.

At the time of hydroxyurea initiation, the average age of the 171 patients in the discovery cohort was 10.4±4.5 years of age. The average age of the 130 patients in the validation cohort was 8.1±4.0 years. All patients were treated under a similar dose escalation to MTD regimen according to protocol, or similar institutional guidelines 18, 19. After a minimum of 6 months on hydroxyurea therapy, all patients reached a stable MTD (average 25.1±4.5 mg/kg/day in the discovery cohort, 27.1±4.3 mg/kg/day in the validation cohort) with predictable laboratory benefits (Table 1). The mean increase in HbF was 19.5±6.6% in the discovery cohort and 13.9±7.0% in the validation cohort, reflecting slight differences between the two groups of patients. There was evidence of consistent myelosuppression across both cohorts, however. The baseline HbF, distribution of ΔHbF at MTD and final HbF at MTD were all similar to prior reports (Figure 1, A–C). [15,20].

Whole exome sequencing

All 171 samples in the discovery cohort passed stringent WES quality control parameters with an average of 92% of the targeted

Table 1. Comparison of discovery and validation cohorts.

	Discovery Cohort	Validation Cohort	Discovery Cohort	Validation Cohort
Age (years)	10.4 ±4.5	8.1 ±4.0	-	-
WBC ($\times 10^9$/L)	13.5 ±4.2	13.1 ±5.7	6.5 ±2.0	6.9 ±2.0
ANC ($\times 10^9$/L)	7.2 ±3.2	6.2 ±4.3	3.0 ±1.2	2.7 ±0.9
Hb (g/dL)	9.1 ±0.9	8.0 ±1.7	9.4 ±1.0	9.5 ±1.3
ARC ($\times 10^9$/L)	0.28 ±0.13	0.29 ±0.12	0.17 ±0.09	0.12 ±0.05
MCV (fL)	86.1 ±4.8	82.1 ±8.3	116.4 ±13.0	97.7 ±11.1
HbF (%)	8.0 ±4.9	11.9 ±5.9	27.6 ±7.3	25.8 ±8.2
ΔHbF (%)	-	-	19.5 ±6.6	13.9 +7.0
HU dose (mg/kg/day)	-	-	25.1 ±4.5	27.1 ±4.3

WBC: white blood cell count; ANC: absolute neutrophil count; ARC: absolute reticulocyte count; MCV: mean corpuscular volume; HU: hydroxyurea.
The discovery cohort was composed of 120 patients from HUSTLE and 51 from SWITCH. The validation cohort was collected from patients treated at TCCH.

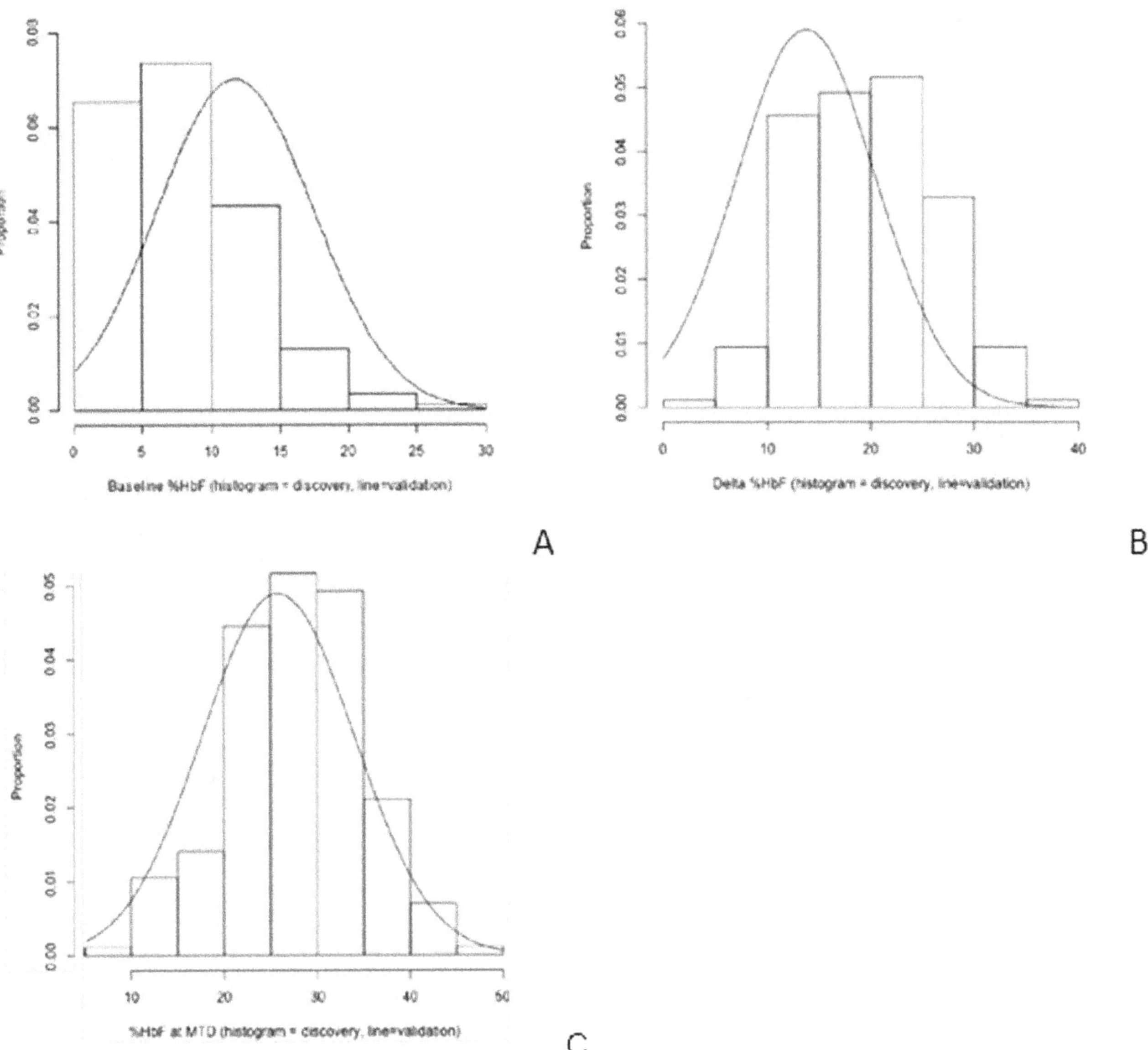

Figure 1. Comparison of discovery and validation cohorts. A, Baseline, or endogenous HbF for the discovery cohort is shown in binned histogram, and distribution of baseline HbF in validation cohort by a line plot. B, Delta HbF for the discovery cohort is shown in binned histogram, and distribution of delta HbF in validation cohort by a line plot. C, Final, or MID HbF for the discovery cohort is shown in binned histogram, and distribution of final, or MID in validation cohort by a line plot.

exonic regions sequenced at greater than 20× coverage per individual. We identified a total of 278,639 autosomal variants, and 127,238 of these variants were non-synonymous or splice site variants expected to introduce an amino acid change in their encoded proteins (Table S1). For single variant association testing, we further filtered the non-synonymous variants (n = 127,238) for those with a minor allele frequency (MAF) greater than or equal to 2% (n = 38,012). We corrected for any population stratification using principal component analysis (PCA) performed by the EIGENSTRAT method.

As our phenotypes of interest are continuous variables, we used linear regression analysis to test the association of the 38,012 common (MAF≥2%) non-synonymous variants using final HbF, and ΔHbF as independent, continuous variables. In addition, we attempted to find rare variants with MAF<2% associated with drug response by performing burden analysis with SKAT and T2 tests using the ΔHbF and final HbF phenotypes, but none of the gene level p-values were significant.

We identified 12 variants associated with ΔHbF with a p-value less than 5×10^{-4} (Table 2). In addition, we identified 13 variants associated with final HbF, also with a p-value less than 5×10^{-4} (Table 3). Although none of the p-values achieved genome wide significance level ($p<1.3X10^{-6}$), these results offered suggestive signals of potential associations. We used the existing methods of SIFT and PolyPhen2 [21] for predicting the functional impact of each non-synonymous variant to estimate which of the 25 variants had a predicted damaging or benign effect on encoded protein function (Tables 2 and 3).

From these 25 variants, we identified 13 variants with strongest association with response to hydroxyurea and predicted to

Table 2. Variants associated with ΔHbF on hydroxyurea.

Gene	SNP ID	Amino Acid Change	Protein Function Prediction	MAF (%)	Function	Beta Value	SE	P-value
EML1	rs141631682	Gly109Asp	Damaging	2	Microtubule assembly	10.9	2.7	7.41×10^{-5}
SESN1	rs2273668	Leu103Ile	Damaging	2	Peroxiredoxin reduction	9.3	2.3	8.88×10^{-5}
PAPLN	rs17126352	Val416Ile	Benign	3	Metalloprotease	7.1	1.8	1.35×10^{-4}
DCHS2	rs61746132	Pro1676Lys	Damaging	12	Calcium dependent cell adhesion	3.9	1.0	1.73×10^{-4}
KRT80	rs61749462	Arg364Ser	Damaging	3	Keratin 80	8.0	2.1	1.80×10^{-4}
SALL2	rs61743453	Pro840Arg	Damaging	4	Transcription factor	6.7	1.8	2.37×10^{-4}
NOM1	rs61742645	Arg779Cys	Benign	2	PP1 interacting protein	8.7	2.3	2.43×10^{-4}
N4BP2L2	rs35108810	Asp246Val	Damaging	15	*ELA2* transcription inhibitor	−3.3	0.9	3.47×10^{-4}
RNF113B	rs16955011	Val92Met	Damaging	18	Ring finger protein	3.1	0.8	3.76×10^{-4}
FTSJ2	rs55904231	Ser11Phe	Benign	7	RNA methyltransferase	5.2	1.4	3.76×10^{-4}
RHPN2	rs28626308	Arg70Gln	Damaging	7	Rho GTPase binding protein	5.2	1.4	3.91×10^{-4}
ADAR	rs17843865	Tyr587Cys	Benign	4	Adenosine deaminase	−6.4	1.8	4.65×10^{-4}

Variants selected were predicted damaging, with a p-value <0.001 in the discovery cohort, n = 171, composed of patients from HUSTLE and SWITCH trials.

introduce an amino acid change that has a damaging effect on protein structure or function. We genotyped these 13 variants by TaqMan PCR in our independent validation cohort of 130 patients with SCA. We found that one of the 13 variants, located in the *SALL2* gene, maintained association with hydroxyurea response. In the discovery cohort, the P840R variant in the *SALL2* gene (rs61743453) was associated with a higher change in HbF in response to hydroxyurea ($p = 2.37\times10^{-4}$, beta value 6.7). In the validation cohort, this same P840R variant was associated with a higher final HbF, with a p-value of 0.05, and a beta value of 4.2. Using Fisher's combined probability test method, a meta analysis of the association of the *SALL2* variant with ΔHbF in the discovery and validation sample groups (n = 301) leads to a combined p-value of 8.30×10^{-4}. The meta analysis of the association of *SALL2* with final HbF in the discovery and validation sample groups resulted in a combined p-value of 1.48×10^{-4}.

Discussion

Many individuals with SCA are prescribed hydroxyurea, and there is evidence that genetic modifiers affect individual response [17,22]. In order to identify novel candidate genes and variants associated with hydroxyurea response, we sequenced the exomes of 171 individuals enrolled in two prospective clinical trials and related their sequence variant data to HbF response. This discovery cohort was obtained from patients treated on protocol, with the highest level of drug compliance supervision, including monthly pill counts. Our validation cohort (n = 130) was treated under guidelines similar to that of the discovery cohort. As expected, individual MTD was achieved at different hydroxyurea doses, within a range of 10–35 mg/kg/d, reflecting the typical range in bioavailability among patients. There was no correlation between hydroxyurea dose and HbF response (p = 0.56), supporting the conclusion that differences in pharmacokinetics and pharmacodynamics affect HbF levels achieved on hydroxyurea [22].

Whole exome sequencing permitted analysis of genes beyond a usual set of *a priori* biologic candidate genes for this phenotype and variants across a broad allele frequency spectrum. We identified multiple non-synonymous variants associated with ΔHbF or final HbF (Tables 2 and 3) in the discovery cohort. We then performed genotyping on a validation cohort for 13 candidate variants with the lowest p-values and were also predicted to be damaging. Of the 13 variants genotyped, the variant in SALL2 was associated with a higher HbF in the discovery cohort, and a higher final HbF at MTD in the discovery cohort. The validated variant in *SALL2* represents a novel variant not previously implicated in -globin expression or HbF response to hydroxyurea. Further studies of other sickle cell cohorts treated with hydroxyurea are needed to confirm this promising association.

SALL2 is a multi-zinc finger transcription factor implicated in hematopoietic cell maturation and cell cycle arrest [23]. It contains the same conserved 12 amino acid N-terminal motif as BCL11A [24,25]. This motif has been shown to be essential for binding of the nucleosome remodeling and deacetylase co-repressor complex, or NuRD, which includes the histone deacelylases HDAC1 and HDAC2. Both HDAC1 and HDAC2 have been shown to act as co-repressors of gamma globin [26]. The variant identified here (rs61743453), causes a proline to arginine change at residue 840 and is predicted to bedamaging to protein function. This P840R SALL2 variant was associated with a higher HbF response to hydroxyurea (Figure 2). Further function-

Table 3. Variants associated with final HbF on hydroxyurea.

Gene	SNP ID	Amino Acid Change	Protein Function Prediction	MAF (%)	Function	Beta Value	SE	P-value
RSPH3	rs61750777	Ala154Val	Damaging	6	Radial spoke protein	−6.5	1.6	6.55×10^{-5}
OLR1	rs11053646	Lys167Asn	Benign	2	Opioid receptor	3.4	0.9	1.22×10^{-4}
SEC31B	rs11819496	Arg478Thr	Damaging	2	ER transport	−12.0	3.1	1.55×10^{-4}
COPE	rs34510432	Arg85 His	Damaging	2	ER transport	9.9	2.6	1.88×10^{-4}
RNF113B	rs16955011	Val92Met	Damaging	18	Ring finger protein	3.4	0.9	1.93×10^{-4}
CDHR3	rs6967330	Cys529Tyr	Benign	29	Calcium dependent cell adhesion	3.1	0.8	2.58×10^{-4}
ETAA1	rs3770655	Pro771Ser	Benign	89	Ewing's tumor associated antigen	4.3	1.2	2.84×10^{-4}
TTLL10	rs113596156	Arg35Gln	Benign	2	Polyglycylase	9.8	2.7	2.91×10^{-4}
DOCK1	rs869801	Ala1793Thr	Benign	21	Cytokinesis	−3.5	1.0	3.60×10^{-4}
MYBBP1A	rs899441	Lys637Glu	Benign	6	MYB associated	−5.4	1.5	4.26×10^{-4}
MARCH10	rs116835087	Gly587Ser	Damaging	6	Membrane-associated ring finger	−6.0	1.7	4.33×10^{-4}
PKD1L1	rs11972142	Thr879Ala	Benign	15	Polycystic kidney disease like	3.6	1.0	4.78×10^{-4}
ADCY10	rs16859886	Thr234Met	Benign	12	Adenyl cyclase	3.9	1.1	4.96×10^{-4}

Variants selected were predicted damaging, with a p-value <0.001 in the discovery cohort, $n = 171$, composed of patients from HUSTLE and SWiTCH trials.

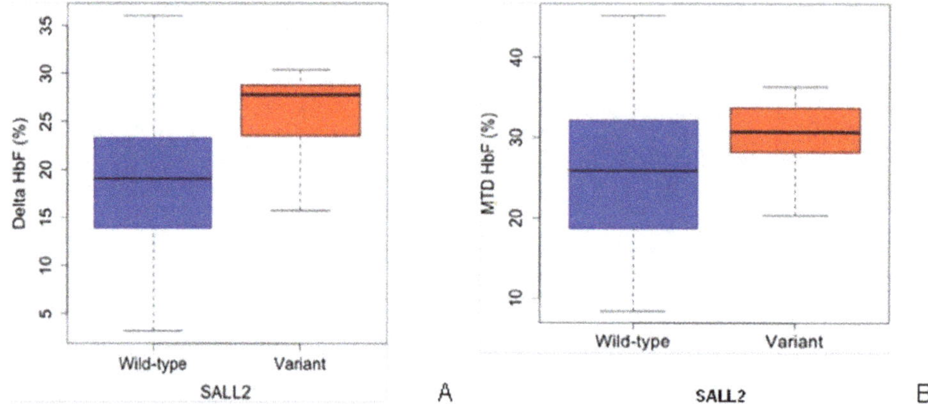

Figure 2. Effect of *SALL2* variant rs61743453 on HbF response to hydroxyurea. A, Effect of rs61743453 on delta HbF in discovery cohort. B, Effect of rs61743453 on MTD HbF in validation cohort. Variant refers to the Pro840Arg variant; no individuals were homozygous for this change.

al studies will help establish the role of SALL2 in HbF induction in the context of hydroxyurea.

Despite the relatively small sample size, we used the best genotype-phenotype pairs available from prospectively treated pediatric patients from two clinical trials for the discovery cohort. We assembled a validation cohort from patients treated with hydroxyurea according to standard of care and expert guidelines in a pediatric hematology center with an established sickle cell program.

This study may have failed to detect loci with modest effects because of low statistical power and some associations identified in the discovery cohort may have failed validation given the small size of the validation cohort. Accordingly, all of the mutations identified in the discovery cohort may represent coding variants worth pursuing in future studies. The data presented here bodes well for the success of larger collaborative efforts aimed at identifying genetic modifiers of hydroxyurea response, and serves as a call for coordinated collaboration among pediatric sickle cell centers to increase sample size and increase the odds for novel discovery and translational potential.

Methods

Subjects

The discovery cohort was composed of 171 unrelated children with SCA; 120 were enrolled in the Hydroxyurea Study of Long-Term Effects (HUSTLE, NCT00305175); and 51 were enrolled in the NHLBI-sponsored Stroke with Transfusions Changing to Hydroxyurea (SWiTCH, NCT00122980). HUSTLE was a single center trial investigating long term effects of hydroxyurea in SCA, while SWiTCH was a multi-center trial investigating the use of hydroxyurea on stroke prevention. HUSTLE and SWiTCH study patient samples were used with approval from the Baylor College of Medicine Internal Review Board, protocol H-29047. Patients and their families in both clinical trials provided written consent for DNA sample collection, storage and sequencing. Texas Children's Hospital Hematology Center patients and their families provided written consent to whole exome sequencing, posting of sequences to dbGAP, and data collection under BCM Internal Review Board protocol H31356. All DNA samples and data in this study were denominalized for analysis. All 171 individuals had a known baseline HbF level measured at greater than 3 years of age, were initially treated with hydroxyurea at 20 mg/kg, and then dose-escalated to mild myelosuppression using a standardized regimen [18,19].

The validation cohort contained 130 unrelated children with SCA followed at the Texas Children's Hospital Hematology Center (TCHHC). All patients receiving hydroxyurea at TCHHC were approached for enrollment in an Internal Review Board-approved protocol for genetic analysis. They were treated with hydroxyurea using institutional guidelines rather than a specific protocol, but all were escalated to MTD following a standardized regimen as previously described [19]. All patients were treated with hydroxyurea for at least 6 months prior to the designated MTD timepoint. Total HbF levels for both discovery and validation cohorts were measured by HPLC.

Ethics Statement

All patients and their families gave informed consent for genomic DNA sample collection, storage, and sequencing. The WES genomic analyses were approved by the Baylor College of Medicine Institutional Review Board. All DNA samples and data in this study were denominalized for analysis.

Whole exome sequencing

DNA concentrations were quantified using picogreen fluorescent detection method (Quant-iT, Invitrogen). For each DNA sample, the entire exome was captured using the NimbleGen VCRome 2.1 capture reagent followed by sequencing on an Illumina platform using standard chemistries. The sequencing reads were mapped to Hg19 reference genome using the BWA [27]. Sample level genome variants were identified and annotated using the Human Genome Sequencing Center's integrated Mercury pipeline which includes quality score recalibration and insertion/deletion (Indel) realignment, genome variant identification by AtlasSNP [28], and annotation using Cassandra software. A project level variant call format (VCF) was generated for all the samples, and included variants that were present in at least one sample. Variants with more than 5% missed genotyping calls were excluded from analysis. Error threshold for alignment was two base errors per read with penalties for indels (maximum of 1) are much more costly than the penalties for SNVs (maximum of 2). We allowed for read-trimming to 35 bp.

WES genotyping of variants of interest with heterozygosity scores less than 0.45 were verified by TaqMan genotyping. TaqMan genotyping assays were performed on an Applied Biosystem's StepOne instrument (AB, Foster City, CA). After 40 amplification cycles, threshold cycle values were automatically calculated, and the individual SNP genotypes were called by the StepOne v2.0 software (AB, Foster City, CA).

Statistical Analysis

Linear regression analysis was used to test the association of the filtered variants using final HbF and ΔHbF as independent, continuous variables. The ΔHbF and final HbF phenotypes both had normal distributions, indicating they were suitable for linear regression analysis (Figure 1); values were adjusted for age and gender. Principal component analysis (PCA) was performed using the EIGENSTRAT method, and applied to all models. Quality control filtering steps, including SNP missingness check, removal of sex chromosomes, monomorphic site, synonymous and intronic variant removal, excess heterozygosity filter and minor allele frequency (MAF) cut-off of 2% and the impact of these filtering steps on the total number of SNPs, are described in Table S1.

To analyze the effect of rare variants (MAF<2%) on the phenotypes ΔHbF and final HbF, we used two gene based tests, a simple burden test (T2) and SKAT [29,30]. In SKAT and T2 testing, a collection of rare variants within a single gene are tested for association with the phenotype. The T2 considers those rare variants with MAF less than 2% and assumes that the effects of all variants are in the same direction. SKAT is a kernel-based test that considers rare variants having effects in either direction [29,31]. Both tests considered only non-synonymous variants.

Validation

Genomic DNA from 130 patients from TCHHC collected as a validation cohort were genotyped by TaqMan or Sanger sequencing for 13 SNPs with the lowest p-values that were identified as associated with HbF response to hydroxyurea, non-synonymous, and damaging. The relationship between genotype and HbF response to hydroxyurea was analyzed with a one directional t-test.

Supporting Information

Table S1 Quality control filters used in WES analysis. Sex chromosomes were removed, as gender did not impact HbF response to hydroxyurea. Sites with heterzygousto homozygous ration>0.4 were removed.Variants with MAF<2% were analyzed by burden testing.

Acknowledgments

We thank all the patients and families, as well as the clinical investigators and research staff, for their participation in the SWiTCH and HUSTLE trials. We would like to thank the patients, their families, and the research staff at Texas Children's Hematology Center for their participation in FWES, which provided the validation cohort.

Author Contributions

Conceived and designed the experiments: VAS JMF EB RAG REW. Performed the experiments: TAH AS DMM SDP. Analyzed the data: JRC EB. Contributed reagents/materials/analysis tools: RAG EB. Wrote the paper: VAS JMF REW EB. Clinical trial data analysis and sample collection: BA KAN NAM REW.

References

1. Platt OS, Brambilla DJ, Rosse WF, Milner PF, Castro O, et al. (1994) Mortality in sickle cell disease. Life expectancy and risk factors for early death. N Engl J Med 330: 1639–1644.
2. Cheetham RC, Huehns ER, Rosemeyer MA (1979) Participation of haemoglobins A, F, A2 and C in polymerisation of haemoglobin S. J Mol Biol 129: 45–61.
3. Powars DR, Weiss JN, Chan LS, Schroeder WA (1984) Is there a threshold level of fetal hemoglobin that ameliorates morbidity in sickle cell anemia? Blood 63: 921–926.
4. Steinberg MH, McCarthy WF, Castro O, Ballas SK, Armstrong FD, et al. (2010) The risks and benefits of long-term use of hydroxyurea in sickle cell anemia: A 17.5 year follow-up. Am J Hematol 85: 403–408.
5. Voskaridou E, Christoulas D, Bilalis A, Plata E, Varvagiannis K, et al. (2010) The effect of prolonged administration of hydroxyurea on morbidity and mortality in adult patients with sickle cell syndromes: results of a 17-year, single-center trial (LaSHS). Blood 115: 2354–2363.
6. Lobo CL, Pinto JF, Nascimento EM, Moura PG, Cardoso GP, et al. (2013) The effect of hydroxcarbamide therapy on survival of children with sickle cell disease. Br J Haematol 161: 852–860.
7. Lebensburger J, Johnson SM, Askenazi DJ, Rozario NL, Howard TH, et al. (2011) Protective role of hemoglobin and fetal hemoglobin in early kidney disease for children with sickle cell anemia. Am J Hematol 86: 430–432.
8. Lebensburger JD, Pestina TI, Ware RE, Boyd KL, Persons DA (2010) Hydroxyurea therapy requires HbF induction for clinical benefit in a sickle cell mouse model. Haematologica 95: 1599–1603.
9. Steinberg MH, Barton F, Castro O, Pegelow CH, Ballas SK, et al. (2003) Effect of hydroxyurea on mortality and morbidity in adult sickle cell anemia: risks and benefits up to 9 years of treatment. JAMA 289: 1645–1651.
10. Smith WR, Ballas SK, McCarthy WF, Bauserman RL, Swerdlow PS, et al. (2011) The association between hydroxyurea treatment and pain intensity, analgesic use, and utilization in ambulatory sickle cell anemia patients. Pain Med 12: 697–705.
11. Maier-Redelsperger M, de Montalembert M, Flahault A, Neonato MG, Ducrocq R, et al. (1998) Fetal hemoglobin and F-cell responses to long-term hydroxyurea treatment in young sickle cell patients. The French Study Group on Sickle Cell Disease. Blood 91: 4472–4479.
12. Kinney TR, Helms RW, O'Branski EE, Ohene-Frempong K, Wang W, et al. (1999) Safety of hydroxyurea in children with sickle cell anemia: results of the HUG-KIDS study, a phase I/II trial. Pediatric Hydroxyurea Group. Blood 94: 1550–1554.
13. Zimmerman SA, Schultz WH, Davis JS, Pickens CV, Mortier NA, et al. (2004) Sustained long-term hematologic efficacy of hydroxyurea at maximum tolerated dose in children with sickle cell disease. Blood 103: 2039–2045.
14. Ware RE, Aygun B (2009) Advances in the use of hydroxyurea. Hematology Am Soc Hematol Educ Program: 62–69.
15. Ware RE, Eggleston B, Redding-Lallinger R, Wang WC, Smith-Whitley K, et al. (2002) Predictors of fetal hemoglobin response in children with sickle cell anemia receiving hydroxyurea therapy. Blood 99: 10–14.
16. Green NS, Ender KL, Pashankar F, Driscoll C, Giardina PJ, et al. (2013) Candidate sequence variants and fetal hemoglobin in children with sickle cell disease treated with hydroxyurea. PLoS One 8: e55709.
17. Steinberg MH, Voskaridou E, Kutlar A, Loukopoulos D, Koshy M, et al. (2003) Concordant fetal hemoglobin response to hydroxyurea in siblings with sickle cell disease. Am J Hematol 72: 121–126.
18. Ware RE, Helms RW (2011) Stroke With Transfusions Changing to Hydroxyurea (SWiTCH). Blood 119: 3925–3932.
19. Ware RE (2009) How I use hydroxyurea to treat young patients with sickle cell anemia. Blood 115: 5300–5311.
20. Steinberg MH (2001) Modulation of fetal hemoglobin in sickle cell anemia. Hemoglobin 25: 195–211.
21. Flanagan SE, Patch AM, Ellard S (2010) Using SIFT and PolyPhen to predict loss-of-function and gain-of-function mutations. Genet Test Mol Biomarkers 14: 533–537.
22. Ware RE, Despotovic JM, Mortier NA, Flanagan JM, He J, et al. (2011) Pharmacokinetics, pharmacodynamics, and pharmacogenetics of hydroxyurea treatment for children with sickle cell anemia. Blood 118: 4985–4991.
23. Chai L (2011) The role of HSAL (SALL) genes in proliferation and differentiation in normal hematopoiesis and leukemogenesis. Transfusion 51 Suppl 4: 87S–93S.
24. Sankaran VG, Menne TF, Xu J, Akie TE, Lettre G, et al. (2008) Human fetal hemoglobin expression is regulated by the developmental stage-specific repressor BCL11A. Science 322: 1839–1842.
25. Lauberth SM, Rauchman M (2006) A conserved 12-amino acid motif in Sall1 recruits the nucleosome remodeling and deacetylase corepressor complex. J Biol Chem 281: 23922–23931.
26. Bradner JE, Mak R, Tanguturi SK, Mazitschek R, Haggarty SJ, et al. (2010) Chemical genetic strategy identifies histone deacetylase 1 (HDAC1) and HDAC2 as therapeutic targets in sickle cell disease. Proc Natl Acad Sci U S A 107: 12617–12622.
27. Li H, Durbin R (2009) Fast and accurate short read alignment with Burrows-Wheeler transform. Bioinformatics 25: 1754–1760.

28. Challis D, Yu J, Evani US, Jackson AR, Paithankar S, et al. (2012) An integrative variant analysis suite for whole exome next-generation sequencing data. BMC Bioinformatics 13: 8.
29. Lee S, Wu MC, Lin X (2012) Optimal tests for rare variant effects in sequencing association studies. Biostatistics 13: 762–775.
30. Li B, Leal SM (2008) Methods for detecting associations with rare variants for common diseases: application to analysis of sequence data. Am J Hum Genet 83: 311–321.
31. Morgenthaler S, Thilly WG (2007) A strategy to discover genes that carry multi-allelic or mono-allelic risk for common diseases: a cohort allelic sums test (CAST). Mutat Res 615: 28–56.

23

Prolonged Seasonality of Respiratory Syncytial Virus Infection among Preterm Infants in a Subtropical Climate

Chyong-Hsin Hsu[1]*, Chia-Ying Lin[1], Hsin Chi[2], Jui-Hsing Chang[1], Han-Yang Hung[1], Hsin-An Kao[1], Chun-Chih Peng[1], Wai-Tim Jim[1]

1 Department of Pediatrics, Division of Neonatology, Mackay Memorial Hospital, Taipei, Taiwan, **2** Department of Pediatrics, Division of Infectious Disease, Mackay Memorial Hospital, Taipei, Taiwan

Abstract

Objective: There is limited epidemiological data on the seasonality of respiratory syncytial virus (RSV) infection in subtropical climates, such as in Taiwan. This study aimed to assess RSV seasonality among children ≤24 months of age in Taiwan. We also assessed factors (gestational age [GA], chronologic age [CA], and bronchopulmonary dysplasia [BPD]) associated with RSV-associated hospitalization in preterm infants to confirm the appropriateness of the novel Taiwanese RSV prophylactic policy.

Study Design: From January 2000 to August 2010, 3572 children aged ≤24-months were admitted to Taipei Mackay Memorial Hospital due to RSV infection. The monthly RSV-associated hospitalization rate among children aged ≤24 months was retrospectively reviewed. Among these children, 378 were born preterm. The associations between GA, CA, and BPD and the incidence of RSV-associated hospitalization in the preterm infants were assessed.

Results: In children aged ≤24 months, the monthly distribution of RSV-associated hospitalization rates revealed a prolonged RSV season with a duration of 10 months. Infants with GAs ≤32 weeks and those who had BPD had the highest rates of RSV hospitalization ($P<0.001$). Preterm infants were most vulnerable to RSV infection within CA 9 months.

Conclusions: Given that Taiwan has a prolonged (10-month) RSV season, the American Academy of Pediatrics' recommendations for RSV prophylaxis are not directly applicable. The current Taiwanese guidelines for RSV prophylaxis, which specify palivizumab injection (a total six doses until CA 8–9 months) for preterm infants (those born before $28^{6/7}$ weeks GA or before $35^{6/7}$ weeks GA with BPD), are appropriate. This prophylaxis strategy may be applicable to other countries/regions with subtropical climates.

Editor: Oliver Schildgen, Kliniken der Stadt Köln gGmbH, Germany

Funding: The authors received no specific funding for this work.

Competing Interests: The authors have declared that no competing interests exist.

* Email: t200441@mmh.org.tw

Introduction

Respiratory syncytial virus (RSV) is the major pathogen of acute lower respiratory tract infection (ALRTI) in infancy and childhood [1,2]. Of note, premature infants are ten-fold more likely than term infants to develop complicated RSV [3] and experience higher rates of hospitalization and mortality [4]. As there is no effective etiopathogenetic treatment once an infant is infected by RSV, effective RSV prophylaxis is extremely important [5].

Since 1998, the American Academy of Pediatrics (AAP) has recommended the use of palivizumab for passive immunization against RSV [6]. The AAP recommendations account for seasonality of RSV infection ie, in temperate climates, RSV infection rates typically peak during the cold season, whereas in tropical climates RSV infection rates typically peak during the rainy season [7]. To date, however, there is limited information regarding RSV seasonality in subtropical climates [6,8]. As RSV surveillance is a globally important issue, a thorough understanding of RSV epidemiology in subtropical climates, such as that in Taiwan, is important for the optimization of global RSV prevention strategies. The current Taiwanese recommendations (published in 2010 December) for RSV prophylaxis specify six doses of palivizumab, targeting preterm infants born before $28^{6/7}$ weeks gestational age (GA) or those born before $35^{6/7}$ weeks GA with bronchopulmonary dysplasia (BPD), until a chronologic age (CA) of 8–9 months.

The purpose of this study was to determine the seasonality of RSV infection among children aged ≤24 months in Taiwan, a subtropical area. We also examined the effects of gestational age (GA), CA, and BPD on the incidence of RSV infection in preterm infants to confirm the appropriateness of the novel RSV prophylactic policy for premature infants in Taiwan.

Methods

Study Design and Data Collection

This retrospective single-center cohort study was conducted at Taipei Mackay Memorial Hospital, a tertiary medical center serving the greater Taipei metropolitan area in Northern Taiwan. Eligible participants were children aged ≤24 months who had a discharge diagnosis of RSV-associated bronchiolitis and/or pneumonia (ICD-9 CM Codes 466.11, 480.1, or 079.6) from January 2000 to August 2010. Preterm infants were included in the study if they were born in Taipei Mackay Memorial Hospital, had a GA <37 weeks, and were discharged alive from the neonatal intensive care unit (NICU) from 1 January 2000 to 31 August 2010. Prematurity was defined as birth before 37 weeks of GA (ie, GA ≤36 weeks and 6 days) in accordance with ICD-9 codes 765.10~765.19 and 765.01–765.09. Infants were excluded from the study if they had congenital heart disease, other than patent ductus arteriosus or a septal defect that was hemodynamically insignificant, or any congenital anomaly. Repeat admission infants were also excluded because repeated admission may be related to other potentially confounding factors (aside from GA, CA, and BPD) eg, the level of neutralizing antibodies in the serum, etc.

A case manager from the Premature Baby Foundation of Taiwan assisted with the contact of preterm babies with very low birth weight (≤1500 g), almost all of whom had regular outpatient department follow-up visits after their discharge from Taipei Mackay Memorial Hospital. Note: for reasons of convenience, most preterm infants return to Taipei Mackay Memorial Hospital for any additional care requirements after discharge.

The diagnosis of RSV infection was confirmed by examination of nasopharyngeal specimens using either RSV antigen-specific direct immunofluorescence assay or virus culture. We defined a respiratory illness as being attributable to RSV if the patient had RSV infection necessitating hospitalization and was for positive the RSV-specific antigen or had a positive virus culture between 7 days before and 3 days after admission [8]. As the incubation period for RSV is typically 3 to 5 days, patients who had symptoms that appeared ≥5 days after admission were considered to have nosocomial RSV infection [7–9]. In addition to RSV testing, patients underwent throat virus cultures after admission (no comorbid viruses were detected).

We obtained the following information from neonatal chart records: GA, birth weight, gender, dates of nursery admission and discharge, and time on oxygen in the NICU. The presence of BPD was also recorded. BPD was defined as persistent oxygen dependency 28 days after birth [10], the need for oxygen at 36 weeks postmenstrual age [11], and the presence of a characteristic chest roentgenographic finding in accordance with ICD-9 code 770.7. De-identified patient data were collated by a single neonatologist. All links between the final data analyzed and the original data were removed. The study was approved by the local Study Review Board and Ethics Committee of Taipei Mackay Memorial Hospital. Written informed consent was given by next of kin of the participants.

Outcome Measures

The monthly incidence of RSV-associated hospitalization for children aged ≤24 months was calculated for the study period to determine the seasonal activity of RSV infection at Taipei Mackay Memorial Hospital. We used the surveillance model for seasonality proposed by the Taiwan Centers for Disease Control (CDC) (Taiwan-CDC) [12,13] as well as the seasonality model of the US CDC [14] to determine RSV seasonality in Taiwan. The RSV season was defined as a period of two or more consecutive months in which the RSV-associated hospitalization rate was above the baseline rate. The baseline RSV-associated hospitalization rate was calculated by firstly determining the monthly RSV-associated hospitalization rate for children aged ≤24 months old as follows:

$$X_i = \frac{\text{Number of RSV hospitalizations}}{\text{Total number of hospitalizations}},$$

$$i = 1, 2, ..., 12 \text{ (from January to December).}$$

The average monthly RSV-associated hospitalization rate was then calculated as follows: $\frac{1}{12}\sum_{i=1}^{12} X_i = 29.67$ (‰)

The months with RSV-associated hospitalization rates <29.67 ‰ were defined as "non-epidemic months". The average monthly RSV-associated hospitalization rate of "non-epidemic months" was defined as the "baseline rate".

Infants who were born preterm were categorized into three GA-based groups for comparison of RSV-related hospitalization: ≤28, 29–32, and 33–36 weeks.

Children who were born preterm with RSV infection were further stratified into three subgroups according to their CA of onset for comparison: ≤9, 10–15, and 16–24 months.

RSV-infected premature infants with underlying BPD were identified for subgroup data analyses.

Statistical Analyses

Categorical variables are presented as counts and percentages, and were compared by chi-square test. Birth weight data are presented as median and full range. Statistical analyses were two-sided and carried out using SPSS software, version 20 (SPSS Inc., Chicago, IL). Statistical significance was indicated by $P<0.05$.

Results

Study Population

From January 2000 to August 2010, a total of 123,975 children aged ≤24 months were admitted to Taipei Mackay Memorial Hospital, 3,572 for RSV infection (Figure 1). Of these 5,572 children who were born premature (boys: n = 3048; girls: n = 2524; median birth weight: 1848 g [range: 522–3386 g]), 413 were admitted for RSV infection. After the exclusion of repeated admissions and infants who had nosocomial infections (Figure 1), 378 preterm infants were included in the study (boys: n = 230; girls: n = 148; median birth weight: 1859 g [range: 522–2864 g]). Of these infants, 67 had underlying BPD and 311 did not. Hence, 10.6% (378/3572) of the admissions due to RSV infection were preterm infants. The attributable mortality rate for RSV infection among the preterm infants was 7.9 ‰ (n = 3) in our study population.

Monthly Incidence of RSV-Associated Hospitalization and Assessment of Seasonality

The monthly incidence of RSV-associated hospitalization among children aged ≤24 months in the study period is shown in Figure 2. Figure 2A summarizes the monthly RSV-associated hospitalization rate for the entire observation period. Figure 2B summarizes the average monthly RSV-associated hospitalization rate from January to December for the observation period. The baseline monthly RSV-related hospitalization rate was 18.52 ‰. The RSV season was defined as a period of two or more

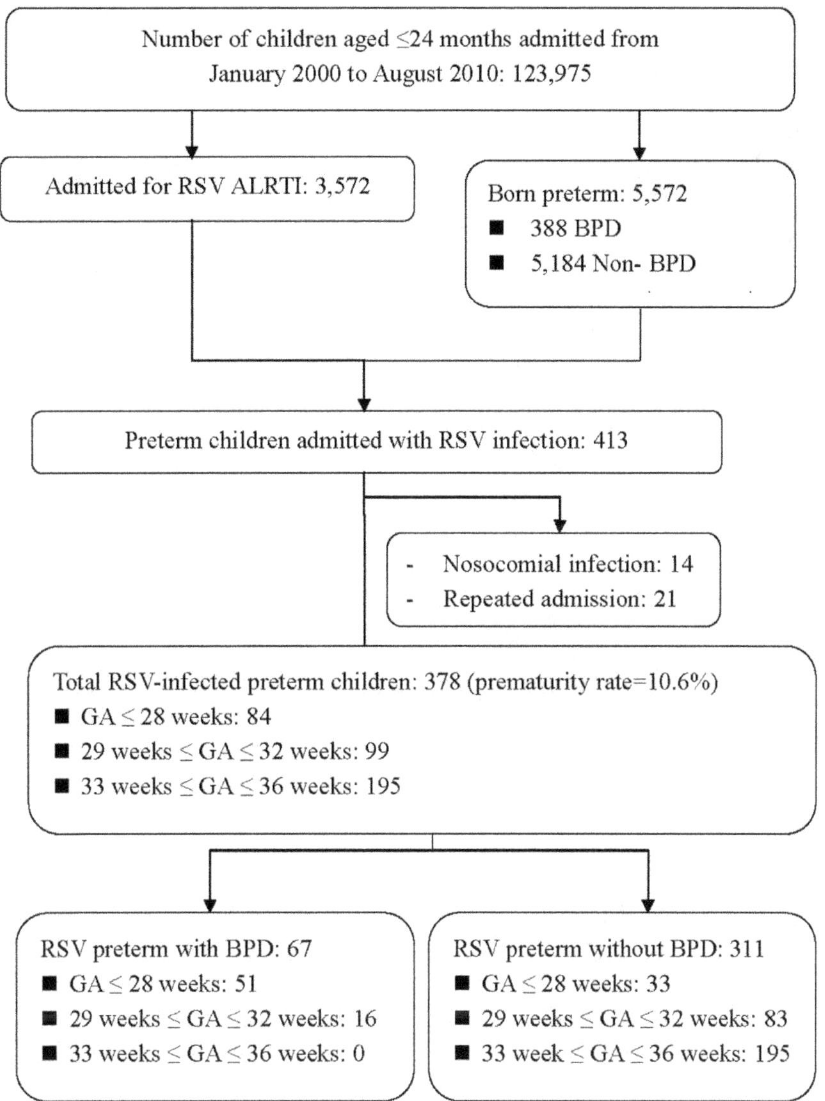

Figure 1. Flow chart of infants aged ≤24 months included in the study. ALRTI, acute lower respiratory tract infection; BPD, bronchopulmonary dysplasia; GA, gestational age; RSV, respiratory syncytial virus.

consecutive months, in which the RSV-associated hospitalization rate was above the basal rate. In our study, there was a prolonged, continuous RSV season lasting 10 months.

The Impact of Gestational Age (GA) on RSV-Associated Hospitalization

The proportion of infants with RSV infection by GA (among the 5,572 infants who were born preterm) is summarized overall and by BPD status in Table 1. There were no differences in the rate of RSV infection by GA among infants who had underlying BPD. Of the non-BPD infants, those with GAs ≤28 weeks and 29–32 weeks had a significantly higher rate of RSV-associated hospitalization compared with those with a GA 33–36 weeks ($P<0.001$).

Effect of BPD on RSV Infection

Of the 5,572 premature infants, 388 had BPD and 5184 did not. A significantly higher proportion of infants who had BPD experienced RSV infection compared infants who did not have BPD (67/388; 17.3% vs 311/5184; 6.0%, $P<0.001$).

Trends in RSV-Related Hospitalization by CA and Prematurity

The proportion of infants hospitalized due to RSV infection by CA of onset (categorized by GA and BPD status) is presented in Figure 3. As most extremely low birth weight preterm infants (birth weight ≤1000 g) and very low birth weight infants (birth weight ≤1500 g) usually remained in hospital for 2–3 months after birth, we used a CA of 9 months (ie, almost 6 months after discharge) as the first cut-off point, and thereafter stratified the cut-off points by 6-month blocks to assess the timing of when preterm neonates were most vulnerable to RSV infection after discharge. Therefore, RSV-associated hospitalization rates were analyzed for infants grouped into three age cohorts: (≤9 months, 10 to 15 months, and 16 to 24 months). Moreover, the preterm infants with RSV with and without BPD were divided into 3 GA categories to

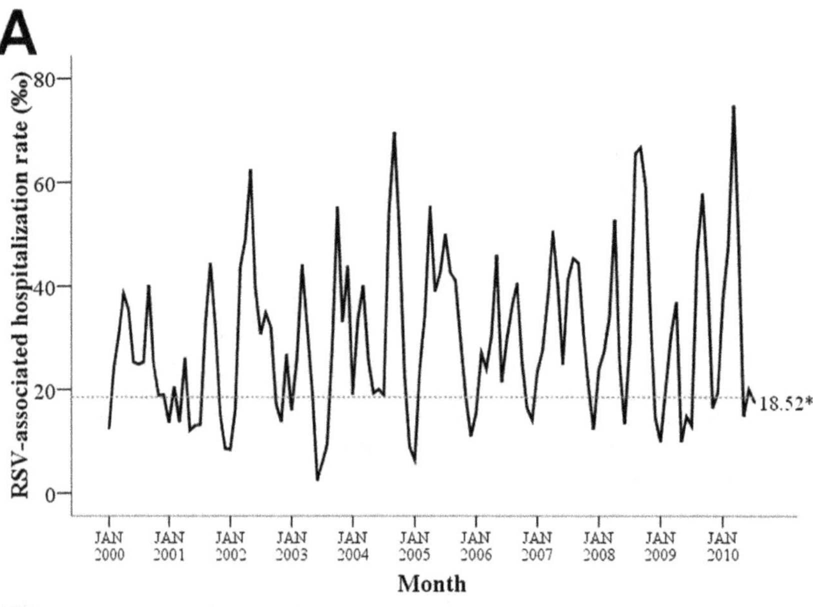

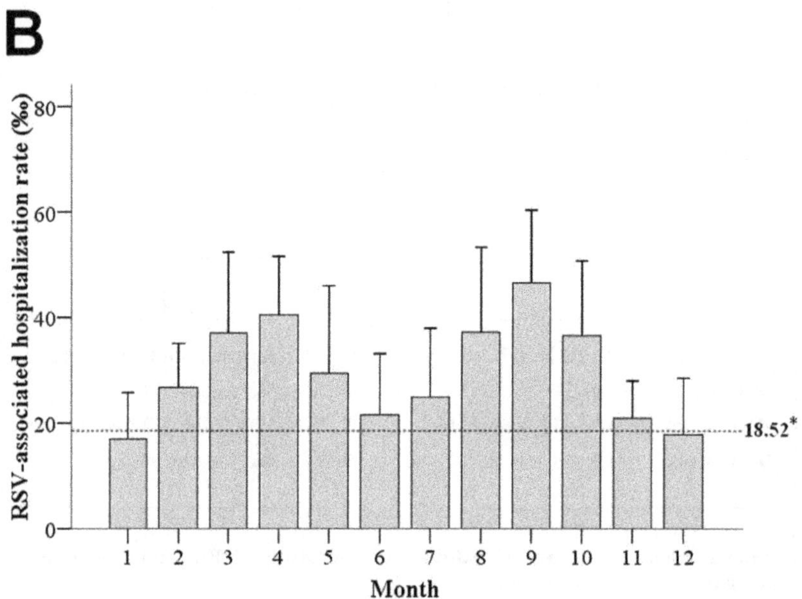

Figure 2. Monthly distribution of the RSV-associated hospitalization rate among all infants aged ≤24 months in the study (from January 2000 to August 2010). *The baseline rate of RSV infection was 18.52 ‰. RSV, respiratory syncytial virus. (A) Monthly RSV-associated hospitalization rates for the entire observation period. (B) Average monthly RSV-associated hospitalization rates from January to December for the observation period.

Table 1. Respiratory syncytial virus infection by gestational age for infants aged ≤24 months who were born premature (overall and by bronchopulmonary dysplasia status).

Infants	Gestational Age			*P* Value
	≤28 weeks	**29–32 weeks**	**33–36 weeks**	
Overall (378/5572), n/N (%)	84/584 (14.4)*	99/935 (10.6)*	195/4053 (4.8)	<0.001
With underlying BPD (67/388), n/N (%)	51/301 (16.9)	16/83 (19.3)	0/4 (0)	0.825
Without underlying BPD (311/5184), n/N (%)	33/283 (11.6)*	83/852 (9.7)*	195/4049 (4.8)	<0.001

BPD, bronchopulmonary dysplasia.
N = total premature babies (by gestational age); n = RSV-infected premature babies (by gestational age).
*Indicates a significant difference compared with gestational age 33–36 weeks.

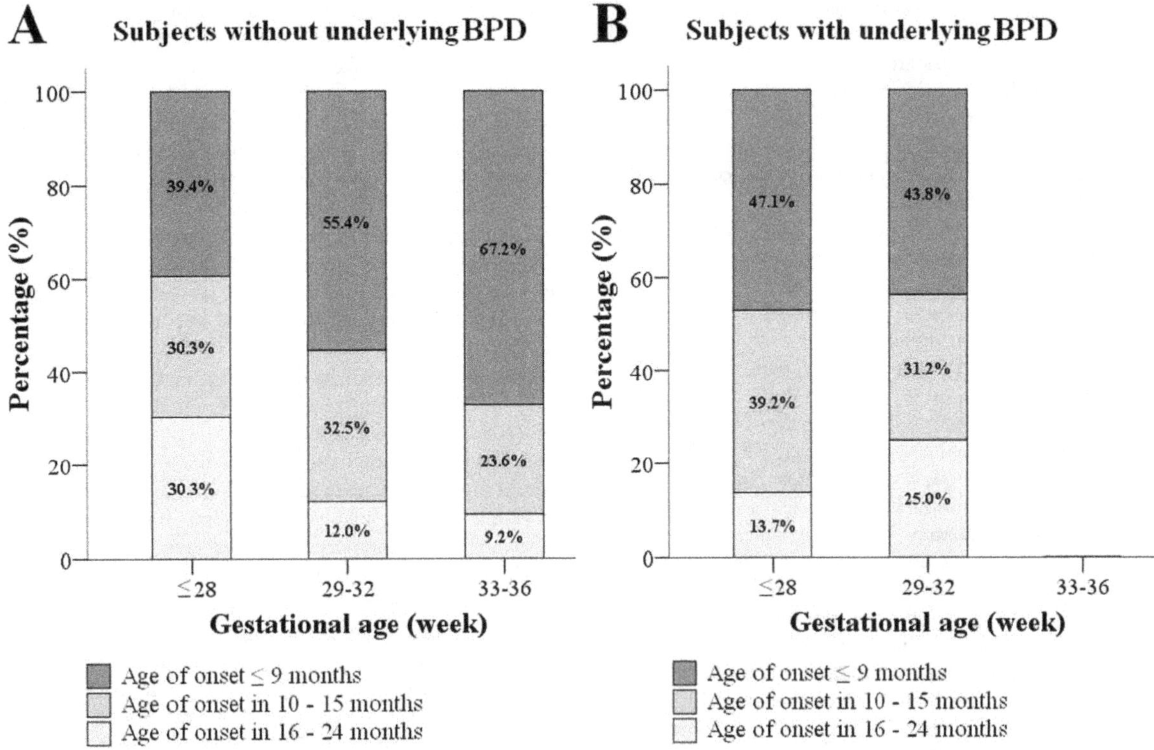

Figure 3. Percentage of infants (born premature) aged ≤24 months-with respiratory syncytial virus infection by age of onset (chronologic age), by gestational age, and BPD status (A: without BPD, n = 311; B: with BPD, n = 67). Note: there were no infants with underlying BPD at gestational age 33–36 months. BPD, bronchopulmonary dysplasia.

facilitate GA comparisons: ≤28 weeks, 29–32 weeks, and 33–36 weeks.

Overall. Overall, 58.5% (221/378) of infants admitted due to RSV infections experienced onset within 9 months, 28.5% (108/378) experienced onset within 10–15 months, and 12.9% (49/378) experienced onset within 16–24 months. Regardless of BPD status and GA, RSV infection most frequently occurred within 9 months, followed by 10–15 months, and 16–24 months.

Without underlying BPD. The results for infants without underlying BPD are summarized in Figure 3A. Regardless of GA, RSV infection was most common within 9 months, followed by 10–15 months, and then 16–24 months.

With underlying BPD. The results for infants with underlying BPD are summarized in Figure 3B. There were no infants born at GA 33–36 weeks with BPD. Regardless of GA, RSV infection was most common within 9 months, followed by 10–15 months, and then 16–24 months.

Discussion

RSV-prophylaxis strategies are globally important given that RSV circulates throughout the world. To the best of our knowledge, this is the first population-based, retrospective cohort study demonstrating prolonged seasonality of RSV infection (duration = 10 months) among children aged ≤24 months in a subtropical climate. This is different from RSV epidemiology data obtained in the United States, Canada, and European countries. The prolonged RSV seasonality makes the establishment of an RSV prevention policy challenging because one of the most important elements of the current RSV prophylactic guideline recommended by AAP is the existence of a distinct RSV season for 5 months from November to March (or from December to April) in temperate climate zones [15]. Other countries located in subtropical climate regions, such as Hong Kong, Northern Vietnam, and southern China [16,17] are also faced with the potential problem of RSV being present throughout the year, which complicates the development of effective prophylactic programs.

Taiwan is located at 23°0′N~25°5′N latitude and 120° 39' E~121° 33' E longitude; hence, the entire country is located in a subtropical climate region. Our result confirmed that there is a prolonged RSV season in Taiwan. In a previous report, Huang et al [6]reported that there was RSV infection year-round in Taiwan. Two previous retrospective studies [3,18] also reported an apparent biannual pattern of RSV infection in Taiwan. The explanation for the disparate study findings may relate to differences in study design, unequal-aged based populations, population characteristics, and sample size. The prolonged seasonality in our study may be explained by the lack of marked seasonal changes in temperature and the lack of any profound effect of rainfall in Taiwan [19].

Given our finding of prolonged RSV seasonality, the AAP guideline on RSV prophylaxis with palivizumab are not directly applicable in Taiwan. The AAP guidelines specify a total of 5 doses (as the maximum) of monthly palivizumab to prevent RSV infection because the average duration of RSV season in temperate climates is 5 months [15]. The AAP guidelines also specify that palivizumab should be given during the RSV season to protect high-risk groups such as premature infants (GA $\leq 28^{6/7}$ weeks) or infants with BPD. Such an approach is not practical in a subtropical area with an RSV season lasting 10 months. Indeed, high-risk preterm infants would require 10 doses of palivizumab during the RSV season in Taiwan according to the AAP guidelines; this is not economically feasible. Hence, factors aside from seasonality must be considered in developing a reasonable and practical prophylaxis strategy in Taiwan (and presumably other countries in subtropical climate regions). Our findings suggest that GA, CA, and BPD are three important factors that should be considered in the establishment of cost–effective palivizumab prophylaxis strategies.

Our finding that preterm infants who have BPD have an increased risk for RSV infection are consistent with those determined in the IMpact RSV and other studies [5,18,20–22]. Our findings are also in keeping with those of the IRIS study group [21] who reported that preterm infants with either a GA ≤ 32 weeks or those with BPD have a very high risk of RSV-associated hospitalization. Of note, we found that CA ≤9 months was the most susceptible period for RSV infection among preterm infants in a subtropical climate with prolonged RSV seasonality. Only one previous report has examined this relationship and found that RSV-related hospitalization was most commonly observed among (predominantly term-born) infants aged 3–6 months [23]. Different to the findings from the IRIS and FLIP studies, which indicate that the risk of RSV infection is highest among infants with a CA <3 or 6 months at the start of the RSV season, our findings suggest that once preterm infants are discharged, monthly palivizumab should be administered for a total 6 doses until CA 8–9 months. There are several potential explanations for our finding regarding CA and the risk of RSV infection. First, preterm infants typically remain in the intensive care unit during the first 2–3 months after birth, so the risk of infection is highest within the first 6 months after discharge ie, 8–9 months of CA. Second, before CA 9 months, parents may become less vigilant about the potential risks of infection due to the relatively improved physiological conditions of their premature infants. Third, infants with underlying BPD (or other co-morbidities) often require frequent outpatient follow-up visits or interventions before CA 9 months, which may increase their likelihood of exposure to RSV. Finally, in Taiwan, infants' mothers return to work around this time and infants are typically cared for by babysitters thereafter. These babysitters usually look after more than one infant, thus increasing the risk of cross-infection. Our findings indicate that CA ≤9 months is a critical period for re-admission of preterm infants; hence, the first dose of palivizumab should be given 3–4 days before discharge and monthly thereafter until CA 8–9 months.

Although we employed a number of measures to minimize potential bias, our study does have several limitations. First, palivizumab was not widely available until 2010 December in Taiwan; hence, we could not conduct a prospective study to assess seasonality before 2010. Widespread prophylaxis with palivizumab from 2010 will make it difficult to collect the necessary epidemiologic data to analyze the risk factors for RSV-induced ALRTI in the future. For the same reason, there was no control group in our study. Despite being retrospective in nature, our study did encompass a significant (10-year) period of time and thus, we believe, contributes important epidemiological information. Second, although the RSV screening method used had very high sensitivity (93%) and specificity (98%), it is possible that some relevant cases of RSV infection were missed. Third, not all infants with ALRTI underwent RSV rapid test or throat virus culture. Hence, the RSV infection rate may have been underestimated. Fourth, as this study was carried out at a single institution, an additional population-based study acquiring data from multiple centers is warranted to confirm our findings and provide valuable information that could be used to optimize RSV prophylaxis. Despite the aforementioned limitations, we suggest that the data presented herein are extremely important, and provide a reasonable representation of RSV infection among children aged ≤24 months in a subtropical climate.

In our study, both GA≤28 weeks and GA 29–32 weeks were high-risk groups for RSV infection. Since December 2010, the Taiwan Society of Neonatology advised the Bureau of National Health Insurance in Taiwan to provide a total six monthly doses of palivizumab injections to premature infants with a GA $\leq 28^{6/7}$ weeks or prematurity with BPD and born before GA $35^{6/7}$ weeks, including the first dose before discharge and continuing until five months after discharge. Therefore, eligible infants will be protected by CA of 8–9 months, the most critical period of susceptibility to RSV infection. The current policy in Taiwan, subtropical climate country with prolonged RSV seasonality, is appropriate and may serve as a reference for other countries in subtropical climates in which the AAP guideline may not be applicable for RSV prophylaxis.

Acknowledgments

The authors acknowledge the kind assistance and wonderful team work provided by the staff at Taipei Mackay Memorial Hospital.

Author Contributions

Conceived and designed the experiments: CHH. Performed the experiments: CYL. Analyzed the data: CYL. Contributed reagents/materials/analysis tools: CHH CYL HC JHC HYH HAK CCP WTJ. Wrote the paper: CHH CYL HC JHC HYH HAK CCP WTJ.

References

1. Hall CB, Weinberg GA, Iwane MK, Blumkin AK, Edwards KM, et al. (2009) The burden of respiratory syncytial virus infection in young children. N Engl J Med. 360: 588–598.
2. Nair H, Nokes DJ, Gessner BD, Dherani M, Madhi SA, et al. (2010) Global burden of acute lower respiratory infections due to respiratory syncytial virus in young children: a systematic review and meta-analysis. Lancet. 375: 1545–1555.
3. Chi H, Chang IS, Tsai FY, Huang LM, Shao PL, et al. (2011) Epidemiological study of hospitalization associated with respiratory syncytial virus infection in Taiwanese children between 2004 and 2007. J Formos Med Assoc. 110: 388–396.
4. Tatochenko V, Uchaikin V, Gorelov A, Gudkov K, Campbell A, et al. (2010) Epidemiology of respiratory syncytial virus in children </ = 2 years of age hospitalized with lower respiratory tract infections in the Russian Federation: a prospective, multicenter study. Clin Epidemiol. 2: 221–227.
5. (1998) Palivizumab, a humanized respiratory syncytial virus monoclonal antibody, reduces hospitalization from respiratory syncytial virus infection in high-risk infants. The IMpact-RSV Study Group. Pediatrics. 102: 531–537.
6. Huang YC, Lin TY, Chang LY, Wong KS, Ning SC (2001) Epidemiology of respiratory syncytial virus infection among paediatric inpatients in northern Taiwan. Eur J Pediatr. 160: 581–582.
7. Carbonell-Estrany X, Quero J, Group IS (2001) Hospitalization rates for respiratory syncytial virus infection in premature infants born during two consecutive seasons. Pediatr Infect Dis J. 20: 874–879.
8. Joffe S, Escobar GJ, Black SB, Armstrong MA, Lieu TA (1999) Rehospitalization for respiratory syncytial virus among premature infants. Pediatrics. 104: 894–899.
9. Figueras-Aloy J, Carbonell-Estrany X, Quero-Jimenez J, Fernandez-Colomer B, Guzman-Cabanas J, et al. (2008) FLIP-2 Study: risk factors linked to respiratory syncytial virus infection requiring hospitalization in premature infants born in Spain at a gestational age of 32 to 35 weeks. Pediatr Infect Dis J. 27: 788–793.
10. Northway WH Jr., Rosan RC, Porter DY (1967) Pulmonary disease following respirator therapy of hyaline-membrane disease. Bronchopulmonary dysplasia. N Engl J Med. 276: 357–368.
11. Christine AG, Sherin UD (2012) Avery's disease of the newborn (9th ed). Philadelphia, PA: Elsevier.

12. Chu SC, Wang ET, Liu DP (2013) A review of prevention and control for enterovirus infections in Asia. Taiwan CDC Taiwan Epidemiology Bulletin. 29.
13. Wu TN, Tsai SF, Li SF, Lee TF, Huang TM, et al. (1999) Sentinel surveillance for enterovirus 71, Taiwan, 1998. Emerg Infect Dis. 5: 458–460.
14. US CDC (2013) Overview of influenza surveillance in the US. 17 October 2013.
15. Committee on Infectious Diseases (2009) From the American Academy of Pediatrics: Policy statements–Modified recommendations for use of palivizumab for prevention of respiratory syncytial virus infections. Pediatrics. 124: 1694–1701.
16. Chan PK, Sung RY, Fung KS, Hui M, Chik KW, et al. (1999) Epidemiology of respiratory syncytial virus infection among paediatric patients in Hong Kong: seasonality and disease impact. Epidemiol Infect. 123: 257–262.
17. Stensballe LG, Devasundaram JK, Simoes EA (2003) Respiratory syncytial virus epidemics: the ups and downs of a seasonal virus. Pediatr Infect Dis J. 22: S21–32.
18. Lee JT, Chang LY, Wang LC, Kao CL, Shao PL, et al. (2007) Epidemiology of respiratory syncytial virus infection in northern Taiwan, 2001–2005 – seasonality, clinical characteristics, and disease burden. J Microbiol Immunol Infect. 40: 293–301.
19. Tsai HP, Kuo PH, Liu CC, Wang JR (2001) Respiratory viral infections among pediatric inpatients and outpatients in Taiwan from 1997 to 1999. J Clin Microbiol. 39: 111–118.
20. Kusuda S, Takahashi N, Saitoh T, Terai M, Kaneda H, et al. (2011) Survey of pediatric ward hospitalization due to respiratory syncytial virus infection after the introduction of palivizumab to high-risk infants in Japan. Pediatr Int. 53: 368–373.
21. Carbonell-Estrany X, Quero J, Bustos G, Cotero A, Domenech E, et al. (2000) Rehospitalization because of respiratory syncytial virus infection in premature infants younger than 33 weeks of gestation: a prospective study. IRIS Study Group. Pediatr Infect Dis J. 19: 592–597.
22. Boyce TG, Mellen BG, Mitchel EF Jr., Wright PF, Griffin MR (2000) Rates of hospitalization for respiratory syncytial virus infection among children in medicaid. J Pediatr. 137: 865–870.
23. Fryzek JP, Martone WJ, Groothuis JR (2011) Trends in chronologic age and infant respiratory syncytial virus hospitalization: an 8-year cohort study. Adv Ther. 28: 195–201.

Permissions

All chapters in this book were first published in PLOS ONE, by The Public Library of Science; hereby published with permission under the Creative Commons Attribution License or equivalent. Every chapter published in this book has been scrutinized by our experts. Their significance has been extensively debated. The topics covered herein carry significant findings which will fuel the growth of the discipline. They may even be implemented as practical applications or may be referred to as a beginning point for another development.

The contributors of this book come from diverse backgrounds, making this book a truly international effort. This book will bring forth new frontiers with its revolutionizing research information and detailed analysis of the nascent developments around the world.

We would like to thank all the contributing authors for lending their expertise to make the book truly unique. They have played a crucial role in the development of this book. Without their invaluable contributions this book wouldn't have been possible. They have made vital efforts to compile up to date information on the varied aspects of this subject to make this book a valuable addition to the collection of many professionals and students.

This book was conceptualized with the vision of imparting up-to-date information and advanced data in this field. To ensure the same, a matchless editorial board was set up. Every individual on the board went through rigorous rounds of assessment to prove their worth. After which they invested a large part of their time researching and compiling the most relevant data for our readers.

The editorial board has been involved in producing this book since its inception. They have spent rigorous hours researching and exploring the diverse topics which have resulted in the successful publishing of this book. They have passed on their knowledge of decades through this book. To expedite this challenging task, the publisher supported the team at every step. A small team of assistant editors was also appointed to further simplify the editing procedure and attain best results for the readers.

Apart from the editorial board, the designing team has also invested a significant amount of their time in understanding the subject and creating the most relevant covers. They scrutinized every image to scout for the most suitable representation of the subject and create an appropriate cover for the book.

The publishing team has been an ardent support to the editorial, designing and production team. Their endless efforts to recruit the best for this project, has resulted in the accomplishment of this book. They are a veteran in the field of academics and their pool of knowledge is as vast as their experience in printing. Their expertise and guidance has proved useful at every step. Their uncompromising quality standards have made this book an exceptional effort. Their encouragement from time to time has been an inspiration for everyone.

The publisher and the editorial board hope that this book will prove to be a valuable piece of knowledge for researchers, students, practitioners and scholars across the globe.

List of Contributors

Roy T. Sabo, Miao-Shan Yen and Shumei S. Sun
Department of Biostatistics, School of Medicine, Virginia Commonwealth University, Richmond, Virginia, United States of America

Stephen Daniels
Department of Pediatrics, School of Medicine, University of Colorado, Aurora, Colorado, United States of America

Bart Victor
Owen Graduate School of Management, Vanderbilt University, Nashville, Tennessee, United States of America
Vanderbilt Institute for Global Health, Vanderbilt University, Nashville, Tennessee, United States of America

Meridith Blevins
Vanderbilt Institute for Global Health, Vanderbilt University, Nashville, Tennessee, United States of America
Department of Biostatistics, Vanderbilt University School of Medicine, Nashville, Tennessee, United States of America

Ann F. Green
Vanderbilt Institute for Global Health, Vanderbilt University, Nashville, Tennessee, United States of America

Alfredo E. Vergara
Vanderbilt Institute for Global Health, Vanderbilt University, Nashville, Tennessee, United States of America
Department of Preventive Medicine, Vanderbilt University School of Medicine, Nashville, Tennessee, United States of America

Elisée Ndatimana and Lázaro Gonzá lez-Calvo
Friends in Global Health, Maputo, Mozambique

Edward F. Fischer
Vanderbilt Center for Latin American Studies and Department of Anthropology, Vanderbilt University, Nashville, Tennessee, United States of America

Sten H. Vermund and Troy D. Moon
Vanderbilt Institute for Global Health, Vanderbilt University, Nashville, Tennessee, United States of America
Department of Pediatrics, Vanderbilt University School of Medicine, Nashville, Tennessee, United States of America
Friends in Global Health, Maputo, Mozambique

Omo Olupona
World Vision International, Maputo, Mozambique

Mohsen Besharat Pour, Anna Bergström and Jessica Magnusson
Institute of Environmental Medicine, Division of Epidemiology, Karolinska Institutet, Stockholm, Sweden

Matteo Bottai
Institute of Environmental Medicine, Division of Epidemiology, Karolinska Institutet, Stockholm, Sweden
Institute of Environmental Medicine, Unit of Biostatistics, Karolinska Institutet, Stockholm, Sweden

Inger Kull
Institute of Environmental Medicine, Division of Epidemiology, Karolinska Institutet, Stockholm, Sweden
Department of Clinical Science and Education, Stockholm South General Hospital, Karolinska Institutet, Stockholm, Sweden
Sachs' Children and Youth Hospital, Stockholm South General Hospital, Stockholm, Sweden

Magnus Wickman
Institute of Environmental Medicine, Division of Epidemiology, Karolinska Institutet, Stockholm, Sweden
Sachs' Children and Youth Hospital, Stockholm South General Hospital, Stockholm, Sweden

Tahereh Moradi
Institute of Environmental Medicine, Division of Epidemiology, Karolinska Institutet, Stockholm, Sweden
Centre for Epidemiology and Community Medicine, Stockholm County Council, Stockholm, Sweden

Rachel L. Knowles, Angela Wade, Harvey Goldstein and Carol Dezateux
Population Policy and Practice Programme, Institute of Child Health, University College London, London, United Kingdom

Catherine Bull
Cardiac Unit, Great Ormond Street Hospital for Children NHS Trust, London, United Kingdom

Christopher Wren
Department of Paediatric Cardiology, Freeman Hospital, Newcastle-upon-Tyne, United Kingdom

David W. Lawson
Department of Population Health, London School of Hygiene and Tropical Medicine, London, England, United Kingdom

Monique Borgerhoff Mulder
Department of Anthropology, University of California Davis, Davis, California, United States of America
Savannas Forever Tanzania, Arusha, Tanzania

Susan James
Savannas Forever Tanzania, Arusha, Tanzania

Margherita E. Ghiselli
University of Minnesota, Minneapolis, Minnesota, United States of America

Esther Ngadaya, Bernard Ngowi and Sayoki G. M. Mfinanga
National Institute for Medical Research, Muhimbili Medical Research Centre, Dar es Salaam, Tanzania

Kari Hartwig
St. Catherine University, Minneapolis, Minnesota, United States of America

Jeong-Hyun Kim
Research Institute for Basic Science, Sogang University, Seoul, Republic of Korea
Department of Life Science, Sogang University, Seoul, Republic of Korea

Hyoung Doo Shin
Research Institute for Basic Science, Sogang University, Seoul, Republic of Korea Department of Life Science, Sogang University, Seoul, Republic of Korea
Department of Genetic Epidemiology, SNP Genetics, Inc., Seoul, Republic of Korea

Hyun Sub Cheong
Department of Genetic Epidemiology, SNP Genetics, Inc., Seoul, Republic of Korea

Jae Hoon Sul
Department of Computer Science, University of California Los Angeles, Los Angeles, California, United States of America

Jeong-Meen Seo and Soo-Min Jung
Division of Pediatric Surgery, Department of Surgery, Samsung Medical Center, Sungkyunkwan University School of Medicine, Seoul, Republic of Korea

Dae-Yeon Kim
Department of Pediatric Surgery, Asan Medical Center, University of Ulsan College of Medicine, Seoul, Republic of Korea

Jung-Tak Oh
Department of Pediatric Surgery, Severance Children's Hospital, Yonsei University College of Medicine, Seoul, Republic of Korea

Kwi-Won Park and Hyun-Young Kim
Department of Pediatric Surgery, Seoul National University Children's Hospital, Seoul, Republic of Korea

Kyuwhan Jung
Department of Surgery, Seoul National University Bundang Hospital, Seongnam, Gyeonggi, Republic of Korea

Min Jeng Cho
Department of Surgery, Konkuk University Medical Center, Seoul, Republic of Korea

Joon Seol Bae
Laboratory of Translational Genomics, Samsung Genome Institute, Samsung
Medical Center, Seoul, Republic of Korea

Ying-Piao Wang
Department of Otolaryngology, Head and Neck Surgery, Mackay Memorial Hospital, Taipei, Taiwan
Institute of Public Health and Community Medicine Research Center, National Yang-Ming University, Taipei, Taiwan
Department of Audiology and Speech Language Pathology and School of Medicine, Mackay Medical College, New Taipei City, Taiwan

Mao-Che Wang
Institute of Public Health and Community Medicine Research Center, National Yang-Ming University, Taipei, Taiwan
Department of Otolaryngology, Head and Neck Surgery, Taipei Veterans General Hospital and School of Medicine, National Yang-Ming University, Taipei, Taiwan

Hung-Ching Lin
Department of Otolaryngology, Head and Neck Surgery, Mackay Memorial Hospital, Taipei, Taiwan
Department of Audiology and Speech Language Pathology and School of Medicine, Mackay Medical College, New Taipei City, Taiwan

Pesus Chou
Institute of Public Health and Community Medicine Research Center, National Yang-Ming University, Taipei, Taiwan

Arantza Meñaca
Departmento de Antropología Social, Universidad Complutense de Madrid, Madrid, Spain

Harry Tagbor and Rose Adjei
Malaria in Pregnancy Group, Department of Community Health, School of Medical Sciences, Kwame Nkrumah University of Science and Technology, Kumasi, Ghana

Constance Bart-Plange
National Malaria Control Programme, Ghana Health Service, Accra, Ghana,

Yvette Collymore and Kelsey Mertes
PATH Malaria Vaccine Initiative, Washington DC, United States of America

Antoinette Ba-Nguz
PATH Malaria Vaccine Initiative, Nairobi, Kenya

Allison Bingham
PATH Kenya, Kisumu, Kenya

Kelly Clarke, James Beard, Anthony Costello, Audrey Prost and Edward Fottrell
Institute for Global Health, University College London, London, United Kingdom

Tanja A. J. Houweling
Institute for Global Health, University College London, London, United Kingdom
Department of Public Health, Erasmus MC University Medical Center Rotterdam, Rotterdam, The Netherlands

Kishwar Azad, Abdul Kuddus, Sanjit Shaha, Tasmin Nahar, Bedowra Haq Aumon and Mohammed Munir Hossen
Perinatal Care Project, Diabetic Association of Bangladesh, Dhaka, Bangladesh

Solange Ouédraogo, Blaise Traoré, Zah Ange Brice Nene Bi, Firmin Tiandama Yonli, Donatien Kima, Pierre Bonané, Lassané Congo, Rasmata Ouédraogo Traoré and Diarra Yé
Charles de Gaulle Pediatric University Hospital, Ouagadougou, Burkina Faso

Christophe Marguet
Respiratory Diseases, Allergy and CF Unit, Paediatric Department, Rouen University
Hospital Charles Nicolle, EA3830, Inserm CIC204, Rouen, France

Jean-Christophe Plantier and Marie Gueudin
Laboratory of Virology, GRAM EA 2656 Rouen University Hospital Charles Nicolle, Rouen, France

Astrid Vabret
Laboratory of Human and Molecular Virology, Caen University Hospital Clemenceau, Caen, France

Yi-kuan Chen, Long-zhi Han, Feng Xue, Cong-huan Shen, Jun Lu, Tai-hua Yang, Jian-jun Zhang and Qiang Xia
Department of Liver Surgery and Liver Transplantation, Ren Ji Hospital, School of Medicine, Shanghai Jiao Tong University, Shanghai, P.R. China

Shang-Ming Zhou, Ronan A. Lyons, Owen G. Bodger, Ann John, Kerina Jones, Mike B. Gravenor and Sinead Brophy
Institute of Life Science, College of Medicine, Swansea University, Swansea, United Kingdom

Huw Brunt
Public Health Wales, Temple of Peace and Health, Cathays Park, Cardiff, United Kingdom

Martí Casals
CIBER de Epidemiologı´a y Salud Pu´ blica (CIBERESP), Barcelona, Spain
Bioestadí stica, Departament de Salut Pública, Universitat de Barcelona, Barcelona, Spain
Departament de Ciencies Basiques, Universitat Internacional de Catalunya, Barcelona, Spain
Servei d'Epidemiologia, Agéncia de Salut Pública de Barcelona, Barcelona, Spain

Josep L. Carrasco
Bioestadística, Departament de Salut Pública, Universitat de Barcelona, Barcelona, Spain

Montserrat Girabent-Farrés
Departament de Fisioterápia (unitat de Bioestadística), Universitat Internacional de Catalunya, Barcelona, Spain

Dong-Hee Kim
Department of Nursing, College of Nursing, Pusan National University, Yangsan, Gyeongsangnamdo, South Korea

Hak Sun Yu
Department of Parasitology, School of Medicine, Pusan National University, Yangsan, Gyeongsangnamdo, South Korea
Immunoregulatory therapeutics group in Brain Busan 21 project, Busan, South Korea

Claudia Witte, Benjamin Lange, Christiane Kiese-Himmel, Nicole von Steinbü chel
Institute of Medical Psychology and Medical Sociology, Georg-August-University Gö ttingen, Göttingen, Germany

Ester Villalonga-Olives
Institute of Medical Psychology and Medical Sociology, Georg-August-University Göttingen, Göttingen, Germany
Department of Social and Behavioral Sciences, Harvard School of Public Health, Boston, Massachusetts, United States of America

Ichiro Kawachi
Department of Social and Behavioral Sciences, Harvard School of Public Health, Boston, Massachusetts, United States of America

Josué Almansa
Department of Health Sciences, Community and Occupational Medicine, University of Groningen, University Medical Center Groningen, Groningen, The Netherlands

Marko Wilke
Department of Pediatric Neurology and Developmental Medicine, Children's Hospital, University of Tübingen, Tübingen, Germany
Experimental Pediatric Neuroimaging group, Pediatric Neurology & Department of Neuroradiology, University Hospital, Tübingen, Germany

Susanne Eifer Møller
Institute of Public Health, Epidemiology, Biostatistics and Biodemography, University of Southern Denmark, Odense, Denmark

Teresa Adeltoft Ajslev and Camilla Schou Andersen
Institute of Preventive Medicine, Bispebjerg and Frederiksberg Hospitals, The Capital Region, Denmark

Thorkild I. A. Sørensen
Institute of Preventive Medicine, Bispebjerg and Frederiksberg Hospitals, The Capital Region, Denmark
Novo Nordisk Foundation Centre for Basic Metabolic Research, Faculty of Health and Medical Sciences, University of Copenhagen, Copenhagen, Denmark

Christine Dalgård
Institute of Public Health, Environmental Medicine, University of Southern Denmark, Odense, Denmark

Natalie Carvalho
Global Burden of Disease Group and Center for Health Policy, Melbourne School of Population and Global Health, Melbourne, Australia
Center for Health Decision Sciences, Harvard School of Public Health, Boston, Massachusetts, United States of America

Naveen Thacker
Deep Children Hospital and Research Centre, Gandhidham, Gujarat, India

Subodh S. Gupta
Department of Community Medicine, Mahatma Gandhi Institute of Medical Sciences, Sewagram, Maharashtra, India

Joshua A. Salomon
Department of Global Health and Population, Harvard School of Public Health, Boston, Massachusetts, United States of America

Sten H. Vermund
Vanderbilt Institute for Global Health, Vanderbilt University School of Medicine, Nashville, Tennessee, United States of America
Department of Pediatrics, Vanderbilt University School of Medicine, Nashville, Tennessee, United States of America
Friends in Global Health, Quelimane and Maputo, Mozambique

Lara M. E. Vaz
Vanderbilt Institute for Global Health, Vanderbilt University School of Medicine, Nashville, Tennessee, United States of America
Department of Preventive Medicine, Vanderbilt University School of Medicine, Nashville, Tennessee, United States of America
Friends in Global Health, Quelimane and Maputo, Mozambique

Meridith Blevins and Bryan E. Shepherd
Vanderbilt Institute for Global Health, Vanderbilt University School of Medicine, Nashville, Tennessee, United States of America
Department of Biostatistics, Vanderbilt University School of Medicine, Nashville,
Tennessee, United States of America

José A. Tique
Vanderbilt Institute for Global Health, Vanderbilt University School of Medicine, Nashville, Tennessee, United States of America
Friends in Global Health, Quelimane and Maputo, Mozambique,

Philip J. Ciampa
Vanderbilt Institute for Global Health, Vanderbilt University School of Medicine, Nashville, Tennessee, United States of America
Department of Medicine, Vanderbilt University School of Medicine, Nashville, Tennessee, United States of America

Troy D. Moon
Vanderbilt Institute for Global Health, Vanderbilt University School of Medicine, Nashville, Tennessee, United States of America
Department of Pediatrics, Vanderbilt University School of Medicine, Nashville, Tennessee, United States of America
Friends in Global Health, Quelimane and Maputo, Mozambique,

Eurico José and Linda Moiane
Friends in Global Health, Quelimane and Maputo, Mozambique,

Mohsin Sidat
School of Medicine, Universidade Eduardo Mondlane, Maputo, Mozambique

Paul Schnitzler
Department of Infectious Diseases, Virology, University of Heidelberg, Heidelberg, Germany,

Julia Tabatabai
Department of Infectious Diseases, Virology, University of Heidelberg, Heidelberg, Germany
London School of Hygiene and Tropical Medicine, London, United Kingdom

Christiane Prifert
Institute of Virology and Immunobiology, University of Wu¨ rzburg, Wu¨ rzburg, Germany

Johannes Pfeil
Department of Pediatrics, University of Heidelberg, Heidelberg, Germany
German Centre for Infectious Diseases (DZIF), Heidelberg, Germany

Jürgen Grulich-Henn
Department of Pediatrics, University of Heidelberg, Heidelberg, Germany

Emily H. Stewart
Walter Reed National Military Medical Center, Bethesda, Maryland, United States of America

Brian Davis
University of Texas Southwestern Medical Center, Dallas, Texas, United States of America

B. Lee Clemans-Taylor and Robert M. Centor
The University of Alabama at Birmingham, Huntsville Campus, Huntsville, Alabama, United States of America

Benjamin Littenberg
University of Vermont, Burlington, Vermont, United States of America

Carlos A. Estrada
University of Alabama at Birmingham, Birmingham, Alabama, United States of America, 6 Birmingham Veterans Affairs Medical
Center and Veterans Affairs Quality Scholar Program, Birmingham, Alabama, United States of America

Vivien A. Sheehan and Jonathan M. Flanagan
Hematology Center, Department of Pediatrics, Baylor College of Medicine, Houston, Texas, United States of America

Jacy R. Crosby
The University of Texas Graduate School of Biomedical Sciences at Houston, Department of Biostatistics, Bioinformatics, and Systems Biology, University of Texas, Houston, Texas, United States of America
Human Genetics Center, University of Texas, Houston, Texas, United States of America

Eric Boerwinkle
Human Genetics Center, University of Texas, Houston, Texas, United States of America
Human Genome Sequencing Center, Baylor College of Medicine, Houston, Texas, United States of America

Aniko Sabo, Donna M. Muzny, Shannon Dugan-Perez and Richard A. Gibbs
Human Genome Sequencing Center, Baylor College of Medicine, Houston, Texas, United States of America

Nicole A. Mortier, Thad A. Howard and Russell E. Ware
Division of Hematology, Cincinnati Children's Hospital Medical Center, Cincinnati, Ohio, United States of America

Banu Aygun
Steven and Alexandra Cohen Children's Medical Center of New York, New Hyde Park, New York, United States of America

Kerri A. Nottage
Department of Hematology, St. Jude Children's Research Hospital, Memphis, Tennessee, United States of America

Chyong-Hsin Hsu, Chia-Ying Lin, Jui-Hsing Chang, Han-Yang Hung, Hsin-An Kao, Chun-Chih Peng and Wai-Tim Jim
Department of Pediatrics, Division of Neonatology, Mackay Memorial Hospital, Taipei, Taiwan

Hsin Chi
Department of Pediatrics, Division of Infectious Disease, Mackay Memorial Hospital, Taipei, Taiwan

Index

www.ingramcontent.com/pod-product-compliance
Lightning Source LLC
Chambersburg PA
CBHW061257190326
41458CB00011B/3699
9781632424716